Immunology of the Gastrointestinal Tract

Immunology of the Gastrointestinal Tract

Edited by

Peter Asquith MB ChB (Manch) MD (Birm) MRCP

Consultant Physician and Gastroenterologist,
Alastair Frazer and John Squire Metabolic and Clinical
   Investigation Unit,
East Birmingham Hospital
Honorary Senior Lecturer,
Department of Medicine
Honorary Clinical Senior Lecturer,
Department of Experimental Pathology,
University of Birmingham

Foreword by

P. G. H. Gell FRS MB BChir MRCS (Eng) LRCP (Lond) FRCPath

Former Professor of Experimental Pathology,
University of Birmingham

CHURCHILL LIVINGSTONE

EDINBURGH LONDON AND NEW YORK 1979

CHURCHILL LIVINGSTONE
Medical Division of Longman Group Limited

Distributed in the United States of America by
Longman Inc., 19 West 44th Street, New York,
N.Y. 10036, and by associated companies,
branches and representatives throughout
the world.

First published 1979

ISBN 0 443 01589 9

British Library Cataloguing in Publication Data

Immunology of the gastrointestinal tract.
  1. Digestive organs – Diseases – Immunological
  aspects
  I. Asquith, Peter
  616.3′3′079   RC802   78-40819

Printed in Great Britain by Butler & Tanner Ltd, Frome and London

Foreword

Any person (such as a scientifically inclined archangel) who was around 200 million or so years ago would have been able to observe the development of an interesting mutation among our distant progenitors in the maritime muds – the divergence of the alpha heavy Ig chain from the gamma heavy chain. This is where the subject of this book really starts; the point at which it became clear that something must and could be done about defence at surfaces as well as in fluids, by the then evolving chordates and vertebrates. It was evidently a successful effort, in that it persisted as a major means of defence; but just how the rather elaborate architecture of J chain and secretory piece, as well as the considerable structural differences in the alpha Fc itself, had to be the acquisition of these special powers, is still a bit obscure, at least to me.

Narrowing the time gap a little, the years between about 1920 when oral immunization and coproantibodies were being actively discussed and the early 1960s when Heremans described IgA, and Tomasi, Bienenstock and their colleagues indicated a function for it, marked an era when what went on in the guts was hardly respectable, at least in the eyes of the professional immunochemists who then dominated the field. The great mass of lymphoid tissue in the intestine, and even more that in the appendix (removed with the gayest abandon in that era), remained *terra incognita* except to morbid pathologists. Nevertheless the very first example of immunological tolerance, by the feeding of picryl chloride, was described by Chase about 1943, to sow seeds which have hardly all germinated even now (any gardener knows that seldom do all seeds in a batch germinate simultaneously: so in science). Indeed it would seem that tolerance *per os* is a subject of maximal practical and theoretical interest yet to be exploited. Moreover the complex dance of cells which goes on in the *lamina propria* of the intestine has only recently come under study, under stimuli from two directions – from academic immunologists interested in (and surprised by) the homing thither of labelled lymphocytes, and, to rather greater effect, from clinicians interested in what on earth could be going on in the tissues of coeliacs, in Crohn's disease, in ulcerative colitis and so on. These carry the (almost) unmistakable stamp of immunologically conditioned diseases: but just what precise mechanisms are at work? In particular what role is played by 'ordinary' and what by IgA and IgE antibody and what by the possibly more primitive mechanisms of cellular hypersensitivity? It is to questions of this sort that this book gives an informed, illuminating though inevitably still incomplete answer.

P. G. H. G.

Preface

My purpose in compiling this book has been to provide a comprehensive and up-to-date account of the immunology of the gastrointestinal tract. To this end the book has two parts: the first consists of three chapters on organisational and functional aspects which form an introduction and basis for Part 2. In this second part disorders of the gut from the mouth to the colon and rectum are considered, mainly as they affect man but also some attention is paid to animal diseases. In planning this book I invited a number of internationally known experts to write on their respective fields and I am very grateful to them for providing a series of extensive and authoritative reviews. The current marked and widespread interest in gut immunity is stimulated by attempts at unravelling the complexities of the immunological apparatus of the gut and also by the belief that some, perhaps many, intestinal diseases may have an immunological basis. I hope the book will be of value to clinicians, immunologists and basic scientists.

I would like to acknowledge my indebtedness to Professor Philip Gell FRS and members of his department who stimulated my interest in gut immunology, and to Dr W. T. Cooke who permitted me to study patients under his care. I am also grateful to Mr S. Jenkins and his staff at the Barnes Medical Library, University of Birmingham, who checked the many references, to Mr Roy Steel for checking the manuscripts and to the staff of Churchill Livingstone for their advice and help during the various stages of this book. Finally my thanks are also due to my wife Janet and our children John, Karen and Helen for their indulgence, encouragement and support.

Birmingham, 1978   P. A.

Contributors

P. Asquith
MB ChB (Manch) MD (Birm) MRCP
Consultant Physician and Gastroenterologist,
Alastair Frazer and John Squire Metabolic and Clinical
   Investigation Unit,
East Birmingham Hospital,
Birmingham.
Honorary Senior Lecturer,
Department of Medicine,
Honorary Clinical Senior Lecturer,
Department of Experimental Pathology,
University of Birmingham,
Birmingham.

M. K. Basu
BDS FDS RCS (Edin)
Lecturer,
Department of Oral Pathology,
University of Birmingham,
Birmingham.
Honorary Senior Registrar, in Oral Medicine and Oral
   Pathology,
Alastair Frazer and John Squire Metabolic and Clinical
   Investigation Unit,
East Birmingham Hospital,
Birmingham.

J. Bienenstock
MD
Professor of Medicine,
McMaster University Medical Centre,
Hamilton,
Ontario,
Canada.

E. Bleumink
PhD
Head, Section of Biochemistry of the Skin,
Department of Dermatology,
State University,
Groningen,
The Netherlands.

S. N. Booth
MD MRCP
Consultant Physician,
Kidderminster General Hospital,
Kidderminster.
Honorary Research Fellow,
Department of Experimental Pathology,
University of Birmingham,
Birmingham.

D. Catty
BSc MSc PhD
Senior Lecturer in Immunology,
Department of Immunology,
University of Birmingham,
Birmingham.

William F. Doe
MSc MRCP
Senior Lecturer in Medicine,
University of Sydney,
Australia.
Honorary Physician (Gastroenterology),
Royal North Shore Hospital,
St Leonards,
New South Wales,
Australia.

P. W. Dykes
MD FRCP FRACP
Consultant Physician,
General Hospital,
Birmingham.
Honorary Senior Lecturer,
Department of Experimental Pathology,
University of Birmingham,
Birmingham.

R. Ferguson
MD MRCP
Senior Registrar in Medicine,
General Hospital,
Nottingham.

M. R. Haeney
MSc MB BCh MRCP
Senior Registrar,
Regional Immunology Laboratory,
East Birmingham Hospital,
Birmingham.

Sumner C. Kraft
MD FACP
Professor of Medicine and Committee on Immunology,
The University of Chicago,
Chicago,
U.S.A.

B. P. Maclaurin
MD MRCP (Lond) FRACP
Associate Professor of Medicine,
University of Otago Medical School,
New Zealand.

D. B. L. McClelland
MB ChB BSc MD (Leiden) MRCP
Consultant,
South-East Scotland Blood Transfusion Service.
Part-time Senior Lecturer,
University Department of Therapeutics and Clinical
    Pharmacology,
Edinburgh.

J. Morley
PhD MRCPath
Director,
Department of Clinical Pharmacology (Asthma Research
    Council),
Cardiothoracic Institute,
University of London,
London.

P. Porter
BSc PhD DSc
Head of the Department of Immunology,
Unilever Research,
Colworth House,
Sharnbrook,
Bedford.
Lecturer in Immunology,
University of Nottingham,
Postgraduate Supervisor,
Open University.

I. N. Ross
MSc MRCS LRCP MB BS MRCP (UK)
Clinical Research Fellow,
Department of Experimental Pathology,
    University of Birmingham.
Present address:
Wellcome Research Unit,
Christian Medical College Hospital,
Vellore,
India.

R. A. Thompson
MBE MB BS BSc MRCP MRCPath
Consultant Immunologist,
Director of the Regional Immunology Laboratory,
East Birmingham Hospital,
Birmingham.
Senior Clinical Lecturer,
Department of Experimental Pathology,
University of Birmingham,
Birmingham.

J. K. Visakorpi
MD
Professor of Paediatrics,
University of Tampere,
Tampere,
Finland.

Contents

PART 1 Organizational and functional aspects

1. The physiology of the local immune response

J. Bienenstock

INTRODUCTION

In 1919 Besredka published his findings showing that oral immunization of rabbits provided protection against otherwise fatal Shiga bacillus infection, regardless of the serum antibody level. In fact, his subsequent monograph entitled 'Local immunization', published in 1927, showed that he had developed theories of immunity, based on such experimental observations, before and during the First World War which he subsequently put into practice in the immunization of thousands of army personnel. The data recorded in his book clearly showed the efficacy of oral immunization in prevention of dysentery. Also at that time Davies (1922) showed that faecal antibody was present in the stools of patients with bacillary dysentery before serum antibody was present. It was some 40 years later that Heremans (1960) described a new immunoglobulin in serum different from those already known, gamma G and gamma M, and termed it gamma A or β_2A. Tomasi and his co-workers (1965), soon afterwards, showed that the IgA class of immunoglobulins predominated in several external secretions, that IgA-containing plasma cells were to be found in large numbers in the salivary gland, and that the secretory IgA in saliva and colostrum differed immunochemically from that found in serum, in being larger, and in having an extra polypeptide chain known at that time as secretory piece. From these observations came a renewed interest in mucosal immunity, a topic which has been the subject of several extensive reviews (Tomasi and Bienenstock, 1968; Heremans, 1968, Dayton, Small, Chanock, Kaufman and Tomasi, 1970; Tomasi and Grey, 1972; Mestecky and Lawton, 1974).

Evidence exists for the presence of IgG, IgM, IgA and IgE in external secretions, particularly if the mucosa is involved by an inflammatory process allowing the egress of serum proteins. The IgA immunoglobulin molecule predominates in external secretions, but it should also be recognized that IgG and IgM may play important roles in terms of local antibody production (*vide infra*). The IgE class of immunoglobulin has been shown to be synthesized locally, particularly in mucosal surfaces (Tada and Ishizaka, 1970). However, the IgE found in secretions does not differ from that found in serum, as it appears not to contain either a J chain or secretory component (Brandtzaeg, 1973).

IgA

STRUCTURE

Tomasi *et al.* (1965) first showed that IgA predominated in certain external secretions and that the IgA molecule differed from its serum counterpart. It is now known that the secretory IgA molecule in its classical 11S form consists of four light chains, four heavy chains, one secretory component and one J chain. The whole molecule has a molecular weight of approximately 385 000. In humans, the secretory component (SC) has a molecular weight of about 60 000 and the J chain about 15 000. The J chain has an enormously increased axial ratio, much higher than other molecules of similar molecular size (Koshland and Wilde, 1974). The J chain appears to be linked to the penultimate cysteine residue of the C terminal octapeptide of the alpha chain and potentially also the same octapeptide of the μ chain (Mestecky, Schrohenloher, Kulhavy, Wright and Tomana, 1974). The SC and J chain do not appear to be interconnected by disulphide bonds; however, the J chain may be necessary for the attachment of the SC (Eskeland and Brandtzaeg, 1974) rather than for the polymerization of the molecule (Halpern and Koshland, 1970). The SC is an unusual protein in that it appears to be totally deficient in methionine (Kobayashi, 1971). The J chain is clearly also found in other polymeric immunoglobulins such as IgM as shown by Metstecky, Ziram and Butler (1971), and Brandtzaeg (1973), and is thus not peculiar to secretory IgA or polymeric IgA molecules.

The SC in human secretory IgA is linked in the main to the IgA polymer by disulphide bridges (Tomasi and Bienenstock, 1968) whereas in the rabbit much of the secretory component is bound by non-covalent bonds. The SC is found in most secretions both in the free and bound forms. Antisera to the free form show antigenic (I) determinants (Brandtzaeg, 1971) which are inaccessible in the bound form and therefore such antisera can be used to identify free versus bound SC.

One version of the structure of the secretory IgA molecule is shown diagrammatically, in Figure 1.1 which is a composite drawing of data presented by a large number of workers in this field. This double Y configuration has been observed using electron-microscopy by Bloth and Svehag (1971) as the predominant form of secretory IgA in human colostrum. In gastrointestinal secretions such as small intestinal fluid, approximately 33 per cent of the IgA is in the 7S IgA form (Bull and Tomasi, 1968) whereas parotid saliva usually contains less than 10 per cent of 7S IgA. It is important to understand that any attempt to estimate the amount of IgA and other immunoglobulins present in such secretions is fraught with a number of technical difficulties. Thus it is difficult to find a standard of satisfactory size; it is

total cellular immunoglobulin content of the spleen. This lymphoid mass produces some 3 g of IgA per day, 50 per cent of which is secreted. The majority of the IgA-containing cells are found towards the bases of the villi, amongst the glands as well as near the Peyer's patches. The average half life of an IgA cell has been calculated at 4.7 days in the mouse (Mattioli and Tomasi, 1973).

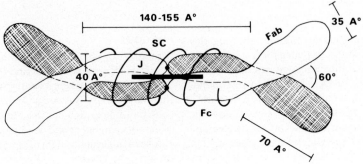

Fig. 1.1 Colostral 11S sIgA.

hard to retard proteolytic digestion or prevent losses in storage and during concentration; the external secretions particularly contain substances giving rise to non-immunologic precipitin lines and, if inflammation supervenes in the local mucosal surfaces, leakage of serum proteins may cause results which may be wrongly interpreted (Tomasi and Bienenstock, 1968, and Tomasi and Grey, 1972).

SYNTHESIS, ASSEMBLY AND TRANSPORT

IgA-containing cells predominate in the gastrointestinal tract as first shown by Crabbé and Heremans (1966). Heremans (1975) has estimated that the human gastrointestinal tract may contain 50 g of immunoglobulin containing lymphoid tissue, equivalent to the

The IgA appears to be synthesized as a dimer in most animals and in man, and to be locally synthesized in the adjacent mucosa in most tissues so far examined. The secretory component is thought to be synthesized by glandular epithelial cells but not goblet cells (Poger and Lamm, 1974; Brandtzaeg, 1974) and is probably concentrated by the Golgi apparatus (Van Munster, 1971). The J chain seems to be synthesized by the same cells as those making IgA (O'Daly and Cebra, 1971). The J chain may act as a clasp rather than a bracelet in joining two μ chains together, and a similar mechanism is suggested for the IgA polymer since only one mole of J chain appears to be present per mole of polymer (Koshland and Wilde, 1974).

The route of transport of the secretory IgA molecule

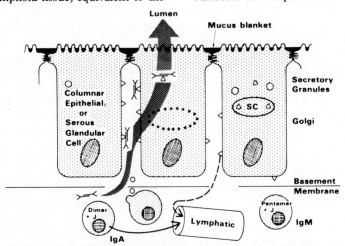

Fig. 1.2 Transport of immunoglobulins into external secretions.

is shown schematically in Figure 1.2. The IgA appears to pass between gaps found in the basement membrane (Tourville, Adler, Bienenstock and Tomasi, 1969) and is probably transported via a receptor mechanism consisting of secretory component on the outside of the cell membrane (Brandtzaeg, 1973) and is then transmitted to the luminal surface across the apical portion of the cell by exocytosis. Alternatively, membrane-bound packages of IgA follow the same route as has been suggested in the pig (Allen, Smith and Porter, 1973). There is some evidence that J chain may determine the selective combination not only of IgA but also IgM with secretory component (Eskeland and Brandtzaeg, 1974). Indeed further support that IgM may share a pathway with IgA comes from the observation that IgM purified from several secretions is 70 per cent saturated with secretory component (Brandtzaeg, 1973). In IgA deficiency, IgM often replaces IgA both in the experimental models of this condition and in man. The mode of transport of IgE into secretions is unknown. However, IgE does not bear secretory component when isolated from secretions. (Newcomb and Ishizaka, 1970).

In-vitro experiments have suggested a feedback control mechanism of the synthesis of the secretory IgA molecule (Lawton, Asofsky, Mage, 1970) since dimeric IgA stimulates synthesis of secretory component by rabbit mammary tissue in culture. Much of the locally synthesized IgA in most mammals, and possibly also in humans, may enter the lymphatics and be found in the circulation (Heremans and Vaerman, 1971). It is not clear whether the dimer in man or in animals has a special transport advantage especially since the predominant form of serum IgA in man is monomeric. However, Thompson and Asquith (1970) have shown secretory IgA in human serum, and an increased level of this in diseases associated with inflammation of mucous membranes. In most animals the majority of serum IgA is in the dimeric form and Dive and co-workers have shown that 50 per cent of biliary IgA in the dog emanates from serum (Heremans, 1975). Strober, Blaese and Waldmann (1970) have clearly shown that 96 per cent of salivary IgA is synthesized at local sites. Although small quantities of 7S serum IgA could pass into saliva, transport from serum to this secretion appeared to account for only a very small amount of the total. Thus most published evidence supports the view of local synthesis although some evidence exists to contradict it. The major IgA class exists in the form of two subclasses in the human: IgA1 and IgA2. In serum, IgA1 is the predominant subclass occupying approximately 80 per cent to 90 per cent of the total IgA, whereas in colostrum Grey, Able, Yount and Kunkel (1968) have shown that there was a relatively high percentage of IgA2. Whether this observation reflects a selective increase in IgA2 synthesizing cells in the breast, or some form of selective transport advantage of the IgA2 subclass, is not known.

ONTOGENY AND PHYLOGENY

Human newborn peripheral lymphoid intestinal tissue appears to lack IgA producing capacity (Van Furth, Schuit and Hijmans, 1965) and the same has been found to apply to rodents and the bovine species. The amount of IgA in cord blood is only 1 per cent of the normal adult serum level while that of IgM is about 20 per cent. Indeed, elevations of either IgM or IgA in cord blood have been considered as useful screening tests for the possibility of intra-uterine infections. Synthesis of IgG occurs as early as 10 weeks of gestation in the human foetus; synthesis of IgM by 12 weeks but no detectable IgA synthesis was found by Gitlin and Biasucci (1969) up to 32 weeks. The role of the intestinal contents in establishing the normal complement of immunoglobulin-containing cells in the intestine has clearly been shown by Crabbé, Nash, Bazin, Eyssen and Heremans (1970) in a study of conventionalization of germ-free mice. Even germ-free mice possess IgA-containing cells since dietary antigenic stimulation still occurs in such animals. There is no similar information available on ontogeny of development of the IgE class of immunoglobulin in terms of the aspects just discussed.

It is thought that IgA may be important in determining resistance to infection of mucosal surfaces. It has been recently suggested that the alpha chain may have diverged from the μ chain in evolution some 200 million years ago. This suggestion has been made on the basis of a comparison of amino acid sequences of human alpha, gamma and mu C terminal regions by Chuang, Capra and Kehoe (1973). Since mammals are considered to have appeared about 175 million years ago and birds diverged from reptiles about the same time this would place the IgA system further back than has been thought heretofore. The demonstration that chickens possess an IgA system supports this view (Lebacq-Verheyden, Vaerman and Heremans, 1972).

It is of further interest that the J chain appears to be a polypeptide of great evolutionary stability since Vaerman, Kobayashi and Heremans (1974) have shown extensive cross-reactivity of J chain across many species, including fish.

FUNCTIONS OF SECRETORY IgA

Antibody activity in this class has been shown to exist with specificity to bacteria, viruses, autoantigens, toxins and a variety of other antigens used to immunize experimental animals. The molecule has four combining sites and is more efficient in agglutination than IgG or the 7S IgA (Taubman and Genco, 1971). Human and rabbit secretory IgA surprisingly does not precipitate multivalent antigen, and although there are some differences in this ability between these two species no really satisfactory explanation has yet been brought forward to account for these findings (Newcomb and Sutoris, 1974).

There is controversy over the ability of secretory IgA to opsonize (Zipursky, Brown and Bienenstock, 1973) a variety of antigens for phagocytosis (Kaplan, Dalmasso and Woodson, 1972). Most evidence currently weighs against opsonization either by peripheral blood phagocytes or by alveolar macrophages (Reynolds and Thompson, 1973). Secretory IgA will not activate complement by the classical pathway (Colten and Bienenstock, 1974), but the only study of 11S IgA antibodies so far reported in which human antiblood group A substance antibody was used has shown no activation of the alternate pathway (Colton and Bienenstock, 1974). Secretory IgA antibody blocks bacterial adherence to mucosal surfaces and thereby prevents colonization (Williams and Gibbons, 1972). It also may inhibit bacterial growth and change growth characteristics of bacteria (Brandtzaeg, Fjellanger and Gjervldsen, 1968). The molecule is markedly resistant to proteolysis (Tomasi and Bienenstock, 1968). This property in probably endowed by combination with SC, and is clearly an advantage in a proteolytic enzyme environment such as the gastrointestinal tract. The secretory IgA molecule binds to a variety of serum proteins, and the significance in this regard of the frequent combination with α-1-antitrypsin (Tomasi and Hauptman, 1974) is not known. It has been shown that IgA may act as a blocking antibody in terms of allergic reactions in nasal secretions (Turk, Lichtenstein and Norman, 1970) and that blocking of bacteriolysis may also be mediated in the same way (Hall, Manion and Zinneman, 1971). Adinolfi, Glynn, Lindsay and Milne (1966) have shown that together with a source of complement and lysozyme the antibody was effective in enhancement of bacteriolysis and recently this has been confirmed (Burdon, 1973; Hill and Porter, 1974). The secretory IgA antibody prevents absorption of albumin by rats after intragastric immunization (Heremans, 1975) and extensive studies by Walker, Isselbacher and Bloch (1973) have now elegantly shown that rat intestinal IgG1 is also effective in prevention of absorption of luminal antigen. In IgA-deficient humans, increased levels of serum antibody against dietary antigens have been recorded (Buckley and Dees, 1969) and infantile deficiency has been associated with subsequent atopy (Taylor *et al.*, 1973). It is quite possible that the function of secretory IgA to block or partially control antigen access to the organism may be an important modulating influence in human health and disease.

EPITHELIUM

Burnett (1959) first proposed the concept, later expanded by Heremans and Crabbé (1967), that antibodies lining the gastrointestinal tract may be regarded as an 'antiseptic paint'. It has recently been shown (Heremans, 1975) that mucin possesses cystein residues which may be available for protein interactions and that through this mechanism antibodies especially of the IgA class may be bound to the luminal surface of the epithelial cells of the intestine. In immunofluorescent studies of mucosal surfaces this layer of secretory IgA has clearly been demonstrated adherent to the apical surface of the columnar epithelial cells. The importance of this layer has been emphasized by experiments in which the action of a reducing agent on the mucous coat of immunized rat intestine allowed increased access of antigen across the epithelial layer (Walker and Bloch, personal communication).

The columnar epithelial layer consists of cells renewed in the crypts. The cells have microvilli on the luminal surface and synthesize and excrete into the lumen a number of proteins, one of which is the secretory component. The cells are capable of transporting luminal substances including carbohydrate, protein, fat, viruses and bacteria across the cell and basement membrane. It has long been known that in this cell layer are found cells variously referred to as lymphocytes and termed by Fichtelius (1968) thelio-lymphocytes. In the adult animal the ratio of these cells to epithelial cells in the small intestine is about 1:10. These cells are found in the intercellular spaces and can be recognized by their nuclei which are below the basal epithelial nuclei. The cell population is present in germ-free animals and in foetal intestine transplanted under the kidney capsule of syngeneic recipients (Ferguson and Parrott, 1972). In the chicken it is diminished in number by thymectomy or bursectomy (Bäck, 1970). Many of these cells possess granular inclusions (Collan, 1972) although they structurally resemble lymphocytes (Rudzik and Bienenstock, 1974). It has been suggested that some of these cells may be derived from mast cells on the basis of ultrastructural characteristics (Murray, Miller and Jarrett, 1968). These cells in the rabbit can be degranulated by PHA or Con A with the consequent release of histamine (Day and Bienenstock, unpublished). They may have a half life which differentiates them from the epithelial cells between which they reside (Darlington and Rogers, 1966) and from the lymphocytes in the lamina propria, and they therefore have been thought to represent a closed population. Whatever their derivation they have a resemblance both to lymphocytes and to mast cells and may act as specific passively sensitized sentinel cells at the mucosal surface. In hyperimmune pigs when antigen is placed into the lumen of a ligated segment of intestine a massive emigration of granulocytes appears within a few hours (Bellamy and Nielson, 1974) which does not leave any subsequent morphological evidence of permanent damage. The initiation of this stimulus is unknown but could conceivably be through the granular lymphocytes. This may also be the mechanism whereby pathotopic potentiation of mucosal surfaces occurs. This phenomenon originally observed and documented by Fazekas de St Groth and Donnelley (1950a and b) describes the influx of serum-borne immunity to a non-specifically stimulated site. Whether such cells indeed may be sensitized by IgE locally synthesized in the mucosa is not known. The older literature contains references to the importance of the intestinal tract in elimination of a variety of white cells (Ambrus and Ambrus, 1959; Teir, Rytömaa, Cederberg and Kiviniemi, 1963) and this aspect of immunity and defence has received little attention.

ORAL IMMUNIZATION

Oral immunization with a variety of antigens leads to local IgA antibody. Continued local feeding of protein antigens such as BSA in man and in animals eventually leads to a serum antibody response which in amount, class and affinity is indistinguishable from that seen following parenteral immunization (Rothberg, Kraft and Farr, 1967). The dissociation between serum and local antibody following oral immunization has been noted for more than 50 years (Davies, 1922). Oral immunization in man with Sabin vaccine led to a predominant IgA response in the intestinal secretions whereas parenteral immunization (Salk) did not lead to intestinal antibody (Ogra, Karzon, Righthand and MacGillivray, 1968). Both routes led to serum antibody. Similar results have been obtained with *Shigella* in monkeys and man, and with typhoid and cholera vaccines in man and animals (Shearman, Parkin and McClelland, 1972). The weight of this evidence suggests that the local response depends on the amount of antigen given orally and that attenuated live vaccines are effective in promoting resistance to infection, whereas killed local vaccines may be ineffective unless given repeatedly (Freter, 1962). Depending on the dose, parenteral immunization may lead to the appearance of local antibody in the intestine presumably due to dissemination of sufficient amounts of antigen to reach the intestinal lymphoid system (Shearman *et al.*, 1972).

The nature of the antigen used may also be highly significant. Hunter (1972) has shown that flagellin but not ovalbumin or bovine gammaglobulin will localize in the lamina propria of the unimmunized intestine and bronchus. Surprisingly, feeding of hapten (such as DNCB or picryl chloride) leads to tolerance and not immunity (Chase, 1946). However, feeding of ferritin to germ-free mice (Crabbé, Nash, Bazin, Eyssen and Heremans, 1969) led to a predominant IgA response in the

serum, peripheral lymph nodes and intestine. Similar observations have been made following sheep red blood cell administration to germ-free (Bazin, Levi and Doria, 1970) as well as conventional animals (Andre, Bazin and Heremans, 1973). However, feeding of conventional animals with ferritin or BSA does not result in a predominant IgA response (Dolezel and Bienenstock, 1971a). The existence of prior immunity may well result in blocking of antigen uptake by the bowel and may influence the distribution and amount of antigen which is taken up into the portal circulation rather than the lymph.

ANTIGEN HANDLING

Oral feeding of BSA to hamsters (Dolezel and Bienenstock, 1971b) results in early appearance of antigen inside presumed intestinal macrophages. The observation that antigens will cross the intestinal wall and can be recovered intact in the circulation was first documented by Uhlenhuth (1900). Since then a wide variety of substances, which include bacteriophage, botulinus toxin, starch granules, ferritin, horse-radish peroxidase and BSA have been recorded in either portal or systemic circulation or lymph after oral feeding. The route for such absorption appears to be anatomically the reverse of that taken in the secretion of IgA (Warshaw, Walker, Cornell and Isselbacher, 1971). It is possible that secretion of proteins including antibody may share a common pathway (Kagnoff, Serfilippi and Donaldson, 1973) with absorption of proteins. Thus the antigen load could theoretically regulate antibody secretion.

S. typhi obtains entrance into the lamina propria and then passes to the draining lymph nodes via the regional Peyer's patches (Carter and Collins, 1974). Extensive parenteral immunization or oral immunization in rats has shown the formation of luminal immune complexes in the blockade of intestinal uptake (Walker, Wu, Isselbacher and Bloch, 1975) and luminal degradation. IgA (Heremans) and IgG1 (Walker, Isselbacher and Bloch, 1973) have similarly been incriminated in the rate of this process by two independent groups of observers. Removal of the mucous blanket by reducing agents led to increased uptake in preimmunized animals (Walker and Bloch, personal communication).

The mechanism of antigen handling may be crucial to the development or non-development of immunity. Oral administration of DNCB produces systemic tolerance in guinea-pigs. Such animals also have local mucosal tolerance and do not react to antigen introduced into the mucosal wall whereas following systemic sensitization a delayed type of hypersensitivity response occurs (Strauss and Bienenstock, unpublished). In this case the antigen appears mainly confined to the small intestine (Silverman and Pomeranz, 1972). Similarly, tolerance has been achieved by the introduction of minute amounts of hapten into the portal system (Battisto and Miller, 1962). In dogs with porta-caval shunts the same experiment results in a systemic immune response (Cantor and Dumont, 1967). Similar experiments with analogous results have been performed with sheep red blood cells and hepatotoxins (Triger, Cynamon and Wright, 1973). The partitioning of antigen at the epithelial level either to the portal system or lymph, which may depend on the chemical nature of the antigen as well as other unknown factors, thus appears crucial in determining the nature of the immune response after oral immunization. Soluble antigen–antibody ratios favouring antigen cause increasingly inefficient removal of such complexes by the liver (Thomas and Vaez-Zadeh, 1974). Such compartmentalization in lymph or portal blood is well known to occur for lipids with more or less than 10–12 carbon atoms. Intragastric admini-stration of sheep red cells to BALB/c mice for 4 days led to splenic tolerance for 12 weeks (Crabbé, Nash, Bazin, Eyssen and Heremans, 1969), and a primary type of response on secondary gastric immunization. The role of the Sulzberger–Chase phenomenon, effect of in-testinal antibody, and partitioning of antigen between lymph and portal blood, result in a balance between immunity and tolerance. A better knowledge of this normal balance and maintenance of immunity is essential to understand how immune defences and control of bacterial flora of the intestine are maintained.

CELLULAR BASIS OF THE INTESTINAL IMMUNE RESPONSE

One of the most likely mechanisms whereby a local immune response occurs is that oral immunization results in the generation of immune competent cells in the intestine, and that these return after circulation. However, the oral immunization of rabbits by daily administration of 0.1 per cent to 2.0 per cent BSA in the drinking water produced no antigen reactive cells in the blood (Goldberg, Kraft, Peterson and Rothberg, 1971). These cells were found in the spleen whence they could be mobilized (Rothberg, Kraft, Asquith and Michalek, 1973). Such a circulation of cells following local immunization has also been suggested following BSA feeding of hamsters (Dolezel and Bienenstock, 1971a), sheep red blood cell administration to rats (André, Bazin and Heremans, 1973) and ferritin to germ-free mice (Crabbé, Nash, Bazin, Eyssen and Heremans, 1969). Following oral immunization sequential examina-tion showed antibody-containing cells appeared earliest in the intestinal lamina propria followed by the mesen-teric lymph node and spleen (André, Bazin and Heremans, 1973; Rothberg, Kraft and Michalek, 1973; Robertson and Cooper, 1973).

Blast cells in the thoracic duct (TD) consist mainly of non-recirculating cells (Moore and Hall, 1972) which home to the lamina propria of the intestine. Recent evidence suggests that the majority of these cells contain IgA, possess cell surface IgA and/or IgM, and synthesize almost exclusively dimeric IgA (Jensenius and Williams, 1974; Bienenstock, Rudzik, Clancy and Perey, 1974; Uhr and Vitetta, 1974). The majority of these cells may go on to IgA production. T-cell TD blasts also mainly home to the intestinal epithelium (Sprent and Miller, 1972; Guy-Grand, Griscelli and Vasalli, 1974). Although some homing occurs on the basis of antigen, TD blast cells home to neonatal unsuckled intestine (Halstead and Hall, 1972), as well as to subcutaneous transplants of isogeneic foetal intestine (Moore and Hall, 1972) in the same order as to normal intestine. Vitetta, Grundke-Iqbal, Holmes and Uhr (1974) have suggested that activated T-cells may be necessary for the switch to occur from IgM to other classes of immunoglobulins. Circumstantial evidence suggests that the thymus is im-plicated in IgA production since nude mice have little IgA, neonatal thymectomy of rabbits leads to depressed IgA and serum IgA antibody responses, and thymectomy added to bursectomy of neonatal chickens leads to total depletion of IgA (Perey and Bienenstock, 1973). Uhr and Vitetta (1974) found that in axenic mice most TD cells synthesized only IgM. Since axenic guinea-pigs are incapable of expressing delayed hypersensitivity (Lev and Battisto, 1970) they may lack the appropriate sub-population of T-cells which when activated allow the switch from IgM to IgA to occur. Although there is still controversy as to whether or not IgM can switch directly to IgA, much circumstantial evidence supports this as one possibility (Martin and Leslie, 1974). However, the alternative suggestion of a switch from IgM to IgG to IgA (Cooper, Lawton and Kincade, 1972) has certainly not been excluded. The above synthesis would account for the repopulation of the intestinal lamina propria with IgM-containing cells in the chicken and human models of IgA deficiency and is supported by the frequent clinical observation of T-cell deficits in IgA deficiency. The discrepancy between two chicken models of IgA deficiency (bursectomy alone [Kincade and Cooper, 1973] as opposed to bursectomy and thymectomy [Perey and Bienenstock, 1973] at hatching) may be due to maturation differences in separate strains.

ROLE OF MUCOSAL LYMPHOID AGGREGATES

The Peyer's patches consist of multiple lymphoid aggre-gates covered by a specialized lymphoepithelium infiltrated with lymphocytes. Immediately below the epithelium lies the dome and below that the lymphoid follicle (Waksman, Ozer and Blythman, 1973). In between the follicles is a thymus-dependent area. The lymphoepithelium appears to preferentially sample the luminal contents by pinocytosis (Bockman and Cooper, 1973). Normally very few cells with evidence of cytoplasmic immunoglobulin are seen. The membranes of the majority of the cells stain with either IgA or IgM antisera (Moore and Hall, 1972), and lateral to the follicles are collections of IgA-containing cells. The presence of bacteria in the dome, sometimes intracellular but often intercellular, suggests a lack of normal macrophage handling which is supported by the observation of the lack of a primary immune response with this tissue *in vivo* (Bienenstock and Dolezel, 1971). An *in-vitro* primary response was obtained (Kagnoff and Campbell, 1974) by the addition of 2-mercaptoethanol and the suggestion was made that this tissue lacks a sufficient number of competent adherent cells, presumed macrophages. A secondary response can be found (Veldkamp, Van Der Graag and Willers, 1973) in this tissue *in vivo*.

Small B-lymphocytes from the TD tend to home to the dome (Howard, Hunt and Gowans, 1972) and thymidine labelled, presumed B-cells, also go to the dome, whereas thymic cells go to the thymus-dependent area as well as to the dome epithelium (Waksman, 1973). Scanning electron-microscopy of rabbit Peyer's patches shows some with sheets of relatively smooth lymphocytes (Bienenstock and Johnston, 1976) overlying the domes on the luminal surface so that one route of such cells may be destined for the lumen of the intestine, as suggested by Waksman (1973).

Craig and Cebra (1971) showed that Peyer's patch cells transferred into lethally irradiated rabbits within 6 days, repopulated the lamina propria of the intestine and spleen with predominantly IgA-producing cells. Subsequent experiments have confirmed these results (Bienenstock, Rudzik, Clancy, Day and Perey, 1974) and have shown that the results in the spleen may have been primarily due to the allogeneic difference and that Peyer's patches contained evidence of repopulation by cells with membranes staining for IgA. Pronase digestion of these cells, and examination before infusion, showed that only μ-negative b-positive α-negative cells in patches caused subsequent repopulation with IgA (Cebra and Jones, 1974). Subsequent studies have shown the IgA precursors to possess α on their cell surface.

Mesenteric lymph-node blast cells tend to return to the intestine (Griscelli, Vassalli and McCluskey, 1969) as do thoracic duct lymphoblasts. Peyer's patch cells by and large tend to return to Peyer's patches and peripheral lymph nodes. These homing results were obtained at 24

to 48 hours and the repopulation results at 6 days. Additional factors potentially affecting lymphocytes in the Peyer's patch are endotoxin from the lumen, enzymes (particularly proteolytic enzymes which can enhance lymphocytotoxic activity as well as responses to PHA [Clancy and Bienenstock, submitted]), or unknown microenvironmental factors such as the local stroma. The Peyer's patches may serve as unusual draining lymphoid aggregates to local regions of the intestine (Carter and Collins, 1974) and because they appear unable to retain antibody-producing cells presumably act as the school where education of cells committed to specific IgA antibody, and to some extent other classes of immunoglobulin-producing cells, occurs. Contact with either macrophages and/or activated T-cells may then occur elsewhere. Such a postulated recirculation may occur several times before cells seen as blasts appear in the thoracic duct.

CONCLUSION, A COMMON MUCOSAL IMMUNOLOGICAL SYSTEM

In the irradiated rabbit repopulation model, Peyer's patch cells repopulate the bronchial lamina propria (Bienenstock, Rudzik, Clancy, Day and Perey, 1974) with IgA as well as the intestine. Bronchus-associated lymphoid tissue (Bienenstock, Johnston and Perey, 1973a, b), morphologically very similar to Peyer's patches, repopulates the intestinal lamina with IgA-containing cells. Feeding of rabbits with DNP-pneumococci (Montgomery, Rosner and Cohn, 1974) led to a high IgA antibody in the colostrum and no association between antibody class in serum and secretions. Similar results have been reported by Bohl (1973) with transmissible gastroenteritis in pigs. It seems that sensitized cells educated in mucosal aggregates, be they in the lung or the intestine, have the potential to home to other mucosal sites. Although this suggestion is at variance with some of the studies of local immunization and immunity (Ogra and Karzon, 1969) the differences may be solely one of sensitivity of the techniques used for assay of antiviral antibodies versus the presence of antibody-containing cells. This system is suggested to apply to B-cells and their precursors but it is conceivable that it also may apply to a T-cell effector system as has been suggested by Behelak and Richter (1972). However, this aspect is far from clear, and although cell-mediated local immune responses may well occur in the intestine, as has been reported for the respiratory tract (Waldman, Spencer and Johnson, 1972), this has yet to be demonstrated.

Such a common mucosal system (Bienenstock, Johnston and Perey, 1973) interposed at sentinel sites along the bronchus and intestine would have a major advantage for the survival of the organism. This hypothetical system would account for the presence of high titres of colostral IgA antibody to blood group substances presumably engendered by cross-reacting bacteria in the intestine.

REFERENCES

Adinolfi, M., Glynn, A. A., Lindsay, M. & Milne, C. M. (1966) Serological properties of γA antibodies to *Escherichia coli* present in human colostrum. *Immunology*, **10**, 517–526.

Allen, W. D., Smith, C. G. & Porter, P. (1973) Localization of intracellular immunoglobulin A in porcine intestinal mucosa using enzyme-labelled antibody. *Immunology*, **25**, 55–70.

Ambrus, C. M. & Ambrus, J. L. (1959) Regulation of the leukocyte level. *Annals of the New York Academy of Science*, 77, 445–486.

André, C., Bazin, H. & Heremans, J. F. (1973) Influence of repeated administration of antigen by the oral route on specific antibody-producing cells in the mouse spleen. *Digestion*, 9, 166–175.

Bäck, O. (1970) Studies on the lymphocytes in the intestinal epithelium of the chicken. IV. Effect of bursectomy. *International Archives of Allergy and Applied Immunology*, 39, 342–351.

Battisto, J. R. & Miller, J. (1962) Immunological unresponsiveness produced in adult guinea pigs by parenteral introduction of minute quantities of hapten or protein antigen. *Proceedings of the Society for Experimental Biology and Medicine*, 111, 111–115.

Bazin, H., Levi, G. & Doria, G. (1970) Predominant contribution of IgA antibody-forming cells to an immune response detected in extra-intestinal lymphoid tissues of germ-free mice exposed to antigen by the oral route. *Journal of Immunology*, 105, 1049–1051.

Behelak, Y. & Richter, M. (1972) Cells involved in cell-mediated and transplantation immunity. III. The organ source(s) of the cells in the normal rabbit which mediate a reaction of cellular immunity in vitro. *Cellular Immunology*, 3, 542–558.

Bellamy, J. E. C. & Nielsen, N. O. (1974) Immune-mediated emigration of neutrophils into the lumen of the small intestine. *Infection and Immunity*, 9, 615–619.

Besredka, A. (1919) La vaccination contre les états typhoides par la voie buccale. *Annales de l'Institut Pasteur*, 33, 882–903.

Besredka, A. (1927) In *Local Immunization*. Baltimore: Williams & Wilkins.

Bienenstock, J. & Dolezel, J. (1971) Peyer's patches: lack of specific antibody-containing cells after oral and parenteral immunization. *Journal of Immunology*, 106, 938–945.

Bienenstock, J., Johnston, N. & Perey, D. Y. E. (1973a) Bronchial lymphoid tissue. I. Morphologic characteristics. *Laboratory Investigation*, 28, 686–692.

Bienenstock, J., Johnston, N. & Perey, D. Y. E. (1973b) Bronchial lymphoid tissue. II. Functional characteristics. *Laboratory Investigation*, 28, 693–698.

Bienenstock, J. & Johnston, N. (1976) A morphologic study of rabbit bronchial lymphoid aggregates and lymphoepithelium. *Laboratory Investigation*, 35, 343–348.

Bienenstock, J., Rudzik, O., Clancy, R. L. & Perey, D. Y. E. (1974) Bronchial lymphoid tissue. In *The Immunoglobulin A System*, ed. Mestecky, J. & Lawton, A. R., pp. 47–56. New York: Plenum Publishing.

Bienenstock, J., Rudzik, O., Clancy, R., Day, R. & Perey,

D. Y. E. (1974) Rabbit IgA: reconstitution experiments with bronchus associated lymphoid tissue (BALT) and Peyer's patches (GALT). *Federation Proceedings*, 33, 594.

Bloth, B. & Svehag, S-E. (1971) Further studies on the ultrastructure of dimeric IgA of human origin. *Journal of Experimental Medicine*, 133, 1035–1042.

Bockman, D. E. & Cooper, M. D. (1973) Pinocytosis by epithelium associated with lymphoid follicles in the bursa of fabricius, appendix and Peyer's patches. An electron microscopic study. *American Journal of Anatomy*, 136, 455–477.

Bohl, E. H., Saif, L. J., Gupta, R. K. P. & Frederick, G. T. (1974) Secretory antibodies in milk of swine against transmissible gastroenteritis virus. In *The Immunoglobulin A System*, ed. Mestecky, J. & Lawton, A. R., pp. 337–342. New York: Plenum Publishing.

Brandtzaeg, P. (1971) Human secretory immunglobulins. VI. Association of free secretory piece with serum IgA *in vitro*. *Immunology*, 21, 323–332.

Brandtzaeg, P. (1973) Structure synthesis and external transfer of mucosal immunoglobulins. *Annales d'Immunologie (Institut Pasteur)*, **124C**, 417–438.

Brandtzaeg, P. (1974) Mucosal and glandular distribution of immunoglobulin components: differential localization of free and bound SC in secretory epithelial cells. *Journal of Immunology*, 112, 1553–1559.

Brandtzaeg, P., Fjellanger, I. & Gjeruldsen, S. T. (1968) Adsorption of immunoglobulin A onto oral bacteria *in vivo*. *Journal of Bacteriology*, 96, 242–249.

Buckley, R. H. & Dees, S. C. (1969) Correlation of milk precipitins with IgA deficiency. *New England Journal of Medicine*, 281, 465–468.

Bull, D. M. & Tomasi, T. B. (1968) Deficiency of immunoglobulin A in intestinal disease. *Gastroenterology*, 54, 313–320.

Burdon, D. W. (1973) The bactericidal action of immunoglobulin A. *Journal of Medical Microbiology*, 6, 131–139.

Burnet, Sir MacFarlane (1959) *The Clonal Selection Theory of Acquired Immunity*, p. 86. London: Cambridge University Press.

Cantor, H. M. & Dumont, A. E. (1967) Hepatic suppression of sensitization to antigen absorbed into the portal system. *Nature*, 215, 744–745.

Carter, P. B. & Collins, F. M. (1974) The route of enteric infection in normal mice. *Journal of Experimental Medicine*, 139, 1189–1203.

Cebra, J. & Jones, P. P. (1974) Phytogenetic aspects of the secretory immunoglobulin system: Its implications as a mechanism of defense. In *The Immune System and Infectious Diseases*, pp. 306–321. Basel: Karger.

Chase, M. W. (1946) Inhibition of experimental drug allergy by prior feeding of the sensitizing agent. *Proceedings of the Society for Experimental Biology and Medicine*, 61, 257–259.

Chuang, C-Y., Capra, J. D. & Kehoe, J. M. (1973) Evolutionary relationship between carboxyterminal region of a human alpha chain and other immunoglobulin heavy chain constant regions. *Nature*, 244, 158–160.

Clancy, R. & Bienenstock, J. (submitted).

Collan, Y. (1972) Characteristics of non-epithelial cells in the epithelium of normal rat ileum. *Scandinavian Journal of Gastroenterology*, 7, suppl. 18, 5–66.

Colten, H. & Bienenstock, J. (1974) Lack of C3 activation through classical or alternate pathways by human secretory IgA anti-blood group A antibody. In *The Immunoglobulin A System*, ed. Mestecky, J. & Lawton, A. R., pp. 305–308. New York: Plenum Publishing.

Cooper, M. D., Lawton, A. R. & Kincade, P. W. (1972) A two-stage model for development of antibody-producing cells. *Clinical and Experimental Immunology*, 11, 143–149.

Crabbé, P. A. & Heremans, J. F. (1966) The distribution of immunoglobulin-containing cells along the human gastrointestinal tract. *Gastroenterology*, 51, 305–316.

Crabbé, P. A., Nash, D. R., Bazin, H., Eyssen, H. & Heremans, J. F. (1969) Antibodies of the IgA type in intestinal plasma cells of germ-free mice after oral or parenteral immunization with ferritin. *Journal of Experimental Medicine*, 130, 723–738.

Crabbé, P. A., Nash, D. R., Bazin, H., Eyssen, H. & Heremans, J. F. (1970) Immunohistochemical observations on lymphoid tissues from conventional and germ-free mice. *Laboratory Investigation*, 22, 448–457.

Craig, S. W. & Cebra, J. J. (1971) Peyer's patches: an enriched source of precursors for IgA-producing immunocytes in the rabbit. *Journal of Experimental Medicine*, 134, 188–200.

Darlington, D. & Rogers, A. W. (1966) Epithelial lymphocytes in the small intestine of the mouse. *Journal of Anatomy*, 100, 813–830.

Davies, A. (1922) An investigation into the serological properties of dysentery stools. *Lancet*, ii, 1009–1012.

Day, R. P. & Bienenstock, J. (unpublished).

Dayton, D. H., Small, P. A., Chanock, R. M., Kaufman, H. E. & Tomasi, T. B. (1970) In *The Secretory Immunologic System*. U.S. Department of Health, Education and Welfare.

Dolezel, J. & Bienenstock, J. (1971a) Immune response of the hamster to oral and parenteral immunization. *Cellular Immunology*, 2, 326–334.

Dolezel, J. & Bienenstock, J. (1971b) γA and non-γA immune response after oral and parenteral immunization of the hamster. *Cellular Immunology*, 2, 458–468.

Eskeland, T. & Brandtzaeg, P. (1974) Does J chain mediate the combination of 19S IgM and dimeric IgA with the secretory component rather than being necessary for their polymerization? *Immunochemistry*, 11, 161–163.

Fazekas De St Groth, S. & Donnelley, M. (1950a) Studies in experimental immunology of influenza. III. The antibody response. *Australian Journal of Experimental Biology and Medical Science*, 28, 45–60.

Fazekas De St Groth, S. & Donnelley, M. (1950b) Studies in experimental immunology of influenza. V. Enhancement of immunity by pathotopic vaccination. *Australian Journal of Experimental Biology and Medical Science*, 28, 77–85.

Ferguson, A. & Parrot, D. M. V. (1972) The effect of antigen deprivation on thymus-dependent and thymus-independent lymphocytes in the small intestine of the mouse. *Clinical and Experimental Immunology*, 12, 477–488.

Fichtelius, K. E. (1968) The gut epithelium – a first level lymphoid organ? *Experimental Cell Research*, 49, 87–104.

Freter, R. (1962) Detection of copro-antibody and its formation after parenteral and oral immunization of

human volunteers. *Journal of Infectious Diseases*, 111, 37–48.

Gitlin, D. & Biasucci, A. (1969) Development of γG, γA, γM, βIc/βIa, C'1 esterase inhibitor, ceruloplasmin, transferrin, hemopexin, haptoglobin, fibrinogen, plasminogen, αl-antitrypsin, orosomucoid, β-lipoprotein, α2-macroglobulin, and prealbumin in the human conceptus. *Journal of Clinical Investigation*, 48, 1433–1446.

Goldberg, S. S., Kraft, S. C., Peterson, R. D. A. & Rothberg, R. M. (1971) Relative absence of circulating antigen-reactive cells during oral immunization. *Journal of Immunology*, 107, 757–765.

Grey, H. M., Abel, C. A., Yount, W. J. & Kunkel, H. G. (1968) A subclass of human γA-globulins (γA2) which lacks the disulfide bonds linking heavy and light chains. *Journal of Experimental Medicine*, 128, 1223–1236.

Griscelli, C., Vassalli, P. & McCluskey, R. T. (1969) The distribution of large dividing lymph node cell in syngeneic recipient rats after intravenous injection. *Journal of Experimental Medicine*, 130, 1427–1451.

Guy-Grand, D., Griscelli, C. & Vassalli, P. (1974) The gut-associated lymphoid system: nature and properties of the large dividing cells. *European Journal of Immunology*, 4, 435–443.

Hall, W. H., Manion, R. E. & Zinneman, H. H. (1971) Blocking serum lysis of *Brucella abortus* by hyperimmune rabbit immunoglobulin A. *Journal of Immunology*, 107, 41–46.

Halpern, M. S. & Koshland, M. E. (1970) Novel subunit in secretory IgA. *Nature (London)*, 228, 1276–1282.

Halstead, T. E. & Hall, J. G. (1972) The homing of lymph-borne immunoblasts to the small gut of neonatal rats. *Transplantation*, 14, 339–346.

Heremans, J. F. (1960) *Les globulines sériques du système gamma, leur nature et leur pathologie*. Brussels: Arcia.

Heremans, J. F. (1968) Immunoglobulin formation and function in different tissues. *Current Topics in Microbiology*, 45, 131–203.

Heremans, J. F. (1975) In *The Immune System and Infectious Diseases*. Basel: Karger.

Heremans, J. F. & Crabbé, P. A. (1967) Immunohistochemical studies on exocrine IgA. In *Killander Nobel Symposium 3, Gamma globulins; structure and control of biosynthesis*, p. 129. Stockholm: Almquist & Wiksell.

Heremans, J. F. & Vaerman, J-P. (1971) In *Progress in Immunology*, ed. Amos, B., p. 875. New York: Academic Press.

Hill, I. R. & Porter, P. (1974) Studies of bactericidal activity to *Escherichia coli* of porcine serum and colostral immunoglobulins and the role of lysozyme with secretory IgA. *Immunology*, 26, 1239–1250.

Howard, J. C., Hunt, S. V. & Gowans, J. L. (1972) Identification of marrow-derived and thymus-derived small lymphocytes in the lymphoid tissue and thoracic duct lymph of normal rats. *Journal of Experimental Medicine*, 135, 200–219.

Hunter, R. L. (1972) Antigen trapping in the lamina propria and production of IgA antibody. *Journal of the Reticuloendothelial Society*, 11, 245–252.

Jensenius, J. C. & Williams, A. F. (1974) Total immunoglobulin of rat thymocytes and thoracic duct lymphocytes. *European Journal of Immunology*, 4, 98–105.

Kagnoff, M. F. & Campbell, S. (1974) Functional characteristics of Peyer's patch lymphoid cells. *Journal of Experimental Medicine*, 139, 398–406.

Kagnoff, M. F., Serfilippi, D. & Donaldson, R. M. (1973) *In vitro* kinetics of intestinal secretory IgA secretion. *Journal of Immunology,* **110,** 297–300.

Kaplan, M. E., Dalmasso, A. P. & Woodson, M. (1972) Complement-dependent opsonization of incompatible erythrocytes by human secretory IgA. *Journal of Immunology,* **108,** 275–278.

Kincade, P. W. & Cooper, M. D. (1973) Immunoglobulin A: Site and sequence of expression in developing chicks. *Science,* **179,** 398–400.

Kobayashi, K. (1971) Studies on human secretory IgA. Comparative studies of the IgA-bound secretory piece and the free secretory piece protein. *Immunochemistry,* **8,** 785–800.

Koshland, M. E. & Wild, C. E. (1974) Mechanism of immunoglobulin polymer assembly. In *The Immunoglobulin A System,* ed. Mestecky, J. & Lawton, A. R., pp. 129–138. New York: Plenum Publishing.

Lamm, M. E. & Greenberg, J. (1972) Human secretory component. Comparison of the form occurring in exocrine immunoglobulin A to the free form. *Biochemistry,* **11,** 2744–2750.

Lawton, A. R., Asofsky, R. &. Mage, R. G. (1970) Synthesis of secretory IgA in the rabbit. III. Interaction of colostral IgA fragments with T chain. *Journal of Immunology,* **104,** 397–408.

Lebacq-Verheyden, A. M., Vaerman, J. P., Heremans, J. F. (1972) Immunohistologic distribution of the chicken immunoglobulins. *Journal of Immunology,* **109,** 652–654.

Lev, M. & Battisto, J. R. (1970) Impaired delayed hypersensitivity in germ-free guinea pigs. *Immunology,* **19,** 47–54.

Martin, L. N. & Leslie, G. A. (1974) IgM-forming cells as the immediate precursor of IgA-producing cells during ontogeny of the immunoglobulin-producing system of the chicken. *Journal of Immunology,* **113,** 120–126.

Mattioli, C. A. & Tomasi, T. B. (1973) The life span of IgA plasma cells from the mouse intestine. *Journal of Experimental Medicine,* **138,** 452–460.

Mestecky, J. & Lawton, A. R. (Eds.) (1974) *The Immunoglobulin A System,* pp. 1–555. New York: Plenum Publishing.

Mestecky, J., Ziran, J., & Butler, W. T. (1971) Immunoglobulin M and secretory immunoglobulin A: presence of a common polypeptide chain different from light chains. *Science,* **171,** 1163–1165.

Mestecky, J., Schrohenloher, R. E., Kulhavy, R., Wright, G. P. & Tomana, M. (1974) Association of S-IgA subunits. In *The Immunoglobulin A System,* Ed. Mestecky, J. & Lawton, A. R., pp. 99–109. New York: Plenum Publishing.

Montgomery, P. C., Rosner, B. R. & Cohn, J. (1974) The secretory antibody response. Anti-DNP antibodies induced by dinitrophenylated type III pneumococcus. *Immunological Communications,* **3,** 143–156.

Moore, A. R. & Hall, J. G. (1972) Evidence for a primary association between immunoblasts and small gut. *Nature,* **239,** 161–162.

Murray, M., Miller, H. R. P. & Jarrett, W. F. H. (1968) The globule leukocyte and its derivation from the subepithelial mast cell. *Laboratory Investigation,* **19,** 222–234.

Newcomb, R. W. & Sutoris, C. A. (1974) Comparative studies on human and rabbit exocrine IgA antibodies to an albumin. *Immunochemistry,* **11,** 623–632.

O'Daly, J. A. & Cebra, J. J. (1971) Rabbit secretory IgA. I. Isolation of secretory component after selective dissociation of the immunoglobulin. *Journal of Immunology,* **107,** 436–448.

Ogra, P. L. & Karzon, D. T. (1969) Distribution of poliovirus antibody in serum, nasopharynx and alimentary tract following segmental immunization of lower alimentary tract with poliovaccine. *Journal of Immunology,* **102,** 1423–1430.

Ogra, P. L., Karzon, D. T., Righthand, F. & MacGillivray, M. (1968) Immunoglobulin response in serum and secretions after immunization with live and inactivated poliovaccine and natural infection. *New England Journal of Medicine,* **279,** 893–900.

Perey, D. Y. & Bienenstock, J. (1973) Effects of bursectomy and thymectomy on ontogeny of fowl IgA, IgG and IgM. *Journal of Immunology,* **111,** 633–637.

Poger, M. E. & Lamm, M. E. (1974) Localization of free and bound secretory component in human intestinal epithelial cells – a model for the assembly of secretory IgA. *Journal of Experimental Medicine,* **139,** 629–642.

Reynolds, H. Y. & Thompson, R. E. (1973) Pulmonary host defenses. II. Interaction of respiratory antibodies with *Pseudomonas aeruginosa* and alveolar macrophages. *Journal of Immunology,* **111,** 369–380.

Robertson, P. W. & Cooper, G. N. (1973) Immune responses in intestinal tissue to particulate antigens. Development of cells forming different classes of antibody in primary and secondary responses. *Australian Journal of Experimental Biology and Medical Science,* **51,** 575–587.

Rothberg, R. M., Kraft, S. C. & Farr, R. S. (1967) Similarities between rabbit antibodies produced following ingestion of bovine serum albumin and following parenteral immunization. *Journal of Immunology,* **98,** 386–395.

Rothberg, R. M., Kraft, S. C. & Michalek, S. M. (1973) Systemic immunity after local antigenic stimulation of the lymphoid tissue of the gastrointestinal tract. *Journal of Immunology,* **111,** 1906–1913.

Rothberg, R. M., Kraft, S. C., Asquith, P. & Michalek, S. M. (1973) The effect of splenectomy on the immune responses of rabbits to a soluble protein antigen given parenterally or orally. *Cellular Immunology,* **7,** 124–133.

Rudzik, O. & Bienenstock, J. (1974) Isolation and characteristics of gut mucosal lymphocytes. *Laboratory Investigation,* **30,** 260–266.

Shearman, D. J. C., Parkin, D. M. & McClelland, D. B. L. (1972) The demonstration and function of antibodies in the gastrointestinal tract. *Gut,* **13,** 483–499.

Silverman, A. S. & Pomeranz, J. R. (1972) Studies on the localization of hapten in guinea pigs fed picryl chloride. *International Archives of Allergy and Applied Immunology,* **42,** 1–7.

Sprent, J. & Miller, J. F. A. P. (1972) Interaction of thymus lymphocytes with histoincompatible cells. II. Recirculating lymphocytes derived from antigen-activated thymus cells. *Cellular Immunology,* **3,** 385–404.

Strauss, H. & Bienenstock, J. (unpublished).

Strober, W., Blaese, R. M., & Waldmann, T. A. (1970) The origin of salivary IgA. *Journal of Laboratory and Clinical Medicine,* **75,** 856–862.

Tada, T. & Ishizaka, K. (1970) Distribution of γE-forming cells in lymphoid tissues of the human and monkey. *Journal of Immunology,* **104,** 377–387.

Taubman, M. A. & Genco, R. J. (1971) Induction and properties of rabbit secretory γA antibody directed to group A streptococcal carbohydrate. *Immunochemistry,* **8,** 1137–1155.

Taylor, B., Norman, A. P., Orgel, H. A., Stokes, C. R.

Turner, M. W. & Soothill, J. F. (1973) Transient IgA deficiency and pathogenesis of infantile atopy. *Lancet*, **ii**, 111–116.

Teir, H., Rytömaa, T., Cederberg, A. & Kiviniemi, K. (1963) Studies on the elimination of granulocytes in the intestinal tract in rat. *Acta Pathologica et Microbiologica Scandinavica*, **59**, 311–324.

Thomas, H. C. & Vaez-Zadeh, F. (1974) A homeostatic mechanism for the removal of antigen from the portal circulation. *Immunology*, **26**, 375–382.

Thompson, R. A. & Asquith, P. (1970) Quantitation of exocrine IgA in human serum in health and disease.. *Clinical and Experimental Immunology*, **7**, 491–500.

Tomasi, T. B., Tan, E. M., Solomon, A. & Prendergast, R. A. (1965) Characteristics of an immune system common to certain external secretions. *Journal of Experimental Medicine*, **121**, 101–124.

Tomasi, T. B. & Bienenstock, J. (1968) Secretory immunoglobulins. In *Advances in Immunology*, ed. Dixon, F. J. & Kunkel, H. G. Vol. 9, pp. 1–96. New York: Academic Press.

Tomasi, T. B. & Grey, H. M. (1972) Structure and function of immunoglobulin A. *Progress in Allergy*, **16**, 81–213.

Tomasi, T. B. & Hauptman, S. P. (1974) The binding of α-1 antitrypsin to human IgA. *Journal of Immunology*, **112**, 2274–2277.

Tourville, D. R., Adler, R. H., Bienenstock, J. & Tomasi, T. B. (1969) The human secretory immunoglobulin system: immunohistological localization of γA, secretory 'piece', and lactoferrin in normal human tissues. *Journal of Experimental Medicine*, **129**, 411–423.

Triger, D. R., Cynamon, M. H. & Wright, R. (1973) Studies on hepatic uptake of antigen. I. Comparison of inferior vena cava and portal vein routes of immunization. *Immunology*, **25**, 941–956.

Turk, A., Lichtenstein, L. M. & Norman, P. S. (1970) Nasal secretory antibody to inhalent allergens in allergic and non-allergic patients. *Immunology*, **19**, 85–95.

Uhlenhuth, D. (1900) Neuer Beitrag 2 um specifischen nachweis von eiereiweiss auf bioligischen wege. *Med. Wchnschr.*, **26**, 734–735.

Uhr, J. W. & Vitetta, E. S. (1974) Cell surface immunoglobulin. VIII. Synthesis, secretion and cell surface expression of immunoglobulin in murine thoracic duct lymphocytes. *Journal of Experimental Medicine*, **139**, 1013–1018.

Vaerman, J. P., Kobayashi, K. & Heremans, J. F. (1974)

Precipitin cross-reactions between human and animal J-chains. In *The Immunoglobulin A System*, ed. Mestecky, J. & Lawton, A. R., pp. 251–255. New York: Plenum Publishing.

Van Furth, R., Schuit, H. R. E. & Hijmans, W. (1965) The immunological development of the human foetus. *Journal of Experimental Medicine*, **122**, 1173–1188.

Van Munster, P. J. J. (1971) De secretair component. Thesis, Univ. Nijmegen.

Veldkamp, J., Van der Graag, R. & Willers, J. M. N. (1973) The role of Peyer's patch cells in antibody formation. *Immunology*, **25**, 761–771.

Vitetta, E. S., Grundke-Iqbal, I., Holmes, K. V. & Uhr, J. W. (1974) Cell surface immunoglobulin. VII. Synthesis, shedding and secretion of immunoglobulin by lymphoid cells of germ-free mice. *Journal of Experimental Medicine*, **139**, 862–876.

Waksman, B. H. (1973) The homing pattern of thymus-derived lymphocytes in calf and neonatal mouse Peyer's patches. *Journal of Immunology*, **111**, 878–884.

Waksman, B. H., Ozer, H. & Blythman, H. E. (1973) Appendix and γM-antibody formation. VI. The functional anatomy of the rabbit appendix. *Laboratory Investigation*, **28**, 614–626.

Walker, W. A. & Bloch, K. J. (personal communication).

Walker, W. A., Isselbacher, K. J. & Bloch, K. J. (1973) Intestinal uptake of macromolecules. II. Effect of parenteral immunization. *Journal of Immunology*, **111**, 221–226.

Walker, W. A., Wu, M., Isselbacher, K. & Bloch, K. J. (1975) Intestinal uptake of macromolecules. III. Studies on the mechanism by which immunization interferes with antigen uptake. *Journal of Immunology*, **115**, 854–861.

Waldman, R. H., Spencer, C. S. & Johnson, J. E. (1972) Respiratory and systemic cellular and humoral immune responses to influenza virus vaccine administered parenterally or by nose drops. *Cellular Immunology*, **3**, 294–300.

Warshaw, A. L., Walker, W. A., Cornell, R. & Isselbacher, K. J. (1971) Small intestinal permeability to macromolecules. *Laboratory Investigation*, **25**, 675–684.

Williams, R. C. & Gibbons, R. J. (1972) Inhibition of bacterial adherence by secretory immunoglobulin A: a mechanism of antigen disposal. *Science*, **177**, 697–699.

Zipursky, A., Brown, E. J. & Bienenstock, J. (1973) Lack of opsonization potential of 11S human secretory γA. *Proceedings of the Society for Experimental Biology and Medicine*, **142**, 181–184.

2. Immunological mechanisms

R. A. Thompson

INTRODUCTION

The gastrointestinal tract is exposed to a great variety of potentially harmful substances ranging from the enzymes of its own secretions to microorganisms, and substances ingested or derived from the breakdown of food. The sequence of events in the development of gastrointestinal pathology may therefore be difficult to ascertain. Immunological factors may play a primary role or they may be involved secondarily, as a result of initial damage from other causes. The role of immunological mechanisms in the gastrointestinal disease must also be considered in the light of the normal physiology of immunity. In general disease may be due to failure, or imbalance, of normal immune mechanisms. This may be congenitally determined or acquired as the result of the operation of environmental factors, although the strict separation of these two types of influence is often difficult.

Failure of normal mechanisms occurs in the syndromes of immunodeficiency, which are marked by an increased susceptibility to infections. On the other hand, an imbalance or over-action of the system may lead to one or other of the various hypersensitivity reactions. This chapter considers in theoretical terms immunodeficiency syndromes and hypersensitivity reactions with respect to the gastrointestinal tract.

IMMUNODEFICIENCY

OVERALL DEFECTS

Three broad types of non-specific overall immunological defects are recognized. These are based on the concepts of the normal immune response, during which antigen stimulates responding cells from two distinct populations of immunocompetent lymphocytes. Both populations are derived from primitive stem cells of the reticuloendothelial system, but one population passes through the thymus gland during maturation (T-cells) after which the cells are able to participate in cell-mediated reactions, such as delayed hypersensitivity, homograft rejection, and the processing of certain antigens, forming the cellular arm of the immune response. Cells which produce antibodies are derived from a second population of lymphocytes (B-cells),

found mainly in the bone marrow in adult animals. Recovery from infection and immunity from reinfection are the result of the physiological response of both populations of cells to antigens of invading microorganisms, although for certain infections the role of one type of response may be of predominant importance. For instance, T-cells are particularly important in recovery from virus infections and in defence against fungal and mycobacterial infections, while B-cell responses (i.e. antibodies) are necessary to prevent reinfection by viruses and the commoner gram positive and gram negative bacteria.

B-cell deficiency

A failure of immunoglobulin production, and therefore of antibody production, due to absent or nonfunctional B-cells, is the commonest type of deficiency to be recognized clinically, in the various forms of dys- and hypogammaglobulinaemia (Rosen and Janeway, 1966; Martin, 1971), and it is these latter conditions which have received the most attention from a gastrointestinal point of view. Similar syndromes may occur secondarily as a result of antibody loss through the kidney or the gastrointestinal tract, or due to depression of synthesis by cytotoxic drugs or by reticuloendothelial neoplasia.

Selective absence or deficiency of IgA in the serum and external secretions is probably the most common form of dysgammaglobulinaemia, affecting 1 in 700 individuals (Bachmann, 1965), but it occurs more frequently among those with conditions such as rheumatoid arthritis and coeliac disease, and also among individuals with an increased susceptibility to respiratory, especially upper-respiratory, infections. However, this disability affects only a minority of those with selective IgA deficiency, and although IgA is an important part of the defence mechanisms of mucous surfaces, no evidence exists linking its selective deficiency specifically with increased susceptibility to gastrointestinal infection, or for that matter, causally implicating this deficiency in any gastrointestinal disorder. Lack of IgA in serum and secretions, although the most apparent abnormality, may be associated with other subtle defects that are more difficult to evaluate, and which may account for the variable clinical picture with which it is associated. Many individuals without IgA show a compensatory increase in IgM in their secretions (Brandtzaeg, Fjellanger and Geruldsen, 1968), and a proportion of this is linked to secretory component (Thompson, 1970). Whether this plays an important role in the function of local antibody is not known. Also in patients with ataxia telangiectasia, those susceptible to infections have been found to lack both IgA and IgE in their secretions, while IgA-deficient subjects able to cope with infections have normal levels of IgE (Amman et al., 1969).

T-cell deficiency

Failure to develop cell-mediated reactions due to absent or non-functional T-cells is very rare in its pure form, occurring in the Di George syndrome in which thymic aplasia or hypoplasia is associated with hypoparathyroidism and congenital abnormalities of the great vessels (Di George, 1965) and in a syndrome described by Nezalof et al. (1964) in which there is thymic hypoplasia.

Mixed T- and B-cell deficiency

Mixed defects of both T- and B-cells are more common, and a variety of different clinical syndromes (Fudenberg et al., 1970) including the Wiscott–Aldrich syndrome and ataxia telangiectasia have been described in which the immune defects are partial or incomplete, and may be associated with other apparently unrelated abnormalities. The rare but severe form of combined immunodeficiency of Swiss-type agammaglobulinaemia is due to an absence of stem cells from which both T- and B-cells develop. Affected children do not usually survive after the first year of life, but suffer severe, recurrent respiratory and systemic infections, diarrhoea, and fail to thrive (Glanzmann and Riniker, 1950; Gitlin, Vawter and Craig, 1964).

SPECIFIC DEFECTS

In addition to overall defects of immunological mechanisms, operating against a wide range of antigens, there have been recently recognized specific defects in responsiveness to certain types of antigen. This has been more clearly elucidated in experimental animals, where it has been shown that the response to synthetic polypeptide antigens is under genetic control – the genes responsible being called the immune response (Ir) genes (McDevitt and Benacerraff, 1969). In man there are also likely to be Ir genes controlling immune responsiveness, and it is possible that genetically determined failure in immune responsiveness to certain microbial antigens may be a cause of increased susceptibility to a specific type of infection. More probably, partial impairment may lead to poor antigen clearance and chronic persistence of a microorganism, with the consequent development of 'soluble complex' disease. Conversely,

there is the possibility that some Ir genes may result in a heightened response to certain common extrinsic antigens, and produce one or other of the hypersensitivity reactions. These genes are closely linked to genes controlling the expression of the major histocompatibility antigens (including the HL-A system), and the mapping of these in man is proving to be of extreme interest and importance in the whole field of medicine. Already a marked association of certain HL-A antigens has been reported in several diseases (McDevitt and Bodmer, 1974), and of particular interest in the context of gastrointestinal disease is their association with coeliac disease (Falchuk, Rogentine and Strober, 1972; Stokes et al., 1972).

In general the way in which hypofunction of immune mechanisms operates to cause gastrointestinal disease is far from clear. Recurrent diarrhoea, malabsorption and failure to thrive are commonly seen in infants with severe combined immunodeficiency syndrome, but less so in other forms of immunological defect. About 20 per cent of patients with hypogammaglobulinaemia, either the adult acquired form or the more clearly defined sex-linked Bruton's disease, have gastrointestinal symptoms of diarrhoea and malabsorption (Hill, 1971). Overt intestinal giardiasis may be found, as may positive bacterial cultures of duodenal aspirates, with a decrease in gastrointestinal symptoms following chemotherapeutic eradication of the infection. On the contrary, in other individuals with clinical immune deficiency and diarrhoea, the gastrointestinal symptoms are not apparently related to chronic infection, but to other factors, such as gluten enteropathy (Ch. 9).

The intestinal lumen is a hostile enough environment for most pathogenic microorganisms, so that immune mechanisms probably play a minor role in preventing common gastrointestinal infections, although they come into play when invasion of the mucosal surface occurs. Local antibody may function primarily in blocking viruses from entering epithelial cells, and in minimising the uptake and systemic dissemination of antigenic material, resulting from the pinocytosis of incompletely digested proteins.

HYPERSENSITIVITY REACTIONS

Hypersensitivity reactions have been conveniently classified (Coombs and Gell, 1975) into four types (Fig. 2.1), although in any particular disease process more than one mechanism may operate and it may be difficult to define the extent of the contribution of each type.

TYPE I REACTIONS

Type I (immediate hypersensitivity) reactions occur when antigen combines with reaginic or homocytotropic

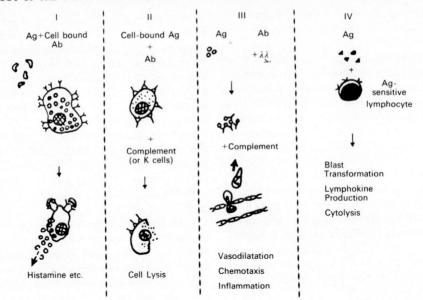

Fig. 2.1 Diagrammatic illustration of the 4 types of allergic reaction. Ag = antigen. Ab = antibody.

antibody on the surface of tissue mast cells. These antibodies appear not to have a physiological role in the circulation but are fixed to cells by means of a site on the Fc portion of the molecule. Combination with antigen sets off a sequence of intracellular reactions resulting in the release of histamine and other vasoactive substances, which produce increased capillary permeability, vasodilation and smooth muscle contraction and sometimes systemic anaphylaxis (Ch. 3). When the reaction occurs following intradermal injection of antigen, it takes the form of a local wheal and flare. IgE-containing plasma cells have been demonstrated in the nasal mucosa, in the tonsils (Tada and Ishizaka, 1970) and in the intestine (Savilahti, 1972), and IgE has been found in nasal fluid, saliva, and sputum (Waldman, Virchow and Rowe, 1973). In the nose, the reaction between antigen and specific IgE-sensitized cells causes mucosal congestion and rhinorrhoea characteristic of hay fever; in the conjunctiva it produces a prickling sensation and increased lacrimation, while in the bronchi it causes the reversible bronchial constriction, symptomatic of asthma. In some respiratory disorders and possibly in some types of allergic rhinorrhoea, homocytotropic IgG antibodies play a role (Parish, 1971). The differences in the pathophysiology of the types of antibody are not clear, but it is possible that IgG antibodies are less susceptible to treatment by 'hyposensitization' procedures. The factors which bring about the predominance of a reaginic antibody response to certain antigens are not well understood, but individuals who develop this type of hypersensitivity tend to occur in families and are referred to as atopic subjects.

The role of Type I reactions in gastrointestinal dis-

orders in man is uncertain. In animals they appear to play a part in bringing about the spontaneous recovery from some worm infestations, with massive worm expulsion (Ogilvie and Jones, 1973); but whilst intestinal worm infestation in man is associated with high circulating levels of total IgE, which decrease after successful chemotherapeutic eradication (Johansson, Melbin and Vahlquist, 1968), there is no evidence that IgE antibodies act against these worms. Clinical reactions which quickly follow the ingestion of specific proteins have been frequently reported (Ch. 11) and are usually ascribed to hypersensitivity reactions. These may take the form of acute diarrhoea and vomiting, or sometimes more general symptoms of urticaria and asthma. Occasionally in atopic subjects, there is an abrupt and brisk reaction, often involving swelling of the mouth and lips with which food was in contact, clearly indicating the action of reaginic antibody. More often, however, the symptoms come on at any time from a few minutes to a few hours after intake, and the causative mechanisms are seldom obvious.

TYPE II REACTIONS

Type II (cytotoxic) hypersensitivity reactions occur between complement-fixing antibodies, and antigens which form an integral part of, or become attached to, the surface of the individual's own cells. The resultant activation of complement causes the destruction or at least a decreased life span of the cells concerned. In addition certain types of IgG antibody convert cells into targets for cytotoxic lymphocytes. These reactions have almost exclusively been described clinically as affecting the cellular elements of the circulation, and they result in haemolytic anaemia, or agranulocytosis, or thrombocytopenia, depending on the cell type involved. This can be a true autoimmune process due to the proliferation of clones of cells which produce antibodies against self-antigens, or it can occur because of an immune response against a drug or chemical such as penicillin, which becomes tightly bound to proteins on the surface of the cells, which are passively lysed as a consequence. In many diseases, e.g. Hashimoto's thyroiditis, idiopathic Addison's disease, etc., 'autoantibodies' are detected; nevertheless there is no evidence that they are responsible for the pathology, and indeed it is possible that they occur as epiphenomena secondary to the main disease process.

So far there is little evidence that Type II mechanisms operate in gastrointestinal disease. Autoantibodies to mucosal antigens have been described in a variety of chronic diseases affecting the intestine, particularly in ulcerative colitis (Broberger and Perlmann, 1959) (Ch. 7). However, the latter are frequently removed by absorption with coliform bacteria, and are undoubtedly the result of cross-reaction. There is no evidence that they play a role in the pathogenesis of this disease, although this evidence would be difficult to obtain, as it is in many putative autoimmune diseases, the definitive test being the transfer of the disease to unaffected individuals, or experimental animals by means of antibodies. Locally produced autoantibodies, or antibodies against drugs or other haptenic substances which adhere to the surface of epithelial cells, may produce pathological reactions but would not necessarily be detectable in the circulation.

Autoantibodies reacting with gastric parietal cells are seen in a high proportion of patients with pernicious anaemia as well as those with simple atrophic gastritis (Ch. 5). IgG antibodies which complex with intrinsic factor also occur in the serum of patients with pernicious anaemia. These antibodies block the uptake of B_{12}, and there are also antibodies to the B_{12}-intrinsic factor complex which block its uptake by intestinal cells (Chanarin, 1975), both types of antibody action being independent of complement. They can thus interfere with the normal physiological mechanisms for B_{12} absorption and might contribute towards the clinicopathological state of B_{12} deficiency.

TYPE III REACTIONS

Type III (Arthus-type) hypersensitivity reactions occur between soluble or microparticulate antigens and complement-fixing antibodies, which form antigen/antibody/complement complexes. In the tissues these produce increased capillary permeability and the ingress of phagocytes (particularly polymorphs) due to the generation of chemotactic and other complement-mediated factors. The complexes are ingested and produce disruption of the polymorphs and release of their lysosomal enzymes, which cause tissue destruction and enhancement of the inflammatory process. This reaction, seen when antigen is injected intradermally in the presence of sufficient circulating antibody, is called an Arthus reaction. It takes 4–6 hours to develop fully, producing an appreciable area of erythema and oedema, which subsides within 24 hours. If the reaction is severe enough, then generalized symptoms can result with hypotension, collapse and bronchospasm.

If an antigen is introduced systemically in the absence of circulating antibody, then, as an immune response develops, the resulting antigen–antibody complexes may be present in antigen excess, fixing complement poorly as a consequence. If the complexes do not reach a sufficient size, they will be poorly eliminated by the reticuloendothelial system, and continue to circulate. They then tend to be deposited more gradually in the walls of small vessels – usually endarterioles on seromucous surfaces and in the renal glomeruli, resulting in an inflammatory vasculitis. This produces the symptoms of joint pain, polyserositis and glomerulitis, which characterize serum sickness as well as many other soluble complex diseases.

Role of complement

The biological function of complement appears, in part at least, to enhance the clearance from the body of antigens. In the case of microbial pathogens, this involves their opsonization and/or lysis. However, the activation of complement is associated with the generation of phlogistic peptides, which cause vasodilatation, increased capillary permeability, and attract and disrupt neutrophil polymorphonuclear leucocytes. These inflammatory processes are necessary for the removal of pathogens, but if occurring on a wide scale throughout a particular organ, they impair the function of that organ and produce disease. This can happen following exposure of an individual to antigens to which complement-fixing antibodies exist (e.g. the reaction between the antigens of M. faeni and antibodies in Farmer's lung), and if constantly repeated may produce structural damage and eventual fibrosis.

Failure of antigen clearance may occur if the antibody or complement system is defective, in which case circulating complexes remain relatively small and, instead of being removed by the reticuloendothelial system, lodge in the walls of small vessels (particularly in the kidneys), where low-grade complement fixation, if sufficiently widespread, will similarly impair physiological function and cause tissue destruction. These pathological processes are usually subacute, taking months or even years to develop, in contrast to the rapid inflammation associated with efficient complement activation.

Most Type II and III reactions depend on the activation of the complement system, and in experimental animals, both are prevented or considerably reduced in intensity by prior decomplementation of the animal. The nature of the antibody formed is of prime importance in the development of these reactions. IgM antibodies, and, in man, those of IgG1, IgG2, and IgG3 subclasses, are capable of fixing complement by the classical pathway (Fig. 2.2). That is, under the appropriate ratios of antigen and antibody, the first component of complement, C1 becomes attached by means of its

The activation of the later components, from C5 through to C9, then follows with the release of further chemotactic factors, and, if the antigen–antibody complex is on the surface of a cell, it can result in cell lysis due to the attachment of later-acting components which damage the cell membrane. Although the haemolysis of sensitized sheep erythrocytes is the system by which complement has been defined, recognized and studied for decades, this lytic process is probably not of major biological significance, since strains of laboratory animals

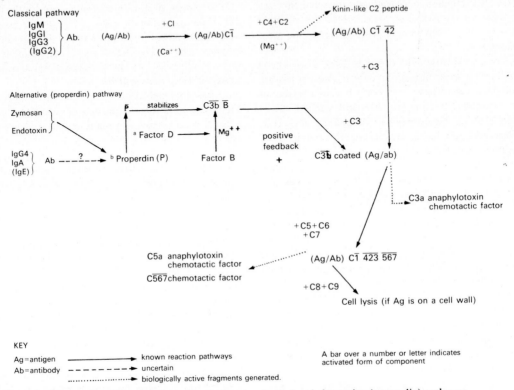

Fig. 2.2 Mechanisms of the activation of complement by the classical and alternative (properdin) pathways.
[a] Factor D is thought to exist in serum in an activated form.
[b] Properdin stabilizes to $\overline{C3b}\ \overline{B}$ complex which is the alternative pathway 'C3 convertase', $\overline{C42}$ being the classical pathway C3 convertase.

C1q subcomponent, and is then activated to an esterase on the C1s subcomponent, which itself acts on the next two components, C2 and C4, to form an enzyme ($\overline{C42}$) called C3 convertase. The activation of the system results in the sequential activation of inactive components to generate this important enzyme, which acts on the major component of the complement system, C3, to release chemotactic and anaphylactic fragments, as well as cause the attachment of C3 molecules in considerable quantity to the complex. This promotes the phagocytosis of the molecule, and is the stage of prime biological importance, resulting in elimination of antigens, including of course invading pathogenic microorganisms.

exist which are genetically deficient in C5 or C6, and which remain in apparent good health, although their serum cannot lyse antibody-coated cells. Also there have been case reports of C6- and C7-deficient humans also in good health. The sera in all these situations is, however, able to fix adequate C3 onto antigen–antibody complexes, which ensures their *in-vivo* removal.

It is now clear that C3 fixation can be promoted by a mechanism, which is known as the alternative pathway of complement fixation (Götze and Muller-Eberhard, 1971). Some such mechanism was first suggested by Pillemer and his associates (1954), who, studying the inactivation of complement by the yeast cell wall polysaccharide zymosan, postulated the intermediate action of a substance called properdin, but this concept fell into disrepute, from which it has only recently emerged. The elements of the system and the way in which they work are still under investigation although proteins termed Factor B and Factor D and properdin itself (Factor P) are recognized; but it appears that the alternative pathway (or the properdin pathway) is itself driven by fixed C3 in a kind of positive feedback resulting in a massive coating of this component onto the surface of antigen–antibody complexes (Nicol and Lachmann, 1973). This reaction is modulated normally by the C3b inhibitor. The pathway can also be activated independently of the classical pathway by certain classes of antibody, notably IgG4 and IgA (and possible IgE), as well as other substances such as bacterial endotoxin and solid polysaccharides like zymosan, inulin and dextran (Ruddy, Gigli and Austen, 1973), through the intermediate action of properdin. Fixation of C3 by the alternative pathway can then be followed by activation of the later components and cell lysis if the reaction is made to take place under appropriate conditions on the surface of a cell.

During the activation of C3 by any pathway, the molecule is split into two fragments, C3a and C3b; only a small proportion of the activated C3b fragments attaches to the initiating agent (antigen–antibody complex, cell surface, zymosan particle, etc.), while none of the smaller C3a, which is the chemotactic and anaphylotoxic fragment, attaches. The bulk of the fragments are released into the supernatant where they are quickly acted upon by inactivators. The C3b inactivators splits C3b further into C3c and C3d. These breakdown products are detectable by immunoelectrophoresis against an anti-C3 antiserum, since they have a more anodal mobility than native C3. While C3b and C3c are rapidly removed from the circulation, C3d appears to be cleared more slowly, and can be seen on electrophoresis of fresh plasma from patients with complement-consuming diseases.

An intact alternative pathway apparently compensates biologically for a deficient classical pathway, in that individuals with a genetic deficiency of C2, whose sera cannot lyse sensitized erythrocytes, are not particularly susceptible to infections although they possibly eliminate antigen–antibody complexes less well than normal. On the other hand, their sera show a normal capacity for promoting *in-vitro* bacterial killing and phagocytosis (Gewurz *et al.*, 1966), due to the adequate fixation of C3 via the alternative pathway. Similarly, a strain of C4-deficient, but apparently healthy guinea-pigs has been described, in which the alternative pathway mechanism operates to promote bacterial killing and also to produce complement-dependent local Arthus reactions, on injection of endotoxin or antigen–antibody complexes (Frank, May and Gaither, 1971).

Any speculation as to the operation of complement-mediated Type II or III hypersensitivity mechanisms in disorders of the gastrointestinal tract must be done in the face of some major theoretical considerations. Firstly, there is the nature of the antibody. IgA antibody, apparently of major importance in the gastrointestinal tract, is unable to fix complement by the classical pathway. However, Adinolphi, Glynn, Lindsay and Milne (1966) reported that bacteria could be lysed by IgA antibody in the presence of complement and lysozyme, and this somewhat controversial finding can now be explained on the basis of the fixation of complement by IgA using the alternative pathway. Nevertheless, this mechanism is probably less efficient at promoting lysis than the classical pathway, and in conditions of limited complement availability, the reaction, if it occurred, would be more likely to generate phlogistic complement-derived factors, rather than cause cell death.

The other objections concern the facts that little if any complement is present in the external secretions of the gastrointestinal tract and, moreover, the complement components are extremely sensitive to inactivation by proteolytic enzymes. Once antigen had penetrated the mucosa, however, complement and other systemically operating factors could be brought into play, giving rise to submucosal reactions. On the other hand IgA auto-antibodies to complement in saliva and other external secretions have been described in normal subjects (Lachmann and Thompson, 1970). These antibodies are different from the normal serum immunoconglutinins, in that they are inhibited by native C3, and are also cation dependent, so that it is possible that they arise as a result of different factors.

Possible roles of IgA

Local IgA probably acts to limit the entry of foreign antigens through the epithelium rather than expedite their removal from the body. Thus a relatively small antigenic molecule penetrating the surface epithelium might stimulate local IgA antibodies, which would prevent the antigen's subsequent re-entry by complexing with it in the lumen and effectively increasing its size. Similarly IgA antibodies could neutralize toxins, or limit the mobility (and hence the penetration) of potential pathogens at external surfaces. An imperfect IgA response, on the other hand, would allow the entry of antigens and stimulate systemic antibodies resulting in mucosal or submucosal hypersensitivity reactions on subsequent exposure. Antigen present in excess (possibly from a non-lethal virus replication in epithelial cells) could also form soluble complexes with IgA antibody, which would escape into the general circulation and cause systemic effects. There appears to be a natural requirement for some modulation of the antigenic load from the gut as increased levels of antibodies to food antigens are found in individuals with selective IgA deficiency and also in patients with cirrhosis and a disordered portal circulation; these latter also show increased antibody titres to bacterial and viral antigens (Bjorneboe, Prytz and Orskov, 1972; Triger, Alp and Wright, 1972).

The possibility exists that this antigenic load might outstrip these protective mechanisms, for either local anatomical reasons or because of a genetic deficiency in immune responsiveness, so producing immunologically mediated disease. It has been shown (Taylor et al., 1973) that children with a defective secretory IgA system in early life are more likely to develop extrinsic allergies later; an ineffective IgA response allows ingress of antigens and the development of a predominant IgE response. Also chronic disorders of the gut, such as ulcerative colitis and Crohn's disease, frequently have systemic complications of iritis, dermatitis and arthritis which are the hallmarks of diseases due to circulating antigen–antibody complexes. It is possible that other 'immune complex' diseases, such as some forms of nephritis and rheumatoid arthritis, may also be due to a primary defect in control of the release of antigens from the intestine.

Some acute gastrointestinal reactions to the ingestion of specific foods are accompanied by evidence of complement consumption (Matthews and Soothill, 1970). This has been reported in patients with milk protein sensitivity; milk challenge usually results in acute episodes of diarrhoea and vomiting occurring in the course of a few hours, over which time there is a concomitant fall in the serum complement levels, as well as the appearance in the circulation of complement breakdown products. These patients have appreciable amounts of circulating IgG anti-milk antibodies, and it is most likely that the symptoms are due to Type III reactions occurring in the submucosa, once the protein has gained entry. It is probable that the massive complement-fixing reaction is made possible by initial reaction with IgE antibody which increases capillary permeability and allows the ingress of larger amounts of serum antibodies and complement. This has been postulated as operating in allergic pulmonary disease (Pepys, 1969).

TYPE IV REACTIONS

Type IV (delayed hypersensitivity) reactions involve the interaction between antigen and antigen-sensitive lymphocytes; these are usually carried out as intradermal skin tests, which take 24–48 hours to become positive. Histologically the lesion is characterized by the perivascular accumulation of mononuclear cells, mainly macrophages and lymphocytes. The most familiar Type IV reaction is the tuberculin (Mantoux) skin text, while the best-recognized clinical condition resulting from the operation of this mechanism is contact dermatitis. During the formation of the clinical lesion the reacting lymphocytes are thought to release large amounts of soluble mediators or lymphokines. These are small molecular weight peptides having a diverse effect, not only on other lymphocytes and macrophages, but also on tissues, by altering capillary permeability, etc. (Ch. 3). The formation of certain types of granulomata is thought to be one of the consequences of cell-mediated immune reactions, although the precise requirements for granuloma formation have not been elucidated.

Evidence for the operation of Type IV hypersensitivity to produce gastrointestinal disease is not strong and is largely circumstantial. Lymphocytes are plentiful in the lamina propria and the epithelial cell layer of the intestine (Ch. 1). Also in certain diseases, for example in Crohn's disease, the histological picture includes granuloma formation in the bowel wall, and this is evidence of accompanying impaired cellular immunity (Jones et al., 1972). On the other hand, in coeliac disease, evidence has been produced of increased cellular reactivity to gluten (see review by Haeney and Asquith, 1976), especially involving cells from mesenteric lymph nodes, (Housley, Asquith and Cooke, 1969). Still, the problems of interpreting such data (Haeney and Asquith, 1976), and distinguishing cause from effect, are great.

Another type of cellular mechanism, which appears to be part of the immune response, involves the ability of lymphocytes directly to kill target cells by a little-understood process of cytolysis, independent of complement. T-lymphocytes do this directly against cells bearing antigens to which they are sensitive – and also non-specifically when stimulated by certain mitogens such as phytohaemagglutinin. Other lymphocyte-like cells can kill target cells which have been sensitized or reacted with IgG antibody. This antibody-dependent cytotoxicity was thought to be a property of a subpopulation of B-cells, but these cells are now known as K- (Killer) cells. Normal lymphocytes with sera from patients with coeliac disease have been shown to attach to intestinal epithelial cells in tissue culture, suggesting that this mechanism may be important in producing the disease (Fakhri and Hobbs, 1972; Ezeoke et al., 1974).

CONCLUSION

The special immunological requirements of the gastrointestinal tract relate to its unique role in being subject to a considerable antigenic load, which must be excluded from the milieu interior, while at the same time it must allow the selective absorption of all that is useful for life. These requirements are met by the secretory immune system, and many gastrointestinal disorders are likely to have their roots in the aberrant action of this system.

Defects in its operation may lead on the one hand to a decreased resistance to microbial infection, or on the other, to any of the various hypersensitivity syndromes, because of inappropriate stimulation of more centrally operating immunocompetent cells, by antigens which would otherwise fail to gain entry. Some of these reactions may involve the complement system, acting perhaps via the alternative pathway. The role of cell-mediated immune responses could be of considerable importance but requires further evaluation. The mechanisms have been difficult to elucidate, partly because of the inaccessibility of the gastrointestinal surfaces to examination and experimentation, but also because of the inaccessibility of the portal circulation, which forms the vascular drainage of the intestinal tract. The application of modern endoscopic procedures and experimental techniques of tissue culture and intestinal loop isolation will undoubtedly produce more definitive information.

REFERENCES

Adinolfi, M., Glynn, A. A., Lindsay, M. & Milne, C. M. (1966) Serological properties of gamma-A antibodies to *Escherichia coli* present in human colostrum. *Immunology*, **10**, 517–526.

Amman, A. J., Cain, W. A., Ishizaka, K., Hong, R. & Good, R. A. (1969) Immunoglobulin E deficiency in ataxia-telangiectasia. *New England Journal of Medicine*, **281**, 469–472.

Backmann, R. (1965) Studies on the serum gamma-A-globulin level. III. The frequency of agamma-A-globulinaemia. *Scandinavian Journal of Clinical and Laboratory Investigation*, **17**, 316–320.

Bjørneboe, M., Prytz, H. & Ørskov, F. (1972) Antibodies to intestinal microbes in serum of patients with cirrhosis of the liver. *Lancet*, **i**, 58–60.

Brandtzaeg, P., Fjellanger, I. & Gjeruldsen, S. T. (1968) Immunoglobulin M; local synthesis and selective secretion in patients with immunoglobulin A deficiency. *Science*, **160**, 789–791.

Broberger, O. & Perlmann, P. (1959) Autoantibodies in human ulcerative colitis. *Journal of Experimental Medicine*, **110**, 657–674.

Chanarin, I. (1975) The stomach in allergic diseases. In *Clinical Aspects of Immunology*, 3rd edn, ed. Gell, P. G. H., Coombs, R. R. A. & Lachmann, P. J., pp. 1429–1440. Oxford: Blackwell Scientific.

Coombs, R. R. A. and Gell, P. G. H. (1975) Classification of allergic reactions responsible for clinical hypersensitivity and disease. In *Clinical Aspects of Immunology*, 3rd edn, ed. Gell, P. G. H., Coombs, R. R. A. & Lachmann, P. J., pp. 761–781. Oxford: Blackwell Scientific.

DiGeorge, A. M. (1965) A new concept of the cellular basis of immunity. *Journal of Paediatrics*, **67**, 907–908.

Ezeoke, A., Ferguson, N., Fakhri, O., Hekkens, W. Th. J. M. & Hobbs, J. R. (1974) Antibodies in the sera of coeliac patients which can coopt K-cells to attack gluten-labelled targets. In *Coeliac Disease: Proceedings of the Second International Coeliac Symposium*, ed. Hekkens, W. Th. J. M. & Peña, A. S., pp. 176–186. Leyden: Stenfert-Kroese.

Fakhri, O. & Hobbs, J. R. (1972) Detection of antibodies which can cooperate with lymphocytes. *Lancet*, **ii**, 403–406.

Falchuk, Z. M., Rogentine, G. N. & Strober, W. (1972) Predominance of histocompatibility antigen HL-A8 in patients with gluten-sensitive enteropathy. *Journal of Clinical Investigation*, **51**, 1602–1605.

Frank, M. M., May, J., Gaither, T. & Ellman, L. (1971) *In vitro* studies of complement function in sera of C4-deficient guinea-pigs. *Journal of Experimental Medicine*, **134**, 176–187.

Fundenberg, H. H., Good, R. A., Goodman, H. C., Hitzig, W., Kunkel, H. G., Roitt, I. M., Rosen, F. S., Rowe, D. S., Seligmann, M. & Soothill, J. R. (1970) Primary immunodeficiencies. The cellular basis of immune responses. *Bulletin of the World Health Organisation*, **45**, 125–142.

Gewurz, H., Pickering, R. J., Muschel, L. H., Mergenhagen, S. E. & Good, R. A. (1966) Complement-dependent biological functions in complement deficiency in man. *Lancet*, **ii**, 356–360.

Gitlin, D., Vawter, G. & Craig, J. M., (1964) Thymic alymphoplasia and congenital aleukocytosis. *Pediatrics*, **33**, 184–192.

Glanzmann, E. & Riniker, P. (1950) Essentielle lymphocytaphthise. Ein neues Krankheitsbild aus der Sawglingspathologie. *Annales Paediatrici*, **175**, 1–32.

Götze, O. & Muller-Eberhard, H. J. (1971) The C3-activator system: an alternate pathway of complement activation. *Journal of Experimental Medicine*, **134**, 90s–108s.

Haeney, M. & Asquith, P. (1976) Stimulation of lymphocytes from patients with coeliac disease by subfraction of gluten. *Lancet*, **ii**, 629–630.

Hill, L. E. (1971) Clinical features of hypogamma-globulinaemia. In *Hypogammaglobulinaemia in the U.K. – report of an MRC working party*. London: HMSO.

Housley, J., Asquith, P. & Cooke, W. T. C. (1969) Immune response to gluten in adult coeliac disease. *British Medical Journal*, **ii**, 159–161.

Johansson, S. G. O., Mellbin, T. & Vahlquist, B. (1968) Immunoglobulin levels in Ethiopian pre-school children with special reference to high concentrations of immunoglobulin E (IgND). *Lancet*, **i**, 1118–1121.

Jones, J. V., Housley, J., Ashurst, P. M. & Hawkins, C. F. (1969) Development of delayed hypersensitivity to dinitrochlorobenzene in patients with Crohn's Disease. *Gut*, **10**, 52–56.

Lachmann, P. J. & Thompson, R. A. (1970) Immunoconglutinins in human saliva – a group of unusual IgA antibodies. *Immunology*, **18**, 157–169.

McDevitt, H. O. & Benacerraf, B. (1969) Genetic control of specific immune responses. *Advances in Immunology*, **11**, 31–74.

McDevitt, H. O. & Bodmer, W. F. (1974) HL-A, immune response genes, and disease. *Lancet*, **i**, 1269–1275.

Martin, N. H. (1971) Recognition of the hypogamma-globulinaemia syndrome. In *Hypogammaglobulinaemia in the U.K. – report of an MRC working party*. London: HMSO.

Matthews, T. S. & Soothill, J. F. (1970) Complement activation after milk feeding in children with cow's milk allergy. *Lancet*, **ii**, 893–895.

Nezelof, C., Jammet, M. L., Lortholary, P., Labrune, B. &

Lamy, M. (1964) L'hypoplasie héréditaire du Thymus: Sa place et sa responsabilité dans une observation d'aplasie lymphocytaire, normoplasmocytaire et normoglobulinemique du Nourrisson. *Archives Françaises de Pediatrie (Paris)*, **21**, 897–920.

Nicol, P. A. E. & Lachmann, P. J. (1973) The alternate pathway of complement activation. The role of C3 and its inactivator (KAF). *Immunology*, **24**, 259–275.

Ogilvie, B. M. & Jones, V. E. (1973) Immunity in the parasitic relationship between helminths and hosts. In *Progress in Allergy*, Vol. 17, ed. Kallós, P., Waksman, B. H. & de Weck, A., pp. 93–144. Basel: Karger.

Parish, W. E. (1970) Short-term anaphylactic IgG antibodies in human sera. *Lancet*, **ii**, 591–592.

Pepys, J. (1969) *Hypersensitivity Diseases of the Lungs due to Fungi and Organic Dusts*. Basel: Karger.

Pillemer, L., Blum, L., Lepow, I. H., Ross, O. A., Todd, E. W. & Wardlaw, A. C. (1954) The Properdin system and immunity: I. Demonstration and isolation of a new serum protein, properdin, and its role in immune phenomena. *Science*, **120**, 279–285.

Rosen, F. S. & Janeway, C. A. (1966) The gamma-globulins III. The antibody deficiency syndromes. *New England Journal of Medicine*, **275**, 709–715 & 769–775.

Ruddy, S., Gigli, I. & Austen, K. F. (1972) The complement system of man. *New England Journal of Medicine*, **287**, 489–495, 545–549, 642–646.

Savilahti, E. (1972) Immunoglobulin-containing cells in the intestinal mucosa and immunoglobulins in the intestinal juice in children. *Clinical and Experimental Immunology*, **11**, 415–425.

Stokes, P. L., Asquith, P., Holmes, G. K. T., Mackintosh, P. & Cooke, W. T. (1972) Histocompatibility antigens associated with adult coeliac disease. *Lancet*, **ii**, 162–164.

Tada, T. T. & Ishizaka, K. (1970) Distribution of γE-forming cells in lymphoid tissues of the human and monkey. *Journal of Immunology*, **104**, 377–387.

Taylor, B., Norman, A. P., Orgel, H. A., Stokes, C. R., Turner, M. W. & Soothill, J. F. (1973) Transient IgA deficiency and pathogenesis of infantile atopy. *Lancet*, **ii**, 111–113.

Thompson, R. A. (1970) Secretory piece linked to IgM in individuals deficient in IgA. *Nature*, **226**, 946–948.

Triger, D. R., Alp, M. H. & Wright, R. (1972) Bacterial and dietary antibodies in liver disease. *Lancet*, **i**, 60–63.

Waldman, R. H., Virchow, C. and Rowe, D. S. (1973) IgE levels in external secretions. *International Archives of Allergy and Applied Immunology*, **44**, 242–248.

3. Mediators of allergic inflammation

J. Morley

INTRODUCTION

It is generally accepted that in allergic responses there is release or secretion of materials whose biological activities can account for many of the features of allergic inflammation. These materials are not products of antigen degradation, nor are they substances showing immunological reactivity or specificity towards the sensitizing antigen. Their potent pharmacological actions and local release could justify their designation as autacoids (Douglas, 1970), but they are usually referred to under the term mediator.

Characterization and chemical identification of mediators of allergic inflammation are of clinical interest for two reasons. Firstly, in a number of diseases, including those affecting the intestine, pathological events may be due to allergic responses that are excessive in their magnitude or duration. Thus, hypersensitivity responses occurring in the intestine to exogenous or endogenous agents may result in acute or chronic inflammation, as for example in food allergy (Ch. 11) or in inflammatory bowel disease (Ch. 7) respectively. It is considered that precise identification of mediators in such reactions would considerably assist efforts to devise drugs capable of specifically suppressing the actions of these mediators (Brocklehurst, 1976). Secondly, it is apparent that some mediators of allergic inflammation share identity with mediators of totally unrelated physiological processes. For example, histamine is involved in a central position both in Type I allergic responses (Rocha e Silva, 1966) and in gastric acid secretion (Lundell, 1975). This latter phenomenon poses a dilemma, for suppression of allergic mediator production in inflammation may impair the normal physiology of the gastrointestinal tract. Conversely, suppression of gastrointestinal function, for example the use of the histamine (H_2) antagonist cimetidine in the treatment of peptic ulceration, may impair those allergic responses which maintain the integrity of the intestine against attack from exogenous and endogenous substances.

For these reasons, mediators are regarded in this chapter in the context of their action in physiological allergic responses as well as the more usual situation in which emphasis is placed upon their contribution to pathology.

THE MEDIATOR CONCEPT

The clinical manifestations of allergic inflammation are consequent upon the modification of the behaviour of a particular cell type (the immunological effector cell), following the reaction of the host to a specific antigen. This reaction with antigen can be on the effector cell itself, as for example when antigen interacts with reaginic antibody on a mast cell (Ch. 2). Alternatively, the reaction can be with preformed immunologically specific material, for example, circulating immunoglobulin, with the formation of immune complexes. These in turn may then modify the behaviour of cell types which do not show immunological specificity, such as the neutrophil. The effector cells most clearly identified are the mast cell, basophil, eosinophil and platelet in Type I reactions, the neutrophil and platelet in Type III reactions, and the small lymphocyte and macrophage in Type IV reactions. It is likely that other cells which are identified in allergic reactions may have greater significance than that often accorded to them. The uncertainty as to the identity of the effector cell in particular reactions is amply illustrated by the Jones–Mote reaction, a mild delayed response, that was widely regarded as a typical Type IV reaction until the recent demonstration that the most abundant cell type in such lesions is, in fact, the basophil (Richerson, Dvorak and Leskowitz, 1970; Dvorak *et al.*, 1970).

It is the ability of immunological effector cells to markedly affect, and even kill, unrelated cell types in adjacent tissue that endows them with their considerable pathogenic potential. This property is compounded by the phenomenon of hypersensitivity, that is, the ability of an organism to alter its reactivity to an antigen, often by several orders of magnitude, following a single exposure to the antigen. The possession by an animal of such powerful amplification devices can be regarded as advantageous in evolutionary terms, as they provide mechanisms for the speedy elimination of potentially hazardous microorganisms. Yet situations clearly arise in which this potentially beneficial system will produce deleterious rather than advantageous effects. Thus, in guinea-pigs exhibiting Type I reactivity, local challenge in the skin with substantial doses of antigen may evoke a systemic reaction in the form of bronchospasm which is of such severity that it completely overshadows the local skin reaction. Alternatively, in Type III and IV hypersensitivity, skin reactions in response to a substantial antigenic dose can result in local necrosis. Whilst this could be viewed as a device for physical elimination of antigen in skin (by shedding antigen in the sloughed necrotic tissue), it is evident that in tissues not so amenable to necrosis, for example in synovium, the result could be severe loss of function of the joint, a catastrophe for non-domestic animals. An adverse effect of interaction between antigen and the host's immunological defences was first appreciated by Portier and Richet (1902). They observed that repeated treatment of a dog with a venom derived from *Physalia sp.* resulted in exacerbation and alteration of its response to venom, so that Richet coined the term 'anaphylaxis', as opposed to prophylaxis, to describe the phenomenon (Rocha e Silva, 1966). Richet attempted to interpret the phenomenon on the basis of production of a toxic material, but mediation by an antigen–antibody product was the preferred explanation at that time. On the contrary, it has progressively become apparent that in the Type I response as in the other major responses (Types III and IV), there is release of potent biologically active substances lacking immunological specificity; their responses do not depend upon interaction with antigen (i.e. non-antibody) and they are not antigen-degradation products. These materials (mediators) include agents such as histamine, 5-hydroxytryptamine, slow reacting substance of anaphylaxis (SRS-A), kinins, prostaglandins and lymphokines as well as many less identifiable factors.

fact the dominance of contemporaneous immunological theories (such as the antibody concept at the turn of the century or the small lymphocyte involvement in Type IV reactions in the fifties and sixties) has ensured that a role for autacoids (i.e. biologically active molecules without immunological specificity) in such reactions has been slow in securing acceptance. Indeed, in Type IV responses current evidence continues to favour direct cell–cell contact rather than secretion of a lymphotoxin in cytoxic manifestations of Type IV hypersensitivity (Cerottini and Brunner, 1974). Nonetheless, it is apparent that many features of allergic reactions can be mimicked by endogenous, biologically active material in the absence both of antigen and of the recognition mechanism (Table 3.1). These include the classical features of the inflammatory reaction, such as increased vascular permeability, vasomotor changes, haematogenous cell accumulation and pain. The ready accessibility of skin in mammalian species has resulted in widespread use of skin reactions to study mediator involvement in allergic responses *in vivo*. This is despite its obvious unsuitability for certain aspects of the response exhibited in other organs, for example, the degradation of bone and cartilage in joints. Isolated intestinal smooth muscle has been the principal preparation for the study of smooth muscle spasmogens, yet alteration in smooth muscle tone provides only one facet of the allergic response in the intestine. Modification in other features, for example, the composition and duration of digestive and mucous secretion, the absorption of materials or the cell turnover at the luminal surface, may be more deci-

Table 3.1

Allergic response	Recognition mechanism	Primary effector elements	Secondary effector elements	Mediators released or generated
Type I	Cell bound IgE or IgG	Mass cell, Basophil	Eosinophil, Platelet	Histamine, 5-HT, SRS-A, kinins, PGs, thromboxanes
Type III	Circulating IgG or IgM	Neutrophil, Platelet		Complement components C3a and C5a, kinins, PGs, thromboxanes
Type IV	Small lymphocyte surface receptor	Small lymphocyte	Macrophage	Lymphokines, PGE$_2$, thromboxanes

Table 3.1 illustrates the basic concept of mediator release, in which antigen interacts with a recognition mechanism to result in activation of the effector cell with production of biologically active materials.

INVOLVEMENT OF MEDIATORS IN ALLERGIC REACTIONS

It is not axiomatic that mediators must be directly responsible for all features of allergic inflammation. In

sive than erythema and altered vascular permeability in affecting normal physiology of the alimentary tract.

CRITERIA FOR MEDIATOR EVALUATION

In physiology, the emergence of the concept that neurotransmitter substances and endocrine secretions were intermediaries for communication between cells has resulted in the formulation of criteria which potential mediators should satisfy (Dale, 1933). These criteria may be summarized in the context of allergic inflammation as follows:

1. The tissue (in this case the proposed effector cell) must be capable of producing or releasing the mediator.
2. Mechanisms must exist for the destruction or elimination of the mediator.
3. Local application of the mediator released should mimic the endogenous allergic response both quantitatively and qualitatively.
4. The time course of mediator release should correspond with the time course of the endogenous allergic response.
5. Depletion of precursors of the mediator or suppression of mediator production should produce an appropriate reduction in the allergic response.
6. Suppression of mediator destruction should result in an augmentation of the allergic response.
7. Specific antagonists should suppress both responses due to local application of the mediator and the endogenous allergic response.

During the period in which these criteria emerged there was some application to mediators of allergic inflammation, with Dale himself exhibiting a sustained interest in this problem (Feldberg, 1970). Despite this fact, it is clear that criteria for mediator identification are orientated more towards the problem of synaptic transmission and endocrine identification. For example, the first criterion would appear to be unnecessary to immunologists, as most would assume that the obvious location to search for a mediator would be at the site of an allergic response, or, its *in-vitro* equivalent (for example, isolated intestinal tissue or cultures of particular cell types associated with the allergic response). However, in the search for synaptic transmitters, attention was originally focussed upon material with many of the requisite properties for a synaptic transmitter that existed in certain natural (i.e. biological) products, but which had not been demonstrated as components of the mammalian nervous system. Thus the first biological material shown to contain acetylcholine was ergot (Dale, 1914) and it was several years before its isolation from the mammalian tissues, ox and horse spleen (Dale and Dudley, 1929).

Similarly the last criterion appears almost superfluous, in that existence of specific antagonists seems to presuppose satisfaction of other criteria so that such drugs merely provide confirmatory evidence of mediator identity, of interest mainly because of their therapeutic implications. In fact, in the search for synaptic transmitters, use of naturally occurring antagonists (for example, nicotine, curare and atropine) which would interfere with synaptic transmission long preceded

mediator identification. These drugs served initially to focus attention upon particular compounds as potential transmitters as well as subsequently to complement other evidence of mediator identification.

When allergic responses are viewed in the light of such criteria, it is apparent that few have been studied as comprehensively as nerve transmitter substances or hormones. Histamine is a notable exception which interestingly enough resembles acetylcholine in first being isolated from ergot (Barger and Dale, 1910). Its failure to achieve status as a mediator of allergic inflammation comparable to acetylcholine as a neurotransmitter stems largely from the initial absence of specific antagonists to histamine. Thus, clinically effective histamine (H_1) and histamine (H_2) antagonists were not recognized until 1942 (Halpern, 1942) and 1972 (Black *et al.*, 1972) respectively. The deflection of interest from histamine following the failure of histamine (H_1) antagonists (for example, mepyramine) to suppress allergic responses, and the resurgence of interest in histamine following the demonstration of H_2 receptors by the use of H_2 antagonists on allergic effector cells, are clear indications of the critical role specific pharmacological antagonists play in mediator identification.

MEDIATORS OF ALLERGIC INFLAMMATION

The principal substances considered as mediators of allergic inflammation are the vasoactive amines, SRS-A, kinins, prostaglandins and allied compounds with an assemblage of additional active materials usually designated as 'factors'. These latter have received less attention. The order given is 'chronological', each mediator having experienced phases of popularity and decline, with prostaglandins currently receiving much attention.

VASOACTIVE AMINES

Histamine, the amine derivative of histidine, and serotonin or 5-hydroxytryptamine, the amine derivative of tryptophan, have both been considered as mediators of various aspects of allergic inflammation.

Histamine

Soon after its isolation from ergot (Barger and Dale, 1910) histamine was found to be a constituent of intestinal mucosa (Barger and Dale, 1911). It was shown to produce hypotension, capillary dilatation and increased vascular permeability (Dale and Richards, 1918). Dale suggested its identity with the 'H-substance', the vasoactive material responsible for the triple response in skin (Lewis, 1927). Histamine is widely distributed throughout mammalian tissues and an association between mast cells and tissue histamine has been established

(Riley, 1959). However, histamine available for release in inflammation is not restricted to mast cells, being found also in platelets, basophils and eosinophils, and considerable changes in histidine decarboxylase in cells other than mast cells can accompany inflammation (Kahlson and Rosengren, 1970).

In the context of allergic inflammation, the most striking features of histamine as a potential mediator are its vasoactive properties, i.e. the production of local vasodilatation and increased vascular permeability. Nevertheless, it has additional pharmacological properties of relevance to inflammation, for example the production of pruritis in skin, the induction of gastric acid secretion and the alteration of gastrointestinal motility by a spasmogenic action on intestinal smooth muscle.

The most penetrating arguments levelled against it as a mediator of allergic inflammation have been its relative ineffectiveness in the rat and mouse. Also histamine (H_1) antagonists fail to modify many allergic responses (e.g. Type I and Type IV reactions in guinea-pig skin), in contrast to their effectiveness in selectively abolishing responses to intradermal injection of histamine (for full review see Kahlson and Rosengren, 1970; Rocha e Silva, 1966).

5-Hydroxytryptamine

5-Hydroxytryptamine (5-HT) was investigated as enteramine, a constituent of the enterochromaffin cells of the gastrointestinal tract, and independently as serotonin, a vasoconstrictor formed in defibrinated blood (Erspamer, 1954). In the gastrointestinal tract, 5-HT is associated with chromaffin cells, and with carcinoid tumours, the latter containing, and releasing, substantial amounts of the material. It is also a constituent of blood platelets from which it can be released by immune complexes (Humphrey and Jacques, 1955) and, in rats and mice, it is a notable constituent of mast cells (Riley, 1959). Its potential as an inflammatory mediator stems in part from its potency in evoking increased vascular permeability (Rowley and Benditt, 1956), so fulfilling the need for a mediator insensitive to the histamine (H_1) antagonists. The ability of the latter to suppress responses to exogenous histamine but not endogenous allergic responses had precluded histamine as a sole mediator of many inflammatory responses. The 5-HT antagonists (for example, lysergic acid diethylamide) are effective in suppressing permeability responses to 5-HT, but like the histamine (H_1) antagonists they have proved relatively ineffectual in experimental allergic reactions (for full review see Lewis, 1958; Erspamer, 1966).

SLOW REACTING SUBSTANCE OF ANAPHYLAXIS

SRS-A is a lipid soluble material, released in Type I allergic reactions, that is characterized by its ability to cause a slow, protracted contraction in certain isolated smooth muscle preparations, for example guinea-pig ileum (Bocklehurst, 1960). In the rat, SRS-A is released from IgE-sensitized mast cells, whilst in IgG-mediated release, complement and neutrophils are involved in SRS-A formation (Orange, Stechschulte and Austen, 1970). The identification and assay of SRS-A is achieved by reference to its biological as opposed to its chemical properties. SRS-A can be distinguished from prostaglandins by differential inhibition of release by cromoglycate and eicosatetraynoic acid (Dawson and Tomlinson, 1974). The sensitivity of SRS-A to arylsulphatases and the sulphur content of purified preparations suggest the presence of a sulphate ester group (Orange, Murphy and Austen, 1974) but further chemical identification has not been achieved.

In addition to causing slow contraction of smooth muscle, SRS-A potentiates responses to other agonists (Orange and Austen, 1969); it is able to contract human bronchial smooth muscle at low concentrations without tachyphylaxis (Brocklehurst, 1962) and crude preparations produce increased vascular permeability unrelated to mast cell degranulation. This inflammatory effect is most marked in the guinea-pig and monkey and increased doses produce localized haemorrhagic necrosis (Orange and Austen, 1969). The lack of readily available partially purified SRS-A has restricted its evaluation in comparison to chemically defined potential mediators, for example the prostaglandins (for extensive review see Brocklehurst, 1962; Orange and Austen, 1969; Austen, 1974).

THE KININS

The kinins are a group of peptides with potent pharmacological properties including a hypotensive action, contraction of a range of smooth muscles, production of pain and production of increased vascular permeability. Kinins are released from a substrate in mammalian plasma by enzymes in various biological fluids, including blood. The kinin released by serum kininogenase was termed kallidin (Werle and Berek, 1948), a nonapeptide of identical structure to bradykinin, the kinin produced by the action of trypsin on serum globulin (Rocha e Silva, Beraldo and Rosenfeld, 1949). The evidence favouring bradykinin as an inflammatory mediator is primarily circumstantial. The kinins exhibit high potency in evoking features of inflammation; an abundance of substrate (kininogen) is present in plasma and lymph and the enzymes capable of kinin release can be rapidly activated, the kininogenase activation system being closely linked to activation of the clotting cascade (Colman, 1974; Brocklehurst and Movat, 1975). Technical difficulties, such as the lability of the peptide in blood and lymph, the ease with which kininogenases may be activated by surfaces or dilution, and the absence of specific antagonists of kinins, have precluded their unequivocal establishment as primary inflammatory mediators. Nevertheless, there is evidence of their release in Type I (Brocklehurst and Lahiri, 1962; Jonasson and Becker, 1966) and Type III (Eisen and Smith, 1970) responses. Relevant to the intestine is the ability of trypsin to act both as a prekininogenase activator and as a kinin-releasing enzyme. This fact must make the kinins presumptive mediators in situations in which intestinal contents are in intimate contact with plasma proteins. The kinins have been extensively reviewed by Erdos (1970), Rocha e Silva and Garcia Leme (1972), while their role in pathology has been reviewed by Lewis (1964), Webster and Innerfeld (1965), Eisen (1969), Schachter (1969) and Colman (1974).

PROSTAGLANDINS

The prostaglandins are a group of 20-carbon unsaturated fatty acids of related structure. Initially they were investigated as possible smooth muscle stimulants of the female reproductive tract (Eliasson, 1959). Prostaglandins were not widely favoured as potential inflammatory mediators until it was demonstrated that non-steroidal anti-inflammatory drugs (NSAIDs) were potent inhibitors of prostaglandin synthetase enzymes (Vane, 1971; Flower, 1974). E-type prostaglandins are vasodilator smooth muscle stimulants. Their ability to reproduce features of the inflammatory response may in certain situations require interaction with other agonists, for example in the production of increased vascular permeability in the guinea-pig (Williams and Morley, 1973) and in the production of protracted pain or of hyperalgesia in man (Ferreira, 1972). Such phenomena may reflect their potent action as modulators of other agonists in a variety of physiological systems (Bergström, 1967; Horton, 1969). This basic property of prostaglandins facilitates explanation of adverse side effects of NSAIDs such as bleeding from gastric erosions (Vane, 1973); the gastric erosions produced by NSAIDs providing an example of the interrelationships between mediators in normal gastrointestinal physiology and mediators of allergic responses. Prostaglandins show adequate potency for effecting a number of features of the inflammatory response in the intestine, including stimulation of gastrointestinal motility, inhibition of sodium and water absorption, and the production of pain (Nakano and Koss, 1973). Prostaglandins are at present strongly favoured as inflammatory mediators and in allergic responses there is evidence of their production in Type I (Piper and Vane, 1969; Gréen, Hedqvist and Svanborg, 1974) and Type IV responses (Bray, Gordon and Morley, 1974), in the latter situation the cellular origin of PGE_2 production having been identified as the macrophage (Gordon, Bray and Morley, 1976).

An introduction to the subject of prostaglandins is provided by Ramwell and Pharris (1972) and Bergström and Bernhard (1973) whilst their participation in inflammatory responses has been recently reviewed by Willoughby Giroud, Di Rosa and Velo (1973), Zurier (1974) and Ferreira and Vane (1974). A more recent development in this field is the identification of thromboxanes as major products from cyclic endoperoxides (Samuelsson and Vane, 1976), particularly in platelets, and it appears that these highly active compounds of short biological half life may prove quantitatively more important than PGs in certain situations.

LYMPHOKINES

Lymphokines are non-antibody products of *in-vitro* lymphocyte activation that exhibit a range of biological activities in non-sensitized animals or tissues. The association of such biologically active material with Type IV hypersensitivity was first appreciated by Bloom and Bennett (1966) and David (1966) who referred to the active material as 'macrophage migration inhibition factor' or MIF. Subsequently, an increase in a host of other biological activities was detected in the products of lymphocyte activation, each being referred to as a corresponding factor, for example, mitogenic factor and inflammatory factor. It is still not apparent to what extent these various activities may reflect the properties of particular molecular species, hence the term lymphokine has been introduced as a generic term for the products of lymphocyte activation (Dumonde *et al.*, 1969). Nevertheless, current evidence suggests that lymphokines are a heterogeneous group of substances (Bray *et al.*, 1975). The evidence for these materials serving as mediators of Type IV allergic responses is based primarily upon their ability to produce appropriate effects *in vitro* and *in vivo*. Quantitative investigation, comparable to that directed towards neurotransmitters or hormones is insubstantial (Morley, Wolstencroft and Dumonde, 1973; Morley 1974b). Bloom and Glade (1971) and Morley (1977) have described techniques used in lymphokine measurement whilst reviews of the background and biological significance of these materials are provided by Bloom (1971), David and David (1972), Dumonde and Maini (1971).

REGULATION OF IMMUNE RESPONSES

Endocrine substances achieve their specificity of action because of distinctive features of their target cells. Classical neurotransmitters behave similarly, but their specificity of action is also dependent upon their very restricted release, namely at the synaptic junction. By comparison, in allergic reactions the inflammatory response must be localized, but at the same time it must also alter the *potential* reactivity of the whole organism without producing systemic reactions. This implies the existence of control mechanisms serving to limit the extent and duration of allergic reactions.

Two devices, of relevance to this objective, result in the release of substances whose properties do not fulfil the accepted criteria for classical transmitters. The first of these is 'potentiation', where two agents produce an effect of considerably greater magnitude than the sum of their independent actions. This is clearly illustrated by the action of PGE_1 on guinea-pig skin. The intradermal injection of PGE_1 alone is relatively ineffective in evoking increased vascular permeability (Horton, 1963), hence PGE_1 would be excluded by classical mediator criteria. Yet this compound is able to effect a considerable potentiation of the action of other agonists, for example histamine and bradykinin (Williams and Peck, 1977). A similar phenomenon is shown by the glucocorticosteroids in a number of tissues where the action of an agonist is only manifest in the presence of glucocorticosteroids (the 'permissive' effect of steroids). Such systems as 'potentiation' achieve the capacity for overall reactivity by the systemic release of one component of the inflammatory response. However, actual inflammation is confined to the site of antigenic stimulation because it is *only* at that site that the co-factor is released. Mechanisms involving potentiation also reduce the risk of incidental activation of the inflammatory response.

A second device is the liberation of materials which regulate or modulate mediator release by the effector cells. This regulation may take the form of positive feedback systems in which the regulatory material (which may also be a mediator of some aspects of the inflammatory response) intensifies the production of mediators by other potential effector cells. Lymphokines, the proposed mediators of Type IV reactions, fall into this category. Thus it can be anticipated that lymphokines, released by antigen activation of sensitized lymphocytes, as well as causing macrophage activation, stimulate non-sensitized lymphocytes to produce additional lymphokines. In the face of such a powerful positive feedback mechanism it is clearly desirable to have negative feedback control systems. Four classes of endogenous compounds have been shown to inhibit components of allergic responses: glucocorticosteroids, prostaglandins, β-adrenergic agents and vasoactive amines. Examples of this type of process are seen in each class of allergic response. Thus in Type I hypersensitivity reactions, following antigenic exposure, *in-vitro* release of histamine from the basophil can be inhibited by histamine (Lichtenstein and Gillespie, 1973). In Type III reactions the release of lysosomal enzymes in response to phagocytic stimuli is inhibited by high concentrations of PGE_1 (Weissmann, Dukor and Zurier, 1971) whilst in Type IV reactions lympho-

kine formation is inhibited by E-type prostaglandins (Bray, Gordon and Morley, 1974) and glucocorticosteroids (Wahl, 1974). It has been proposed that the regulatory actions of these different substances are achieved by a common mechanism, namely the modification of cyclic nucleotide levels in the effector cell appropriate to the particular type of allergic response (Bourne *et al.*, 1974). Whilst evidence for this unifying theory is incomplete it provides a useful framework for considering drug actions on allergic effector mechanisms. The efficacy of these regulatory materials in inhibiting mediator release *in vitro* is not doubted, but it is less certain that they are generally released in adequate concentrations for this to represent a physiological as opposed to a pharmacological phenomenon. Nonetheless, such a theory could reconcile long-standing and somewhat paradoxical observations. Thus, histamine has long been considered as a possible inflammatory mediator in Type IV reactions. In support of this is the observation of elevated histamine synthesis in Type IV lesions in the rat (Graham and Schild, 1967), but in contradiction is the failure of local or systemic treatment with histamine (H_1) receptor antagonists (e.g. mepyramine) to affect permeability changes in established Type IV reactions.

Finally, regulation of immune reactions can also be achieved by more indirect mechanisms with greater latency. An example of this type of regulatory device has emerged from the investigations of the chemical properties of SRS-A. It was shown that this mediator is particularly susceptible to enzymic degradation by aryl sulphatase and that the eosinophil possesses a potent aryl sulphatase (Orange, Murphy and Austen, 1974). Hence, in Type I responses the release of eosinophil chemotactic tetrapeptide would result in the accumulation of cells in the lesions which then eliminate the actions of an unrelated mediator (i.e. SRS-A).

MEDIATORS IN ALLERGIC INFLAMMATION

It seems likely that valid models of allergic responses will inevitably be complex, their complexity being a consequence of the devices necessary to assure synchrony of a preordained sequence of events. To this end the distribution of receptors to regulatory molecules on the surface of effector cells (e.g. H_2 distribution in T-dependent lymphocytes (Plaut, Lichtenstein and Henney, 1973)) is of central importance to this process. However, in spite of this alleged complexity the basic sequence of events illustrated in Figures 3.1–3.3 continues to be instructive as a format for experimental investigation and clinical interpretation.

Following cellular activation by interaction with

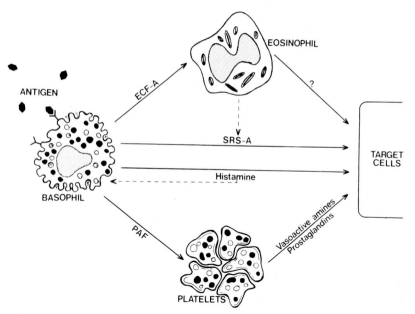

Fig. 3.1 Diagrammatic representation of mediator release in Type I hypersensitivity reaction. ECF-A, eosinophil chemotactic factor; SRS-A, slow reacting substance of anaphylaxis; PAF, platelet activating factor. Solid lines indicate mediator production. Dotted lines indicate an inhibitory action of histamine on mediator secretion and destruction of SRS-A by eosinophil aryl sulphatase. Target cells are classically smooth muscle cells but will include other cell types.

antigen in Type I and IV responses or by phagocytosis of antigen–antibody complexes in Type III responses there is initiation of secretory activity, resulting in release of cell products, a process generally regarded as being regulated by cyclic nucleotide levels. (Bourne *et al.*, 1974). Thus in Type I reactions, the sensitized mast cell or basophil releases the biogenic amines, histamine and 5-hydroxytryptamine together with heparin. Addi-

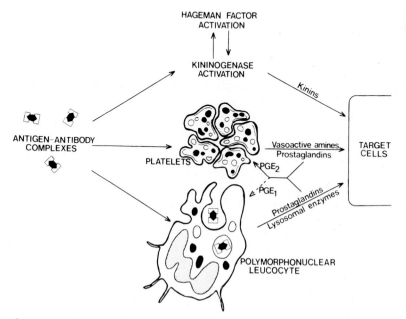

Fig. 3.2 Diagrammatic representation of mediator release in a Type III hypersensitivity response. PGE_1 and PGE_2, prostaglandins E_1 and E_2. Solid lines indicate mediator production. Dotted lines indicate an inhibitory action of PGE on mediator secretion. Target cells are classically smooth muscle cells but will include other cell types.

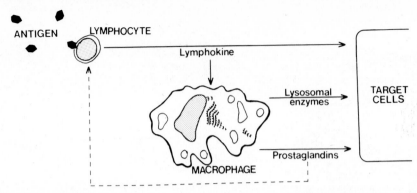

Fig. 3.3 Diagrammatic representation of mediator release during a Type IV hypersensitivity reaction. Solid lines indicate mediator secretion. Dotted lines indicate inhibitory action of E-type prostaglandin on lymphocyte activation.

tional smooth muscle spasmogenic material is released in the form of SRS-A and prostaglandins as well as material chemotactic for eosinophils. In Type III reactions, the phagocytic neutrophil releases lysosomal enzymes, as well as other biologically active agents such as prostaglandins, neutral peptides, and proteins producing increased vascular permeability (Weissmann and Dukor, 1970). In Type IV reactions the lymphocyte responds to antigen by releasing lymphokines, agents with a range of properties of relevance to chronic inflammation. These actions include production of increased vascular permeability, stimulation of DNA synthesis in lymphocytes, modification of macrophage migration *in vitro*, macrophage chemotaxis and macrophage activation. Furthermore, as a consequence of macrophage activation there is increased production and release of lysosomal enzymes (Allison and Davies, 1974; Pantalone and Page, 1975) and production of substantial amounts of PGE$_2$ (Bray *et al.*, 1974).

As a general principle it seems likely that most hypersensitivity reactions will be mixed; for example, Types I and III might occur together so that division into these taxonomic compartments should be regarded as no more than a convenience for experimental analysis. These divisions should not be allowed to obscure the possible consequences of interactions between each type of response, as such interactions may provide the dominant feature of the inflammatory reaction; for example, in mixed Type I and Type III responses the release of platelet aggregating factors from basophils results in extravascular accumulation of immune complexes (Cochrane and Koffler, 1973).

CONCLUSION

Interest in mediation of the allergic responses is substantially motivated by consideration of their relevance to the pathogenesis of disease, with the attendant implica-

tion of pharmacological manipulation of the response. A practical example of this in the field of gastroenterology is the use and reported beneficial effect of sodium cromoglycate in patients with inflammatory bowel disease (Heatley *et al.*, 1974). Elaboration of models of the physiological allergic response of increasing complexity is a consequence of the need to accommodate new experimental observations. Nevertheless, their complexity is offset by the provision of an improved basis for explanation of drug actions. Thus, the concept of an intracellular final common path in Type I reactions permits an explanation of synergism between unrelated agents inhibiting mediator release, for example theophylline and isoprenaline. In addition, a consequence of improved models of the allergic response is the development of new models of pathogenic mechanisms in allergic inflammation. For example, the concept of effector cell secretions serving as regulators allows alternative theories of pathogenesis (i.e. for certain common diseases such as asthma and rheumatoid arthritis). Thus, it has been proposed that in bronchial asthma there is a defective action of adenyl cyclase following stimulation of β-adrenergic receptors by endogenous adrenaline (Szentivanyi, 1968). In the case of rheumatoid arthritis the basis for chronicity could be a result of defective regulation of lymphokine secretion by lymphocytes recruited into the synovial tissue (Morley, 1974b) and evidence of this defect has been reported in patients with multiple sclerosis (Kirby *et al.*, 1976). In these diseases such defects in regulation have been proposed to accommodate models of pathogenesis based on over-production of classical mediators for which no satisfactory alternative explanation has emerged. It seems reasonable to suggest that these concepts might also be applied to diseases of the intestine. For example, coeliac disease and inflammatory bowel disease may be explained on the basis of classical mediator release following antigenic challenge of the intestinal mucosa (Chs. 6 and 7). However, there are many difficulties in such hypotheses and it is possible that defective regulation of mediator release may be impor-

tant in the pathogenesis of these and other intestinal diseases.

REFERENCES

Allison, A. C. & Davies, P. (1974) Mechanisms underlying chronic inflammation. In *Future Trends in Inflammation*, ed. Velo, G. P., Willoughby, D. A. & Giroud, J. P., pp. 449–480. Padua & London: Piccin.

Austen, K. F. (1974) Reaction mechanisms in the release of mediators of immediate hypersensitivity from human lung tissue. *Federation Proceedings*, 33, 2256–2262.

Barger, G. & Dale, H. H. (1910) The presence in ergot and physiological activity of β-imidazolylethylamine. *Journal of Physiology*, 40, Proc. xxxviii.

Barger, G. & Dale, H. H. (1911) β-imidazolylethylamine: a depressor constituent of intestinal mucosa. *Journal of Physiology*, 41, 499–503.

Bergström, S. (1967) Prostaglandins: members of a new hormonal system. *Science*, 157, 382–391.

Bergström, S. & Bernhard, S. (1973) *Advances in the Biosciences*, Vol. 9. Oxford: Pergamon.

Bloom, B. R. (1971) *In vitro* approach to the mechanisms of cell mediated immunity. *Advances in Immunology*, 13, 101–208.

Bloom, B. R. & Bennett, B. (1966) Mechanism of a reaction *in vitro* associated with delayed-type hypersensitivity. *Science*, 153, 80–82.

Bloom, B. R. & Glade, P. R. (1971) *In-vitro Methods in Cell-Mediated Immunity*. New York: Academic Press.

Bourne, R. E., Lichtenstein, L. M., Melmon, K. L., Henney, C. S., Weinstein, Y. & Shearer, G. (1974) Modulation of inflammation and immunity of cyclic AMP. *Science*, 184, 19–28.

Bray, M. A., Gordon, D. & Morley, J. (1974) Role of prostaglandins in reactions of cellular immunity. *British Journal of Pharmacology*, 52, 453 P.

Bray, M. A., Dumonde, D. C., Hanson, J. M., Morley, J. & Wolstencroft, R. A. (1976) Heterogeneity of lymphokines. *Clinical and Experimental Immunology*, 223, 333–346.

Brocklehurst, W. E. (1960) Slow-reacting substance and related compounds. *Progress in Allergy*, 6, 539–558.

Brocklehurst, W. E. (1962) The release of histamine and formation of a slow-reacting substance (SRS-A) during anaphylactic shock. *Journal of Physiology*, 151, 416–435.

Brocklehurst, W. E. (1976) Many facts, but insufficient knowledge: the story of asthma. *Journal of Pharmacy and Pharmacology*, 28, 361–368.

Brocklehurst, W. E. & Lahiri, S. C. (1962) Formation and destruction of bradykinin during anaphylaxis. *Journal of Physiology*, 165, 39–40.

Brocklehurst, W. E. & Movat, H. (1975) Pharmacological mediators of immediate hypersensitivity. II. Plasma factors. In *Progress in Immunology II*, ed. Brent, L. & Holborow, J., Vol. 4, pp. 298–301. Amsterdam: North-Holland.

Cerottini, J. C. & Brunner, K. T. (1974) Cell-mediated cytotoxicity, allograft rejection and tumour immunity. *Advances in Immunology*, 18, 67–132.

Cochrane, C. G. & Koffler, D. (1973) Immune complex disease in experimental animals and man. *Advances in Immunology*, 16, 185–264.

Colman, R. W. (1974) Formation of human plasma kinin. *New England Journal of Medicine*, 291, 509–515.

Dale, H. H. (1914) The occurrence in ergot and action of acetyl-choline. *Journal of Physiology*, 48, Proc. iii.

Dale, H. H. (1933) Progress in autopharmacology: a survey of present knowledge of the chemical regulation of certain functions by natural constituents of the tissues. *Bulletin of the Johns Hopkins Hospital*, 53, 297–347.

Dale, H. H. & Dudley, H. W. (1929) The presence of histamine and acetylcholine in spleen of ox and horse. *Journal of Physiology*, 68, 97–123.

Dale, H. H. & Richards, A. N. (1918) The vasodilator action of histamine and of some other substances. *Journal of Physiology*, 52, 110–165.

David, J. R. (1966) Delayed hypersensitivity *in vitro*. Its mediation by cell-free substances formed by lymphoid cell–antigen interaction. *Proceedings of the National Academy of Sciences (Washington)*, 56, 72–77.

David, J. R. & David, R. R. (1972) Cellular hypersensitivity and immunity. *Progress in Allergy*, 16, 300–449.

Dawson, W. & Tomlinson, R. (1974) Effect of cromoglycate and eicosatetraynoic acid on the release of prostaglandins and SRS-A from immunologically challenged guinea-pig lungs. *British Journal of Pharmacology*, 52, 107–108P.

Douglas, W. W. (1970) Autacoids. In *The Pharmacological Basis of Therapeutics*, ed. Goodman, L. S. & Gilman, A., 4th edn, pp. 620–662. London: Macmillan.

Dumonde, D. C. & Maini, R. N. (1971) The clinical significance of mediators of cellular immunity. *Clinical Allergy*, 1, 123–139.

Dumonde, D. C., Wolstencroft, R. A., Panayi, G. S., Matthew, M., Morley, J. & Howson, W. T. (1969) 'Lymphokines'. Non-antibody mediators of cellular immunity generated by lymphocyte activation. *Nature*, 224, 38–42.

Dvorak, H. F., Dvorak, A. M., Simpson, B. A., Richerson, H. B., Leskowitz, S. & Karnovsky, M. J. (1970) Cutaneous basophil hypersensitivity. II. A light and electron microscopic description. *Journal of Experimental Medicine*, 132, 558–582.

Eisen, V. (1969) Kinin formation in human diseases. In *Scientific Basis of Medicine, Annual Reviews*, pp. 146–165. London: Athlone Press.

Eisen, V. & Smith, H. G. (1970) Plasma kinin formation by complexes of aggregated γ-globulin and serum proteins. *British Journal of Experimental Pathology*, 51, 328–331.

Eliasson, R. (1959) Studies on prostaglandin. *Acta Physiologica Scandinavica*, 46 (Supplement 158), 1–73.

Erdos, E. G. (ed.) (1970) Bradykinin, kallidin and kallikrein. In *Handbook of Experimental Pharmacology XXV*. Berlin: Springer-Verlag.

Erspamer, V. (1954) Pharmacology of indolealkylamines. *Pharmacological Reviews*, 6, 425–487.

Erspamer, V. (ed.) (1966) 5-Hydroxytryptamine and related indolealkylamines. In *Handbook of Experimental Pharmacology XIX*. Berlin: Springer-Verlag.

Feldberg, W. S. (1970) Henry Hallett Dale. *Biographical Memoirs of Fellows of the Royal Society*, 16, 77–174.

Ferreira, S. H. (1972) Prostaglandins, aspirin-like drugs and analgesia. *Nature (New Biology)*, 240, 200–203.

Ferreira, S. H. & Vane, J. R. (1974) New aspects of the mode of action of non-steroid anti-inflammatory drugs. *Annual Review of Pharmacology*, 14, 57–73.

Flower, R. J. (1974) Drugs which inhibit prostaglandin biosynthesis. *Pharmacological Reviews*, 26, 33–67.

Gordon, D., Bray, M. A. & Morley, J. (1976) Control of lymphokine secretion by prostaglandins. *Nature,* **262,** 401–402

Graham, P. & Schild, H. O. (1967) Histamine formation in the tuberculin reaction of the rat. *Immunology,* **12,** 725–727.

Gréen, K., Hedqvist, P. & Svanborg, N. (1974) Increased plasma levels of 15-keto-13, 14-dihydro-prostaglandin $F_{2\alpha}$ after allergen-provoked asthma in man. *Lancet,* **ii,** 1419–1421.

Halpern, B. N. (1942) Les antihistaminiques de synthèse: essais de chimiothérapie des états allergiques. *Archives internationales de pharmacodynamie et de thérapie,* **68,** 339–408.

Heatley, R. V., Calcraft, B. J., Rhodes, J., Owen, E. & Evans, B. (1974) Treatment of chronic proctitis with disodium cromoglycate. *Gut,* **15,** 829.

Horton, E. W. (1963) Action of prostaglandin E_1 on tissues which respond to bradykinin. *Nature,* **200,** 892–893.

Horton, E. W. (1969) Hypotheses on physiological roles of prostaglandins. *Physiological Reviews,* **49,** 122–161.

Humphrey, J. H. & Jacques, R. (1955) The release of histamine and 5-hydroxytryptamine (serotonin) from platelets by antigen–antibody reactions (*in vitro*). *Journal of Physiology,* **128,** 9–27.

Jonasson, O. & Becker, E. L. (1966) Release of kallikrein from guinea-pig lung during anaphylaxis. *Journal of Experimental Medicine,* **123,** 509–522.

Kahlson, G. & Rosengren, E. (1970) *Biogenesis and Physiology of Histamine.* Baltimore: Williams & Wilkins.

Kirby, P. J., Morley, J., Ponsford, J. R. & McDonald, W. I. (1976) Defective PGE reactivity in leucocytes of multiple sclerosis patients. *Prostaglandins,* **11,** 621–630.

Lewis, G. P. (ed.) (1958) *5-Hydroxytryptamine.* London: Pergamon Press.

Lewis, G. P. (1964) Plasma kinins and other vasoactive compounds in acute inflammation. *Annals of the New York Academy of Science,* **116,** 847–854.

Lewis, T. (1927) *The Blood Vessels of the Human Skin and their Responses.* London: Shaw.

Lichtenstein, L. M. & Gillespie, E. (1973) Inhibition of histamine release by histamine controlled by H_2 receptor. *Nature,* **244,** 287–288.

Lundell, L. (1975) Elucidation by a H_2-receptor antagonist of the significance of mucosal histamine mobilization in exciting acid secretion. *Journal of Physiology,* **244,** 365–383.

Morley, J. (1974a) Cell migration inhibition: an appraisal. *Acta Allergologica,* **29,** 185–208.

Morley, J. (1974b) Prostaglandins and lymphokines in arthritis. *Prostaglandins,* **8,** 315–326.

Morley, J. (1977) Lymphokines. In *Handbook of Experimental Pharmacology,* eds. Vane, J. R. & Ferreira, S. H. Springer-Verlag: London (in press).

Nakano, J. and Koss, M. C. (1973) Pathophysiologic roles of prostaglandins and the action of aspirin-like drugs. *Southern Medical Journal,* **66,** 709–723.

Orange, R. P. & Austen, K. F. (1969) Slow reacting substance of anaphylaxis. *Advances in Immunology,* **10,** 105–144.

Orange, R. P., Murphy, R. C. & Austen, K. F. (1974) Inactivation of slow reacting substance of anaphylaxis (SRS-A) by arylsulfatases. *Journal of Immunology,* **113,** 316–322.

Orange, R. P., Stechschulte, D. J. & Austen, K. F. (1970) Immunochemical and biologic properties of rat IgE. II. Capacity to mediate the immunologic release of histamine and slow reacting substance of anaphylaxis (SRS-A). *Journal of Immunology,* **105,** 1087–1095.

Pantalone, R. M. & Page, R. C. (1975) Lymphokine-induced production and release of lysosomal enzymes by macrophages. *Proceedings of the National Academy of Sciences of the United States of America* (*Washington*), **72,** 2091–2094.

Piper, P. J. & Vane, J. R. (1969) Release of additional factors in anaphylaxis and its antagonism by anti-inflammatory drugs. *Nature,* **223,** 29–35.

Plaut, M., Lichtenstein, L. M. & Henney, C. S. (1973) Increase in histamine receptors on thymus derived effector lymphocytes during the primary immune response to alloantigens. *Nature,* **244,** 284–287.

Portier, P. & Richet, C. (1902) De l'action anaphylactique de certains venins. *Comptes Rendus Société de Biologie* (*Paris*), **54,** 170–172.

Ramwell, P. W. & Pharriss, B. B. (eds.) (1972) *Prostaglandins in Cellular Biology.* New York: Plenum Press.

Richerson, H. B., Dvorak, H. F. & Leskowitz, S. (1970) Cutaneous basophil hypersensitivity. I. A new look at the Jones-Mote reaction, general characteristics. *Journal of Experimental Medicine,* **132,** 546–557.

Riley, J. F. (1959) *The Mast Cells.* Edinburgh: Livingstone.

Rocha e Silva, M. (1966) Release of histamine in anaphylaxis. In *Histamine and Antihistamine Handbook of Pharmacology XVIII (1),* ed. Rocha e Silva, M., pp. 432–486. Berlin: Springer-Verlag.

Rocha e Silva, M. & Garcia Leme, J. (1972) *Chemical Mediators of the Acute Inflammatory Reaction.* Oxford: Pergammon.

Rocha e Silva, M., Beraldo, W. T. & Rosenfeld, G. (1949) Bradykinin, a hypotensive and smooth muscle stimulatory factor released from plasma-globulin by snake venoms and by trypsin. *American Journal of Physiology,* **156,** 261–273.

Rowley, D. A. & Benditt, E. P. (1956) 5-Hydroxytryptamine and histamine as mediators of the vascular injury produced by agents which damage mast cells in rats. *Journal of Experimental Medicine,* **103,** 399–411.

Samuelsson, B. & Vane, J. R. (1976) *Prostaglandins and Thromboxanes,* New York: Raven Press.

Szentivanyi, A. (1968) The beta adrenergic theory of the atopic abnormality in bronchial asthma. *Journal of Allergy,* **42,** 203–232.

Schachter, M. (1969) Kallikreins and kinins. *Physiological Reviews,* **49,** 509–547.

Vane, J. R. (1971) Inhibition of prostaglandin synthesis as a mechanism of action for aspirin-like drugs. *Nature (New Biology),* **231,** 232–235.

Vane, J. R. (1973) Prostaglandins in the inflammatory response. In *Inflammation Mechanisms and Control,* ed. Lepow, I. H. & Ward, P. A., pp. 261–275. New York: Academic Press.

Wahl, S. (1975) Corticosteroid inhibition of chemotactic lymphokine production by T and B lymphocytes. *Annals of the New York Academy of Sciences,* **256,** 375–385.

Webster, M. E. & Innerfield, I. (1965) Interrelationship of human plasma kallikrein and plasmin in inflammation. *Enzymologia Biologia et Clinica (Basel),* **5,** 129–148.

Weissmann, G. & Dukor, P. (1970) The role of lysosomes in immune responses. *Advances in Immunology,* **12,** 283–331.

Weissmann, G., Dukor, P. & Zurier, R. B. (1971) Effect of cyclic AMP on release of lysosomal enzymes from phagocytes. *Nature (New Biology),* **231,** 131–135.

Werle, E. & Berek, V. (1948) Zur Kenntnis des Kallikreins. *Angew. Chem.,* **60A,** 53.

Williams, T. J. & Morley, J. (1973) Prostaglandins as potentiators of increased vascular permeability in inflammation. *Nature*, **246**, 215–217.

Williams, T. J. & Peck, M. J. (1977) Role of prostaglandin-mediated vasodilatation in inflammation. *Nature*, **270**, 530–532.

Willoughby, D. A., Giroud, J. D., Di Rosa, M. & Velo, G. P. (1973) The control of the inflammatory response with special reference to the prostaglandins. In *Prostaglandins and Cyclic AMP*, ed. Kahn, R. H. & Lands, W. E. M., pp. 187–206. New York: Academic Press.

Zurier, R. B. (1974) Prostaglandins, inflammation, and asthma. *Archives of Internal Medicine*, **133**, 101–110.

PART 2 Disorders of gastrointestinal immunity

4. Immunological aspects of the mouth

M. K. Basu and P. Asquith

INTRODUCTION

The mouth is sterile at birth, but soon afterwards it becomes a habitat for commensal microorganisms (McCarthy, Snyder and Parker, 1965), and also acts as a portal of entry for numerous food and bacterial antigens. It is widely accepted that immunological mechanisms play a major role in preventing and resisting antigenic damage to the oral tissues (Brandtzaeg, 1972; Burnett and Scherp, 1968), and there is increasing evidence to suggest that immunological mechanisms participate in the aetiology and pathogenesis of oral diseases (Lehner, 1972). The purpose of this chapter is to consider immunological mechanisms as they occur in the normal mouth, and to describe changes in oral immunological reactivity in oral disease and certain other diseases including inflammatory bowel disease and coeliac disease.

IMMUNOLOGICAL ASPECTS OF THE NORMAL MOUTH

HUMORAL IMMUNITY

Salivary gland associated immunoglobulins

The saliva which bathes the oral mucosa is synthesized in three pairs of major salivary glands, the parotid, submaxillary and sublingual – and also in numerous minor salivary glands scattered throughout the oral submucosa. In contrast to the glands of the intestinal mucosa, salivary glands are present as discrete structures that are anatomically separate from the stratified squamous epithelium lining the oral cavity. IgA predominates in saliva (Tomasi and Zeigelbaum, 1963; Ishizaka, Dennis

and Hornbrook, 1964; Simons, Weber, Stiel and Grasbeck, 1964; Brandtzaeg, Fjellanger and Gjeruldsen, 1970); indeed in parotid and submaxillary gland saliva (Table 4.1), the IgA to IgG ratio is approximately 400 times greater than that found in serum. The immunoglobulins are produced locally and are derived from serum, thus tissue cultures of human salivary gland have shown that they synthesize IgA, IgG and IgM, the IgA being synthesized in amounts 5 to 10 times greater than IgG (Hurlimann and Zuber, 1968). Also radioactive tracer studies have shown that approximately 96 per cent of the IgA and 20 per cent of the IgG in saliva are synthesized locally (Strober, Blaese and Waldmann, 1970), whilst immunofluorescence techniques have demonstrated a preponderance of IgA-containing plasma cells (Tomasi, Tan, Solomon and Prendergast, 1965).

Not only is IgA the predominant immunoglobulin, but of the total IgA in parotid and submaxillary saliva approximately 90 per cent is present as secretory IgA and has properties similar to the secretory IgA of other mucous membrane secretions and of colostrum (Tomasi *et al.*, 1965). It originates in gland-associated plasma cells which synthesize IgA in the dimeric form (Lawton and Mage, 1969) which then links to secretory piece (SP) derived from the acinar epithelial cells of the parotid gland (Tourville, Adler, Bienenstock and Tomasi, 1969). The immunochemical properties of secretory IgA and SP, and the possible role of the latter in the process of selective transport of IgA by epithelial cells, are discussed in Chapter 1.

With respect to the other immunoglobulin classes, parotid salivary IgM usually predominates over IgG, although the opposite is found in serum and in the

Table 4.1 Immunoglobulin concentrations (mg/100 ml) in saliva and serum of 18 normal individuals (mean and SE)

Sample	Immunoglobulin		
	IgG	IgA	IgM
Stimulated parotid secretion	0·032	3·82 ± 0·27	0·053
Unstimulated whole saliva	7·75 ± 1·84	13·25 ± 2·02	0·56 ± 0·41
Serum	1196·10 ± 131·88	377·20 ± 55·35	84·30 ± 14·86
Submaxillary secretion (Brandtzaeg *et al.*, 1970)	0·04	4·5	0·06

stromal immunoglobulin pool (Brandtzaeg et al., 1970), suggesting that IgM is selectively transferred across the acinar epithelium during the process of saliva secretion. The molecular size and immunochemical characteristics of the IgM are similar to those of the 19S IgM in serum, but recently it has been shown that SP is attached to a proportion of salivary IgM (Coelho, Pereira, Virella and Thompson, 1974). It would appear that the mechanisms responsible for the active secretion of immunoglobulins have a special adaptive capacity to secrete IgM in the absence of IgA; for example, in IgA-deficient patients, the IgM concentration in parotid saliva exhibits a compensatory increase (Table 4.2). This special adaptive capacity of the secretory mechanisms does not extend to IgG, for its concentration is not increased in the saliva of either IgA-deficient or combined IgA- and IgM-deficient patients (Table 4.2).

Table 4.2 Immunoglobulin concentrations (mg/100 ml) in stimulated parotid saliva and serum of two patients with dysgammaglobulinaemia

| Patient | Immunoglobulins | | | | | |
| | Serum | | | Saliva | | |
	IgG	IgA	IgM	IgG	IgA	IgM
GP	747	0.4	0.9	1.8	0.4	0.9
BM	1524	0.4	74	1.8	0.4	3.1

IgG is present in salivary secretions in low concentration, it lacks SP and its physical and immunochemical characteristics are similar to those of serum IgG (Brandtzaeg et al., 1970). Approximately 1 per cent of the plasma cells in the parotid gland contain IgG although relatively large quantities of this immunoglobulin are present in the stromal immunoglobulin pool, suggesting that most of the IgG in the latter is serum derived. Indeed it has been shown that the concentration of IgG in parotid saliva is proportional to its availability from serum (Brandtzaeg, 1971). Very little information is available with regard to glandular synthesis and transfer of IgE and IgD, but Salmon (1970) has reported the presence of traces of IgE in whole saliva which could be attributed to leakage from the oral mucous membranes.

Oral mucosa associated immunoglobulins

Between the numerous discrete minor salivary glands which characterize the oral mucous membrane are relatively large tracts of mucous membrane covered by stratified squamous epithelium. In contrast to the stroma of salivary glands, immunofluorescent studies show very few IgA plasma cells in the lamina propria (Lai, Fat, Cormane and Van Furth, 1974) and no SP in the epithelial cells (Brandtzaeg, 1972). Except in the region of the crevicular epithelium (Fig. 4.1) it is difficult to collect samples from the surface of the stratified squamous epithelium that are uncontaminated by glandular secretion. Hence, the secretions which normally exude from the surface of the crevicular epithelium, that is the crevicular fluid, have been studied almost exclusively when attempting to characterize the mucosa-derived immunoglobulins.

7S IgG, 7S IgA and 19S IgM are present in crevicular fluid in approximately the same proportions and concentrations as in serum (Brandtzaeg, 1965; Holmberg and Killander, 1971; Shillitoe, 1972). Normally these immunoglobulins are mainly derived from serum in that tracer studies have indicated that serum immunoglobulins accumulate in the connective tissue beneath the crevicular epithelium, and part of this pool then leaks through (Cowley, 1966). However,

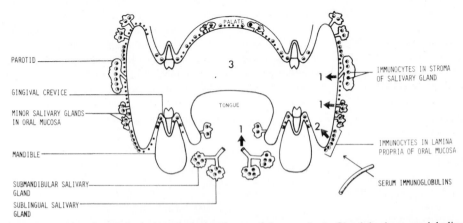

Fig. 4.1 Schematic representation of the immunological make-up of the mouth. 1. Glandular immunoglobulins, predominantly locally produced 11S IgA. 2. Mucosal immunoglobulins, predominantly IgG and which are locally produced as well as serum derived. 3. Immunoglobulins of whole saliva which are a combination of 1 and 2. ◉ = Immunocytes responsible for local synthesis of immunoglobulins. ● = T-lymphocytes responsible for cell-mediated immunity.

a proportion also originates from the plasma cells present in the local connective tissue, the majority of which are IgG producing (Brandtzaeg, 1972; Clark, 1974). During inflammation and following trauma, the overall concentration of immunoglobulins in crevicular fluid shows an increase (Shillitoe, 1972; Brandtzaeg, 1972), but there is a greater increase in IgG concentration over IgA and IgM, and IgA concentration over IgM. Hence, the mucosal stratified squamous epithelium appears to act as a passive molecular sieve favouring transmission of IgG (Brandtzaeg et al., 1970).

Antibody activity in salivary and mucosal immunoglobulins
Natural antibodies and antibodies against exogenous microbiota have been found in salivary and mucosa-derived immunoglobulins (Hanson and Brandtzaeg, 1972) including secretory IgA (Table 4.3). They are

have been demonstrated in human gingival mucous membrane (Berglund, 1971). They are probably derived from the gingival plasma cells; however, the finding of agglutinating and precipitating antibodies to several indigenous oral bacteria in adult serum (Evans, Spaeth and Mergenhagen, 1966; Wilton, Ivanyi and Lehner, 1971) raises the possibility that a proportion are serum derived. In animals local plasma cells synthesize antibodies after antigens have been introduced into the oral mucous membrane (Thonard and Dalbow, 1965; Brandtzaeg, 1972). Furthermore, intramucosal bacterial antigens also provoke antibody production by the immunocompetent cells of the regional lymph nodes and/or spleen, and this cellular response correlates well with the serum antibody titres against the same antigen (Berglund, Rizzo and Mergenhagen, 1969).

In spite of these observations in humans and in

Table 4.3 Antibody activity associated with human salivary IgA (after Brandtzaeg, 1972)

Isohaemagglutinins	N+	Tomasi et al. (1965)
Enterococcus	N++	Sirisinha & Charupatana (1971)
Escherichia coli	N+	Tourville et al. (1968)
Pneumococcus	N+	Mouton et al. (1970)
Salmonella paratyphosi	P+	Sirisinha & Charupatana (1970)
Streptococcus	N++	Sirisinha & Charupatana (1971)
Veillonella	N++	Sirisinha & Charupatana (1971)
Influenza virus	N+	Waldman et al. (1968)
Influenza virus inactivated	P+	Mann et al. (1968)
Mumps virus	I++	Nakao et al. (1970)
Poliovirus	N+	Berger et al. (1967)
Rhinovirus	I+	Cate et al. (1966); Douglas et al. (1967)
Candida albicans	I+	Chilgren et al. (1967)

N = in normal subjects.
I = after infectious disease.
P = after parenteral vaccination.
++ = appreciable titre.
+ = low to moderate titre.

also found following parenteral vaccination (Hanson and Brandtzaeg, 1972). Also whole saliva contains significant concentrations of immunoconglutinins (Lachmann and Thompson, 1970). Salivary secretory IgA, in addition to showing antibody activity against bacteria, also exhibits several other antibacterial functions. Of particular relevance is the finding that parotid secretory IgA inhibits the adherence of *Strep. sanguis*, *Strep. mitis* and *Strep. salivarius* to oral epithelial cells (Williams and Gibbons, 1972). Since bacterial adherence is a prerequisite for colonization of mucous or tooth surfaces, secretory IgA antibodies could prevent oral disease by this mechanism. Nevertheless, *Strep. sanguis*, a common oral bacterium, could jeopardize this mechanism in that it is able to cleave secretory IgA to form Fc and Fab fragments (Plaut, Genco and Tomasi, 1974). With regard to the oral mucosa, antibodies against *Esch. coli* 012:B8, *Fusobacteria* and *Veilonella*

animals, the IgG-class immunoglobulins which constitute a large part of antibodies derived from the oral mucosa are thought not to be protective at mucosal surfaces (Hand, Smith and Sandford, 1971). This concept receives support from the observation that much of the IgG in human dental plaque is present in a degraded form – a fragment of approximately 24 000 molecular weight bearing Fc antigenic determinants (Taubman, 1974).

In summary, humoral mechanisms in the mouth would appear to depend on two functionally distinct components – one, the gland-associated secretory IgA which probably forms a first line of defence, and two, the predominantly IgG mucosal component which constitutes a second line of defence. The former probably acts at the mucosal surface to prevent antigens from entering the mucous membrane (Tomasi and Beinenstock, 1968), while the latter may act within the mucosal epithelium and lamina propria to neutralize antigens and promote their phagocytosis once they have gained entry.

CELL-MEDIATED IMMUNITY

Examination of the normal oral mucous membrane reveals the presence of small lymphocytes which could be T-lymphocytes; these may be involved in cell-mediated mechanisms which prevent disease, but this hypothesis is difficult to substantiate.

Phenomena associated with cell-mediated immunity and delayed hypersensitivity, such as graft rejection and contact hypersensitivity, occur not infrequently in the oral tissue (Fisher, 1973). Studies of cell-mediated mechanisms include the demonstration of a delayed hypersensitivity reaction in the oral mucosa of animals with dinitrochlorobenzene (DNCB) after previous skin sensitization (Adams, Williamson and Dolby, 1969). Furthermore it has been possible to demonstrate passive transfer of delayed hypersensitivity to DNCB in the oral mucous membrane of experimental animals (Dolby, Williamson and Adams, 1969). Also in animals a delayed hypersensitivity reaction has been elicited in the skin with oral bacterial extracts after previous sensitization through the oral mucous membrane (Wilton, 1972). Furthermore, in humans in-vitro studies show that in some oral mucosal diseases extracts of appropriate oral bacteria will induce the patients' lymphocytes to undergo blast transformation and exhibit cytotoxicity and macrophage migration inhibition (Ivanyi, Wilton and Lehner, 1972).

IMMUNOLOGICAL ASPECTS OF COMMON ORAL DISEASES

DENTAL CARIES

Dental caries is considered to be an infective disease caused by microorganisms present in dental plaque, which are aggregations of a large variety and number of microorganisms behaving as a natural microbial ecological system.

Studies on germ-free animals have shown that a number of different plaque organisms, such as Strep. mutans, Strep. sanguis, L. acidophilus and A. viscosus, can, in the presence of a sugar substrate, produce dental caries (Fitzgerald, Jordan and Archard, 1966). In man, Strep. mutans appears to be the most important organism producing dental caries for two reasons: it is capable of rapidly producing enough acid to lower the pH to that required for dissolving human enamel, and it produces glucosyltransferase, the enzyme responsible for the synthesis of the extracellular polysaccharides which form the plaque matrix (Guggenheim, 1970).

Immune reactivity in dental caries

The immunological aspects of dental caries have of necessity been studied in terms of humoral immunity, because dental caries is predominantly a disease of acellular tissue. Geller and Lovelstad (1959) first found an association between high levels of γ-globulins in parotid saliva and a low incidence of caries; however, Kraus and Sirisinha (1962) were unable to confirm these findings. More recently a significantly reduced level of IgA has been found in whole saliva (Lehner, Cardwell and Clarry, 1967) and in submaxillary saliva (Zengo, Mandel, Goldman and Khurana, 1971) of patients with a high incidence of caries compared with individuals with a low incidence. In contrast, the serum IgA levels of the former were found to be higher than the latter (Lehner et al., 1967), suggesting a dissociation between salivary and serum IgA responses.

With respect to antibody activity, patients with a previous history of caries but without active caries at the time of study had higher parotid salivary antibodies to Strep. mutans glucosyltransferase than patients with active caries (Challacombe, Lehner and Guggenheim, 1972). An essentially similar pattern has been obtained in respect of serum antibodies to Strep. mutans glucosyltransferase (Challacombe et al., 1972) and other antigens from allegedly cariogenic bacteria (Kennedy, Shklair, Hayashi and Bahn, 1968; Lehner, Wilton and Ward, 1970; Challacombe, 1971). Based on these observations, Challacombe et al. (1972) postulated that the initial development of caries results in an increase in the levels of serum antibodies against cariogenic oral bacteria and of salivary antibodies against Strep. mutans glucosyltransferase, whilst caries develops when the levels of these antibodies are not sustained. Nevertheless, it should be pointed out that the role of different oral bacteria in the initiation and development of human dental caries is still not clear, which renders the interpretation of results of immunological studies in terms of pathogenesis of caries very difficult.

PERIDONTAL DISEASE

The peridontal tissues consist of the gingiva, periodontal ligament, alveolar bone and cementum. The most common disease affecting these tissues is associated with local irritation which starts as an inflammation of the gingival margin; a mild degree of inflammation of the gingival and deeper periodontal tissues has been reported in most adults, and advanced tissue destruction in about half the middle-aged and elderly (WHO, 1961).

The histological changes seen in periodontal disease include widening of the intercellular spaces, followed by ulceration and hyperplasia of the crevicular epithelium; there is simultaneous infiltration of the gingival lamina propria by neutrophils, lymphocytes, plasma cells and histiocytes. Lymphocytes predominate during the early stages, while at the later stages plasma cells become more prominent (Schroeder, Munzel-Pedrassoli and Page, 1972). Extension of the infiltrate into the deeper tissues is associated with breakdown of the collagen fibres of the periodontal ligament, resorption of alveolar bone, and proliferation of the crevicular epithelium along the root surface to form periodontal pockets.

The aetiological factors responsible for this type of periodontal disease are unknown, but deposition of bacterial plaque near the gingival margin is considered to be important. *Veillonella*, *Fusobacteria*, *Bacteriodes* and *Spirochaetes* are found commonly and in large numbers in plaque (Burnett and Sherp, 1968) and it has been postulated that lipopolysaccharide endotoxins derived from these bacteria induce periodontal tissue damage through a local Schwartzmann reaction, complement activation and the release of mediators (Snyderman, Gewurz and Mergenhagen, 1968). Hyaluronidase and B-glucoronidase produced by plaque *Streptococci* have also been implicated in the initial changes observed in the crevicular epithelium (Schultz-Haudt and Scherp, 1955).

Humoral immunity in periodontal disease

Approximately 75 per cent of the plasma cells in the normal human gingiva produce IgG (Brandtzaeg, 1972). With gingival inflammation there is an increase in the number of IgG- and IgM-class plasma cells (Clarke, 1974), of which IgG-cells show the greatest proportionate increase (Brandtzaeg, 1972). The crevicular fluid of diseased gingivae also contains increased concentrations of IgG, IgA and IgM (Holmberg *et al.*, 1971; Shillitoe, 1972; Brandtzaeg, 1972); again IgG shows the greatest increase.

With regard to salivary immunoglobulins patients with periodontal disease show increased concentrations of secretory IgA in whole saliva compared to clinically healthy controls (Brandtzaeg *et al.*, 1970). But, in a more recent study, the concentration and secretion rate of parotid IgA was found to be independent of the degree of periodontal inflammation (Chandler, Silverman, Lundblad and McFall, 1974).

High serum IgA (Shillitoe, 1972) and raised serum levels of agglutinating antibodies to *F. polymorphum*, *V. alcalescens* and *T. microdentium* have been detected in periodontal disease (Evans *et al.*, 1966; Steinberg and Gershoff, 1968). From presently available evidence (Thonard *et al.*, 1965; Brandtzaeg, 1972) it seems likely that some of these antibodies are produced locally in the lamina propria of the gingiva.

Using a modified Mancini technique (Fahey and McKelvey, 1965) the concentrations of IgG, IgA and IgM in whole saliva of patients with peridontal disease have been studied before and after gingivectomy (Basu, Glenwright, Fox and Becker, 1976). The results showed that pre-operatively the IgG concentration was high, and IgA concentration low, but following gingivectomy, levels of both return towards normal, the increase in IgA being significant ($p < 0.01$) (Table 4.4).

The higher IgG concentrations before gingivectomy can be accounted for on the basis of a local IgG response to the antigenic challenge of bacterial plaque, whereas the low pre-operative IgA concentrations can be explained if in gingivitis the salivary IgA forms large complexes and aggregates with products of bacterial plaque and exudate. IgA is known to form such aggregates and to complex with other proteins (Tomasi and Decoteau, 1970) especially in the presence of free SP, which abounds in saliva (Brandtzaeg *et al.*, 1970). In this event, falsely low IgA estimates could be expected with the modified Mancini technique used. Alternatively, a large proportion of crevicular fluid 7S IgA could be degraded within bacterial plaque before being added to whole saliva; evidence of such degradation has been found recently (Taubman, 1974). Finally, the concentration of IgA in saliva could also be low pre-operatively as a result of dilution from excessive saliva production consequent to gingival inflammation.

Cellular immunity in periodontal disease

Cellular reactivity in this disease has been studied quite extensively (Ivanyi and Lehner, 1970; Ivanyi and Lehner, 1971; Ivanyi *et al.*, 1972; Horton, Liekin and Oppenheim, 1972) and it has been shown that ultrasonicates of autologous and control plaque bacteria induce lymphocyte transformation in patients with mild or moderate periodontal disease. Such transformation could not be obtained in clinically normal individuals or when ultrasonicates from 'non-plaque' bacteria were used.

Table 4.4 IgG, IgA and IgM concentrations (mg/100 ml) in whole saliva of 12 patients before and after gingivectomy (mean and SE)

Immunoglobulins	Before gingivectomy concentration	After gingivectomy concentration	Probability
IgG	22.43 ± 7.55	8.68 ± 2.69	P > 0.05
IgA	5.45 ± 0.78	13.10 ± 2.03	P < 0.01
IgM	3.40 ± 1.26	5.83 ± 1.52	P > 0.05

Other tests of cell-mediated immunity, including macrophage migration inhibition and lymphocyte cytotoxicity against target chicken red cells, have been found to correlate with lymphocyte transformation (Lehner, 1972). It has therefore been suggested that exaggerated cell-mediated immunity against bacterial plaque antigens occurs in periodontal disease, terminating in nonspecific damage to periodontal tissues. Further support for this concept is provided by the findings that human lymphocytes stimulated by plaque antigens release a lymphotoxin which is cytotoxic for human gingival fibroblasts *in vitro*. Further, they release a factor which stimulates osteoclastic bone resorption when added to cultures of foetal rat bones (Horton *et al.*, 1972).

ACUTE ULCERATIVE GINGIVITIS (VINCENT'S INFECTION)

Acute ulcerative gingivitis is characterized by acute ulceration of the interdental and marginal gingivae and occurs in association with certain oral commensal bacteria, especially the Gram-negative obligate anaerobes *F. fusiforme*, *Borellia vincentii* and *B. melaninogenicus*. Whether one or several species are necessary to induce this disease is unknown.

Humoral immunity in Vincent's infection

Parotid salivary IgA concentrations remain unaffected during the onset and convalescent phases of the disease (Wilton, Ivanyi and Lehner, 1971), Whilst in the serum during the active stage IgG is significantly decreased, IgM increased, and IgA remains within normal limits (Lehner, 1969a). It has been suggested that endotoxins from the aforementioned Gram-negative bacteria are responsible for the depression of IgG and elevation of IgM, but antibodies against these bacteria have not been detected in the sera of patients recovering from the disease either by fluorescent antibody methods or by immunoprecipitation techniques (Wilton *et al.*, 1971). Therefore, it could be argued that in acute ulcerative gingivitis changes in serum immunoglobulin levels merely reflect immunological response to the entry of irrelevent antigens through the ulcerated gingival mucous membrane.

Also of interest is the fact that the antigens responsible for lymphocyte transformation in acute ulcerative gingivitis (*vide infra*) have been shown to be capable of provoking a local Schwartmann reaction in the skin of rabbits. Of special interest are the findings that C5b fragments of complement are found in the crevicular fluid in this disease (Mergenhagen, 1972), while high levels of C3 and C5 are found in chronic periodontal inflammation (Shillitoe, 1972; Mergenhagen, 1972). This may denote complement activation in patients with acute ulcerative gingivitis although the possibility of cleavage by bacterial enzymes cannot be ruled out.

Cellular immunity in Vincent's infection

Lymphocytes from patients with acute ulcerative gingivitis when grown *in vitro* show significant stimulation with *F. fusiforme*, *V. alcalescens* and *B. melaninogenicus*, but not with *L. casei* and intestinal *Prot. mirabilis* (Wilton *et al.*, 1971). These results suggest that in such patients a subpopulation of lymphocytes are sensitized to *F. fusiforme*, *V. alcalescens* and *B. melaninogenicus*; subsequent *in-vivo* response of the patients to these bacteria could result in a delayed hypersensitivity reaction with consequent mucosal ulceration.

RECURRENT APHTHOUS ULCERATION

Recurrent aphthous ulceration of the mouth is common, incidences of 19 per cent (Sircus, Church and Kelleher, 1957) and 40 per cent (Ship, Merritt and Stanley, 1962) having been reported. According to their clinical features they have been classified into major, minor and herpetiform types (Truelove and Morris-Owen, 1958; Cooke, 1961). In most patients the ulcers are limited to the mouth, but in some one or more extra oral sites may be affected, giving rise to genital ulceration and iridocyclitis (Behcet's syndrome), while recently cutaneous, vascular, joint, neurological and gastrointestinal lesions have also been described (Monacelli and Nazarro, 1966).

Several possible aetiological agents have been suggested, including infection with herpes simplex virus (but with essentially negative results: Sircus *et al.*, 1957; Farmer, 1958), adenovirus Type 1 (Nasz, Kulcsar, Dan and Sallay, 1971) and *Strep. sanguis* and its L. form (Barile, Francis and Graykowski, 1968). Trauma, folic acid and other vitamin deficiencies, emotional stress, hormonal imbalance and familial factors have also been implicated. Recently, however, immunological mechanisms have received increasing attention.

Humoral immunity in aphthous ulceration

IgA concentrations in whole saliva of patients with major, minor and herpetiform ulcers have been reported as essentially normal, whereas patients with Behcet's syndrome had slightly increased values (Lehner, 1969a). In the serum, IgA and IgG concentrations were found to be increased in patients with major aphthous ulcers and in Behcet's syndrome (Lehner, 1969a), and either normal (Lehner, 1969a; Thomas, Ferguson, McLennan and Mason, 1973) or decreased (Body and Silverman, 1969) in patients with minor and herpetiform aphthous ulcers.

Serum antibody activity against several antigens has also been found in patients with recurrent aphthous ulcers. Thus an increased incidence of antibodies to milk protein and gluten were found by Taylor, Truelove and Wright (1964) in patients with major aphthous ulcers and more recently in patients with minor aphthous ulcers and other oral ulcerative diseases by Thomas *et al.* (1974). The latter authors suggested that local mucosal breakdown, leading to absorption of increased amounts of food antigen, was responsible, implying the food antibodies were secondary to some other pathogenic mechanism. Of relevance, therefore, was the detection of antitissue antibodies in such patients, suggesting that ulcers may have an autoimmune basis. Thus, Oshima *et al.* (1963) reported the presence of haemagglutinating antibodies against foetal oral mucosal extracts in patients with Behcet's syndrome. Similar antibodies against saline homogenates of foetal lip and cheek mucous membrane were detected in 70–80 per cent of patients with major and minor ulceration, and with Behcet's syndrome, but in only 20 per cent of patients with herpetiform ulceration and 10 per cent of normal controls (Lehner, 1964, 1967a). Recently the sera of patients with minor aphthous ulcers have also been found to contain IgG- and IgM-class antibodies against adult oral mucous membrane (Donatsky and Dabelsteen, 1974). A similar autoimmune basis may underly the finding of anti-reticulin antibodies in 18 per cent of aphthous ulcer patients (Wright and Alp, 1971).

Cellular immunity in aphthous ulceration

Extracts from *Strep. sanguis* have been found to induce significant leucocyte migration inhibition in patients with aphthous ulcers (Donatsky and Bendixen, 1972); on this basis a delayed hypersensitivity response to *Strep. sanguis* antigens might occur and lead to ulceration. Foetal oral mucosal extracts have also been found to cause lymphocyte transformation in patients with major and minor ulcers (Lehner, 1967b), the lymphocyte transformation activity correlating well with the clinical features of the ulcers. Further, lymphocytes from patients with minor aphthous ulcers have been found to be cytotoxic for oral epithelial target cells (Dolby, 1969). These findings are again consistent with the view that autoimmunity to oral mucosal antigens plays a part in the pathogenesis of aphthous ulceration. The exact mechanism through which this may be accomplished is not clear, although cross-reactivity between oral mucosa and food or bacterial antigens would seem to be a distinct possibility.

Of possible relevance to this hypothesis is the finding of an increased incidence of HLA-B5 in Behcet's syndrome (Ohno *et al.*, 1973), as on the basis of animal studies such antigens are thought pertinent to the development of autoimmune disease (McDevitt and Bodmer, 1972). In contrast, in a study of 40 patients with major, minor and herpetiform ulceration a normal distribution of HLA antigens has been found (unpublished observations).

Other immunological mechanisms in aphthous ulceration

Some preliminary data have suggested that Levamisole could be useful in aphthous ulcers (Symoens and Brugmans, 1974). We have tried it in a limited number of patients without obvious effect (Asquith and Basu, 1977, unpublished observations). These studies were uncontrolled; recently two double blind studies have also reported benefit (Lehner, Wilton and Ivanyi, 1976; Meyer *et al.*, 1977). Levamisole allegedly activates functionally defective T-cells (Biniaminov and Ramot, 1975). Hence the above benefits provide indirect evidence that patients with recurrent aphthous ulcers have defective cell-mediated immunity to an unidentified antigen(s) (see section on aphthous ulcers in coeliac disease). Levamisole has other immunological effects, including a possible effect on macrophages and on leucocyte function (Janssen Laboratories, personal communication, 1977) and we have found it of marked benefit in one patient with the lazy leucocyte syndrome (Geddes, Thompson and Asquith, 1977, unpublished observations). These latter points suggest that involvement of non-T-cell dependent mechanisms may also, or alternatively, be involved in recurrent aphthous ulcers. Clearly further studies are necessary to resolve this dilemma.

HERPETIC GINGIVO-STOMATITIS

Primary herpetic gingivo-stomatitis is characterized by a sore mouth and throat with fever, malaise, regional lymphadenitis and severe local discomfort due to vesiculation. The base of the vesicle contains giant and multinucleated cells, and many of the nuclei contain the eosinophilic inclusion body. Rupture of the roof of the vesicle leads to ulcer formation. The ulcers are small and occur in crops, but they may coalesce to form large shallow, irregular-shaped ulcers with surrounding erythema.

In contrast, recurrent herpetic infection is limited to the vermilion border of the lip and adjacent skin. The lesion starts as a blister or a crop of blisters which frequently become secondarily infected with *Staph. pyogenes*. It usually lasts between 3 to 10 days and recurs at various intervals over many years.

The mechanisms responsible for the development of recurrent herpetic infection are not completely understood. Clinical evidence indicates that fever, exposure to sunlight, local trauma, emotional stress and menstruation can precipitate recurrences. It has been suggested that during primary infection in the mouth, the virus may ascend along sensory nerve fibres to the trigeminal ganglion (Ellison, Carton and Rose, 1959; Baringer and Swoveland, 1973), to produce a latent non-cytolytic infection of the nerve cells. From this site the virus may descend along the nerve to the area of skin supplied by it. Alternatively, the virus may reside in salivary glands (Kaufman, Brown and Ellison, 1967) with reinfection occurring through the saliva.

Immunology of herpes virus infection

Primary infection

After primary infection with *Herpesvirus hominis* Type 1, complement fixing and neutralizing antibodies are found in the serum against the virion (viral or 'V' antigen) and a soluble component (soluble or 'S' antigen) which is released from the infected cells. They appear about the 5th or 6th day and usually reach a peak in 2 or 3 weeks. In a high proportion of patients, these antibodies persist indefinitely, suggesting continuing infection. In others, the antibody titres drop to low levels (complement-fixing antibodies tending to decline sooner than neutralizing antibodies) or the antibodies disappear, apparently reflecting the elimination of the virus (Scott and Tokumaru, 1964).

With regard to cell-mediated immunity in herpes virus infection, 1 to 4 weeks after the primary infection macrophage migration inhibition activity and lymphocyte-mediated cytotoxicity become evident, also delayed hypersensitivity reactions to the herpes virus antigen can be elicited in the skin of sero-positive subjects (Rose and Molloy, 1947).

Recurrent infection

Typical recurrent herpes virus infection of the lips can occur in individuals with complement-fixing antibodies in the serum and showing *in-vitro* lymphocyte transformation with herpes virus antigen (Wilton, Ivanyi and Lehner, 1972; Russell, 1973). However, Wilton *et al.*, (1972) found evidence of impaired macrophage migration inhibition and impaired lymphocyte-mediated cytotoxicity in these individuals and suggested that a partial deficiency of cell-mediated immunity was responsible for recurrent herpetic infection. Nevertheless, in patients with impaired cell-mediated immunity, for example in Hodgkin's disease, clinical experience suggests that these patients do not have an increased frequency of recurrent herpetic infection of the lip (Chang, 1971; Lopez, Bigger and Park, 1972; Russell, 1973). Furthermore, as recurrent herpetic infection of the lip may occur twelve or more times a year it is highly unlikely that prior waning of cell-mediated immunity can be a major factor. Finally, with regard to the development of intraoral herpetic lesions, their recurrence has also been attributed to low serum IgA levels (Greenberg and Brightman, 1971) and absence of salivary antibodies (Tokumaru, 1966).

ORAL CANDIDIASIS

Candida albicans is part of the normal flora of the mouth, but under certain conditions it is also an oppor-

tunistic pathogen giving rise to mucosal inflammation. Although infection is usually endogenous, cross-infection does occur, as between infants in a nursery. The inflammatory reaction is usually mild and superficial with polymorphs predominating in the exudate. Systemic invasion is seen in drug addicts, patients on immunosuppressive and cytotoxic therapy, or in genetically predisposed individuals.

Four varieties of oral candidiasis have been described, acute pseudomembranous candidiasis (thrush), acute atrophic candidiasis, chronic atrophic candidiasis (denture stomatitis) and chronic mucocutaneous candidiasis (Lehner, 1966).

Patients with chronic mucocutaneous candidiasis may have an associated immunodeficiency syndrome (Swiss-type agammaglobulinaemia, hereditary thymic dysplasia, chronic granulomatous disease and Di George's syndrome), but otherwise they have been subdivided into four groups: familial chronic mucocutaneous candidiasis, diffuse chronic mucocutaneous candidiasis, candida endocrinopathy syndrome and late onset candidiasis (Higgs and Wells, 1973).

Humoral immunity in candidiasis

Raised titres of salivary IgA antibodies against *C. albicans* have been found in patients with chronic atrophic candidiasis (Lehner, 1966; Budtz-Jorgensen, 1972) and with familial mucocutaneous candidiasis (Wells, 1973). However, the presence of these antibodies in asymptomatic carriers (Lehner, 1965) suggests they are merely the result of the presence of candida in the mouth and are not necessarily involved in the pathogenesis of oral lesions (Wells, 1973). Raised titres of agglutinating and precipitating antibodies to candidal extracts are also found in the sera of patients with chronic atrophic candidiasis (Lehner, 1966; Lehner, Buckley and Murray, 1972; Budtz-Jorgensen, 1973); again their occurrence in normal individuals suggests that serum antibody levels reflect a normal humoral immune response. Nevertheless, it has recently been suggested that candida precipitins in human sera (as shown by the technique of counter-immunoelectrophoresis) may be useful in differentiating between colonization and infection with candida (Remington, Gaines and Gilmer, 1972), a hypothesis which is disputed by the occurrence of positive reactions in some healthy subjects as well as subjects with allergic asthma (Hellwege, Fischer and Blaker, 1972).

Cellular immunity in candidiasis

Cell-mediated immunity is assumed to be intact in patients with pseudomembranous and acute atrophic candidiasis (Lehner, 1972). In contrast, based on the results of skin and macrophage migration inhibition tests, Budtz-Jorgensen (1973) has suggested delayed hypersensitivity occurs to candidal antigens in patients with chronic atrophic candidiasis (denture stomatitis). Several defects of cell-mediated immunity have been documented in patients with chronic mucocutaneous candidiasis: skin anergy to candidal extracts, an inability of patients' lymphocytes to produce macrophage migration inhibition (Chilgren *et al.*, 1969; Kirkpatrick, Chandler and Schimke, 1970; Valdimarsson *et al.*, 1970; Lehner, Wilton and Ivanyi, 1972), impaired lymphocyte cytotoxicity towards ^{51}Cr-labelled chicken red cells (Lehner *et al.*, 1972) and impaired lymphocyte response to PHA (Lehner *et al.*, 1972). In addition, a serum inhibitory factor has been found in certain patients which prevents lymphocyte transformation (Canales *et al.*, 1969; Higgs, 1973).

All of these findings suggest a heterogeneous pattern of cell-mediated immunodeficiency in patients with chronic mucocutaneous candidiasis, but the relationship of the defects to the pathogenesis of the different types of the disease is not clear. Thus, sequential *in-vitro* studies in patients with severe diffuse chronic mucocutaneous candidiasis have revealed that defects in cell-mediated immunity were constant, whereas those found in familial chronic mucocutaneous candidiasis were liable to variation (Valdimarsson *et al.*, 1973). Furthermore, at least 40 per cent of these latter patients had no demonstrable defect in lymphocyte function, suggesting that abnormal responses are more likely to be acquired than to constitute the primary defect in this condition. Support for this theory is provided by the observation that a high proportion of patients have latent iron deficiency associated with low iron absorption (Higgs, 1973) and in some patients prolonged iron therapy results not only in improvement of the oral lesions but also in restoration of the delayed skin test to candida antigen. Finally, a restoration of macrophage migration inhibition after antifungal therapy has been observed in patients with denture-associated chronic atrophic candidiasis (Budtz-Jorgensen, 1973).

ORAL CARCINOMA

In western countries 5 per cent of all malignant tumours originate in oral tissues; squamous cell carcinoma is by far the most common, accounting for 90 per cent of oral tumours (Lucas, 1972). By contrast, in certain parts of India, oral carcinoma constitutes almost 50 per cent of all malignant tumours (Paymaster, 1957). Tobacco chewing, smoking, alcohol consumption, dental and oral infection, for example with herpes simplex virus, or with *Candida albicans*, oral melanosis and submucous fibrosis, have all been suggested as significant aetiological factors in oral carcinoma (Lucas, 1972).

Humoral immunity in oral carcinoma

Whole salivary IgA levels have been estimated in patients with oropharyngeal carcinoma and the results compared with levels in individuals with genito-urinary carcinoma, in individuals with inflammatory oral lesions, in smokers, in alcohol consumers and in healthy subjects who were neither smokers, nor alcohol consumers (Mandel, Dvorak and Decosse, 1973). The results showed that patients with oropharyngeal carcinoma had the highest salivary IgA levels, followed by the group with inflammatory oral lesions, the smokers and the alcohol consumers. All of these had higher levels of IgA in their whole saliva than the non-smoking, non-drinking controls, and the group with genito-urinary carcinoma. From this it was suggested that in smokers, alcohol consumers and those patients with oral inflammatory conditions, alterations in the oral environment resulted in increased salivary IgA secretion, wheras in oropharyngeal carcinoma, increased salivary IgA levels represented attempted elimination of neoplastic cells by the local immunological system. However, it is worth recalling that oral carcinoma is frequently complicated by ulceration and candida infection (Cawson, 1969; Lucas, 1972), conditions which would facilitate leakage from the affected mucous membrane with consequent increases in concentration of salivary 7S IgA.

Cellular immunity in oral carcinoma

Oral leukoplakia has been considered a precancerous lesion (King, 1964) and epithelial atypia as preliminary histological evidence of malignant change in oral epithelium (Cooke, 1956). Also infection with Herpes simplex virus (Lucas, 1972) and candida infection have been thought significant in the aetiology of oral carcinoma. On this basis Lehner, Wilton, Shillitoe and Ivanyi (1973) studied cell-mediated and humoral response in three groups of patients: patients with oral leukoplakia showing parakeratosis and acanthosis only, patients with oral leukoplakia showing epithelial atypia, and patients with early oral carcinoma. Lymphocyte transformation and macrophage migration inhibition to *Herpesvirus hominis* Type 1 and *C. albicans* antigens were determined. In addition complement-fixing antibodies to *H. hominis* Types 1 and 2, cytomegalovirus and adenovirus, and fluorescent antibodies to *C. albicans*, were estimated in each patient. The results showed that patients with epithelial atypia tended to have the highest stimulation and migration indices to *H. hominis* Type 1, but not to *C. albicans*. In patients with parakeratosis and acanthosis only, there was no correlation between lymphocyte transformation and migration inhibition with both *H. hominis* Type 1 and *C. albicans*, whereas in patients with oral carcinoma, lymphocyte transformation and migration inhibition with both *H. hominis* Type 1 and *C. albicans* were depressed. Titres of complement-fixing antibodies to *H. hominis* Types 1 and 2, cytomegalovirus and adenovirus, and of fluorescent antibodies to *C. albicans*, failed to show a significant pattern in any one of the three groups of patients.

From these results it was suggested that in patients with leukoplakia showing parakeratosis and acanthosis, there was a defect in cell-mediated immunity. The authors also suggested that the specific increase in cell-mediated immunity to *H. hominis* Type 1 in patients with leukoplakia showing epithelial atypia argues in favour of the participation of the virus in malignant transformation of some oral leukoplakias; and frank malignancy being associated with a non-specific impairment of cell-mediated immunity occurring as a result of prolonged stimulation by *H. hominis* Type 1.

The existence of a specific tumour-directed immune response is now well established (Hellstrom, Hellstrom, Pierce and Young, 1968). Preliminary studies have shown that oral carcinomata have specific antigenic properties (Cannell, 1973) and it has also been shown that effector lymphocytes from patients with oral carcinoma are cytotoxic to target cells derived from oral and laryngeal carcinoma (Cannell, 1974). Evidence for specificity of this cytotoxic action was provided by the following observations: non-significant cytotoxic activity of 'oral carcinoma' effector cells against normal skin cells, low-cytotoxic activity of 'healthy control' effector cells, non-significant cytotoxic activity of 'other malignancy' effector cells against oral and laryngeal carcinoma target cells. Also of interest was the finding that in oral carcinoma, autologous serum caused either blocking or enhancement of the cytotoxic ability of the effector lymphocytes, depending upon the clinical status and tumour burden. The results from these studies suggest that specific assay of cell-mediated immunity may prove useful in predicting the clinical course, and recurrence after treatment of oral carcinomata.

IMMUNOLOGICAL ASPECTS OF ORAL LESIONS ASSOCIATED WITH DISEASES OF OTHER SYSTEMS

Oral lesions are often found in diseases known to be associated with altered immune reactivity; thus they have been described in gastrointestinal diseases such as Crohn's disease, ulcerative colitis and coeliac disease, in skin diseases such as pemphigus vulgaris, bullous pemphigoid, benign mucous membrane pemphigoid and dermatitis herpetiformis, and in diseases of connective tissue such as lupus erythematosus and Sjogren's disease. Studies of oral immunological reactivity have been carried out in several of these diseases and these are described below.

ORAL LESIONS IN CROHN'S DISEASE

A retrospective analysis of the case reports of 382 patients with Crohn's disease showed that 6 per cent had

suffered recurrent oropharyngeal ulceration (Croft and Wilkinson, 1972). There have also been a number of reports of apparently specific oral lesions in Crohn's disease which macroscopically and microscopically resemble those in the gastrointestinal tract (Dudeney and Todd, 1969; Issa, 1971; Schiller, Golding, Peebles and Whitehead, 1972). From a systematic study of 100 patients with intestinal Crohn's disease, 100 age, sex and denture status-matched controls, and 100 ulcerative colitis patients, an increased incidence (P < 0.05) of mouth lesions was found in Crohn's disease (9/100), compared to patients with ulcerative colitis (2/100), and controls (1/100) (Basu, Asquith, Thompson and Cooke, 1975). The mouth lesions in Crohn's patients could be

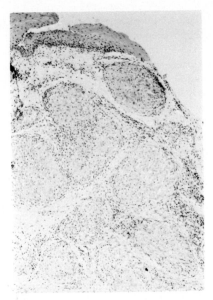

Fig. 4.2 Cobble-stone lesion from Crohn's patients showing epithelioid cell follicles in the lamina propria of the oral mucous membrane. (× 120 H & E.)

classified, according to their macroscopic appearances, into cobble-stone, ulcerative, tag and erythema migrans type lesions.

Of the 9 oral lesions in Crohn's disease, only 1 showed epithelioid cell follicles in the lamina propria (Fig. 4.2) and the rest showed other histological features similar to those described in the intestine of patients with Crohn's disease. No significant differences were found in the mean values, nor in the incidence of low levels, of serum folate, B_{12} or iron between Crohn's patients with, and those without, oral lesions. In contrast, an increased number of Crohn's patients with oral lesions had raised serum seromucoid and low serum albumin levels compared with the incidence in patients without oral lesions (P < 0.05), suggesting that the incidence of oral lesions in Crohn's patients was related to the presence of active bowel disease.

Immunological reactivity

With a view to elucidating the reactivity of the salivary gland based immune system, parotid IgA secretion rates of 20 patients with Crohn's disease was estimated and compared with 20 age and sex matched healthy volunteers (Basu *et al.*, 1975); these showed no significant overall differences. However, Crohn's patients with raised serum seromucoid and low serum albumin levels (that is, patients with active disease) had significantly lower ($P < 0.05$) IgA secretion rates than patients with low serum seromucoid and high serum albumin, and the healthy controls. The parotid IgA secretion rate of patients with Crohn's disease also showed a significant regression ($P < 0.05$) when plotted against their serum albumin levels (Fig. 4.3), suggesting that secretion of IgA by the parotid gland was progressively reduced with increasing activity of the bowel disease.

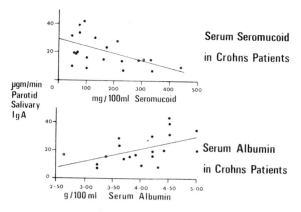

Fig. 4.3 Regression of parotid IgA secretion rate on serum seromucoid and serum albumin in Crohn's patients ($P < 0.05$).

This latter finding could be explained if it is postulated that a transient transepithelial block to IgA develops in the parotid gland; such a blockage has been alleged to occur in diseased epithelium of resected bowel specimens in Crohn's disease (Green and Fox, 1975). An alternative explanation is that in active disease a substantial part of the parotid IgA exists as high polymers or large complexes giving rise to falsely low IgA estimates with the single radial diffusion technique used. It could also be postulated that in patients with active disease, sensitized IgA plasma cells destined for the parotid gland are diverted to the site of maximum antigenic stimulation in the bowel. IgA is thought to be important in the defence of mucosal surfaces (Tomasi and Bienenstock, 1968), so that if the latter explanation is true the relative lack of IgA in the mouth of patients with active bowel disease may allow invasion of the oral mucous membrane by the food or bacterial antigens known to be present (Ivanyi and Lehner, 1970) so producing a mouth lesion.

ORAL LESIONS IN ULCERATIVE COLITIS

Patients with ulcerative colitis, especially those with active disease, suffer from recurrent oral lesions including major aphthous ulcers (Edwards and Truelove, 1964). Pyostomatitis vegetans has also been described (McCarthy and Snyder, 1963), and these authors considered that the oral lesions were part of a syndrome which also included ulcerative colitis.

In a prospective study of oral manifestations of Crohn's disease, Basu *et al.* (1975) found 2 per cent of a 'control group' of 100 ulcerative colitis patients had persistent ulcerative oral lesions and 3 per cent had recurrent aphthous ulceration. Subsequently another 8 ulcerative colitis patients were seen with oral lesions. The lesions in these 13 patients could be classified into 4 groups: aphthous ulceration, lesions analogous to pyoderma gangrenosum, pyostomatitis vegetans and haemorrhagic

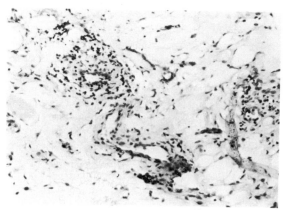

Fig. 4.4 Histology of aphthous ulcer from patient with ulcerative colitis, showing angiitis and perivascular leucocytoclasia. ($\times 120$ H & E.)

ulceration of the skin and oral mucosa (Basu, Asquith, Cooke and Thompson, 1977, submitted for publication). In most cases the presence of the oral lesions correlated with signs and symptoms of active bowel disease.

Histological studies of the oral lesions showed evidence of angiitis or vasculitis with leucocytoclasia in the lamina propria and submucosa (Fig. 4.4).

Immunological reactivity

Secretory IgA concentrations in whole saliva in patients with ulcerative colitis are usually normal (Soltoft, Binder and Gudman-Hoyer, 1973). Although the pathogenesis of the oral lesions in ulcerative colitis and their relationship to the intestinal lesion is not clear, certain immunopathological associations between the two seem possible. Thus, peripheral lymphocytes from patients with inflammatory bowel disease, after challenge by enterobacteria, release lymphotoxins that are cytotoxic for colonic epithelial cells (Shorter, Huizenga and Spencer, 1972; Shorter *et al.*, 1976). Since the cytotoxic effects of lymphotoxins are not tissue specific (Granger, 1970) and enterobacteria can be isolated from the mouths of some normal individuals (Burnett and Scherp, 1968), and patients with inflammatory bowel disease (Basu, 1976), it can be argued that entry of enterobacterial antigens into the oral mucous membrane is responsible for the development of oral lesions in patients with ulcerative colitis. Circulating immune complexes (Hodgson, Potter and Jewell, 1975), and antibodies to *Esch. coli* (Eckhardt, Heinisch and Meyer Zum Buschenfelde, 1976; Sewell, Maxwell, Basu and Asquith, 1977, unpublished observations), have been detected in patients with ulcerative colitis, hence it would seem that the potential exists for Type III hypersensitivity reactions to also occur within the oral mucosal tissues. The histological findings of angiitis and vasculitis (Figure 4.4) could be explained on this latter mechanism.

ORAL LESIONS IN COELIAC DISEASE AND DERMATITIS HERPETIFORMIS

An association between aphthous ulcers and coeliac disease (CD) was noted by Cooke, Peeney and Hawkins (1953), 59 per cent of adults with CD having ulcers at presentation. Also, changes described in CD, such as reduced levels of serum folate and iron, and serum antibodies to gluten, lactalbumin and reticulin (Taylor, Truelove and Wright, 1964; Farmer, 1968), have been reported in patients with aphthous ulceration. In view of these observations, a systemic study of 33 patients presenting with major and minor aphthous ulcers was carried out (Ferguson, Basu, Asquith and Cooke, 1976). Jejunal biopsies were performed and the HLA status, haemoglobin, serum levels of folate, vitamin B_{12}, IgG, IgA and IgM, and parotid saliva IgA levels determined. Biopsies were also obtained from several oral ulcers.

Intestinal biopsies from 8 patients (24 per cent) showed Grade III changes (classified according to the criteria of Roy-Choudhury *et al.*, 1966) consistent with a diagnosis of CD. This incidence of CD in patients with aphthous ulceration is much higher than the reported incidence of CD in the general population (McNeish and Anderson, 1974).

The results of cell counts on jejunal biopsies from these and two other groups of individuals, namely normal controls and patients with CD on a normal diet, showed that in the lamina propria, the plasma cell counts in the non-coeliac group of patients with aphthous ulcers were significantly raised compared with those of normal controls (P 0.001). The numbers of intraepithelial lymphocytes in the non-coeliac group were also raised compared with those in the normal controls (P < 0.05). These changes are similar to, but less pronounced than, those seen in patients with flat jejunal biopsies (i.e. coeliac disease) on a normal diet, with or without aphthous ulcers, suggesting that

aphthous ulcer patients who did not have a flat jejunal mucosa might also have been exhibiting some form of immunological reaction to a dietary factor such as gluten at the intestinal mucosal surface.

The aphthous ulceration in the 8 patients with flat biopsies disappeared on withdrawing gluten from the diet. Recently it has been shown that aphthous ulcers respond to haematinics (Wray *et al.*, 1975). However, haematinics were not given to the 8 patients put on a gluten-free diet. On the basis of these preliminary findings it seems that gluten sensitivity is an aetiological factor in recurrent aphthous ulceration.

The findings of Ferguson *et al.* (1976) have major implications with respect to any patient presenting with recurrent oral aphthous ulceration. Indeed, based on that study it was suggested that all such patients should have intestinal biopsies. Because of that suggestion a further completely separate study has just been completed (Asquith and Basu, 1977, unpublished observations). This study is of a further 50 patients with similar oral manifestations to the Ferguson *et al.* (1976) study. Only 2 patients have been found to have a flat jejunal biopsy, giving an incidence of 'coeliac disease' of 4 per cent. The reasons for the discrepancy between these two studies is being intensively analysed, in considering them one further point is relevant: an association between CD and HLA-B8 has been reported (initially by Stokes *et al.*, 1972; Falchuk, Rogentine and Strober, 1972); 12 of the 33 patients with aphthous ulceration (Ferguson *et al.*, 1976) were found to have HLA-B8, 8 patients with Grade III mucosal changes belonging to this group.

Of additional interest were the concentrations of parotid salivary IgA in patients with CD (Table 4.5), which were significantly lower than the mean levels in patients without CD (P < 0.01). Furthermore, the parotid IgA concentrations were less than 3 mg/100 ml in all patients with CD, while only 29 per cent of patients without CD had such low levels.

These results differ from those of Wallington, Adjukiewicz, Read and Verrier-Jones (1972) who found increased concentrations of IgA in whole saliva of untreated coeliacs compared to controls. In the present study, falls in salivary IgA concentrations could be due to a dilutional effect, if in aphthous ulceration it is postulated that secretion of saliva is reflexly increased. In coeliacs ingesting gluten the number of IgA plasma cells in the jejunum is increased (Savilahti, 1972); in theory a proportion of these cells could migrate there instead of to the salivary gland, resulting in a reduced local secretion of salivary IgA. Finally, with regard to the histology of the actual oral ulcers, patients with CD appear to have a greater number of plasma cells in the lamina propria than patients without CD.

Table 4.5 Serum and salivary immunoglobulin concentrations in patients with recurrent aphthous ulceration (mg/100 ml)

	Overall		With CD		Without CD		
	Mean	SE	Mean	SE	Mean	SE	P
Serum							
IgG (500–1600)	1633.37	86.80	1315.86	176.04	1730.00	92.53	>0.05
IgA (125–425)	353.46	40.59	364.43	74.95	350.35	41.25	>0.05
IgM (47–170)	142.31	16.33	121.57	49.67	150.85	13.18	>0.05
Parotid saliva							
IgA (2–8)	4.29	0.63	2.37	0.15	4.77	0.76	<0.01

CD = coeliac disease.   Figures in parenthesis = normal range.

With respect to dermatitis herpetiformis, in a recent study, 11 out of 15 patients with the disease were found to have typical oral lesions (Fraser, Kerr and Donald, 1973). Immunofluorescent examinations of the oral lesions revealed the presence of granular IgA deposits in the basement membrane region and the walls of blood vessels. Deposits of IgA and complement were also found in the tips of the connective tissue papillae of the uninvolved mucous membrane of some patients (Dabelsteen, 1974).

ORAL LESIONS OF PEMPHIGUS VULGARIS

In 50 per cent of cases of pemphigus vulgaris, the disease presents in the mouth, but the mouth is probably involved at some stage in all. The oral lesions consist of flaccid bullae, erosions and ulcers, and histologically typical intraepithelial bullae containing acantholytic epithelial cells are seen.

Immunological reactivity

Immunofluorescence studies have indicated binding of IgG immunoglobulin in the intercellular region of the oral epithelium. It is possible this immunoglobulin represents autoantibodies to interepithelial antigen which combines with antigens in skin and/or mucous membrane (Chorzelski and Beutner, 1969).

ORAL LESIONS IN LUPUS ERYTHEMATOSUS

Oral lesions occur in both systemic and discoid lupus erythematosus. In fact the criteria proposed for the diagnosis of systemic lupus erythematosus (SLE) by the American Rheumatic Association include oral or naso-pharyngeal ulceration (Cohen and Canoso, 1972). Mouth lesions in SLE appear as erythematous, atrophic or erosive patches, surrounded by elevated, white radiating striae. Histologically, the oral epithelium exhibits atrophy or hyperplasia, hyperkeratosis, keratin plugging and liquefaction of the basal cells, while in the lamina propria, a perivascular mononuclear cell infiltrate and deposits of fibrin are seen (Andreason, 1964).

Immunological reactivity

Reduced salivary IgA levels associated with increases in serum IgA have been reported in SLE (Tomasi et al., 1965). Of possible relevance to this finding is the demonstration of serum antibodies against salivary duct cells (Jablonska and Chorzelski, 1974) and focal lymphocytic sialadenitis in a proportion of patients (Whaley et al., 1973). Of unknown significance in SLE is the detection of a 'fluorescent-band' at the lamina propria-epithelial junction of oral lesions (Schoidt, Dabelsteen, Ullman and Halberg, 1974).

ORAL ASPECTS OF SJOGREN'S SYNDROME

The full triad of Sjogren's syndrome consists of keratoconjunctivitis sicca, xerostomia, and a connective tissue disorder (usually rheumatoid arthritis) with the term 'sicca syndrome' being reserved for cases in which only the first two features occur. In a detailed study of 66 patients with Sjogren's syndrome, xerostomia occurred in 72.7 per cent, oral soreness in 74.2 per cent, and oral ulceration in 36.4 per cent, while focal lymphocytic sialadenitis of labial minor salivary glands was present in 70 per cent (Whaley et al., 1973). With respect to connective tissue disorders, although rheumatoid arthritis is the most common association, scleroderma and polymyositis have also been reported (Hughes and Whaley, 1972).

Immunological reactivity

Salivary IgG is frequently increased in patients with Sjogren's syndrome (Tomasi and DeCoteau, 1970). At least a portion of this IgG appears to be produced locally, in that lip biopsies from patients with Sjogren's syndrome cultured in vitro synthesize greater amounts of IgG, IgA and IgM than biopsies from patients with uncomplicated rheumatoid arthritis (Talal, Asofsky and Lightbody, 1970). Diffuse hypergammaglobulinaemia occurs almost invariably in Sjogren's syndrome and the serum contains a variety of organ-specific and non-organ-specific autoantibodies. Thus, 75–100 per cent of patients have rheumatoid factor (Block, Buchanan, Wohl and Bunim, 1965) while antinuclear antibodies are found in roughly two-thirds of patients (Beck, Anderson, McElwhinney and Powell, 1962). Antibodies to thyroglobulin, thyroid microsomes (Block and Bunim, 1963) and to salivary duct cells (Feltkamp and Van Rossum, 1968) are also fairly common. The latter antibody is not exclusive to patients with Sjogren's syndrome, as it has been found in 26 per cent of patients with uncomplicated rheumatoid arthritis (MacSween et al., 1972). Doubt has been cast on the pathogenic significance of the antibody in Sjogren's syndrome and in rheumatoid arthritis by a lack of correlation between the presence of this antibody and focal lymphocytic and histiocytic adenitis in the labial salivary glands (Whaley et al., 1969). With respect to cell-mediated immunity, a good association has been found between severe lymphocytic and histiocytic sialadenitis and leucocyte migration inhibition to human salivary antigens (Davies et al., 1972), suggesting the occurrence of cell-mediated immunity to salivary glands in Sjogren's syndrome.

CONCLUSION

Immunological mechanisms occurring in the mouth have received increasing attention. Major advances have been made in understanding the normal and abnormal state that have paralleled those made in intestinal research. The accessibility of the oral cavity allows direct study of the immunology of a variety of conditions, many of them common, for example aphthous ulceration. Recently it has become apparent in a significant number of patients with gastrointestinal diseases that the mouth is specifically involved. Currently patients with Crohn's disease, ulcerative colitis and coeliac disease are being studied. It is suggested that detailed immunological investigation of the oral manifestations of these diseases should lead to a better understanding of the aetiology of the intestinal condition.

REFERENCES

Adams, D., Williamson, J. J. & Dolby, A. E. (1969) Delayed hypersensitivity response in guinea-pig oral mucosa. Journal of Pathology, 97, 495–501.

Andreason, J. O. (1964) Oral manifestations in discoid and systemic lupus erythematosus. 1. Clinical investigation. Acta ondontologica Scandinavica, 22, 295–310.

Barile, M. F., Francis, T. C. & Graykowski, E. A. (1968) Streptococcus sanguis in the pathogenesis of recurrent aphthous stomatitis. In Microbial Protoplasts, Spheroplasts and L. Forms, ed. Guze, L. B. Baltimore: Williams & Wilkins.

Baringer, J. R. & Swoveland, P. (1973) Recovery of herpes simplex virus from human trigeminal ganglions. New England Journal of Medicine, 288, 648–650.

Basu, M. K. (1976) Oral manifestations of Crohn's disease: studies in the pathogenesis. Proceedings of the Royal Society of Medicine, 69, 765–766.

Basu, M. K., Asquith, P., Cooke, W. T. & Thompson, H. (1977) Oral lesions in ulcerative colitis (submitted for publication).

Basu, M. K., Asquith, P., Thompson, R. A. & Cooke, W. T. (1975) Oral manifestations of Crohn's disease. Gut, 16, 249–254.

Basu, M. K., Glenwright, H. D., Fox, E. C. & Becker, J. F. (1976) Salivary IgG and IgA before and after periodontal therapy. A preliminary report. Journal of Periodontal Research, 44, 226–229.

Beck, J. S., Anderson, J. R., McElwhinney, A. J. & Powell, N. R. (1962) Antinucleolar antibodies. Lancet, ii, 575–577.

Berglund, S. E. (1971) Immunoglobulins in human gingiva with specificity for oral bacteria. Journal of Periodontology, 42, 546–551.

Berglund, S. E., Rizzo, A. A. & Mergenhagen, S. E. (1969) The immune response in rabbits to bacterial somatic antigen administered via the oral mucosa. Archives of Oral Biology, 14, 7–17.

Biniaminov, M. & Ramot, B. (1975) In vitro restoration by Levamisole of thymus-derived lymphocyte function in Hodgkin's disease. Lancet, i, 464.

Bloch, K. J. & Bunim, J. J. (1963) Sjogren's syndrome and its relation to other connective tissue diseases. Journal of Chronic Diseases, 16, 915–927.

Bloch, K. J., Buchanan, W. W., Wohl, M. J. & Bunim, J. J. (1965) Sjogren's syndrome. A clinical pathological and serological study of 62 cases. Medicine, 44, 187–231.

Brandtzaeg, P. (1965) Immunochemical comparisons of proteins in human gingival pocket fluid, serum and saliva. Archives of Oral Biology, 10, 795–803.

Brandtzaeg, P. (1971) Human secretory immunoglobulins. III. Immunochemical and physicochemical studies of secretory IgA and free secretory piece. Acta pathologica et microbiologica Scandinavica, section B, 79, 189–203.

Brandtzaeg, P. (1972) Local formation and transport of immunoglobulins related to the oral cavity. In Host Resistance to Commensal Bacteria, ed. Macphee, Torquil. Edinburgh: Churchill Livingstone.

Brandtzaeg, P., Fjellanger, I. & Gjeruldsen, S. T. (1970) Human secretory immunoglobulin. I. Salivary secretions from individuals with normal or low levels of serum immunoglobulins. Scandinavian Journal of Haematology, Supplementum 12, 1–83.

Brody, H. A. & Silverman, S. (1969) Studies on recurrent oral aphthae. I. Clinical and laboratory comparisons. Oral Surgery, 27, 27–34.

Budtz-Jorgensen, E. (1972) Denture stomatitis. V. Candida agglutinins in human sera. Acta odontologica Scandinavica, 30, 313–325.

Budtz-Jorgensen, E. (1973) Cellular immunity in acquired candidiasis of the palate. Scandinavian Journal of Dental Research, 81, 372–382.

Burnett, G. W. & Scherp, H. W. (1968) Oral Microbiology and Infectious Disease, 3rd ed. Baltimore: Williams & Wilkins.

Canales, L., Middlemass, R. D., Louro, J. M. & South, M. A. (1969) Immunological observations in chronic mucocutaneous candidiasis. Lancet, ii, 567–571.

Cannell, H. (1973) Oral cancer and immunity. British Journal of Oral Surgery, 11, 171.

Cannell, H. (1974) Cell-mediated and humoral immunity responses to primary oral cancers. Journal of Maxillo-facial Surgery, 2, 108–113.

Cawson, R. A. (1969) Leukoplakia and oral cancer. *Proceedings of the Royal Society of Medicine*, **62**, 610–615.

Challacombe, S. J. (1971) Serum antibodies in subjects with dental caries. *Journal of Dental Research*, **50**, 654–655.

Challacombe, S. J., Lehner, T. & Guggenheim, B. (1972) Serum and salivary antibodies to glucosyltransferase in dental caries. *Nature*, **238**, 219.

Chandler, D. C., Silverman, M. S., Lundblad, R. L. & McFall, W. T. (1974) Human parotid IgA and peridontal disease. *Archives of Oral Biology*, **19**, 733–735.

Chang, T. W. (1971) Recurrent viral infection (reinfection). *New England Journal of Medicine*, **284**, 765–773.

Chilgren, R. A., Meuwissen, H. J., Quie, P. G., Good, R. A. & Hong, R. (1969) The cellular immune defect in chronic mucocutaneous candidiasis. *Lancet*, **i**, 1286–1288.

Chorzelski, T. P. & Beutner, E. H. (1969) Factors contributing to occasional failures in demonstration of pemphigus antibodies by immunofluorescent test. *Journal of Investigative Dermatology*, **53**, 188–191.

Clarke, A. (1974) *Proceedings of Workshop*. London: British Oral Pathology Club.

Coelho, I. M., Pereira, M. T., Virella, G. & Thompson, R. A. (1974) Salivary immunoglobulins in a patient with IgA deficiency. *Clinical and Experimental Immunology*, **18**, 685–699.

Cohen, A. S. & Canoso, J. J. (1972) Criteria for the classification of systemic lupus erythematosus – status 1972. *Arthritis Rheumatism*, **15**, 540–543.

Cooke, B. E. D. (1956) Leukoplakia buccalis and oral epithelial naevi. *British Journal of Dermatology*, **68**, 151–174.

Cooke, B. E. D. (1961) Recurrent Mickulicz's aphthae. *Dental Practitioner*, **12**, 119–124.

Cooke, W. T., Peeney, A. L. P. & Hawkins, C. F. (1953) Symptoms, signs and diagnostic features of steatorrhoea. *Quarterly Journal of Medicine*, **22**, 59–77.

Cowley, G. C. (1966) Fluorescence studies of crevicular fluid. *Journal of Dental Research*, **45**, 655–661.

Croft, C. B. & Wilkinson, A. R. (1972) Ulceration of the mouth, pharynx and larynx in Crohn's disease of the intestine. *British Journal of Surgery*, **59**, 249–252.

Dabelsteen, E. (1974) *Proceedings of Workshop*. London: British Oral Pathology Club.

Davies, D., Berry, H., Bacon, P. A., Issa, M. A. & Schofield, J. J. (1973) Labial sialadenitis in Sjogren's syndrome and in rheumatoid arthritis. *Journal of Pathology*, **109**, 307–314.

Dolby, A. E. (1969) Recurrent aphthous ulceration. Effect of sera and peripheral blood lymphocytes upon epithelial tissue culture cell. *Immunology*, **17**, 709–714.

Dolby, A. E., Williamson, J. J. & Adams, D. (1969) The retest contact hypersensitivity reaction in guinea pig skin and oral mucosa. *British Journal of Experimental Pathology*, **50**, 343–346.

Donatsky, O. & Bendixen, G. (1972) *In vitro* demonstration of hypersensitivity to *Strep. 2A* in recurrent aphthous stomatitis by means of leucocyte migration test. *Acta Allergologica*, **27**, 137–144.

Donatsky, I. & Dabelsteen, E. (1974) An immunofluorescence study on the humoral immunity to adult human oral mucosa in recurrent aphthous stomatitis. *Acta Allergologica*, **29**, 308–318.

Dudeney, T. P. & Todd, I. P. (1969) Crohn's disease of the mouth. *Proceedings of the Royal Society of Medicine*, **62**, 1237.

Eckhardt, R., Heinisch, M. & Meyer zum Buchenfelde, K. H. (1976) Cellular immune reactions against common antigen, small intestine and colon antigen in patients with Crohn's disease, ulcerative colitis and cirrhosis of the liver. *Scandinavian Journal of Gastroenterology*, **11**, 49–54.

Edwards, F. C. & Truelove, S. C. (1964) The course and prognosis of ulcerative colitis. III. Complications. *Gut*, **5**, 1.

Ellison, S. A., Carton, C. A. & Rose, H. M. (1959) Studies of recurrent herpes simplex infections following sections of the trigeminal nerve. *Journal of Infectious Diseases*, **105**, 161–167.

Evans, R. T., Spaeth, S. & Mergenhagen, S. E. (1966) Bacterial antibody in mamalian serum to obligatory anaerobic Gram negative bacteria. *Journal of Immunology*, **97**, 112–119.

Fahey, J. L. & McKelvey, E. M. (1965) Quantitative determination of serum immunoglobulins in antibody–agar plates. *Journal of Immunology*, **94**, 84–90.

Falchuk, Z. M., Rogentine, G. N. & Strober, W. (1972) Predominance of histocompatibility antigen HL-A8 in patients with gluten-sensitive enteropathy. *Journal of Clinical Investigation*, **51**, 1602–1605.

Farmer, E. C. (1958) Recurrent aphthous ulcers. *Dental Practitioner*, **8**, 177–184.

Feltkamp, T. E. W. & Van Rossum, A. L. (1968) Antibodies to salivary duct cells, and other autoantibodies, in patients with Sjorgren's syndrome and other idiopathic autoimmune diseases. *Clinical and Experimental Immunology*, **3**, 1–16.

Ferguson, R., Basu, M. K., Asquith, P. & Cooke, W. T. (1976) Jejunal mucosal abnormalities in patients with recurrent aphthous ulceration. *British Medical Journal*, **i**, 11–13.

Fisher, A. A. (1973) Allergic contact stomatitis cheilitis. In *Dentistry and the Allergic Patient*, ed. Frazier, C. A. Springfield: Charles C. Thomas.

Fitzgerald, R. J., Jordon, H. V. & Archard, H. O. (1966) Dental caries in gnotobiotic rats infected with a variety of *Lactobacillus acidophilus*. *Archives of Oral Biology*, **11**, 473–476.

Fraser, N. G., Kerr, N. W. & Donald, D. (1973) Oral lesions in dermatitis herpetiformis. *British Journal of Dermatology*, **89**, 439–450.

Geller, J. H. & Rovelstad, G. H. (1959) Electrophoresis of saliva. Relationship of protein components to dental caries. *Journal of Dental Research*, **38**, 1060–1065.

Granger, C. A. (1970) Mechanisms of lymphocyte-induced cell and tissue destruction *in vitro*. *American Journal of Pathology*, **60**, 469–481.

Green, F. H. Y. & Fox, H. (1975) The distribution of mucosal antibodies in the bowel of patients with Crohn's disease. *Gut*, **16**, 125–131.

Greenberg, M. S. & Brightman, V. J. (1971) Serum immunoglobulins in patients with recurrent intra-oral herpes simplex infections. *Journal of Dental Research*, **50**, 781.

Guggenheim, B. (1970) Enzymatic hydrolysis and structure of water-insoluble glucan produced by glucosyltransferases from a strain of *Streptococcus mutans*. *Helvetia Odontologica Acta*, **14**, Supplement V, 89.

Hand, W. L., Smith, J. W. & Sandford, J. P. (1971) The antibacterial effect of normal and infected urinary bladder. *Journal of Laboratory and Clinical Medicine*, **77**, 605–615.

Hanson, L. A. & Brandtzaeg, P. (1972). Secretory antibody systems. In *Immunologic Disorders in Infants and Children*, eds. Steihm, E. R. and Fulginiti, V. A. Philadelphia: Saunders.

Hellstrom, I., Hellstrom, K. E., Pierce, G. E. & Young,

J. P. S. (1968) Cellular and humoral immunity to different types of human neoplasms. *Nature*, **220**, 1352–1354.

Hellwege, H. H., Fischer, H. & Blaker, F. (1972) Diagnostic value of Candida precipitins. *Lancet*, **ii**, 386.

Higgs, J. M. (1973) Chronic mucocutaneous candidiasis: iron deficiency and the effects of iron therapy. *Proceedings of the Royal Society of Medicine*, **66**, 802–804.

Higgs, J. M. & Wells, R. S. (1973) Chronic mucocutaneous candidiasis: new approaches to treatment. *British Journal of Dermatology*, **89**, 179–190.

Hodgson, H. J. F., Potter, B. J. & Jewell, D. P. (1975) Complement in inflammatory bowel disease. *Gut*, **16**, 833–834.

Hoffbrand, A. V. (1974) Anaemia in coeliac disease. In *Clinics in Gastroenterology. Coeliac Disease*, ed. Cooke, W. T. & Asquith, P. London: Saunders.

Holmberg, K. & Killander, J. (1971) Quantitative determination of immunoglobulins (IgG, IgA and IgM) and identification of IgA-type in the gingival fluid. *Journal of Peridontal Research*, **6**, 1–8.

Horton, J. E., Leikin, S. & Oppenheim, J. J. (1972) Human lymphoproliferative reaction to saliva and dental plaque deposits. An *in vitro* correlation with periodontal disease. *Journal of Periodontology*, **43**, 522–527.

Horton, J. E., Raisz, L. G., Simmons, H. A., Oppenheim, J. J. & Mergenhagen, S. E. (1972) Bone resorbing activity in supernatant fluid from cultured human peripheral blood leukocytes, *Science*, **177**, 793.

Hughes, G. R. V. & Wahley, K. (1972) Sjogren's syndrome. *British Medical Journal*, **iv**, 533–536.

Hurliman, J. & Zuber, C. (1968) *In vitro* protein synthesis by human salivary glands. I. Synthesis of salivary IgA and serum proteins. *Immunology*, **14**, 809–817.

Ishizaka, K., Dennis, E. G. & Hornbrook, M. (1964) Presence of reagin and 1A-globulin in saliva. *Journal of Allergy*, **35**, 143–148.

Issa, M. A. (1971) Crohn's disease of the mouth. *British Dental Journal*, **130**, 247–248.

Ivanyi, L. & Lehner, T. (1970) Stimulation of lymphocyte transformation by bacterial antigens in patients with periodontal disease. *Archives of Oral Biology*, **15**, 1089–1096.

Ivanyi, L. & Lehner, T. (1971) Lymphocyte transformation by sonicates of dental plaque in human periodontal disease. *Archives of Oral Biology*, **16**, 1117–1121.

Ivanyi, L., Wilton, J. M. A. & Lehner, T. (1972) Cell-mediated immunity in periodontal disease: cytotoxicity, migration inhibition and lymphocyte transformation studies. *Immunology*, **22**, 141–145.

Jablonska, S. & Chorzelski, T. P. (1974) Lupus erythematosus. In *Immunological Aspects of Skin Diseases*, ed. Fry, L. & Seah, P. P. Lancaster: MTP.

Kaufman, H. E., Brown, D. C. & Ellison, E. H. (1967) Recurrent herpes in rabbit and man. *Science*, **156**, 1628.

Kennedy, A. E., Shklair, J. A., Hayashi, J. A. & Bahn, A. N. (1968) Antibodies to cariogenic streptococci in humans. *Archives of Oral Biology*, **13**, 1275–1278.

King, O. H. (1964) Intraoral leukoplakia. *Cancer*, **17**, 131–136.

Kirkpatrick, C. H., Chandler, J. W. & Schimke, R. N. (1970) Chronic mucocutaneous moniliasis with impaired delayed hypersensitivity. *Clinical and Experimental Immunology*, **6**, 375–385.

Kraus, F. W. & Sirisinha, S. (1962) Gammaglobulin in saliva. *Archives of Oral Biology*, **7**, 221–233.

Lachman, P. & Thompson, R. A. (1970)

Immunoconglutinins in human saliva – a group of unusual IgA antibodies. *Immunology*, **18**, 157–169.

Lai, R. F. M., Fat, A., Carmane, R. H. & Van Furth, R. (1974) An immunopathological study on the synthesis of immunoglobulins and complement in normal and pathological skin and the adjacent mucous membranes. *British Journal of Dermatology*, **90**, 123–136.

Lawton, A. R. & Mage, R. G. (1969) The synthesis of secretory IgA in the rabbit. 1. Evidence for synthesis as an 11S dimer. *Journal of Immunology*, **102**, 693–697.

Lehner, T. (1964) Recurrent aphthous ulceration and autoimmunity. *Lancet*, **ii**, 1154–1155.

Lehner, T. (1965) Immunofluorescent investigation of *Candida albicans* antibodies in human saliva. *Archives of Oral Biology*, **10**, 975–980.

Lehner, T. (1966) Immunofluorescent study of *Candida albicans* in candidiasis, carriers and controls. *Journal of Pathology and Bacteriology*, **91**, 97–104.

Lehner, T. (1967a) Behcet's syndrome and autoimmunity. *British Medical Journal*, **i**, 465–467.

Lehner, T. (1967b) Stimulation of lymphocyte transformation by tissue homogenates in recurrent oral ulceration. *Immunology*, **13**, 159–166.

Lehner, T. (1969a) Immunoglobulin estimation of blood and saliva in human recurrent oral ulceration. *Archives of Oral Biology*, **14**, 351–364.

Lehner, T. (1969b) Characterization of mucosal antibodies in recurrent aphthous ulceration and Behcet's syndrome. *Archives of Oral Biology*, **14**, 843–853.

Lehner, T. (1972) Cell-mediated immune responses in oral disease: a review. *Journal of Oral Pathology*, **1**, 39–58.

Lehner, T., Buckley, H. E. & Murray, I. G. (1972) The relationship between fluorescent, agglutinating and precipitating antibodies to *Candida albicans* and their immunoglobulin classes. *Journal of Clinical Pathology*, **25**, 344–348.

Lehner, T., Cardwell, J. E. & Cleary, E. D. (1967) Immunoglobulins in saliva and serum in dental caries. *Lancet*, **i**, 1294–1296.

Lehner, T., Wilton, J. M. A. & Ivanyi, L. (1972) Immunodeficiencies in chronic mucocutaneous candidiasis. *Immunology*, **22**, 775–787.

Lehner, T., Wilton, J. M. A. & Ivanyi, L. (1976) Double blind crossover trial of Levamisole in recurrent aphthous ulceration. *Lancet*, **ii**, 926–929.

Lehner, T., Wilton, J. M. A. & Ward, R. G. (1970) Serum antibodies in dental caries in man. *Archives of Oral Biology*, **15**, 481–490.

Lehner, T., Wilton, J. M. A., Shillitoe, E. J. & Ivanyi, L. (1973) Cell-mediated immunity and antibodies to Herpes virus Hominis type 1, in oral leukoplakia and carcinoma. *British Journal of Cancer*, **27**, 351–361.

Lopez, C., Biggar, W. D. & Park, B. H. (1972) Viral studies of immunodeficient patients. *Federation Proceedings*, **31**, 635.

Lucas, R. B. (1972) *Pathology of Tumours of the Oral Tissues*, 2nd edn. Edinburgh: Churchill Livingstone.

MacSween, R. N. M., Goudie, R. B., Anderson, J. R., Armstrong, E., Murray, M. A., Mason, D. K., Jasani, M. K., Boyle, J. A., Buchanan, W. W. & Williamson, J. (1972) Occurrence of antibody to salivary duct epithelium in Sjogren's disease, rheumatoid arthritis and other arthritides. *Annals of the Rheumatic Diseases*, **26**, 402–411.

McCarthy, P. & Shklar, G. (1963) A syndrome of pyostomatitis vegetans and ulcerative colitis. *Archives of Dermatology*, **88**, 917–919.

McCarthy, C., Snyder, M. L., Parker, R. B. (1965) The

indigenous oral flora of man. 1. The newborn to the 1 year old infant. *Archives of Oral Biology*, **10**, 61–70.

McDevitt, H. O. & Bodmer, W. F. (1972) Histocompatibility antigens, immune responsiveness and susceptibility to disease. *American Journal of Medicine*, **52**, 1–8.

McNair-Scott, T. F. & Tokumaru, T. (1964) Herpesvirus hominis (virus of herpes simplex). *Bacteriological Review*, **28**, 458–471.

McNeish, A. S. & Anderson, C. M. (1974) The disorder in childhood. In *Clinics in Gastroenterology. Coeliac Disease*, ed. Cooke, W. T. and Asquith, P. London: Saunders.

Mandel, M. A., Dvorak, K. & DeCosse, J. J. (1973) Salivary immunoglobulins in patients with oro-pharyngeal and broncho-pulmonary carcinoma. *Cancer*, **31**, 1408–1413.

Mergenhagen, S. E. (1972) In *Host Resistance to Commensal Bacteria*, ed. Macphee, Toquil. Edinburgh: Churchill Livingstone.

Meyer, J. de, Degraeve, M., Clarysse, J., Loose, F. de & Peremans, W. (1977) Levamisole in aphthous stomatitis: evaluation of three regimens. *British Medical Journal*, **i**, 671–674.

Monacelli, M. & Nazzaro, P. (1966) *Behcet's Disease*. New York: Karger.

Nasz, I., Kulcsar, G., Dan, P. & Sallay, K. (1971) A possible pathogenic role for virus-carrier lymphocytes. *Journal of Infectious Diseases*, **124**, 214–216.

Neisengard, R., Beutner, E. H. & Hazen, S. P. (1968) Immunologic studies of periodontal diseases. IV. Bacterial hypersensitivity and periodontal disease. *Journal of Periodontology*, **39**, 23–26.

Ohno, S., Aoki, K., Sugiura, S., Nakayama, E., Itakura, K. & Aisawa, M. (1973) HL-A5 and Behcet's disease. *Lancet*, **ii**, 1383–1384.

Oshima, Y., Shimuzu, T., Yokohari, R., Matsumoto, T., Kano, K., Kagami, T. & Nagaya, H. (1963) Clinical studies on Behcet's syndrome. *Annals of the Rheumatic Diseases*, **22**, 36–45.

Paymaster, J. C. (1957) The problem of oral, oro-pharyngeal and hypopharyngeal carcinoma in India. *British Journal of Surgery*, **44**, 467–471.

Plaut, A. G., Genco, R. J. & Tomasi, T. B. (1974) Isolation of an enzyme from *Streptococcus sanguis* which specifically cleaves IgA. *Journal of Immunology*, **113**, 289–291.

Remington, J. S., Gaines, J. D. & Gilmer, M. A. (1972) Demonstration of *Candida precipitins* in human sera by counter immunoelectrophoresis. *Lancet*, **i**, 143.

Rose, H. M. & Molloy, E. (1947) Cutaneous reactions with the virus of Herpes simplex. *Journal of Immunology*, **56**, 287–294.

Roy-Choudhury, D. C., Cooke, W. T., Tan, D. T., Banwell, J. G. & Smits, B. J. (1966) Jejunal biopsy: criteria and significance. *Scandinavian Journal of Gastroenterology*, **1**, 57–74.

Russell, A. S. (1973) Cell-mediated immunity to Herpes simplex virus in man. *American Journal of Clinical Pathology*, **60**, 826–830.

Salmon, S. E. (1970) Serum and secreted IgE globulin in man. *Clinical Research*, **18**, 432.

Savilahti, E. (1972) Intestinal immunoglobulins in children with coeliac disease. *Gut*, **13**, 958–964.

Schiller, K. F. R., Golding, P. L., Peebles, R. A. & Whitehead, R. (1971) Crohn's disease of the mouth and lips. *Gut*, **12**, 864–865.

Schiodt, M., Dabelsteen, E., Ullman, S. & Halberg, P. (1974) Deposits of immunoglobulins and complement in oral lupus erythematosus. *Scandinavian Journal of Dental Research*, **82**, 603–607.

Schroeder, H. E., Munzel-Pedrassoli, S. & Page, R. (1972) Correlated morphometric and biochemical analysis of gingival tissue. *Archives of Oral Biology*, **18**, 899–923.

Schultz-Haudt, S. D. & Scherp, H. W. (1955) Production of hyaluronidase and beta-glucoronidase by viridans streptococci isolated from the gingival crevices. *Journal of Dental Research*, **34**, 924–929.

Shillitoe, E. J. (1972) Immunoglobulins and complement in crevicular fluid. In *Host Resistance to Commensal Bacteria*, ed. Macphee, Torquil. Edinburgh: Churchill Livingstone.

Ship, I. I., Merritt, A. D. & Stanley, H. R. (1962) Recurrent aphthous ulcers. *American Journal of Medicine*, **32**, 32–43.

Shorter, R. G., Huizenga, K. A. & Spencer, R. J. (1972) A working hypothesis for the etiology and pathogenesis of non-specific inflammatory bowel diseases. *Digestive Diseases*, **17**, 1024–1032.

Shorter, R. G., Tomasi, T. B., Huizenga, K. A., Spencer, R. J. & Stobo, J. D. (1976) The immunology of chronic ulcerative colitis and Crohn's disease. *Annals of the New York Academy of Sciences*, **278**, 586–591.

Simons, K., Weber, T., Stiel, M. & Grasbeck, R. (1964) Immunoelectrophoresis of human saliva. *Acta medica Scandinavica*, Supplementum **412**, 257–264.

Sircus, W., Church, R. & Kelleher, J. (1957) Recurrent aphthous ulceration of the mouth. A study of the natural history, aetiology and treatment. *Quarterly Journal of Medicine*, **26**, 235–249.

Snyderman, R., Gewurz, H. & Mergenhagen, S. E. (1968) Interactions of the complement system with endotoxin lipopolysaccharide. Generation of a factor chemotactic for polymorphonuclear leukocytes. *Journal of Experimental Medicine*, **128**, 259–275.

Soltoft, J., Binder, V. & Gudman-Hoyer, E. (1973) Intestinal immunoglobulins in ulcerative colitis. *Scandinavian Journal of Gastroenterology*, **8**, 293–300.

Steinberg, A. I. & Gershoff, S. N. (1968) Quantitative difference in spirochaetal antibody observed in periodontal disease. *Journal of Periodontology*, **39**, 286–289.

Stokes, P. L., Asquith, P., Holmes, G. K. T., Mackintosh, P. & Cooke, W. T. (1972) Histocompatibility antigens associated with adult coeliac disease. *Lancet*, **ii**, 162–164.

Strober, W., Blaese, R. M. & Waldman, T. A. (1970) The origin of salivary IgA. *Journal of Laboratory and Clinical Medicine*, **75**, 856–862.

Symoens, J. & Brugmans, J. (1974) Treatment of recurrent aphthous stomatitis and herpes with Levamisole. *British Medical Journal*, **4**, 592.

Talal, N., Asofsky, R. & Lightbody, P. (1970) Immunoglobulin synthesis by salivary gland lymphoid cells in Sjogren's syndrome. *Journal of Clinical Investigation*, **49**, 49–54.

Taubman, M. A. (1974) Immunoglobulins of human dental plaque. *Archives of Oral Biology*, **19**, 439–446.

Taylor, K. B., Truelove, S. C. & Wright, R. (1964) Serological reaction to gluten and cow's milk proteins in gastrointestinal disease. *Gastroenterology*, **46**, 99–108.

Thomas, H. C., Ferguson, A., Lennan, J. G. & Mason, D. K. (1973) Food antibodies in oral disease: a study of serum antibodies to food proteins in aphthous ulceration and other oral diseases. *Journal of Clinical Pathology*, **26**, 371–374.

Thonard, J. C. & Dalbow, M. H. (1965) Local cellular antibodies. 1. Plaque formation by sensitized oral mucosal cells from conventional animals. *Journal of Immunology*, **95**, 209–213.

Tokumaru, T. (1966) Possible role of gamma-A immunoglobulin in herpes simplex infection in man. *Journal of Immunology*, **97**, 248–259.

Tomasi, T. B. & Bienenstock, J. (1968) Secretory immunoglobulins. *Advances in Immunology*, **9**, 1–96.

Tomasi, T. B. & DeCoteau, E. (1970) Mucosal antibodies in respiratory and gastrointestinal disease. *Advances in Internal Medicine*, **16**, 401–425.

Tomasi, T. B. & Zeigelbaum, S. (1963) The selective occurrence of γIA-globulins in certain body fluids. *Journal of Clinical Investigation*, **42**, 1552–1560.

Tomasi, T. B., Tan, E. M., Solomon, A. & Prendergast, R. A. (1965) Characteristics of an immune system common to certain external secretions. *Journal of Experimental Medicine*, **121**, 101–124.

Tourville, D. R., Adler, R. H., Bienenstock, J. & Tomasi, T. B. (1969) The human secretory immunoglobulin system: immunohistological localization of γA, secretory piece and lactoferrin in normal human tissues. *Journal of Experimental Medicine*, **129**, 411–429.

Truelove, S. C. & Maurice-Owen, R. M. (1958) Treatment of aphthous ulceration of the mouth. *British Medical Journal*, **i**, 603–607.

Valdimarsson, H., Holt, L., Riches, R. C. & Hobbs, J. R. (1970) Lymphocyte transformation abnormality in chronic mucocutaneous candidiasis. *Lancet*, **i**, 1259–1261.

Valdimarsson, H., Higgs, J. M., Wells, R. S., Yamamura, M., Hobbs, J. R. & Holt, P. J. L. (1973) Immune abnormalities associated with chronic mucocutaneous candidiasis. *Cellular Immunology*, **6**, 348–361.

Wallington, T., Adjukiewicz, A. B., Read, A. E. & Verrier-Jones, J. (1972) Levels of salivary IgA in treated and untreated coeliac disease. *Gut*, **13**, 718–720.

Wells, R. S. (1973) Chronic mucocutaneous candidiasis: a clinical classification. *Proceedings of the Royal Society of Medicine*, **61**, 801–802.

Whaley, K., Williamson, J., Chisholm, D. M., Webb, J., Mason, D. K. & Buchanan, W. W. (1973) Sjogren's syndrome. 1. Sicca components. *Quarterly Journal of Medicine*, **42**, 279–304.

Whaley, K., Chisholm, D. M., Goudie, R. B., Downie, W. W., Dick, W. C., Boyle, J. A. & Williamson, J. (1969) Salivary duct autoantibody in Sjogren's syndrome: correlation with focal sialodenitis in the labial mucosa. *Clinical and Experimental Immunology*, **4**, 273–282.

WHO (1961) Report of an expert committee on dental health. No. 207.

Williams, R. C. & Gibbons, R. J. (1972) Inhibition of bacterial adherence by secretory immunoglobulin A: a mechanism of antigen dispersal. *Science*, **177**, 697–699.

Wilton, J. M. A. (1972) A comparative study of gingival and systemic routes of immunization in the guinea pig. In *Host Resistance to Commensal Bacteria*, ed. Macphee, Torquil. Edinburgh: Churchill Livingstone.

Wilton, J. M. A., Ivanyi, L. & Lehner, T. (1971) Cell-mediated immunity and humoral antibodies in acute ulcerative gingivitis. *Periodontal Research*, **6**, 9–16.

Wilton, J. M. A., Ivanyi, L. & Lehner, T. (1972) Cell-mediated immunity in Herpesvirus hominis infections. *British Medical Journal*, **i**, 723–726.

Wray, D., Ferguson, M. M., Mason, D. K., Hutcheon, A. W. & Dagg, J. H. (1975) Recurrent aphthae: treatment with vitamin B_{12}, folic acid, and iron. *British Medical Journal*, **ii**, 490–493.

Wright, R. & Alp, M. H. (1971) Autoantibodies to reticulin in patients with various gastrointestinal diseases and their relationship to immunoglobulins and dietary antibodies. *Gut*, **12**, 858–859.

Zengo, A. N., Mandel, I. D., Goldman, R. & Khurana, H. S. (1971) Salivary studies in human caries resistance. *Archives of Oral Biology*, **16**, 557–560.

5. The stomach – pernicious anaemia and gastritis

B. P. Maclaurin

INTRODUCTION

There is a very large literature relating to all aspects of gastritis, including those forms which have evidence of associated autoimmunity. A number of recent reviews (Irvine, 1965; Chanarin, 1972; Strictland and MacKay, 1973) have dealt with various aspects of gastric disease associated with autoimmunity, but there is still considerable controversy and lack of knowledge about some features of this disease complex. It is hoped that this chapter will serve to highlight those features requiring further study as well as summarizing current knowledge in this field. The discussion is concluded with an account of some previously unpublished observations on the cellular immune status of pernicious anaemia patients with respect to antigens other than those of the gastric mucosa; emphasis is placed on the possible relation of these findings to the increased gastric cancer incidence in this disorder.

THE HISTOLOGICAL AND ANATOMICAL BASIS OF IMMUNOLOGICAL DAMAGE TO THE STOMACH

In spite of the ready availability of direct-vision gastric biopsy from multiple sites using fibreoptic instruments, many studies on gastritis give only very limited information on the geographic location of the histological abnormalities found in the stomach, with little attempt to differentiate antral from body of stomach specimens. The early descriptions of gastric atrophy in pernicious anaemia (Magnus and Ungley, 1938; Meulengracht, 1939; Cox, 1943) emphasized the localization of the lesion to the body and fundus of the stomach, but more recent studies have suggested that the separation may not always be so clear cut and a few patients with generalized gastritis may ultimately develop overt vitamin B_{12} deficiency.

Strickland and MacKay (1973) in a recent extensive review have advocated classification of all cases of gastritis into two major subgroupings, partly on the presence or absence of gastric autoantibodies and partly on the basis of involvement or sparing of the gastric antrum. Their long-term review of 100 patients with atrophic gastritis has provided considerable support for this approach. Nonetheless, not all patients studied by other writers seem to fit neatly into this classification, often because there is insufficient histological evidence given and only meticulous biopsy studies will allow definite conclusions to be made. Whitehead, Truelove and Gear (1972) have recently described their experience in the reporting of more than 2500 gastric biopsy specimens. The classification they suggest could provide a suitable framework for histological reporting in the future and allow a quantitative assessment of individual histological features.

The presence of autoantibodies directed against gastric parietal cells and against gastric intrinsic factor has been extensively documented (Irvine, Davies and Delamore, 1962; Taylor, Roitt and Doniach, 1962; Taylor, 1959). There is a clear correlation between the presence of parietal cell antibodies (pca) in the serum and the presence of histological damage to the gastric mucous membrane in the great majority of subjects studied (Adams *et al.*, 1964; Wright, Whitehead, Wangel, Salem and Schiller, 1966). Nevertheless, there is no conclusive evidence that this damage is the direct consequence of the presence of such antibodies. However, perfusion studies by Tanaka and Glass (1970) injecting human serum positive for pca into rats has resulted in a reduction of parietal cells and a fall in acid secretion levels. The development of pca in animals immunized with gastric extracts has tended to follow rather than precede the development of histological damage to the gastric mucosa (Krohn and Finlayson, 1973) and the titre of antibody has not correlated directly with the severity of the gastric lesion. However, the presence of antibodies to intrinsic factor in the gastric lumen rather than the serum has clearly been shown in human subjects to diminish the absorption of labelled vitamin B_{12} (Rose and Chanarin, 1971). This was not the case when such antibodies were present only in the serum. Intraluminal intrinsic factor antibody in the presence of gastritis of the gastric body and fundus can therefore be accepted as playing a significant role in the pathogenesis of the macrocytic anaemia of pernicious anaemia. Few would now dispute that this disease should be classed as an autoimmune process. However, intrinsic factor antibodies in the gastric lumen can only be readily detected in a small proportion of pernicious anaemia patients using standard techniques, though, by manipulation designed to dissociate antigen/antibody complexes, it has been shown that intrinsic factor antibodies are present in over half of these patients (Rose and Chanarin, 1969; Goldberg and Bluestone, 1970).

The nomenclature and definition of the gastritis associated with vitamin B_{12} deficiency present some difficulties, since there may be some element of overlap between the gastritis of pernicious anaemia and more generalized gastritis occasionally associated with vitamin B_{12} deficiency. An attempt at classification by Strickland and MacKay (1973) has been briefly mentioned earlier; they suggested that gastritis characterized by absence of antral involvement, a positive pca test, diffuse involvement of the body and fundus mucosa and severe impairment of gastric secretion should be designated as Type A autoimmune gastritis, and this does have some merit. This would be in contrast to a Type B gastritis characterized by antral as well as body and fundus involvement, a negative pca test, mainly focal histological change and only moderate impairment of gastric secretion. However, although prolonged follow up of gastritis in patients in Melbourne showed the development of overt pernicious anaemia only in the Type A group, other workers have noted that a number of patients otherwise entirely typical of pernicious anaemia have not shown a positive pca reaction and a rigid separation is probably not possible. In the Melbourne patients it was noteworthy that some Group A patients did show mild degrees of antral inflammation. One of the main advantages of a classification based on the presence or absence of antral involvement is the finding that serum gastrin levels are markedly elevated in the latter group. This provides an additional parameter in the evaluation of patients with suspected pernicious anaemia (McGuigan and Trudeau, 1970; Korman, Strickland and Hansky, 1971).

For convenience, but with some reservations, the classification into Type A and Type B gastritis will be utilized in the remainder of this discussion. The frequency of gastric autoantibodies should provide some measure of the prevalence of Type A gastritis. In tests on 600 blood donors and apparently healthy members of Elderly Citizens' Clubs, Ungar, Stocks, Martin, Whittingham and Mackay (1968) found positive tests for pca in 5 per cent of females aged 15 to 40, 15 per cent in the 41 to 60 age range and 21 per cent above this age. The figures for males were considerably less below the age of 60, but in the older age group 18 per cent showed positive tests. It is clear that antibody frequency is age and sex dependent, and that in the over-60 age group, roughly one-fifth of the population will show such antibodies. The incidence of intrinsic factor antibodies was very much less in this same study; in 800 normal subjects, none showed antibody below the age of 50 and only 5 in the 51 to 90 age group. The fasting serum gastrin level rises with age in subjects positive for pca (Strickland, Korman and Hansky, 1973) but not in those negative for pca. This observation tends to confirm the validity of pca positivity as a reflection of gastric histology and secretory capacity.

The prevalence of Type B gastritis is much more difficult to assess since there is no marker readily available. Studies reported by Siurala, Isokoski, Varis and Kekki (1968) and Isokoski, Krohn, Varis and Siurala (1969) showed that of 140 'normal' adults submitted to gastric biopsy, 28 per cent showed gastritis but only 8 per cent of the subjects were positive for pca. If the presence of parietal cell antibodies is accepted as the main criterion, these findings would suggest that Type B gastritis is 3 to 4 times more common than Type A. However, it is noteworthy that in a more recent progress report on the same case material (Siurala, Lehtola and Ihamaki, 1974) the degree of round cell infiltration and atrophy was more marked in the body of stomach than in the antrum, with metaplasia about equal in the two sites. Furthermore, the fasting serum gastrin levels of 24 of the 35 patients available for study were above 71 pmol/l compared with only 1 of 24 controls. In 7 cases values above 400 pmol/l were found; parietal cell antibodies were present in only 2 of these 7 cases. It should be noted also that in the Strickland and Mackay material, 5 of 19 patients positive for pca did show mild to moderate changes in the antral mucosa. Hence the distinction between Type A and Type B gastritis on the basis of geographic location of the pathological change in the gastric mucosa is by no means absolute.

Evaluation of the numbers of immunoglobulin-secreting plasma cells in the intestinal mucosa has been well studied in pernicious anaemia but not apparently in patients with Type B gastritis. Odgers and Wangel (1968) found a 90 per cent reduction in the numbers of IgA-containing cells in the gastric mucosa in pernicious anaemia while IgG-containing cells were increased by 15 per cent. However, the levels of serum immunoglobulins were found to be normal and the levels of gastric juice immunoglobulins were unrelated to the numbers of the corresponding mononuclear cells in the gastric mucosa. These observations have been confirmed by Søltoft (1974) who also noted a small but significant increase of jejunal IgG-containing cells and a decrease of jejunal IgA-containing cells in patients with pernicious anaemia. He found no alteration in the rectal mucosa, contrary to the findings of Odgers and Wangel (1969). In pernicious anaemia the immunoglobulin class of parietal cell or intrinsic factor antibodies in gastric juice is frequently IgG rather than IgA (Strickland, Baur, Ashworth and Taylor, 1971).

The above findings indicate that the normal gastric IgA dominance is reduced in pernicious anaemia. Pernicious anaemia in association with selective serum IgA deficiency has been reported in a total of 7 cases (Ginsberg and Mullinax, 1970; Spector, 1974). These cases were all of the juvenile type with gastric atrophy, histamine fast achlorhydria and deficient intrinsic factor secretion. In addition they frequently had parietal cell and intrinsic factor antibodies in the serum.

Pernicious anaemia in association with a more generalized hypogammaglobulinaemia of adult acquired type was first reported by Larsson, Hagelquist and Coster (1961) and a detailed case study of 10 such patients has been made by Twomey et al. (1969). Serum IgA was absent in 9 of their patients and barely detectable in the remaining 1. Plasma cells were absent, or greatly diminished in number, in bone-marrow aspirates and in all other available histological material from these 10 patients. None of the patients had demonstrable serum antibodies to parietal cells or intrinsic factor. This latter observation has been interpreted as indicating that gastric antibodies are not an essential feature of the pathogenesis of the gastritis of pernicious anaemia, since the majority of these patients were shown to have marked gastric atrophy. However, the location of the biopsies in the stomach was not stated and subsequent reports have suggested that such patients may have gastritis of generalized type rather than one limited to the body and fundus (Hughes, Brooks and Conn, 1972).

These patients were also unusual in that the gastric lesion presented at a young age (mean age 34 years) and the individuals frequently showed diarrhoea and sometimes overt malabsorption and with an unusually high frequency of giardiasis. The existence of a generalized gastritis in these patients is supported by the observation (Hughes et al., 1972) that individuals with primary hypogammaglobulinaemia with or without pernicious anaemia showed levels of serum gastrin similar to the normal population and significantly lower than patients with uncomplicated pernicious anaemia. Twomey et al. (1969) demonstrated that at least some of their patients were capable of developing positive delayed cutaneous responses to antigens and of giving a mitotic response to phytohaemagglutinin. One possibility that arises from these studies is that the gastric lesion in these patients might relate to a cellular immune response to gastric constituents rather than antibody-induced damage.

ASSOCIATED FEATURES IN AUTOIMMUNE GASTRITIS AND PERNICIOUS ANAEMIA

Humoral aspects of gastric autoimmunity have been extensively reviewed (Irvine, 1965; Chanarin, 1972). There is a close relationship between various organ-specific autoimmune diseases involving the stomach, the thyroid and the adrenal in particular but also including vitiligo and insulin-dependent diabetes mellitus. The relationship is manifest either by coexisting overt disease or the presence of autoantibodies directed against more than one of these organs. Thus in Graves' disease, pernicious anaemia has been reported to occur with a frequency of 3.1 per cent (Chanarin, 1969). Pernicious anaemia was noted in 6 of 118 patients with Addison's disease reported by Blizzard, Chee and Davis (1967) and in 7 of 74 patients with idiopathic hypoparathyroidism (Blizzard, Chee and Davis, 1966). About 50 per cent of patients with pernicious anaemia show thyroid autoantibodies; in thyroid autoimmune disease 30 per cent show gastric autoantibodies and 20 per cent of their healthy relatives also show gastric autoantibodies. Similarly, in Addison's disease, hypoparathyroidism and vitiligo, about 20 per cent of subjects show parietal cell antibodies.

Doniach, Roitt and Taylor (1965) have demonstrated that 36 per cent of healthy relatives of patients with pernicious anaemia show autoantibodies against gastric parietal cells. Also, Wangel, Callender and Spray (1968) have presented evidence that pernicious anaemia, achlorhydria with atrophic gastritis and vitamin B_{12} malabsorption are all more common in the first-degree relatives of patients with pernicious anaemia than in the general population. Other family studies have strongly supported this genetic tendency (Irvine, 1965). Velde et al. (1964) have suggested that the development of pca is controlled by a dominant autosomal gene which is also responsible for the processes leading to atrophic gastritis, gastric achlorhydria and impairment of vitamin B_{12} absorption.

It is clear that some degree of gastric autoimmunity is common in the relatives of patients with pernicious anaemia and to a lesser degree in the community at large, yet overt pernicious anaemia appears to develop in only a very small proportion of these subjects. Various follow-up studies of patients with achlorhydria secondary to autoimmune atrophic gastritis have been reported (Irvine, Cullen and Mawhinney, 1974; Rose, Chanarin, Doniach, Brostoff and Ardeman, 1970). In the former study, of 90 patients followed for a 1 to 15 year period (mean 6 years), 17 patients developed malabsorption of vitamin B_{12}. This occurred more commonly, but not exclusively, in subjects showing the presence of serum intrinsic factor antibody. Nevertheless, such antibody titres were of no value in predicting which patients would develop malabsorption. In follow-up studies there is considerable evidence that intrinsic factor antibody in the gastric juice is much more important than antibody in the serum in determining which patients will develop overt vitamin B_{12} malabsorption (Rose et al., 1970).

The antibody to parietal cells is a 7S gammaglobulin and specific fluorescent staining of parietal cells can be demonstrated equally well with the patient's own gastric mucosa as well as with allogeneic mucosa, indicating the true autoantibody nature of this material (Irvine, 1965). The pca has been found to localize in the microvillus structure of the cell membrane of the parietal cell (Hoedemaker and Ito, 1970). It can be absorbed by an extract of gastric body mucosa and the immunofluorescence of the parietal cell cytoplasm can be inhibited in the indirect Coons' technique by a positive serum (Irvine, 1965). The serum antibody to intrinsic factor is also usually of the IgG class (Chanarin, 1972), but when present in the gastric lumen it is sometimes of the IgA class (Rose et al., 1969) with a secretory end piece (Goldberg, Shuster, Stuckey and Fudenberg, 1968).

In patients with pernicious anaemia various workers have attempted to improve vitamin B_{12} absorption and the appearance of the gastric mucosa by prolonged corticosteroid therapy but with only very limited and transient success. The results obtained have been reviewed and summarized by Baggett and Welsh (1970). In a proportion of subjects the Schilling test showed improvement and a number showed increased gastric juice intrinsic factor and diminution of serum levels of intrinsic factor antibodies. Improvement in gastric histology occurred only occasionally and there was no correlation between improvement in these various parameters. Essentially similar findings have been reported more recently by Strickland, Fisher, Lewin and Taylor (1973).

CELLULAR IMMUNE MECHANISMS IN PERNICIOUS ANAEMIA AND IN EXPERIMENTAL MODELS – *IN-VIVO* AND *IN-VITRO* FINDINGS

Most of the preceding discussion has emphasized the presence of autoantibodies to gastric components in patients with Type A gastritis, and in the elucidation of immune mechanisms in pernicious anaemia this has historically been the dominant theme of studies undertaken. However, in a considerable number of putative autoimmune diseases including pernicious anaemia, the evidence that the multiplicity of autoantibodies demonstrated are actually responsible for the tissue damage observed remains circumstantial. Increasing emphasis is being placed upon the possible role of cellular immune mechanisms. As previously mentioned, a pernicious anaemia-like syndrome occurs in a significant number of patients with acquired agammaglobulinanaemia and with no demonstrable autoantibodies to gastric constituents (Twomey et al, 1969). This fact and the evidence that some degree of cellular immune competence was maintained in some of these patients

have provided considerable stimulus to the study of cellular immunity directed against gastic constituents.

Gastric hyposecretion and gastric atrophy can be produced in rats by repeated injections of human gastric autoantibodies (Tanaka et al., 1970; Inada and Glass, 1972). A more recent, very detailed study (Inada and Glass, 1975) also showed that human intrinsic factor antibody injected serially into rats can produce a significant reduction of intrinsic factor output. However, other experimental animal models have suggested that the development of gastric mucosal damage after immunization precedes by 2 to 4 weeks the ability to demonstrate any autoantibodies. Thus in dogs (Hennes et al., 1962) immunization by repeated injections of gastric juice combined with Freund's adjuvant, produced gastritis at the same time as delayed skin reactivity to the gastric antigen, whereas antibodies to gastric components were not demonstrable until 2 to 4 weeks later. These findings were confirmed by Fixa, Vejbora, Komárková, Langr and Pařízek (1964). The lesion demonstrated was associated with the development of achlorhydria, but the whole process was reversible and the mucosa appeared normal 9 months later. In monkeys, Andrada, Rose and Andrada (1969) were also able to produce a definite histological gastritis by repeated immunization and reported autoantibodies against microsomal and soluble gastric fractions. However, only limited assessment of delayed skin reactivity was made, in a single animal.

The dog studies were confirmed and extended by Krohn and Finlayson (1973). These authors demonstrated the development of cellular immunity to gastric juice antigens by assessment of delayed skin reactivity and by inhibition of peripheral leucocyte migration in the presence of these antigens. They again noted that the evidence of cellular immunity preceded the detection of pca (using the immunofluorescence test) and coincided with the development of histological damage. They further commented that in the leucocyte migration test several gastric antigens appeared to be involved and cellular immunity in this test system could still be shown in the absence of intrinsic factor. This work was performed in dogs, but the same group (Finlayson, Fauconnet and Krohn, 1972) have also shown that migration-inhibition of peripheral leucocytes from patients with pernicious anaemia can be detected in the presence of a variety of gastric juice antigens, and the presence or absence of antibody to parietal cells or intrinsic factor showed no correlation with the migration-inhibition findings. Tai and McGuigan (1969) had earlier shown that the lymphocytes of a proportion of patients with pernicious anaemia undergo blast transformation in the presence of a variety of gastric antigens. They found no correlation between the presence or absence of transformation and the presence or absence of serum antibodies to the parietal cell antigen, but transformation was not found in patients whose serum contained blocking antibodies to intrinsic factor. In about 50 per cent of cases Goldstone, Calder, Barnes and Irvine (1973) have also shown inhibition of migration by pernicious anaemia leucocytes in the presence of extracts of gastric mucosa, stomach mitochondria and stomach microsomes. This compares with only 14 per cent in subjects with atrophic gastritis and pca but without intrinsic factor antibodies and without evidence of vitamin B_{12} malabsorption. Rose et al. (1970) obtained similar findings in pernicious anaemia patients and again noted that patients with atrophic gastritis and gastric autoantibodies but without overt pernicious anaemia, when followed over a 3 to 7 year period, seldom showed evidence of cellular immunity to gastric antigens. The only exception was one patient who had intrinsic factor antibody in gastric juice as well as in serum and showed evidence of migration-inhibition.

Simultaneous assessment of pernicious anaemia subjects by both the inhibition of macrophage migration and lymphocyte transformation techniques gave positive results by one or other method in 85 per cent of 35 patients (James, Asherson, Chanarin, Coghill, Hamilton, Himsworth and Webster, 1974). The same authors noted that 4 out of 9 patients with hypogammaglobulinaemia and 'pernicious anaemia', but with no antibodies detectable against parietal cell antigen or intrinsic factor, did show cellular immunity against these constituents by one or both tests. If hog instead of human intrinsic factor is used to test for cellular immunity, almost 100 per cent of human subjects are claimed to give a positive response (Weisbart, Bluestone and Goldberg, 1975).

In summary, it would seem that cellular immunity to several gastric constituents can be demonstrated in vitro in at least 85 per cent of patients with established pernicious anaemia but only rarely in Type A gastritis not associated with B_{12} malabsorption. In animal models, cellular immunity can also be demonstrated by delayed skin reactivity as well as by inhibition of macrophage migration and develops at the same time as the evidence of histological damage to the gastric mucosa. The evidence suggests but does not conclusively prove that cellular immunity is of greater importance than autoantibody production in the pathogenesis of Type A gastritis. It is of some interest that in a small proportion of pernicious anaemia patients, blast transformation of their lymphocytes has been found in response to gastric antral antigens as well as fundal antigens (Salupere, Nutt and Jarve, 1972). This might suggest that the cellular immune response is not directed exclusively against mucosal components of the body and fundus.

CANCER INCIDENCE IN AUTOIMMUNE GASTRITIS AND RELEVANCE OF CELLULAR IMMUNE STATUS

It has been known for a considerable period that pernicious anaemia is associated with an increased risk of gastric malignancy (Magnus et al., 1938; Rigler and Kaplan, 1945). The degree of risk has been variously assessed from 5 to 10 per cent of patients followed over a period of years (Mosbech and Videbaek, 1950; Blackburn et al., 1968). Furthermore Shearman, Finlayson, Wilson and Samson (1966) have emphasized that a proportion of patients with gastric cancer showing no evidence of overt pernicious anaemia may, nonetheless, show diminished levels of serum B_{12}. Some such patients show autoantibodies to gastric constituents and can be classified as in a 'prepernicious' stage of pernicious anaemia. In a series of 35 consecutive patients with gastric cancer admitted to the Royal Infirmary in Edinburgh, 4 had known pernicious anaemia but a further 3 had gastric autoantibodies and low serum B_{12} levels.

There is evidence of an association between gastric cancer and idiopathic late-onset immunoglobulin deficiency (Hermans and Huizenga, 1972) with an incidence of 7.7 per cent in the cases reported. Twomey et al. (1969) reported a further case and this patient also showed evidence of pernicious anaemia but without autoantibodies.

It is tempting to speculate that the increased cancer incidence in these patients may relate to a diminished immune surveillance capacity as proposed by Burnet (1968) and by others. Although Twomey et al. (1969) found some evidence of maintained cellular immune competence in a proportion of their patients, the tests employed might not have demonstrated subtle diminution in lymphocyte functions. In a more extensive study of a mother and twin daughters with pernicious anaemia and immunoglobulin deficiency (Gelfand et al., 1972), it was shown that although both daughters lacked demonstrable IgA, one of them also showed virtually complete absence of cellular immune responsiveness as measured by a variety of techniques and with multiple antigens including intrinsic factor. Finally the diminution of IgA-secreting plasma cells in the gastric mucosa in the majority of patients with pernicious anaemia (Odgers et al., 1968) may reflect a limited immune deficiency state.

It has been suggested (Allison, Denman and Barnes, 1971) that the development of autoimmune disease results from an impairment of T-lymphocyte (thymus-derived) function, with failure of feedback control upon B-lymphocyte (bone-marrow-derived) production of antibodies to self-antigens. If such an impairment of T-cell function was present in pernicious anaemia, it might contribute to the increased incidence of gastric cancer. Accordingly, a study of cellular immunity has recently been made in a series of patients with pernicious anaemia, uncomplicated by serum immunoglobulin deficiency. Delayed skin reactivity to a battery of test antigens and *in-vitro* mixed lymphocyte responsiveness to an allogeneic lymphoma cell line were selected as being of relevance to immune surveillance capacity and the results obtained have tended to confirm the concept of impaired T-cell function in gastric autoimmune disease. The details of this study are given below.

CELLULAR IMMUNITY TO NON-GASTRIC ANTIGENS IN PERNICIOUS ANAEMIA
(In association with Dr N. Matthews, Research Officer)

METHODS:

A total of 18 patients with proven pernicious anaemia were studied, of whom 8 had been only recently diagnosed (recent treatment group) and had received vitamin B_{12} therapy for from 1 to 10 weeks. The remainder were of long standing, with a mean treatment duration of 6.7 years (prolonged treatment group). Prior to treatment, all patients had been shown to have a megaloblastic bone marrow. Diagnosis was based upon a positive Schilling test – gross impairment of B_{12} absorption improved by intrinsic factor – or upon achlorhydria after pentagastrin stimulation together with gastric autoantibodies. Fourteen of the 18 subjects were shown to have pca by immunofluorescence or complement fixation tests and 10 subjects had thyroid autoantibodies. Estimation of serum IgG, IgA and IgM levels in this patient group showed only minor deviations from the normal range.

Intradermal skin tests were performed with tuberculin, mumps, candida and streptococcal antigens (Forbes, 1971) on patients and closely age-matched controls, as described previously (Broom and Maclaurin, 1973). The skin-tested patients were in both the recent treatment and prolonged treatment groups but the

former patients had all received treatment with vitamin B_{12} for at least 3 months prior to skin testing.

In-vitro lymphocyte responsiveness to allogeneic tumour cell antigens was assessed by mixed culture of lymphocytes from patients or from controls with mitomycin-C-treated cells from a Burkitt lymphoma cell line, EB_2, in a one-way reaction. Triplicate mixed cultures were prepared in Eagle's medium supplemented with 10 per cent pooled normal human serum and with corresponding unstimulated cultures for both patients and controls and set up on the same day and in an identical manner. Proliferative response was assessed by measuring incorporation of tritiated thymidine (^{3}HTdr) into DNA at the end of the 6-day culture period. The methods used have been described in detail in previous papers (Maclaurin, Cooke and Ling, 1971; Broom et al., 1973).

RESULTS:

(a) Delayed skin sensitivity
The results are set out in Table 5.1. One-third of the patients tested showed complete anergy to all four antigens in the doses used, whereas none of the age matched controls and none of a larger series of younger controls showed overall anergy. For the matched pairs, this difference was statistically significant and this was true also for reactivity to tuberculin alone. A similar trend for reactivity to mumps antigen was noted, but for the numbers tested, the difference was not significant. Skin testing on all patients was carried out at least 3 months after B_{12} treatment had been commenced.

(b) *In-vitro* lymphocyte antigenic challenge with allogeneic tumour cell line
In Figure 5.1 these results have been expressed as the stimulation index: i.e. the number of times by which isotope incorporation into DNA in the mixed cultures exceeds that obtained from unstimulated lymphocytes cultured alone. There was a significant depression of

Table 5.1 Comparison of skin test results for treated patients and age matched controls

Test antigens	Mean age		Proportion of negative responses		Level of significance (Fisher's exact test)
	Patients	Controls	Patients	Controls	
All 4 antigens[a]	74	68 (37)	4 of 12	0 of 12 (0 of 20)	p = 0.05
Tuberculin only	74	68 (37)	11 of 12	6 of 12 (9 of 20)	p = 0.03
Mumps only	74	68 (37)	10 of 12	6 of 12 (4 of 18)	p = 0.1

[a] Refers to tuberculin, mumps, candida and streptococcal antigens.
(Results in brackets are from a larger series of younger normal subjects for comparison. Broom and Maclaurin, 1973.)

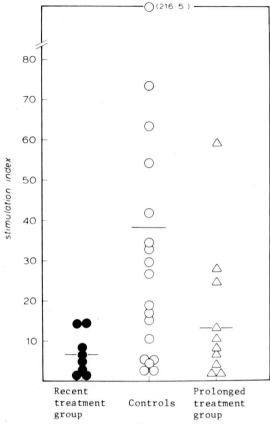

Fig. 5.1 *In-vitro* response of lymphocytes from 18 control individuals and 18 patients with pernicious anaemia (8 of the latter had been recently treated and 10 had received prolonged treatment) to allogeneic tumour cells (EB$_2$ cells).

response in the recent treatment group compared to the paired controls ($0.001 < P < 0.01$ by the Wilcoxon matched-pairs, signed-ranks test) and for the whole patient group compared to all paired controls ($P < 0.05$) However, the prolonged treatment group alone failed to show significant depression in comparison with matched controls.

Control subjects for the recent treatment patient series were mostly healthy blood donors whereas those for the inactive group were mostly drawn from hospitalized old people in an attempt to improve age matching. The latter subjects frequently suffered from complicating illnesses of varying severity and where possible these were matched with pernicious anaemia patients having similar additional diseases.

(c) Comparison of *in-vitro* lymphocyte response in the same test system with previous findings in coeliac disease and sarcoidosis

This is shown in Table 5.2. There is a striking similarity between the results in the patient categories listed.

DISCUSSION:

The depression of delayed skin reactivity to the battery of test antigens used is remarkably similar to the findings in a study on sarcoidosis carried out in the same community and over the same time period (Broom *et al.*, 1973). Furthermore, reactivity to tuberculin as compared to age matched controls also showed a similar reduction in these two disease states. This relative skin anergy was detected at a time when all pernicious anaemia patients had been on treatment for at least 3 months and cannot therefore be attributed to persisting B$_{12}$ deficiency.

Table 5.2 Comparison of results of one-way MLC with lymphoma cells in pernicious anaemia, sarcoidosis and coeliac disease.

	Recent treatment pernicious anaemia group	Corresponding controls	Active sarcoidosis[b]	Corresponding controls	Quiescent coeliac[c] disease	Corresponding controls
No. of cases	8	18	6	14	8	22
Mean stim. index	6.8	38	4.8	21.9	8.3	37
Level of significance[a]	$p < 0.01$		$p < 0.02$		$p < 0.001$	
Mean DPM increment[d]	8742	30 000	5486	33 288	6560	39 000
Level of significance	$p < 0.01$		$p < 0.02$		$p = 0.001$	

[a] Statistical comparison of each patient group with corresponding controls by the Mann-Whitney 'U' test.
[b] Data from study by Broom and Maclaurin (1973).
[c] Data from study by Maclaurin *et al.* (1971).
[d] DPM. increment = disintegrations per minute in mixed cultures minus DPM of the corresponding lymphocytes cultured alone.

No depression of *in-vitro* lymphocyte response was observed in the prolonged treatment group and this observation has been confirmed in a further series of *in-vitro* tests. However, in recently treated pernicious anaemia, the significant depression of *in-vitro* lymphocyte responsiveness in the mixed lymphocyte reaction test system employed was closely comparable to that previously demonstrated in active sarcoidosis (Broom *et al.*, 1973), and for coeliac disease following treatment and prolonged clinical recovery (Maclaurin *et al.*, 1971). The latter result implies a defect of lymphocyte responsiveness of very long standing and this may relate to the well-documented increased incidence of lymphoma and gut cancer in adult coeliac disease (Gough, Read and Naish, 1962; Harris, Cooke, Thompson and Waterhouse, 1967). The same reasoning could also apply to autoimmune gastric atrophy prior to the development of overt pernicious anaemia.

The trend towards greater mixed lymphocyte reactivity (but not skin responsiveness) following treatment may indicate that part of the immune defect relates to interference with lymphocyte function secondary to B_{12} deficiency. It is of interest that Joynson, Jacobs, Murray Walker and Dolby (1972) have reported significant diminution of ^{3}HTdr incorporation into DNA by lymphocytes from iron-deficient patients challenged with tuberculin. These subjects showed impaired tuberculin skin reactivity which was restored by iron therapy to levels found in controls.

Age matching of our simultaneous controls for lymphocyte testing was not ideal. However, since the results for the younger, recent treatment group (mean age 64) were depressed as compared to the older prolonged treatment group (mean age 72) and to the whole control group (mean age 58), and since no fall off with age has been noted in our laboratory in a larger group of normal controls in this test system, the statistical comparisons made appear valid.

The *in-vitro* impairment in function of washed pernicious anaemia lymphocytes was unrelated to the patients' serum and culture of normal lymphocytes in pernicious anaemia serum failed to produce any consistent alteration in their performance in this culture system. This is in contrast to the findings in coeliac disease in which a depressive serum factor in addition to a lymphocyte defect was noted in the majority of subjects (Maclaurin *et al.*, 1971). One pernicious anaemia subject was found to have a lymphocytotoxic factor present temporarily in her serum, but lymphocyte viability in the remainder of the cultures was comparable with that of the controls.

Mild elevation of unstimulated lymphocyte ^{3}HTdr incorporation into DNA was noted for the patients (mean distintegrations per minute 1999) compared to the controls (mean DPM 1574). This may relate to increased antigenic challenge by bacterial products in the upper small intestine and stomach as a consequence of achlorhydria. Alternatively it may reflect prolonged stimulation by autoantigens.

Das and Hoffbrand (1970) have claimed that phytohaemagglutinin response is increased in *untreated* pernicious anaemia as judged by incorporation of ^{3}HTdr into DNA, but total DNA and numbers of blast cells per culture did not differ between patients and controls. They interpreted their results as suggesting normal cellular immunity in untreated cases, but this conclusion may be questioned, since they also showed obvious abnormal morphology of phytohaemagglutinin-transformed 'megaloblastic' lymphocytes and evidence of an altered metabolic pathway for DNA synthesis in B_{12}-deficient lymphocytes. MacCuish, Urbaniak, Goldstone and Irvine (1974) found evidence suggesting impairment of the capacity of pernicious anaemia lymphocytes to incorporate tritiated thymidine into DNA. In their experiments, a significant reduction of lymphocyte responsiveness to phytohaemagglutinin appeared to be present as judged by thymidine-incorporation into DNA, but on radioautography the percentage lymphoblast transformation showed little difference between patients and controls. The patients tested were all on maintenance treatment with vitamin B_{12}, and prior to treatment more marked disturbance of DNA synthesis might well have been observed. We suggest that the mixed lymphocyte response enables detection of an impairment of T-cell responsiveness related to histocompatibility cell surface antigens and possibly of more relevance to tumour cell homeostasis *in vivo*. The results obtained are consistent with the hypothesis that partial impairment of T-cell function may be found in human autoimmune disease. Whether this impairment is causally related to the occurrence of autoimmunity or of complicating cancer remains to be determined. The paradox of increased humoral and cellular immunity to several gastric autoantigens in pernicious anaemia but diminished lymphocyte responsiveness to a range of extrinsic antigens raises the possibility that there may be some element of antigenic competition, with autoantigens monopolizing the patient's immune responsiveness.

ACKNOWLEDGEMENT:

The above study was supported by a project grant from the Medical Research Council of New Zealand. Permission to study cases under the care of physicians on the staff of the Dunedin Hospitals is gratefully acknowledged. Schilling tests were performed by courtesy of Professor R. D. H. Stewart of the Nuclear Medicine Department, and autoantibody studies by Mr Couchman of the Palmerston North Medical Research Foundation. We acknowledge the help of Mr G. Spears of the Department of Preventive and Social Medicine for statistical analysis and Mrs H. Paterson for her careful assistance in the laboratory.

CONCLUSION

The anatomical and immunological classification of gastritis into Type A and Type B as advocated by Strickland and Mackay (1973) has some merit in emphasizing the importance of precise histological assessment, but the distinction between these two types is often difficult and by no means absolute. There is ample evidence that the gastritis of pernicious anaemia is a consequence of autoimmune damage. However,

from studies in experimental animals, it seems that a cellular immune response directed against gastric constituents is at least as important as antibody mechanisms in causing this damage.

In pernicious anaemia, the reduced numbers of IgA-secreting immunocytes in the gastric mucosa and occasional association with acquired hypogammaglobulinaemia suggest that the occurrence of gastric cancer in pernicious anaemia may in part relate to an impairment of immune surveillance. This conclusion is supported by evidence of some T-cell impairment in pernicious anaemia as manifest by the diminished delayed skin test reactivity and mixed lymphocyte reactivity reported in this chapter.

REFERENCES

Adams, J. F., Glen, A. I. M., Kennedy, E. H., Mackenzie, I. L., Morrow, J. M., Anderson, J. R., Gray, K. G. & Middleton, D. G. (1964) The histological and secretory changes in the stomach in patients with autoimmunity to gastric parietal cells. Lancet, i, 401–403.

Allison, A. C., Denman, A. M. & Barnes, R. D. (1971) Cooperating and controlling functions of thymus-derived lymphocytes in relation to autoimmunity. Lancet, ii, 135–140.

Andrada, J. A., Rose, N. R. & Andrada, E. C. (1969) Experimental autoimmune gastritis in the Rhesus monkey. Clinical and Experimental Immunology, 4, 293–310.

Baggett, R. T. & Welsh, J. D. (1970) Observations on the effects of glucocorticoid administration in pernicious anaemia. The American Journal of Digestive Diseases, 15, 871–881.

Blackburn, E. K., Callender, S. T., Dacie, J. V., Doll, R., Girdwood, R. H., Mollin, D. L., Saracci, R., Stafford, J. L., Thompson, R. B., Varadi, S. & Wetherley-Mein, G. (1968) Possible association between pernicious anaemia and leukaemia: a prospective study of 1625 patients with a note on the very high incidence of stomach cancer. International Journal of Cancer, 3, 163–170.

Blizzard, R. M., Chee, D. & Davies, W. (1966) The incidence of parathyroid and other antibodies in the sera of patients with idiopathic hypoparathyroidism. Clinical and Experimental Immunology, 1, 119–128.

Blizzard, R. M., Chee, D. & Davis, W. (1967) The incidence of adrenal and other antibodies in the sera of patients with idiopathic adrenal insufficiency (Addison's disease). Clinical and Experimental Immunology, 2, 19–30.

Bor, S., Feiwel, M. & Chanarin, I. (1969) Vitiligo and its aetiological relationship to organ-specific autoimmune disease. British Journal of Dermatology, 81, 83–88.

Broom, B. C. & Maclaurin, B. P. (1973) Sarcoidosis: correlation of delayed hypersensitivity, MLC. reactivity and lymphocytotoxicity with disease activity. Clinical and Experimental Immunology, 15, 355–364.

Burnet, F. M. (1968) A modern basis for pathology. Lancet, i, 1383–1387.

Chanarin, I. (1969) The Megaloblastic Anaemias. Oxford: Blackwell Scientific Publications.

Chanarin, I. (1972) Pernicious anaemia as an autoimmune disease. British Journal of Haematology, 23 (Suppl.), 101–107.

Cheli, R., Santi, L., Ciancamerla, G. & Canciani, G. (1973) A clinical and statistical follow-up study of atrophic

gastritis. American Journal of Digestive Diseases, 18, 1061–1066.

Cox, A. J. (1943) The stomach in pernicious anaemia. American Journal of Pathology, 19, 491–501.

Das, K. C. & Hoffbrand, A. V. (1970) Lymphocyte transformation in megaloblastic anaemia: morphology and DNA synthesis. British Journal of Haematology, 19, 459–468.

Doniach, D., Roitt, I. M. & Taylor, K. B. (1965) Autoimmunity in pernicious anaemia and thyroiditis: a family study. Annals of the New York Academy of Science, 124, 605–625.

Finlayson, N. D. C., Fauconnet, M. H. & Krohn, K. (1972) In vitro demonstration of delayed hypersensitivity to gastric antigens in pernicious anaemia. American Journal of Digestive Diseases, 17, 631–638.

Fixa, B., Vejbora, O., Komárková, O., Langr, F. & Pařizek, J. (1964) On immunologically induced gastric atrophy in dogs. Gastroenterologia (Basle), 102, 331–338.

Forbes, I. J. (1971) Measurement of immunological function in clinical medicine. Australian and New Zealand Journal of Medicine, 1, 160–170.

Gelfand, E. W., Berkel, A. I., Godwin, H. A., Rocklin, R. E., David, J. R. & Rosen, F. S. (1972) Pernicious anaemia, hypogammaglobulinaemia and altered lymphocyte reactivity: a family study. Clinical and Experimental Immunology, 11, 187–199.

Ginsberg, A. & Mullinax, F. (1970) Pernicious anaemia and monoclonal gammopathy in a patient with IgA deficiency. American Journal of Medicine, 48, 787–791.

Goldberg, L. S. & Bluestone, R. (1970) Hidden gastric autoantibodies to intrinsic factor in pernicious anaemia. Journal of Laboratory and Clinical Medicine, 75, 449–456.

Goldberg, L. S., Shuster, J., Stuckey, M. & Fudenberg, H. H. (1968) Secretory immunoglobulin A: autoantibody activity in gastric juice. Science, 160, 1240–1241.

Goldstone, A. H., Calder, E. A., Barnes, E. W. & Irvine, W. J. (1973) The effect of gastric antigens on the in vitro migration of leucocytes from patients with atrophic gastritis and pernicious anaemia. Clinical and Experimental Immunology, 14, 501–508.

Gough, K. R., Read, A. E. & Naish, J. M. (1962) Intestinal reticulosis as a complication of idiopathic steatorrhoea. Gut, 3, 232–239.

Harris, O. D., Cooke, W. T., Thompson, H. & Waterhouse, J. A. H. (1967) Malignancy in adult coeliac disease and idiopathic steatorrhoea. *American Journal of Medicine*, **42**, 899–912.

Hennes, A. R., Sevelius, H., Lewellyn, T., Joel, W., Woods, A. H. & Wolf, S. (1962) Atrophic gastritis in dogs. *Archives of Pathology*, **73**, 281–287.

Hermans, P. E. & Huizenga, K. A. (1972) Association of gastric carcinoma with idiopathic late-onset immunoglobulin deficiency. *Annals of Internal Medicine*, **76**, 605–609.

Hoedemaeker, P. J. & Ito, S. (1970) Ultrastructural localization of gastric parietal cell antigen with peroxidase-coupled antibody. *Laboratory Investigation*, **22**, 184–188.

Hughes, W. S., Brooks, F. P. & Conn, H. O. (1972) Serum gastrin levels in primary hypogammaglobulinaemia and pernicious anemia: studies in adults. *Annals of Internal Medicine*, **77**, 746–750.

Inada, M. & Glass, G. B. J. (1972) Effects of prolonged administration of intrinsic factor antibodies on gastric morphology and secretion in rats. *Federation Proceedings*, **31**, 299.

Inada, M. & Glass, G. B. J. (1975) Effect of prolonged administration of homologous and heterologous intrinsic factor antibodies on the parietal and peptic cell masses and the secretory function of the rat gastric mucosa. *Gastroenterology*, **69**, 396–408.

Irvine, W. J. (1965) Immunologic aspects of pernicious anaemia. *New England Journal of Medicine*, **273**, 432–438.

Irvine, W. J., Cullen, D. R. & Mawhinney, H. (1974) Natural history of autoimmune achlorhydric atrophic gastritis: a 1–15 year follow-up study. *Lancet*, **ii**, 482–485.

Irvine, W. J., Davies, S. H., Delamore, I. W. & Wynn Williams, A. (1962) Immunological relationship between pernicious anaemia and thyroid disease. *British Medical Journal*, **ii**, 454–456.

Isokoski, M., Krohn, K., Varis, K. & Siurala, M. (1969) Parietal cell and intrinsic factor antibodies in a Finnish rural population sample. *Scandinavian Journal of Gastroenterology*, **4**, 521–527.

James, D., Asherson, G. & Chanarin, I., Coghill, N., Hamilton, S., Himsworth, R. L. & Webster, D. (1974) Cell-mediated immunity to intrinsic factor in autoimmune disorders. *British Medical Journal*, **iv**, 494–496.

Joynson, D. H. M., Jacobs, A., Murray Walker, D. & Dolby, A. E. (1972) Defect of cell-mediated immunity in patients with iron-deficiency anaemia. *Lancet*, **ii**, 1058–1059.

Korman, M. G., Strickland, R. G. & Hansky, J. (1971) Serum gastrin in chronic gastritis. *British Medical Journal*, **ii**, 16–18.

Krohn, K. J. E. & Finlayson, N. D. C. (1973) Interrelations of humoral and cellular immune responses in experimental canine gastritis. *Clinical and Experimental Immunology*, **14**, 237–245.

Larsson, S. O., Hagelquist, E. & Cöster, C. (1961) Hypogammaglobulinaemia and pernicious anaemia. *Acta Haematologica*, **26**, 50–64.

MacCuish, A. C., Urbaniak, S. J., Goldstone, A. H. & Irvine, W. J. (1974) PHA responsiveness and subpopulations of circulating lymphocytes in pernicious anaemia. *Blood*, **44**, 849–855.

McGuigan, J. E. & Trudeau, W. L. (1970) Serum gastrin concentrations in pernicious anaemia. *New England Journal of Medicine*, **282**, 358–361.

Maclaurin, B. P., Cooke, W. T. & Ling, N. R. (1971) Impaired lymphocyte reactivity against tumour cells in patients with coeliac disease. *Gut*, **12**, 794–800.

Magnus, H. A. & Ungley, C. C. (1938) The gastric lesion in pernicious anaemia. *Lancet*, **i**, 420–421.

Magnus, H. A. (1937) Observations on the presence of intestinal epithelium in the gastric mucosa. *Journal of Pathology and Bacteriology*, **44**, 389–398.

Meulengracht, E. (1939) Histologic investigation into the pyloric gland organ in pernicious anaemia. *American Journal of the Medical Sciences*, **197**, 201–214.

Mosbech, J. & Videbaek, A. (1950) Mortality from and risk of gastric carcinoma among patients with pernicious anaemia. *British Medical Journal*, **ii**, 390–394.

Odgers, R. J. & Wangel, A. G. (1968) Abnormalities in IgA-containing mononuclear cells in the gastric lesion of pernicious anaemia. *Lancet*, **ii**, 846–849.

Odgers, R. S. & Wangel, A. G. (1969) Immunoglobulin-secreting cells in the alimentary tract (abstract). *Gut*, **10**, 78.

Rigler, L. G., Kaplan, H. S. & Fink, D. L. (1945) Pernicious anaemia and the early diagnosis of tumours of the stomach. *Journal of the American Medical Association*, **128**, 426–432.

Rose, M. S. & Chanarin, I. (1969) Dissociation of intrinsic factor from its antibody: application to study of pernicious anaemia gastric juice specimens. *British Medical Journal*, **i**, 468–470.

Rose, M. S. & Chanarin, I. (1971) Intrinsic-factor antibody and absorption of vitamin B_{12} in pernicious anaemia. *British Medical Journal*, **i**, 25–26.

Rose, M. S., Chanarin, I., Doniach, D., Brostoff, J. & Ardeman, S. (1970) Intrinsic-factor antibodies in the absence of pernicious anaemia, 3–7 year follow up. *Lancet*, **ii**, 9–13.

Salupere, V., Nutt, H. & Järve, E. (1972) Lymphocyte blast-transformation test *in vitro* in cases of chronic gastritis. *Scandinavian Journal of Gastroenterology*, **7**, 215–218.

Shearman, D. J. C., Finlayson, N. D. C., Wilson, R. & Samson, R. R. (1966) Carcinoma of the stomach and early pernicious anaemia. *Lancet*, **ii**, 403–405.

Siurala, M., Isokoski, M., Varis, K. & Kekki, M. (1968) Prevalence of gastritis in a rural population: bioptic study of subjects selected at random. *Scandinavian Journal of Gastroenterology*, **3**, 211–223.

Siurala, M., Lehtola, J. & Ihamäki, T. (1974) Atrophic gastritis and its sequelae. Results of 19–23 years' follow-up examinations. *Scandinavian Journal of Gastroenterology*, **9**, 441–446.

Søltoft, J. (1974) Intestinal immunoglobulins in pernicious anaemia. *American Journal of Digestive Diseases*, **19**, 623–625.

Spector, J. I. (1974) Juvenile achlorhydric pernicious anaemia with IgA deficiency. *Journal of the American Medical Association*, **228**, 334–336.

Strickland, R. G. & Mackay, I. R. (1973) A reappraisal of the nature and significance of chronic atrophic gastritis. *American Journal of Digestive Diseases*, **18**, 426–440.

Strickland, R. G., Korman, M. G. & Hansky, J. (1973) Gastrin, age and the gastric mucosa. *Australian and New Zealand Journal of Medicine*, **3**, 152–156.

Strickland, R. G., Baur, S., Ashworth, L. A. E. & Taylor, K. B. (1971) a correlative study of immunological phenomena in pernicious anaemia. *Clinical and Experimental Immunology*, **8**, 25–36.

Strickland, R. G., Fisher, J. M., Lewin, K. & Taylor, K. B. (1973) The response to prednisolone in atrophic gastritis: a possible effect on non-intrinsic factor-mediated vitamin B_{12} absorption. *Gut*, **14**, 13–19.

Tai, C. & McGuigan, J. E. (1969) Immunologic studies in pernicious anaemia. *Blood*, **34**, 63–71.

Tanaka, N. & Glass, G. B. J. (1970) Effect of prolonged administration of parietal-cell antibodies from patients with atrophic gastritis and pernicious anaemia on parietal-cell mass and hydrochloric acid output in rats. *Gastroenterology*, **58**, 482–494.

Taylor, K. B. (1959) Inhibition of intrinsic factor by pernicious anaemia sera. *Lancet*, **ii**, 106–108.

Taylor, K. B. (1969) Gastritis. *New England Journal of Medicine*, **280**, 818–820.

Taylor, K. B., Roitt, I. M., Doniach, D., Couchman, K. G. & Shapland, C. (1962) Autoimmune phenomena in pernicious anaemia: gastric antibodies. *British Medical Journal*, **ii**, 1347–1352.

Twomey, J. J., Jordan, P. H., Jarrold, T., Trubowitz, S., Ritz, N. D. & Conn, H. O. (1969) The syndrome of immunoglobulin deficiency and pernicious anaemia: a study of ten cases. *American Journal of Medicine*, **47**, 340–350.

Ungar, B., Stocks, A. E., Martin, F. I. R., Whittingham, S. & Mackay, I. R. (1968) Intrinsic-factor antibody, parietal-cell antibody and latent pernicious anaemia in diabetes mellitus. *Lancet*, **ii**, 415–418.

Velde, K. te, Abels, J., Anders, G. J. P. A., Arends, A., Hoedemaeker, Ph. J. & Nieweg, H. O. (1964) A family study of pernicious anaemia by immunologic method. *Journal of Laboratory and Clinical Medicine*, **64**, 177–187.

Wangel, A. G., Callender, S. T., Spray, G. H. & Wright, R. (1968) A family study of pernicious anaemia. I. Autoantibodies, achlorhydria, serum pepsinogen and vitamin B_{12}. *British Journal of Haematology*, **14**, 161–181, 183–204.

Weisbart, R. H., Bluestone, R. & Goldberg, L. S. (1975) Cellular immunity to intrinsic factor in pernicious anaemia. *Journal of Laboratory and Clinical Medicine*, **85**, 87–92.

Whitehead, R., Truelove, S. C. & Gear, M. W. L. (1972) The histological diagnosis of chronic gastritis in fibreoptic gastroscope biopsy specimens. *Journal of Clinical Pathology*, **25**, 1–11.

Wright, R., Whitehead, R., Wangel, A. G., Salem, S. N. & Schiller, K. F. R. (1966) Autoantibodies and microscopic appearance of gastric mucosa. *Lancet*, **i**, 618–621.

6. Coeliac disease

P. Asquith and M. R. Haeney

INTRODUCTION

Coeliac disease has interested clinicians and researchers for centuries. The first clear-cut description of several of the clinical features was probably that of Aretaeus the Cappadocian in the first century A.D. (quoted by Major, 1945). Although now commonly given the name 'coeliac' disease, in the past it has had various others including Gee-Herter's disease, non-tropical sprue, coeliac sprue, idiopathic steatorrhoea, childhood coeliac disease, primary malabsorption, gluten-induced entero-pathy, gluten-sensitive enteropathy and adult coeliac disease. Since the classic clinical description of the 'coeliac affection' by Samuel Gee in 1888, the topic has been of major interest, more so following the unique observation of Dicke (1950) that wheat and rye flour were harmful to children with coeliac disease. Sub-sequently much of the research has been concerned with trying to explain the mechanism of gluten toxicity. Two main hypotheses have usually been considered. The first postulates that the toxicity is related to a specific enzyme defect in the jejunal mucosa which allows the accumulation to harmful levels of a partial gluten digest (Frazer, 1956; Townley, Bhathal, Cornell and Mitchell, 1973). More recently this theory has been modified to consider the possibility of an abnormal rather than a deficient peptidase which catalyses the formation of a toxic peptide (Yeomans, 1974; Cordone *et al.*, 1975). The second hypothesis suggests that the disease is the outcome of an immunological reaction to gluten. Obviously these two theories are not mutually exclusive (Asquith, 1974b). There are other possibilities with respect to the primary defect, including defective secretory IgA, mucus, ionic surface charge, molecular sieving (Asquith, 1970) and more recently the theory that gluten-induced damage depends on the material acting as a lectin (Weiser and Douglas, 1976).

Nevertheless, the immunological theory has gained increasing support and this chapter reviews the evidence. But first it is necessary to consider the definition of coeliac disease, as this is central to any discussion of mechanisms of toxicity.

DEFINITION

This has varied, but included here are only definitions which post-date the recognition of the essential morpho-logical features (Paulley, 1954) and the introduction of the critical technique of jejunal biopsy (Shiner, 1956).

1. Pink and Creamer (1967) maintained that 'it is apparent, however, that whether the flat jejunal mucosa is primary (that is the cause is unknown) or whether it is secondary to some other suspected cause, the effect of gluten withdrawal is similar and must be tried. It would therefore seem to be a useful concept to regard all patients with a flat jejunal mucosa as one group which may, if the symptoms or other findings merit it, require treatment with a gluten-free diet. To avoid confusion we consider all these patients to have the coeliac syndrome, by which we mean any condition with a flat jejunal mucosa.'

2. When reviewing coeliac disease Cooke (1968) con-sidered that 'the histologically flat jejunal mucosa with mosaic pattern on dissecting microscopy is specific for coeliac disease'.

3. According to Rubin, Eidelman and Weinstein (1970), the first essential is the 'demonstration of a characteristic flat mucosal lesion by suction biopsy of the proximal small intestine', and the second essential is the 'demonstration of a dramatic clinical response to the removal of gluten from the diet'.

4. Following a round-table discussion, the European Society of Paediatric Gastroenterology (ESPG) put forward a further definition (Meeuwisse, 1970). The essence of this definition is a complete restitution to clinical and histological normality on a gluten-free diet with subsequent morphological relapse following further challenge with wheat or (wheat) gluten. A gluten-free diet is one which 'must not contain wheat, rye, barley or oats'.

5. In a further review of coeliac disease, Cooke and Asquith (1974) wrote 'for the moment coeliac disease should be defined as any condition with a flat jejunal mucosa and until other more accurate tests are developed (be they enzymatic, biochemical or immunological) one should recognize that response to gluten-free diets may be manifested by minimal changes, such as in lymphocyte or plasma cell counts'.

6. Asquith (1974d) proposed that clinicians faced with a potential coeliac should 'start with a flat or nearly flat mucosa' (as the corner stone for diagnosis) ... 'and then I would suggest that if the patient showed

a significant improvement in clinical and morphological parameters (on a gluten-free diet) then that is sufficient; by significant, I mean a mathematically 'significant' change which minimally might be an improvement in epithelial lymphocyte counts'.

7. There have been other definitions since, but one other has emerged which is brief and could form the foundation of any study. Booth (1974) defined coeliac disease in the adult 'as a condition in which there is an abnormal jejunal mucosa which improved morphologically when treated with a gluten-free diet and again shows abnormalities when gluten is reintroduced'.

It is sometimes not clear which definition has been used by investigators before including patients in the immunological studies which form the basis of this review. It is to be hoped that most researchers used one comparable to the ESPG (Meeuwisse, 1970) or the Booth (1974) definition.

EVIDENCE RELEVANT TO THE IMMUNOLOGICAL THEORY

Indirect

Many of the morphological features of coeliac disease can be cited in support of an immunological explanation for gluten's action. The presence of immunocompetent cells in the lamina propria and epithelial cell layer in the jejunum (Paulley, 1954; Rubin, Brandborg, Phelps and Taylor, 1960; Anderson, 1960) has been thought pertinent, whilst splenic atrophy (Blumgart, 1923; McCarthy, Fraser, Evans and Read, 1966), mesenteric node hypertrophy (Paulley, 1954), peripheral node hypoplasia (McCarthy et al., 1966) and the malignant potential of coeliac disease, especially for lymphoma (Gough, Read and Naish, 1962; Austad, Cornes, Gough, McCarthy and Read, 1967; Harris, Cooke, Thompson and Waterhouse, 1967; Barry and Read, 1973; Asquith, 1974a; Holmes et al., 1976), are also relevant. Further indirect evidence is provided by the occurrence of gliadin shock (Krainick et al., 1958; Immonen, 1967) and the clinical (Aldersberg, Colcher and Drachman, 1951), gross morphological and histochemical improvement (Wall, Douglas, Booth and Pearse, 1970) seen in coeliacs treated with steroids.

Counts of immunocompetent cells

Lymphocytes, including their various sub-populations, and plasma cells have been quantitated in peripheral blood and mucosal tissue in normal-diet and gluten-free-diet coeliacs.

(a) In peripheral blood. Total numbers of peripheral blood lymphocytes have been variously reported as normal (Winter, McCarthy, Read and Yoffey, 1967; O'Donoghue, Lancaster-Smith, Laviniere and Kumar, 1976; Bullen and Losowsky, 1977) or subnormal (Brandt and Stenstam, 1975) in patients with untreated or treated coeliac disease, or even elevated in coeliacs ingesting a normal diet (Holmes, 1974). These changes do not help in deciding whether a humoral or cell-mediated reaction is occurring; counts of lymphocyte sub-populations could be more informative.

Circulating thymus-derived lymphocytes (T-cells) can be quantitated by their ability to form spontaneous rosettes with sheep red cells (Jondal, Holm and Wigzell, 1972). Using this technique, it has been shown that in untreated coeliacs, the proportion and absolute numbers of T-cells in peripheral blood are decreased compared with treated patients, healthy controls and patients with malabsorption not due to coeliac disease (O'Donoghue et al., 1976; Bullen and Losowsky, 1977). Bullen and Losowsky (1977) have additionally shown that untreated coeliacs with functional hyposplenism have particularly low T-cell percentages. O'Donoghue et al. (1976) reported a rise in T-cells following gluten withdrawal and an inverse correlation between circulating T-cell numbers and jejunal intraepithelial lymphocyte counts. These results indirectly support evidence favouring increased enteric loss of lymphocytes in normal-diet coeliacs (Douglas, Weetman and Haggith, 1976).

(b) In jejunal mucosa. *Intraepithelial lymphocytes.* Current data suggest that intraepithelial (IE) lymphocytes are effector T-cells and reflect ongoing cell-mediated immune responses to intraluminal antigen. Hence it is noteworthy that, in untreated coeliac disease, IE lymphocyte counts are increased; their numbers fall towards normal on a gluten-free diet (Ferguson and Murray, 1971; Fry, Seah, McMinn and Hoffbrand, 1972; Kumar, Silk, Marks, Clark and Dawson, 1973; Ferguson, 1974; Holmes, Asquith, Stokes and Cooke, 1974; Lancaster-Smith, Packer, Kumar and Harries, 1976a; Mavromichalis, Brueton, McNeish and Anderson, 1976) and increase on subsequent gluten challenge (Mavromichalis et al., 1976). By contrast, in other conditions associated with villous damage, IE lymphocyte counts are essentially normal (Mavromichalis et al., 1976). These findings support the contention that a local cell-mediated immune reaction occurs in response to intraluminal gluten but do not necessarily imply that this mechanism is the cause of the villous atrophy.

Lamina propria lymphoid cells. Despite differing techniques, counts of sub-populations of cells in the lamina propria in coeliacs have produced similar results (Holmes et al., 1974; Ferguson, Asquith and Cooke, 1974b; Montgomery and Shearer, 1974; Lancaster-Smith et al., 1976a). In untreated coeliac disease the most obvious changes are raised numbers of total cells and plasma cells with reduced lamina propria lymphocyte counts. Following a gluten-free diet, these abnormalities tend to disappear (Holmes et al., 1974; Lancaster-Smith et al., 1976a). The marked increase in plasma cells and their fall on gluten withdrawal suggest that a local humoral reaction to glutten does occur.

(c) **In other tissues.** Splenic atrophy in coeliac disease is well documented (Blumgart, 1923; McCarthy, Fraser, Evans and Read, 1966) and may occur in up to 40 per cent of patients studied by clearance of heat-damaged red cells (Ferguson, Maxwell and Hutton, 1969). This functional defect does not appear to correlate with other clinical or laboratory features of coeliac disease (Ferguson et al., 1969). The cause is unknown, but it has been related to prolonged cell loss in the intestinal lumen (Douglas and Weetman, 1975). The finding of depleted peripheral blood T-cells in hyposplenic coeliacs (Bullen and Losowsky, 1977) is supportive evidence.

Direct

Taken together, the above data and that derived from the study of animal models of coeliac disease (Ch. 8) provide indirect evidence of atypical humoral and cellular responses to gluten in coeliac subjects. However, direct evidence of humoral and cellular reactivity to gluten in such patients is more important.

HUMORAL IMMUNITY IN COELIAC DISEASE

Humoral immunity in coeliac disease can be assessed by (1) skin tests using various gluten subfractions, (2) measuring immunoglobulins and specific antibodies in the blood and in the intestine, (3) measuring complement levels and (4) studying those diseases apparently associated with coeliac disease for evidence of altered humoral reactivity.

Skin tests (Table 6.1)

There are no reports of positive immediate (Type I) hypersensitivity reactions to gluten. In contrast, two reports have documented positive skin tests within eight hours of injection of antigen (Baker and Read, 1976; Anand, Truelove and Offord, 1977a). Baker and Read (1976) noted erythema in over half the untreated coeliacs using a peptic-tryptic digest of gluten. Biopsies of positive reactions revealed a polymorph infiltrate histologically, and immunoglobulin and C3 deposition on immunofluorescence. A strong correlation between serum gluten antibody titres and positive skin reactivity was found. Anand and his colleagues (1977a) found positive reactions in coeliacs on a gluten-free diet using gluten, gluten fraction III and subfraction B2. Both studies favour cutaneous deposition of antigen–antibody complexes, i.e. an Arthus (Type III) reaction.

TOTAL IMMUNOGLOBULINS

In serum

IgA. Many reports indicate serum IgA levels are increased in a proportion of untreated children and adults with coeliac disease (Immonen, 1967; Hobbs and Hepner, 1968; Blecher, Brzechwa-Ajdukiewicz, McCarthy and Read, 1969; Asquith, Thompson and Cooke, 1969; Kenrick and Walker-Smith, 1970; Baklien, Brandtzaeg and Fausa, 1977). The levels usually fall towards normal following gluten withdrawal. In some children and adults the pre-treatment values can be partially explained on coexisting milk sensitivity (Immonen, 1967; Asquith, 1974b). In general, it appears that the rise in serum IgA consists of both monomeric and polymeric IgA (Baklien et al., 1977), presumably from mucosal IgA cells.

IgM. Whereas IgA is often increased in coeliac disease, serum IgM values are usually reduced in the untreated patient, and normalize following gluten withdrawal (Hobbs and Hepner, 1968; Blecher et al., 1969; Asquith et al., 1969; Soltoft and Weeke, 1969; Kenrick and Walker-Smith, 1970). The changes may occasionally be absent (Brown, Ferguson, Carswell, Horne and MacSween, 1973) or unimpressive (Baklien et al., 1977). Low serum IgM values have been attributed to decreased systemic synthesis (Brown, Cooper, Hepner, 1969) and also to increased transmucosal loss of IgM (Jarnum, Jensen, Søltoft and Westergaardh, 1970), the latter presumably reflecting altered mucosal permeability.

IgG. Predictably, serum IgG levels are frequently low (reviewed by Asquith, 1974b) and, like the low IgM results, can be explained on intraluminal loss of systemic immunoglobulin.

IgE and IgD. Little attention has been paid to serum IgE and IgD (Asquith 1974b), but IgE levels are usually normal (Asquith et al., 1969; Hobbs et al., 1969) while IgD deficiency is common in treated and untreated coeliac disease (Asquith et al., 1969).

Secretory IgA. Like total serum IgA, serum secretory IgA (Sec IgA) values are increased in untreated coeliac disease, some of the increase being related to milk sensitivity. The values fall following treatment (Asquith, Thompson and Cooke, 1970b; Asquith, Thompson and Cooke, 1971; Asquith, 1974b). It can be assumed the Sec IgA is produced by the intestinal mucosa.

Other immunoglobulin abnormalities. *Deficiencies.* These have been reviewed previously (Asquith, 1974b) and are further considered in Chapter 9. The most intriguing association is the apparent excess incidence of IgA deficiency in coeliac patients. Why some IgA-deficient individuals develop a flat mucosa, which is apparently gluten-sensitive, while others – even

Table 6.1 Results of skin tests with gluten fractions in coeliacs

Reference	Patients studied	Route	Antigen	Dose	Control antigen	Time at which response read	Results Macroscopic	Results Histological
Alvey et al. (1957)	14 coeliacs – dietary status unknown	Intradermal	2% gluten solution	2 mg	Not stated	Not stated	Negative in all patients	—
Breton et al. (1959)	5 coeliacs 3 atopic controls	Intradermal	Gliadin and gliadin hydrolysates	Not stated	Lactalbumin Casein Vegetable extracts	20 min 24 h	Results at 20 min negative for gliadin compared with controls	—
Housley et al. (1969)	6 coeliacs on GFD	Intradermal	Gluten fr. III	100 μg	Not stated	48 h	Negative in all patients	—
Asquith (1974c)	21 coeliacs (5 ND; 16 GFD) 8 healthy controls	Intradermal	Gluten fr. III	Dose range 250 μg–1 μg	Saline	48 h	Positive in only 1 of 21 coeliacs and 0 of 8 controls	Perivascular mononuclear cell infiltrate seen in majority of coeliacs and controls
Baker and Read (1976)	55 coeliacs (23 ND; 32 GFD) 52 healthy controls	Intradermal and prick tests	1% solution of peptic-tryptic digest of gluten	1 mg	Water	20 min 5–8 h 24 h 46 h	Erythema after 5–8 h only, in 52% of untreated coeliacs and 33% of all coeliacs. No reactions in controls	Polymorph infiltrate present. Immunoglobulin and C_3 deposition seen in some by immunofluorescence. Positive correlation between serum gluten antibodies and positive skin tests
Anand, Truelove and Offord (1977a)	10 coeliacs on GFD 20 healthy controls	Intradermal	Gluten; gluten fr. III, gluten fr. B and subfractions B_1, B_2, B_3	50 μg	Phosphate buffer and phenol	30 min 3–8 h ?48 h	Immediate and delayed reactions negative. Erythema at 3–8 h to: subfraction B_2 in all 10 coeliacs (0 controls), gluten fr. III in 8 coeliacs (0 controls), gluten in 2 coeliacs (0 controls)	—

on the basis of several jejunal biopsies – have a normal mucosa (Asquith, 1970) is unknown (Ch. 9).

Rarely deficiencies of IgA and IgM have been reported (Asquith 1974b). More frequent have been descriptions of flat biopsies, resembling coeliac disease, in patients with generalized hypogammaglobulinaemia – patients with so-called hypogammaglobulinaemic sprue. There is considerable controversy as to whether the mucosal lesion in these latter patients responds to gluten withdrawal; whatever the answer, it is of major interest that a flat mucosa can exist in the face of such gross humoral defects.

Dysgammaglobulinaemia. In addition to the above changes in serum immunoglobulins other abnormalities have been described. Peña *et al.* (1976) described a single case of transient paraproteinaemia in an atopic adult patient with well-documented coeliac disease. The monoclonal IgG (lambda type) disappeared over three years. Although no antigluten activity was demonstrated in the IgG fraction it was suggested that the paraprotein could be related to chronic challenge of the mucosa with gluten. Transient paraproteinaemia is not confined to coeliacs as it has also been reported in tropical sprue (Young, 1969) and in three cases of steatorrhoea and diarrhoea (Cooke, 1969). Cryoglobulinaemia of more than one immunoglobulin class has been found in four coeliac patients with vasculitis (Doe, Evans, Hobbs and Booth, 1972). It was postulated that the cryoglobulins represented circulating immune complexes of gluten-antigluten antibody.

In secretions and produced *in vitro*

There have been several reports on the concentrations of immunoglobulin-containing plasma cells in the jejunal mucosa, on immunoglobulin levels in intestinal fluid and on immunoglobulin production by cultured mucosal tissue.

Jejunal mucosa plasma cells

The results have been reviewed previously (Asquith, 1974b) and critically re-examined (Brandtzaeg and Baklien, 1976, Table 6.2). The immunofluorescent techniques used and the methods of expressing the results have differed markedly, hence it is not surprising that there has been lack of agreement in the literature. This is especially true for the results of IgA cells. In contrast, with the exception of earlier reports (Rubin, Fauci, Sleisenger and Jeffries, 1965; Crabbé, 1967), IgM plasma cells have been found to be increased (Table 6.2). Their numbers fall on gluten withdrawal. The potential for response to treatment appears to be better in children, but this may be more a reflection of stricter dietary control. IgG cells are increased in children (Søltoft and Weeke, 1969; Søltoft, 1970; Savilahti, 1972) and in occasional (Asquith, 1970), or in many, adults (Gasbarrini, Miglio, Serra and Bernardi, 1974; Lancaster-Smith, Kumar, Marks, Clark and Dawson, 1974; Brandtzaeg and Baklien, 1976). Indeed, unlike many previous authors, Brandtzaeg and Baklien (1976) thought the IgG findings were potentially the most important; IgG class antigluten antibodies, being less easily removed than IgA and IgM antibodies, could produce more adverse immune reactions to ingested gluten. Concentrations of IgE and IgD cells have not received much comment.

In general, techniques employing immuno-fluorescence are not easy to control and results should be interpreted with caution. The newer method of

Table 6.2. Class of immunoglobulin containing plasma cells in the proximal jejunum (after Brandtzaeg and Baklien, 1976)

	IgA (%)	IgM (%)	IgG (%)
Normal mucosa			
Crabbé and Heremans (1966)	83.8	12.4	3.8
Söltoft (1969)	58.6	35.4	6.0
Søltoft and Søeberg (1972)	66.5	22.9	10.6
Savilahti (1972)	72.8	21.0	6.2
Jos *et al.* (1972)	86.7	8.0	5.2
Gasbarrini *et al.* (1972)	58.9	23.4	17.7
Brandtzaeg and Baklien (1976)	80.8	16.5	2.6
Coeliac mucosa			
Douglas *et al.* (1970), ND	64.5 (0.9)[a]	33.7 (3.4)	1.8 (0.6)
Douglas *et al.* (1970), GF	64.3 (0.7)	33.7 (82.2)	2.1 (0.5)
Jos *et al.* (1972), ND	84.8 (1.4)	11.5 (2.1)	3.7 (1.0)
Jos *et al.* (1972), GF	88.0 (1.1)	7.6 (1.0)	4.4 (0.9)
Gasbarrini *et al.* (1974), GF	26.0 (0.7)	39.3 (2.6)	34.7 (3.0)
Brandtzaeg and Baklien (1976)	72.1 (1.3)	20.2 (1.8)	7.5 (4.6)

ND = untreated patients.
GF = results following varying periods of gluten-free diet.
[a] = number of times that cell density is increased above normal.

immunoperoxidase staining is more difficult but, if carefully done, has great potential and a recent study successfully employed it using coeliac mucosa (Anand *et al.*, 1977b).

Immunoglobulins in intestinal secretions
Hobbs, Hepner, Douglas, Crabbé and Johannsson (1969) have found higher IgM levels in the intestinal fluid in patients with coeliac disease than in patients with non-coeliac gastrointestinal disease. Asquith, Thompson and Cooke (1970d) confirmed this but also found IgA and IgG to be raised irrespective of dietary status. However, there are difficulties in estimating immunoglobulins in intestinal secretions (Samson, McClelland and Shearman, 1973) and the fluid potentially contains immunoglobulins from several sources, including bile, pancreas and stomach.

In-vitro synthesis of immunoglobulins by intestinal mucosa
Loeb, Strober, Falchuk and Laster (1971) obtained intestinal biopsy specimens from patients before and after oral gluten challenge. The intestinal tissue was then incubated with ^{14}C-leucine. Local synthesis of both IgA and IgM were measured by the incorporation of ^{14}C-leucine into these immunoglobulins with a solid-phase immunoabsorption technique. Gluten challenge produced a 2- to 5-fold increase in incorporation. Falchuk, Gebhard and Strober (1974) then cultured tissues of untreated and treated patients in the same culture chamber in the presence of gluten peptides and produced evidence suggesting that a humoral (?antigluten antibody) substance was liberated from the untreated mucosa which was toxic to the treated mucosa. In view of the immunofluorescence findings of Brandtzaeg and Baklein (1976) with respect to IgG cells, then the *in-vitro* work of Falchuk, Gebhard and Strober (1974) needs to be extended to include measurement of total IgG and specific IgG antigluten antibody synthesis.

SPECIFIC ANTIBODIES

In serum, secretions and produced *in vitro*

Dietary antibodies
    Serum. Interest in antibodies to gluten and other foods, especially to milk proteins, is long standing (Taylor, Thompson, Truelove and Wright, 1961; Alarcon-Segovia *et al.*, 1964; Katz, Kantor and Herskovic, 1968; Kenrick and Walker-Smith, 1970; Ferguson and Carswell, 1972). Techniques have varied and this presumably explains some of the differences in results. Because of antibodies occurring in (1) normal individuals, (2) in non-coeliac gastrointestinal patients, (3) the lack of correlation of these antibodies with disease activity and (4) the presence in coeliac patients of serum antibodies irrelevant to the mechanism of gluten toxicity, the importance of dietary antibodies has been

doubted. Nevertheless, serum antibody titres have been used to determine the degree of small bowel damage (Kumar, Ferguson, Lancaster-Smith and Clark, 1976). Of considerable interest was the early observation of complement-fixing IgM-class antibodies in the serum (Mietens, 1967), which can now be related to the *in-vitro* studies of Falchuk, Gebhard and Strober (1974) if one assumes some back diffusion of locally producing IgM antigluten antibodies.

    Intestinal secretions. A suggestion that precipitating antibodies to gluten fractions in the stools were only found in coeliac children (Katz, Kantor and Herskovic, 1968) promised to be diagnostically useful. Unfortunately, such antibodies have also been found in the upper intestinal fluid of 8 of 21 non-coeliac children (Ferguson and Carswell, 1972).

    Mucosal antibody production. Falchuk, Gebhard and Strober (1974), in their *in-vitro* tissue culture technique, found that approximately 30–75 per cent of the IgA and IgM immunoglobulin synthesized could be accounted for by specific antigluten antibodies; IgG-class antibody was not determined. These findings contrast with an early immunohistochemical sandwich test performed by Rubin, Fauci, Sleisenger and Jeffries (1965) who were unable to show binding of gliadin to immunoglobulin-producing cells in the intestine. Nevertheless, the latter technique is relatively crude. A much more critical analysis was undertaken by Brandtzaeg and Baklien (1976). With a gliadin digest as antigen, scattered antibody-producing cells were seen in the diseased mucosa. Sixty per cent of the antibody-producing cells were IgA, 40 per cent were IgG and only occasional IgM cells were present. The authors estimated approximately 1.6 per cent of the IgA cells and 5.7 per cent of all the IgG cells were forming antibodies to the gluten antigen. This proportion roughly corresponds with data from animals which show that only a fraction of the stimulated lymphoid cells are engaged in specific antibody production (Moticka, 1974) – far fewer than the findings of Falchuk, Gebhard and Strober (1974) would imply. When the results of mucosal studies on coeliac patients are compared and contrasted with those occurring in say Crohn's disease, ulcerative colitis and milk-protein sensitivity, it is clear that the pattern of immunocyte response is not specific for coeliacs ingesting gluten (Asquith, 1974b; Baklien, Brandtzaeg and Fausa, 1977). This is a critical point when considering the relative roles of humoral and cellular reactions to gluten in the mechanism of gluten toxicity.

Specific antibody responses following deliberate immunization
Few normal subjects have pre-existing antibodies to the bacteriophage ØX174 and clear-cut primary and

secondary immune responses can be demonstrated after immunization (Peacock, Verrier Jones and Gough, 1973). Antibody production is measured as the 50 per cent bacteriophage neutralization titre following the intravenous injection of 2.1×10^9 plaque forming units of ØX174. By this method, Baker, Verrier Jones, Peacock and Read (1975) showed variable impairment of primary antibody production in 8 coeliacs, compared with normal subjects. More impressive were the differences in the secondary responses, which were severely reduced in coeliacs but not in controls (Baker et al., 1975), or in ill patients with Crohn's disease (Bucknall, Verrier Jones and Peacock, 1975). In coeliac subjects, the secondary antibody response showed a higher proportion of IgM antibody than normal, suggesting a defect in switching from IgM to IgG antibody production (Baker et al., 1975). These abnormalities were found to correlate both with the clinical state and a small spleen size as estimated from a [99]Technetium scan (Baker et al., 1975). Recently, impaired immunity to this antigen has also been found in ulcerative colitis patients with associated hyposplenism (Ryan, Holdsworth and Verrier Jones, 1977).

Conflicting results have been reported using more common immunization antigens, namely tetanus toxoid and polio vaccine. Pettingale (1970) found a depression in the primary and secondary antibody responses to intramuscular tetanus toxoid in a group of 14 coeliacs compared with age and sex-matched controls. Specific antitoxin titres were measured by passive haemagglutination and by bioassay. In contrast, Beale, Parish, Douglas and Hobbs (1971), using different immunization schedules, noted a normal antibody response to tetanus toxoid by bioassay in all 5 treated and 5 untreated coeliacs studied.

Using an oral poliovaccine containing Type I, II and III virus, Beale et al. (1971) did find that the majority of coeliacs showed an abnormal response. On the basis that local poliovirus antibody is of IgA class, the authors inferred, but did not prove, that there was an impaired qualitative IgA response in coeliacs. Very different conclusions were drawn by Mawhinney and Love (1975) using an indirect immunofluorescent technique to study the incidence and immunoglobulin class distribution of the serum antibody response to Type II oral polio vaccine in 38 coeliacs on a gluten-free diet and matched control subjects. An antibody response was detected in 56 per cent of coeliacs and 18 per cent of controls. Polio virus-specific IgA responses were seen in 42 per cent of coeliacs and 18 per cent of controls, while polio virus-specific IgG responses were observed in 26 per cent of coeliacs and 11 per cent of controls. No specific IgM responses were found. The pre-immunization virus-specific IgA titres of those subjects showing an antibody response were significantly higher in the coeliac group than in controls, suggesting an enhanced IgA response in coeliac subjects.

Reticulin antibodies

Seah, Fry, Hoffbrand and Holborow (1971a) first reported the detection of an IgG autoantibody directed against certain connective tissue components in 36 per cent of patients with adult coeliac disease and in 17 per cent of patients with dermatitis herpetiformis. Similar findings were published by Alp and Wright (1971). The reactivity appeared to be directed against reticulin and was demonstrated in between 54 per cent and 74 per cent of children with coeliac disease (Seah et al., 1971b; Alp and Wright, 1971; Von Essen, Savilahti and Pelkonen, 1972; Brown et al., 1973). Initially this specificity was thought to be characteristic of sera from patients with coeliac disease (Seah et al., 1971a), but subsequently it was shown to occur in 25 per cent of patients with Crohn's disease and to a lesser extent in other diseases (Alp and Wright, 1971; Seah et al., 1973a). The reactivity was found in the sera of coeliacs on a normal diet more frequently than in patients maintained on a gluten-free diet (Alp and Wright, 1971; Seah et al., 1971b; Von Essen et al., 1972). In 6 children re-challenged with gluten, Alp and Wright (1971) recorded the development of reactivity in four and persistence of reactivity in a fifth and this appeared to correlate with the detection of antibodies to gluten fraction III. Cross reactivity with gluten was considered a likely explanation for these findings (Seah et al., 1972). Fry, Seah and Hoffbrand (1974) reported that they were able to remove anti-reticulin reactivity from the sera of patients with dermatitis herpetiformis using gluten. This has not been the experience of others (Brown et al., 1973; Magalhaes, Peters and Doe, 1974; Asquith, 1974b) and the formation of similar staining patterns with sera from patients with Crohn's disease suggests an alternative mechanism which may be no more than a non-specific reflection of tissue damage. Initially, Seah et al. (1971a) described three types of staining pattern in the sera of patients with coeliac disease, but subsequently they did not differentiate between these (Seah et al., 1971b). The overall reactivity, regardless of minor differences in pattern, appears to correspond to the anti-reticulin specificity described by Alp and Wright (1971), Von Essen et al. (1972) and Brown et al. (1973). Also it seems likely that the basement membrane antibody found in the sera of patients with selective IgA deficiency in coeliac disease (Ammann and Hong, 1971) is of similar specificity.

A further, major study was that of Rizzetto and Doniach (1973). In the course of examining 8000 different sera they described five staining patterns which they assumed to be against distinct antigens of intra- and extra-cellular components of mesenchyme. The overall incidence of these antibodies was established in 3628 sera from various diseases, including coeliac disease. However, they did not report the relative incidence of each staining pattern in relation to the different disease category studied. This was done in a second large series, that of Williamson et al. (1976). They looked at over 1600 patients with a variety of conditions, including 138 with coeliac disease. Serum IgG specificity directed against various components of basement membrane and reticulin were described. The anti-reticulin specificities were subdivided into different groups according to their distinctive histological staining patterns. Specificity directed primarily against endothelial basement membrane was found most frequently in the sera of patients with hiatus hernia (35 per cent) or coeliac disease (22 per cent). The same specificity was also observed in patients with myasthenia gravis and to a lesser extent in Crohn's disease and in a mixed group of patients with unspecified organic gastrointestinal disease. An epithelial basement membrane reactivity was found in patients with rheumatoid arthritis but only rarely in other conditions. Staining of perivascular connective tissue represented a third type of anti-reticulin specificity. Although uncommon, in coeliac disease this reactivity was found more frequently in combination with other connective tissue specificities.

Although the biological significance of reticulin antibodies is still in doubt it seems that their chief relevance will be as a preliminary screening test on large populations prior to jejunal biopsy. The interesting observation by Magalhaes et al. (1974) that IgA-class antireticulin antibodies only occurred in coeliac disease would appear to have additional potential in this respect. Even so, it still remains to be seen whether antibody detection will prove more useful as a preliminary screening test than, say, serum folate or genetic markers.

Other tissue antibodies

Patients with coeliac disease have an increased incidence of autoantibodies compared with normal subjects (Seah, Fry, Hoffbrand and Holborow, 1971a; Lancaster-Smith, Perrin, Swarbrick and Wright, 1974b; Williamson et al., 1976) (Table 6.3). In one series, 20 autoantibodies were detected in 12 of 31 patients tested and autoantibodies to thyroid and gastric antigens seemed common (Lancaster-Smith et al., 1974b). In the study of Williamson et al. (1976) referred to above, the authors found antinuclear antibodies and smooth muscle antibodies in relatively high proportions (18 per cent and 12 per cent respectively) of an in-patient control group, compared with 8 per cent and 3 per cent of patients with coeliac disease and only 0 per cent and 1 per cent of the normal blood donors. The predominant pattern

of antinuclear-antibody staining seen in patients with coeliac disease was of the homogeneous type.

ASSOCIATION OF COELIAC DISEASE AND 'AUTO-ALLERGIC' CONDITIONS

In addition to the occurrence of autoantibodies, putative 'autoallergic' disease may be clinically apparent in some coeliac patients (Table 6.4). Although these associations have been recently reviewed (Bayless, Yardley and Hendrix, 1974; Scott and Losowsky, 1975), their real frequency is largely unknown. In some instances a positive interrelationship is suggested, but many other proposed associations are based on isolated case reports. The most commonly related diseases include thyroid disease, insulin-dependent diabetes mellitus and chronic liver disease (Lancaster-Smith et al., 1974b; Scott and Losowsky, 1975). In one series, 11 of 57 patients (19 per cent) had evidence of past or present diseases thought to be of 'autoallergic' aetiology (Lancaster-Smith et al., 1974b). Of particular interest is the association between coeliac disease and diffuse interstitial lung disease. Initial descriptions of villous atrophy in two patients with allergic alveolitis due to avian exposure (bird fancier's lung) (Hood and Mason, 1970) were followed by reports of sarcoidosis (Scadding, 1970) and fibrosing alveolitis (Lancaster-Smith, Benson and Strickland, 1971) occurring in coeliac disease. Lancaster-Smith et al. (1971) found 3 cases of fibrosing alveolitis among a group of 24 coeliacs. Conversely, 5 out of 16 patients with bird fancier's lung had total or sub-total villous atrophy (Berrill et al., 1975), while precipitins to various avian antigens can be found in sera from coeliac patients (Morris, Read, Jones, Cotes and Edwards, 1971). More recently, 2 patients with allergic alveolitis due to antigens from mouldy hay (farmer's lung) have been shown to have malabsorption and villous atrophy (Robinson, 1976).

Continued interest in disease relationships might be expected to yield further insight into the pathogenesis of coeliac disease and its genetic aspects. The need for strict disease definitions is obvious in any such study, but unfortunately the diagnosis of coeliac disease is questionable in several publications. Some reports are of patients with villous atrophy in whom the diagnosis of coeliac disease was not considered or a gluten-free diet was not tried, or in whom there was no apparent response to a gluten-free diet of undefined strictness and duration (Scott and Losowsky, 1975). Although it is currently impossible to say whether the finding of autoallergic disease in coeliac patients is anything more than chance, it is known that many of the associated conditions are, like coeliac disease, linked to inheritance of the HLA-B8 antigen (Albert, 1976). This has led Scott and Losowsky (1975) to hypothesize that circulating immune complexes originating from the intestine

Table 6.3 Autoantibodies in patients with coeliac disease

Reference	Subject group	Total number studied	Rheumatoid factor	Antinuclear antibody	Number with positive autoantibodies					
					Thyroglobulin antibody	Thyroid microsomal antibody	Gastric parietal cell antibody	Smooth muscle antibody	Anti-mitochondrial antibody	
Seah et al. (1971)	Coeliac	31	NT	2	1	3	4	0	2	
	Control	28	NT	1	NS	1	0	0	0	
Lancaster-Smith et al. (1974)	Coeliac	31	3	3	5	4	1	4	0	
	Control	31	1	1	1	1	0	1	0	
Williamson et al. (1976)	Coeliac: normal diet	42	NT	0	NT	NT	4	2	1	
	Coeliac: GFD	91	NT	11	NT	NT	7	3	1	
	Normal blood donors	100	NT	0	NT	NT	6	1	0	
	Matched controls	110	NT	20	NT	NT	13	13	2	

NT = not tested.
NS = not stated.

Table 6.4 Coeliac disease and reported 'autoallergic' associations

Endocrine:	Thyroid disease Insulin-dependent diabetes mellitus Addison's disease
Gastrointestinal:	Chronic liver disease Ulcerative colitis
Rheumatic:	Systemic lupus erythematosus Rheumatoid arthritis Sjogren's syndrome Polyarteritis nodosa and undefined connective tissue disease
Pulmonary:	Fibrosing alveolitis Allergic alveolitis Sarcoidosis Idiopathic pulmonary haemosiderosis
Dermatological:	Cutaneous vasculitis Psoriasis Vitiligo

may cause other diseases by deposition in the relevant organ. The antigen involved may be derived from the damaged jejunal mucosa, or may be a gluten product.

DERMATITIS HERPETIFORMIS

Characteristically, the skin lesions of dermatitis herpetiformis (DH) are vesicular, produce intense irritation and occur on the elbows, knees, buttocks and shoulders, but can be generalized. Affected and adjacent unaffected skin shows IgA, complement and fibrin below the epithelial basement membrane (Seah *et al.*, 1972; Seah *et al.*, 1973b). The skin improves dramatically with dapsone therapy, irrespective of the dietary status of the individual (Fry, Seah and Hoffbrand, 1974).

The gastrointestinal interest of DH lies in the fact that the majority of patients have a coeliac-like lesion of the proximal intestine, 60 per cent on a single biopsy (Marks, Shuster and Watson, 1966) and more than 90 per cent on the basis of multiple biopsies (Brow, Parker, Weinstein and Rubin, 1971). The intestinal morphology improves on a gluten-free regime and it seems that, if the diet is strict enough, the skin lesions also remit on gluten withdrawal (Fry, Seah, Riches and Hoffbrand, 1973); this includes the degree of IgA staining (Harrington and Read, 1977). The genetic backgrounds of DH and coeliac disease are similar (Katz, Falchuk, Dahl, Rogentine and Strober, 1972; Gebhard, Falchuk, Katz, Sessoms, Rogentine and Strober, 1974; Keunning, Peña, Van Leewen, Van Hooff and Van Rood, 1976; Mann, Katz, Nelson, Abelson and Strober, 1976).

Currently it seems reasonable to assume that the skin lesions in DH represent damage by circulating immune complexes which originate in the mucosa following gluten ingestion. The nature of the receptor site localiz-

ing the complex to the skin is unknown. Also it is not clear why the majority of non-DH coeliacs do not develop vesicular skin lesions.

COMPLEMENT CHANGES

The hypothesis that complement activation by immune complexes formed in the jejunal mucosa is responsible for tissue damage in coeliac disease has been tested in three ways: (1) by measurement of serum complement components and breakdown products, (2) by searching for complement deposition in the mucosa following gluten challenge and (3) by detection of circulating immune complexes.

1. Serum complement levels

Doe, Henry and Booth (1974) found lower C3 and C4 levels in untreated coeliacs than in normal controls and higher C3 and C4 levels in coeliac patients taking a gluten-free diet compared with those on a normal diet. Following oral (Doe, Henry, Holt and Booth, 1972) or intraduodenal (Doe, Henry and Booth, 1974) gluten challenge, coeliacs previously maintained on a gluten-free diet showed an acute fall in serum haemolytic complement and C3 levels which was maximal between 1 and 6 hours after challenge. Others have confirmed complement consumption and the appearance of complement breakdown products 8 hours following gluten challenge (McNeish, Rolles and Thompson, 1974). Conversely, low complement component levels have been found in children with untreated coeliac disease, which gradually rise to normal 2 to 3 weeks following the start of a gluten-free diet (Rossipal, 1974).

2. Mucosal complement deposition

The timing of the serum complement changes correlates with the early morphological changes found in the jejunal mucosa and the endothelial lining of small blood vessels following comparable challenge experiments (Schmerling and Shiner, 1970; Shiner, 1973). Immunofluorescent studies have shown an increased IgA and C3 deposition in the basement membrane region of untreated coeliacs, compared with coeliacs on a gluten-free diet and non-coeliac subjects (Scott, Scott and Losowsky, 1977). Lancaster-Smith, Packer, Kumar and Harris (1976b) also found basement membrane staining with anti-IgA serum in coeliacs, particularly those on a normal diet, but found no evidence of C3 deposition in either coeliac or control biopsies. Gluten challenge of treated coeliacs results in extracellular deposition of fibrinogen, IgM and C3 in the lamina propria, occurring maximally at 4 hours (Doe, Henry and Booth, 1974) and variable staining of the basement membrane with conjugated antisera to IgA and C3 (Shiner and Ballard, 1972), or IgA, IgM and C3 (Doe, Henry and Booth, 1974).

3. Circulating immune complexes

Using the C1q precipitation test for detecting complement binding antigen-antibody complexes, Doe, Booth and Brown (1973) found complexes in the serum of 60 per cent of untreated coeliacs compared with 10 per cent of coeliacs who had been on a gluten-free diet for over 6 months. Complexes were also found in patients with Crohn's disease (57 per cent) and ulcerative colitis (20 per cent) but rarely in controls (3 per cent). Sera from 4 of 6 treated coeliacs gave positive C1q precipitation results 4 to 24 hours after acute gluten challenge (Doe, Henry and Booth, 1974). Immune complexes were not detected in pre-challenge sera. Other workers have detected immune complexes by the same method in 2 of 6 coeliacs (Mowbray, Hoffbrand, Holborow, Seah and Fry, 1973). In patients with dermatitis herpetiformis, circulating complexes were detected in 12 of 15 patients on a normal diet and 4 of 11 taking a gluten-free diet using an anticomplementary assay (Mowbray et al., 1973). In contrast, only 3 of the 25 patients gave positive results by C1q precipitation (Mowbray et al., 1973).

When evaluating these results it should be noted that there are disadvantages to both the techniques used for detecting immune complexes in coeliac disease. Immune complexes with complement already attached may not be anticomplementary, and may be missed in this assay system (Verrier Jones and Cumming, 1977). Conversely, the anticomplementary activity of aggregated IgG present in aged or heat-denatured samples may seriously interfere with interpretation (Thompson, 1974). In addition to precipitating with immune complexes, C1q will also react in this system with DNA, C-reactive protein, heparin, protamine, bacterial lipopolysaccharide and phosphoryl choline (Verrier Jones and Cumming, 1977). C1q reactivity and anticomplementary activity cannot therefore be regarded as completely specific for immune complexes.

CELL-MEDIATED IMMUNITY IN COELIAC DISEASE

An additional, or possible alternative, mechanism for the pathogenesis of coeliac disease is a cell-mediated immune (CMI) response to an immunogenic fragment of gluten (Asquith, 1974b). Cell-mediated (or delayed hypersensitivity) reactions are commonly defined as those immune reactions transferable by viable cells but not by serum. In vivo they include allograft rejection and graft-versus-host disease in addition to classical cell-mediated protective immunity to pathogenic organisms. The term is also applied to in-vitro models of lymphocyte activity which are thought to be analogues of the above in-vivo reactions. Evidence from extirpation experiments has shown that CMI responses are mediated by thymus-derived (T) lymphocytes (Miller, 1962). Responsiveness may be assessed indirectly by quantitation of resting lymphocyte numbers, and directly in vitro by lymphokine generation (MIF and LIF assay), T-cell cytotoxicity and blastogenesis as measured morphologically or by DNA synthesis (Fig. 6.1) or in vivo by delayed-type skin tests.

The experimental evidence relating to cell-mediated immunity in coeliac disease is often inconsistent and sometimes controversial.

NON-SPECIFIC CMI IN COELIAC DISEASE

Lymphocyte counts
Results of quantitation of lymphocytes in the blood, the intestine and in other tissues have already been presented as indirect evidence.

Skin tests
In one series, only 22 per cent of coeliac patients had positive Mantoux tests compared with 85 per cent of a control population (Scott and Losowsky, 1976a). No difference was seen between treated and untreated coeliacs, suggesting a depression of in-vivo CMI in coeliac disease.

Lymphocyte transformation to
Mitogens
Several groups have studied non-specific lymphocyte transformation responses to the plant mitogen phytohaemagglutinin (PHA) (Table 6.5). As PHA preferentially stimulates T-lymphocytes (Ling and Kay, 1975) this test is commonly used in assessing T-cell responsiveness in man (Brostoff, 1976). Results of PHA stimulation in coeliacs are conflicting (Table 6.5). Discrepancies may be due to differences in the experimental methods used. Cultured cells have usually been leucocyte-rich suspensions, but purified lymphocytes and even whole blood have been tried. Potential weaknesses in many reports include (1) the lack of PHA dose-response curves, since it is well recognized that there are individual variations in the optimum dose which will elicit a response (Ling and Kay, 1975), (2) the lack of sufficient replicates and (3) the use of differing methods of quantitation of results – isotope incorporation into DNA is the most sensitive and most easily quantitated technique but lacks morphological correlation, while autoradiographic or morphological estimates are subjective and thus less accurate (Ling and Kay, 1975).

Nevertheless, the majority of reports support the contention that in untreated coeliac disease there is impairment of PHA stimulation which may be variably improved by treatment with a gluten-free diet. This depression of CMI could be partly explained by the unidentified inhibiting serum factor reported by several workers (Table 6.5), by malnutrition in untreated coeliac

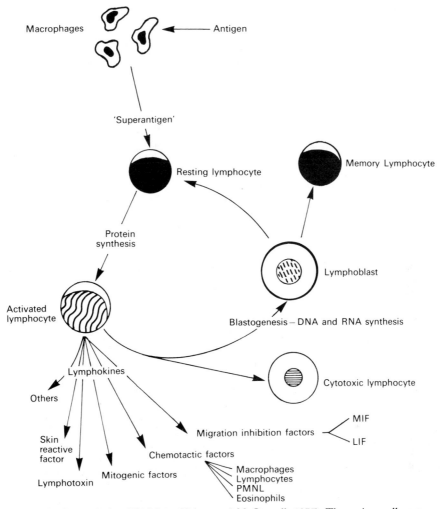

Fig. 6.1 T-lymphocyte activation cycle (modified from Hobart and McConnell, 1975). The various cells, e.g. macrophages, activated and cytotoxic lymphocytes, and some of their products, e.g. lymphokines, are thought to be of varying relevance to the immune theory of gluten toxicity.

disease, or by the increased enteric loss of lymphocytes in this condition (Douglas, Weetman and Haggith, 1976). It is therefore relevant that there are no comparisons of PHA responsiveness in untreated coeliacs and other patients with chronic malabsorptive states, particularly as impaired responses are also found in Crohn's disease (Ch. 7).

Antigens

Transformation of lymphocytes by mitogens reflects a non-specific response of T-lymphocytes. A more physiological appraisal of CMI would be obtained using lymphocyte stimulation by specific antigens provided that prior antigenic exposure is known to have occurred. The information is scant; Housley, Asquith and Cooke (1969) found that peripheral blood and mesenteric node lymphocytes from two coeliacs transformed normally in the presence of purified protein derivative of mycobacterium tuberculosis.

Lymphoid cell lines

Cells of lymphoid cell lines (LCL) are abnormal lymphocytes transformed to a continuously dividing state by Epstein-Barr (EB) virus or other agents. Normal lymphocytes show intense proliferation when grown in mixed culture with viable Burkitt lymphoma cells from an EB_2 LCL (Hardy and Ling, 1969; Hardy, Knight and Ling, 1970). Maclaurin, Cooke and Ling (1971) showed that the proliferative response of coeliac lymphocytes to EB_2 lymphoma cells, as measured by tritiated-thymidine (^{3}H-Tdr) incorporation into DNA, was significantly depressed compared with the response of normal

Table 6.5 Reported studies of PHA induced lymphocyte transformation in coeliac disease

| Reference | Transformation by PHA | | Controls | Cells/replicates | Cell concentration | Culture method | | Expression of results | Serum factor |
	Coeliacs on ND	Coeliacs on GFD				Dose range of PHA	Quantitation		
Winter et al. (1967)	↓↓ 6*(9**)	↓↓ 4 (4)	Healthy adults	Leucocytes – no replicates	NS	1 dose	Morphology	% blasts	+
Housley et al. (1969)	↓ 1 (1)	↓ 2 (5)	Healthy adults Patients with GI disease	Leucocytes – triplicate cultures	3 × 10⁶ cells per culture	1 dose	Morphology; 3H-Tdr incorporation into DNA	% blasts; DPM	–
Blecher et al. (1969)	↓ 5 (10)		Healthy adults	Leucocytes – no replicates	NS	1 dose	Morphology	% blasts	+
Ansaldi et al. (1970)		Normal 6 (6)		Leucocytes – no replicates	NS	1 dose	Morphology	% blasts	NS
Popovic et al. (1970)	↓ 1 (1)	Normal 1 (1)	NS	NS	NS	NS	Morphology	% blasts	NS
Maclaurin et al. (1971)	Mean responses in coeliacs lower than controls, but not significantly (15)		Healthy adults	Leucocytes – triplicates	1 × 10⁶ cells per culture	1 dose	3H-Tdr – incorporation into DNA	DPM	+
Morganroth et al. (1972)	–	Normal 12 (12)	Healthy adults Patients with GI disease. Immunized rabbits	Leucocytes – no replicates	3 × 10⁶ cells per culture	1 dose	Morphology	% blasts	NS
Holmes (1974)	(14) Mean responses in coeliacs lower than controls, but not statistically significant	(21)	Healthy adults	Leucocytes – duplicate cultures	1 × 10⁶ cells per culture	1 dose	3H-Tdr – incorporation in DNA	DPM	+
Scott and Losowsky (1976a)	↓↓ group (10) mean	↓ group (14) mean	Healthy adults	Whole blood – quadruplicates	NS	6 doses	3H-Tdr – incorporation into DNA	CPM per 10⁶ lymphocytes	+
Sikora et al. (1976)	–	No significant group differences from (19) controls	Medical patients GI patients	Lymphocytes – triplicates	1 × 10⁵ cells per culture	NS	125IUDR – incorporation into DNA	Stimulation indices	NS

↓↓ or ↓ = extent of reduction in response as compared with control population.
*/** Refer to number of patients showing reduced responses* out of the total number studied** (in brackets).
NS = Not stated.
ND = untreated coeliacs.
GFD = coeliacs ingesting a gluten-free diet for varying periods.
CPM = counts per minute.
DPM = disintegrations per minute.

lymphocytes. Dietary gluten restriction did not influence this response. The reaction of lymphocytes to LCL in mixed culture has been regarded as a specialized immune surveillance mechanism which is highly effective in removal of aberrant lymphoid cells (Ling, 1973). If the functional capacity of thymus-derived lymphocytes is depressed in coeliac disease this immune surveillance mechanism would inevitably be impaired.

Cytotoxicity tests *in vitro*

Fresh blood lymphocytes activated by mixed culture with cells from a LCL acquire the capacity to kill cells of the line used to induce the activation and are also cytotoxic to cells of other human lymphoid cell lines (Hardy, Ling, Wallin and Aviet, 1970) (Fig. 6.1). This cytotoxic capacity can be assessed by measuring the release of radioactivity from radio-labelled EB cells added to cultures of unstimulated lymphocytes and lymphocytes pre-stimulated for 5 days with irradiated, unlabelled EB cells. Maclaurin, Cooke and Ling (1971) showed that the cytotoxicity of pre-stimulated coeliac lymphocytes was significantly depressed as compared with similarly treated normal lymphocytes. The impaired proliferative and cytotoxic capacity of coeliac lympho-cytes against lymphoid cell lines could be one explana-tion of the increased frequency of lymphomas observed in coeliac disease (see below).

Malignancy in coeliac disease

Until 1962, the malabsorption associated with malignant lymphoid tumours of the gastrointestinal tract was usually considered to be secondary to the reticulosis. Gough, Read and Naish (1962) suggested that intestinal lymphoma was a direct complication of adult coeliac disease and postulated that the mucosal atrophy might be a pre-malignant condition. This concept has been supported by a number of reports (Austad *et al.*, 1967; Harris, Cooke, Thomson and Waterhouse, 1967; Asquith, 1974a; Petreshock, Pessah and Menachemi, 1975; Holmes *et al.*, 1976). The increase in lymphoma was shown to be statistically valid by Harris *et al.* (1967) in a review of 201 patients with idiopathic steatorrhoea and coeliac disease. Malignancy is not confined to lymphoma but includes increased frequencies of adeno-carcinoma of the jejunum (Petreshock *et al.*, 1975), and carcinoma of the oesophagus (Harris *et al.*, 1967) and pharynx (Holmes *et al.*, 1976). There is no good evidence that patients failing to respond clinically to gluten withdrawal are more prone to develop malignancy or that a gluten-free diet is effective in preventing this complication (Holmes *et al.*, 1976).

The combination of impaired CMI and an increased incidence of malignancy in coeliac disease has led to the theory that coeliacs could have defective immune surveil-lance mechanisms (Stokes and Holmes, 1974). The immune surveillance hypothesis was developed by Burnet (1970) from a suggestion by Thomas (1959). The argument is that neoplastic transformation must be a frequent result of somatic cell replication; however, since transformed neoplastic variants are antigenic, they are rapidly eliminated by the immune response. Only rarely, and for unknown reasons, can a neoplastic clone escape this defence mechanism, and thus the vast majority of neoplasms are thought to be eliminated by the immunological surveillance mechanism at a very early stage in their evolution. The increased incidence of neoplastic disease (particularly malignant lymphoma) in patients with immunodeficiency states or receiving exogenous immunosuppressive therapy (e.g. renal allo-graft recipients) is evidence in support of this concept (Burnet, 1970), but the pattern of malignancy in these situations does not reflect their incidence in the general population, and means that the general validity of the surveillance theory may be unsound (Schwartz, 1974). Similarly, the immune surveillance hypothesis does not take into account the decreased incidence of malignancy in some immunosuppressed (Martinez, 1964) or con-genitally athymic (Stutman, 1974) animals. It seems likely that the immunodepression claimed to be present in coeliac disease is one element in the patient's pre-disposition to lymphoreticular malignancies. Other factors are probably also involved (Asquith, 1974a). Proliferation of lymphoid cells by persistent antigenic stimulation in the presence of partial immunosuppres-sion often culminates in malignant lymphomas in experi-mental animals (Krueger, 1972) and may do so in patients with coeliac disease; the work of Maclaurin, Cooke and Ling (1971) supports this.

SPECIFIC CMI IN COELIAC DISEASE

Skin tests (Table 6.1)

To date, skin test reactions to gluten and its subfrac-tions have very largely suggested a humoral Type III hypersensitivity response and have been discussed pre-viously. Delayed responses have been macroscopically positive in only one patient (Asquith, 1974c). Although Asquith (1974c) reported a perivascular mononuclear cell infiltrate and oedema in most coeliacs following intradermal injection of gluten fraction III, the finding was non-specific, being seen equally frequently in healthy adult controls.

Lymphocyte transformation to

Gluten and gluten subfractions
In-vitro activation of peripheral blood lymphocytes from coeliac patients by gluten subfractions is a con-troversial subject (Table 6.6). Initially, Housley, Asquith and Cooke (1969) suggested that, in coeliacs, responses to gluten fraction III occurred only with mesenteric

Table 6.6 Reported studies of gluten-induced lymphocyte transformation in patients with coeliac disease

Reference	Source of lymphocytes	Replicates	Experimental method employed		Quantitation of results	Expression of results
			Cell concentration	Antigen and dose range		
Housley et al. (1969)	Leucocytes	Triplicates	3×10^6 cells per culture	Gluten fr. III 12 mg – 125 μg per culture	Morphology; 3H-Tdr – incorporation into DNA	% blasts dpm
Asquith, et al. (1969)	Leucocytes	Duplicates	3×10^6 cells per culture	Gluten fr. III 1 dose only – 2 mg per culture	3H-Tdr – incorporation into DNA	Transformation ratios
Holt (1969)			Experimental details unpublished			
Ansaldi et al. (1970)	Leucocytes	No replicates	NS	Gluten fr. III	Morphology	% blasts
Morganroth et al. (1972)	Leucocytes	No replicates	3×10^6 cells per culture	Gliadin 1 dose only – 100 μg per culture	Morphology	% blasts
Asquith (1974c)	Leucocytes	Duplicates	1×10^6 cells per culture	Gluten fr. III 10 mg – 7 μg per culture	3H-Tdr – incorporation into DNA	Transformation ratios
von Büllow et al. (1974)		Details not stated		Gliadin and gluten fr. III 1–100 μg per culture	3H-Tdr – incorporation into DNA	cpm
Nelson et al. (1974)			Experimental details unpublished			
Scott (1975)	Whole-blood	Quadruplicates	NS	Gluten fr. III 2 mg–40 μg per culture	3H-Tdr – incorporation into DNA	Transformation ratios
Holmes et al. (1976)	Leucocytes	Duplicates	1×10^6 cells per culture	Gluten fr. III 8 mg–7 μg per culture	3H-Tdr – incorporation into DNA	Transformation ratios
Sikora et al. (1976)	Purified lymphocytes	Triplicates	1×10^5 per culture	Gluten fr. III subfraction B_2 100–0.5 μg per culture	^{125}IUDR – incorporation into DNA	Transformation ratios

ND = untreated coeliacs.
GFD = coeliacs ingesting a gluten-free diet for varying periods.
NS = not stated.

dpm = disintegrations per minute.
cpm = counts per minute.

node lymphocytes. Further and progressively more extensive experiments on peripheral lymphocytes suggested that the response could be generalized in some patients (Asquith, Housley and Cooke, 1969; Asquith, 1970; Asquith, 1974b). Of particular interest was the finding of significantly greater stimulation in gluten-free coeliacs compared with normal-diet coeliacs (Asquith, Housley and Cooke, 1969; Asquith, 1970; Asquith, 1974b; Holmes, Asquith and Cooke, 1976). More recently, von Büllow and colleagues (1974) reported significant transformation with gliadin but not gluten fraction III, although Scott (1975) and Holmes, Asquith

and Cooke (1976) have been able to stimulate coeliac lymphocytes with gluten fraction III. Sikora and others (1976) have demonstrated a positive response using their B_2 subfraction of gluten which is known to be both clinically toxic and to cause positive skin reactions (Anand, Truelove and Offord, 1977). In contrast, other workers have failed to show any transformation of coeliac lymphocytes, either by morphological criteria (Ansaldi, de Sanctis, Fabris and Ponzone, 1970; Morganroth, Watson and French, 1972) or by unstated methods (Holt, 1969; Nelson and Strober, 1974).

The techniques outlined in these various reports have

Table 6.6 (*continued*) Results of lymphocyte transformation

Reference	No. patients studied and results		Controls	Other comments
	Coeliacs – ND	Coeliacs – GFD		
usley et al. (1969)	1	5	Healthy adults Patients with GI disease	Transformation of mesenteric node lymphocytes from coeliacs in response to 2 mg gluten per culture
	No transformation seen			
quith, et al. (1969)	4	15	Healthy adults	
	Increased transformation in gluten-free coeliacs only			
at (1969)	17	19	NS	
	No transformation seen			
aldi et al. (1970)	6	6	NS	
	No transformation seen			
rganroth et al. (1972)	0	12	Healthy adults Patients with GI disease Immunized rabbits	Rabbit controls showed +ve transformation
	No transformation seen			
uith (1974c)	14	27	Healthy adults	Maximum response seen with 2 mg or 4 mg gluten fr. III per culture
	Increased transformation in 17%	Increased transformation in 34%		
Büllow et al. (1974)	1	9	NS	Transformation seen with gliadin but not gluten fr. III
	Increased transformation in 3 patients			
son et al. (1974)	No transformation seen		NS	
tt (1975)	Increased transformation in 3 of 11 coeliacs		Healthy adults	
mes et al. (1976)	14	21	Healthy adults	Maximum response seen with 2 mg or 4 mg gluten fr. III per culture
	Increased transformation in 29%	Increased transformation in 52%		
ora et al. (1976)	0	19	Medical patients Patients with GI disease	48 h culture optimal
	Increased transformation seen			

differed widely, as has the nature and dose of the antigens used (Table 6.6). Yet critical attention to detail in this situation is mandatory. The nature of the growth media, serum supplements, methods of lymphocyte isolation, cell concentrations and culture conditions are all relevant (Ling and Kay, 1975). In addition it is important that a uniform method of quantitation of transformation should be used, and the commonly used 'transformation ratios' may be misleading (Ling and Kay, 1975; Haeney and Asquith, 1976). The discrepancy between different reports is therefore not surprising, but the weight of evidence now indicates that lymphocyte stimulation by gluten subfractions does occur in patients with coeliac disease but not in healthy controls. The specificity of this cell-mediated response is largely untested, although Jos (1974) has found that lymphocytes of some coeliac children without clinical cow's milk intolerance also transform in the presence of cow's milk proteins.

Small intestinal mucosa
Using a whole-blood method of lymphocyte transformation, Scott and Losowsky (1976b) showed that 3 out of 15 coeliacs demonstrated significant transformation to a crude freeze-dried preparation of whole jejunal mucosa. This interesting report requires confirmation since it suggests that a cell-mediated autoallergic reaction to jejunal mucosa may exist in some coeliacs. This could perpetuate mucosal damage even after gluten restriction.

Lymphokine production

By peripheral blood lymphocytes

LIF assay. Lymphocytes from subjects exhibiting delayed hypersensitivity can, when incubated with the sensitizing antigen *in vitro*, release a number of biologically active substances into the culture medium (Fig. 6.1). These products of activated lymphocytes, the lymphokines (Ch. 3), have been regarded as possible mediators of cellular immunity (Dumonde *et al.*, 1969). One such lymphokine, macrophage migration-inhibition factor (MIF), affects the migration of normal macrophages from capillary tubes *in vitro* and has been extensively reviewed (David and David, 1972). An adaptation of this technique for use in human diseases utilizes peripheral blood leucocytes packed into capillary tubes and incubated with specific antigen (Bendixen and Søborg, 1970). Rocklin (1974) has shown that this leucocyte inhibitory factor (LIF) is distinct from MIF in that it inhibits the migration of polymorphonuclear leucocytes but does not affect the migration of guinea-pig macrophages or human monocytes. Both leucocyte and macrophage migration systems have been accepted as *in-vitro* correlates of cellular immunity (David and David, 1972).

Recently, evidence has been presented to show that leucocyte migration inhibition to gluten occurs in patients with coeliac disease. Bullen and Losowsky (1976) briefly reported significantly impaired leucocyte migration in the presence of gluten fraction III in treated, but not untreated, coeliacs compared with controls. Approximately 40 per cent of their treated patients were below the normal range. Detection of leucocyte migration inhibition was related to the time since gluten withdrawal, serial measurements showing a progressive fall in migration over a 6-month period following the start of a gluten-free diet. Douwes (1976), using a Clausen (1973) modification of the leucocyte migration-inhibition test, also demonstrated migration inhibition in the presence of a gluten fraction in a group of 12 patients with coeliac disease. Patients with a variety of other gastrointestinal diseases showed no such lymphokine release.

Leucocyte adherence. Inhibition of the leucocyte adherence reaction in the presence of gliadin has been studied by Allardyce and Shearman (1975). Peripheral blood leucocytes, incubated for 30 minutes at 37°C in the presence and absence of gliadin, were counted and then recounted one hour later, following the gentle removal of non-adherent cells. Adherence of leucocytes was not inhibited in the majority of normal controls (16), but significant inhibition of adherence was observed in groups of patients with dermatitis herpetiformis (20) and coeliac disease (11). It has been suggested that inhibition of leucocyte adherence to glass following

in-vitro exposure to specific antigen may be functionally related to lymphokine-mediated reactions (Halliday, Malhuish and Isbister, 1974). However, the T-lymphocyte mediation of this test has not yet been conclusively demonstrated.

By jejunal mucosa in organ culture. More relevant to any possible involvement of cell-mediated immune reactions in the pathogenesis of coeliac disease is the demonstration of local cellular immunity to gluten fractions within the small intestinal mucosa. Ferguson, MacDonald, McClure and Holden (1975) cultured 2–4 mg fragments of jejunal biopsy specimens, in the presence and absence of gliadin for 5 hours, and then assayed the culture-medium for its capacity to inhibit the migration of normal human peripheral blood leucocytes. In 6 control patients, culture with gliadin did not generate leucocyte inhibitory activity into the culture-medium, but did so in 5 of 6 patients with untreated coeliac disease. In 2 gluten-free diet-treated patients with coeliac disease, migration was not inhibited by culture with gliadin. Ferguson *et al.* (1975) thought that the leucocyte inhibitory factor found in these studies was produced by activated T-lymphocytes but alternative explanations are equally possible. Leucocyte migration may be inhibited by specific and non-specific release of lymphokines, or by unrelated factors. The normal migration of peritoneal exudate cells derived from unstimulated guinea-pigs can be inhibited by passively sensitizing the cells with various antigen–antibody complexes (Spitler, Huber and Fudenberg, 1969). This is particularly relevant since other workers (Falchuk, Gebhard and Strober, 1974; Falchuk, Gebhard, Sessoms and Strober, 1974), also using an *in-vitro* organ culture system, have shown that gluten challenge induces an increase in immunoglobulin production within the jejunal mucosa of coeliacs but not of controls. A major part of this immunoglobulin increase is composed of antigliadin antibodies (Falchuk, Laster and Strober, 1971). On this basis, gliadin–antigliadin complexes could explain the leucocyte inhibitory activity found by Ferguson *et al.* (1975).

Alternative explanations for LIF-like activity include the presence of macrophages/monocytes coated with cytophilic antibody, or the possible release of LIF from non-lymphoid cells. Spontaneous synthesis by fibroblast cell culture lines of material inhibiting leucocyte migration is known to occur (Tubergen, Feldman, Pollock and Lerner, 1972). Finally, studies on mediator production by highly purified human T- and B-lymphocytes suggest that both T- and B-cells can produce MIF in response to a specific antigenic stimulus (Rocklin, McDermott, Chess, Schlossman and David, 1974). It is apparent that leucocyte migration inhibition may be due to factors other than activation of T-lymphocytes.

Cytotoxicity testing

Killer (K) cells are a distinct subpopulation of mononuclear cells capable of killing target cells sensitized with IgG antibodies. This killing does not require the presence of sensitized effector cells, but is mediated by lymphoid cells carrying membrane receptors for the Fc region of IgG (Perlmann and Holm, 1969). Cytotoxic activity is probably induced when these receptors react with the Fc part of the antibodies coating the target cells. K-cells are the subject of controversy (MacLennan and Harding, 1974) and antibody-dependent K-cell-mediated cytotoxicity is not strictly a cell-mediated immune effector mechanism since neither T-lymphocytes (MacLennan and Harding, 1970; Van Boxel, Stobo, Paul and Green, 1972) nor conventional phagocytes (Perlmann, 1976) are involved, and the specificity is provided by antibodies. However, B-lymphocytes are not the killer cells as removal of immunoglobulin-bearing lymphocytes does not affect cytotoxic capacity of lymphoid suspensions (Greenberg, Shen and Roitt, 1973). It is a matter of speculation whether K-cells are a distinct type of fully differentiated effector cell or an immature form of lymphocyte or mononuclear phagocyte.

mental factors, and coeliac disease is no exception. Genetic factors are involved (Stokes, Asquith and Cooke, 1973) and gluten is a necessary environmental agent. An important link between genetic factors and an adverse reaction to a common environmental hazard, namely gluten, could be the occurrence of a highly significant increase in the incidence of HLA-A1 and HLA-B8 in coeliac disease (initially described by Falchuk, Rogentine and Strober, 1972, and Stokes et al., 1972). In animals, genes determining HLA antigens are closely associated with those responsible for determining immune responses, the so-called IR genes (McDevitt and Bodmer, 1972; Morris, 1975; Fig. 6.2). Therefore the altered frequency of HLA antigens in coeliac disease may be relevant to the initial process of immunization or to the quality of that response. HLA antigens on cell surfaces (for example, intestinal epithelial cells) may either allow specific binding to gluten with resultant cell damage or share antigenic determinants with gluten, so making the individual unable to mount an adequate immune response to the material. Alternatively a specific gene which is influenced by the HLA system may determine the patient's response to gluten (Asquith, 1975). In

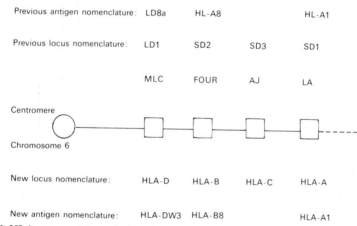

Fig. 6.2 HLA system with particular reference to coeliac disease – WHO nomenclature (1975).

In this respect it has been shown that sera from coeliacs in relapse contains lymphocyte-dependent antibodies (LDA) to α gliadin (Ezeoke, Ferguson, Fakhri, Hekkens and Hobbs, 1974). In the presence of α-gliadin-labelled target cells, these antibodies induce K-cell cytotoxicity of that target. Ezeoke et al. (1974) postulated that antibody-dependent K-cell cytotoxicity could be an important in-vivo mechanism of mucosal damage in coeliac disease.

GENETIC FACTORS

In any disease we can assume that the disease is dependent upon the interaction of genetic and environ-

coeliacs the particular HLA antigen found may reduce the efficiency of an immune response to gluten mounted by such a gene. Nevertheless, other factors must be relevant as HLA-A1 and -B8 exist in 20 per cent of the normal population, and these individuals do not have coeliac disease by any current criteria. Faced with the starting fact that approximately 80 per cent of patients have HLA-B8 two questions immediately arise: (1) do the remaining 20 per cent non-HLA-B8 individuals really have the condition and (2) is the mechanism of their sensitivity to gluten the same as in the HLA-B8 positive individuals? A side issue to these questions, but nevertheless very interesting, is the noting by Scott and his colleagues (1975) that the majority of non-HLA-B8 coeliacs were HLA-B12 positive. However, the answer to question (1) above is that non-HLA-B8 'apparent' coeliacs do have coeliac disease (Ferguson, Asquith and Cooke, 1974a) while the answer to the second is still not clear (Ferguson *et al.*, 1974a; Nelson *et al.*, 1975).

The problem of the 20 per cent HLA-B8 positive, non-coeliac normal population remains; it has been raised before (Asquith, 1974c). To illustrate the point, if we start with a hypothetical population, say 3000 individuals, and assume that the frequency of coeliac disease is that seen in the West of Ireland, which is one in 300 (McCarthy *et al.*, 1974), that would give us 10 coeliacs in that 3000 starting population. On our current data, of those 10, approximately 8 will have HLA-B8. However, 20 per cent of that starting population, that is 600 individuals, will have HLA-B8 and not have coeliac disease. In other words for every 8 patients whose coeliac disease is associated with HLA-B8 we have 600 individuals with HLA-B8 who do not have coeliac disease! Hence could it be that those 8 coeliacs in our hypothetical population really have a lack of some factor which is protective against coeliac disease (Asquith, 1974c). This remains a distinct possibility and the finding of an apparent decrease in the incidence of HLA-B7 in 149 patients with coeliac disease (Harms *et al.*, 1974) could be relevant to this point.

The recent findings of a series of additional genetic markers in a high percentage of coeliacs has added a further exciting dimension to the search for 'coeliac-specific' genetic markers. Two other markers have now been identified: (1) coeliac disease-associated B-cell antigen (Mann *et al.*, 1976) and (2) HLA-DW3 antigen (Keunning *et al.*, 1976) (Fig. 6.2). Furthermore the family occurrence of these markers has been determined (Peña *et al.*, 1977). The latter study included the following: 17 control individuals, 20 patients with coeliac disease and 37 members of 7 unrelated families of patients with coeliac disease. The HLA-DW3 antigen was present in 75 per cent of the patients and in 35.2 per cent of the controls. The coeliac disease-associated B-cell antigen (B-1) was present in 70 per cent of the patients and in 5.9 per cent of the controls. From their family studies Peña *et al.* (1977) concluded that DW3 antigen and coeliac disease-associated B-cell antigen are non-identical and under control of separate genes, the former being dominant, the latter recessive. This is fascinating as it suggests cell-surface specific antigens associated with coeliac disease could form all or part of a genetically determined receptor site on the surface of lymphoid cells which result in cell activation and immune responses upon exposure to gluten.

Two final points on the question of coeliac disease and genetics are worthy of mention. Firstly, there is the reporting of coeliac disease in one member of identical twin pairs where the genetic identity of the twins was thoroughly examined (Hoffman, Wollaeger and Greenberg, 1966; Walker-Smith, 1973). Secondly, there is the fact that coeliac disease occurs more frequently in women than men (Cooke, 1968). Taken together, these two points at least suggest the operation of important environmental and also hormonal factors in the pathogenesis of coeliac disease.

IDENTITY OF THE DAMAGING MATERIAL

Relevant to any immunological hypothesis is the nature of the fragment or fragments of gluten which are toxic. It is possible that by knowing the exact molecular structure (primary, secondary and tertiary) of the material(s) one could predict the likely mechanism of its toxicity. The suggestion that the essential material may have a molecular weight as low as 1000 to 1500 (Kowlessar, 1967) might imply that it is unlikely to be immunogenic (Watson, 1969). However, synthetic polypeptides of this approximate size or even smaller have been shown to be immunogenic in guinea-pigs (Borek, Stupp and Sela, 1965). Alternatively, by combining with one or more substances to produce a more active molecule the relevant material may be acting as a hapten. In this latter respect, Falchuk, Sessoms and Strober (1972) have shown *in vitro* that gluten is not directly toxic to biopsy samples from patients with coeliac disease, but that some endogenous factor also seemed necessary. This observation was extended to include other non-gliadin materials in a series of important and elegant studies (Jos, Lenair, de Ritis and Rey, 1974). One of the several possible explanations of these observations (Falchuk *et al.*, 1972; Jos *et al.*, 1974) is that the endogenous factor is a component of the B- or T-cell arm of the coeliacs' immune apparatus, but a non-immunological host factor might also be operating.

Concerning the identification of the toxic material, the meticulous work of Kasarda, Nimmo and Bernardin (1974); Hekkens *et al.* (1974); Phelan *et al.* (1974); Schneider, Kendall and Hawkins (1974); and Cornell (1974) should also be cited. Different starting materials, techniques for fractionation and systems for testing toxicity were used and hence the experiments are difficult to compare exactly. The suggestion that the toxic material could be made harmless by its exposure to specific carbohydrases (Phelan *et al.*, 1974) is particularly noteworthy.

Since 1974, separation and identification of the relevant fragment have been extended considerably in a series of painstaking experiments at Oxford (Dissanayake, Jerrome, Offord, Truelove and Whitehead, 1974; Sikora, Anand, Truelove, Ciclitira and Offord, 1976; Anand, Truelove and Offord, 1977a; Anand, Offord, Piris and Truelove, 1977b). In addition to doing fractionation

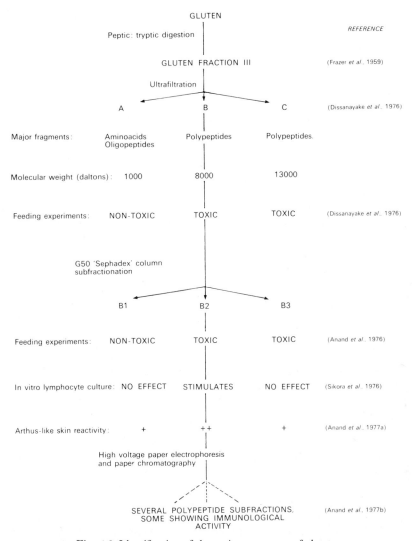

Fig. 6.3 Identification of the toxic component of gluten.

experiments they also performed a parallel series of studies to elucidate the mechanism of the toxic material isolated. Their work is summarized in Figure 6.3, and it leaves one with the impression that the elusive peptide will soon be identified.

CONCERNING IMMUNOLOGICAL MECHANISMS AND PATHOGENESIS

AFFECTOR ARM

On the basis of the accumulated data presented and summarized above, it is clear that abnormalities of humoral and cellular immunity are detectable in many patients with coeliac disease. However, two initial points should be made: (1) the percentage of patients exhibiting an abnormality differs according to the parameter under investigation, for example the number of coeliacs showing lymphocyte stimulation with gluten, compared to the number showing positive Arthus-like skin reactivity, and (2) for a given test the percentage showing the abnormality differs from one laboratory to another. There are several possible explanations of these two facts, including heterogeneous patient groups, differing patient selection criteria or merely varying laboratory techniques.

Accepting this, it is next pertinent to consider the relative merits of data on differing types of immunological reactivity. A widely accepted classification of immunological reactions divides them into Types I, II, III and IV (Coombs and Gell, 1976). Of these, Types I, II and III are broadly considered humoral reactions, and Type IV cellular.

Humoral mechanisms

Of humoral reactions relevant to gluten toxicity the current information on Type III reactions seems the most impressive. Nevertheless, it must be remembered that evidence implicating Type I and to a lesser extent Type II reactions would be more difficult to accumulate purely on current availability of techniques. This may have an artificial bias favouring Type III reactions, so distorting the 'rank order' of humoral responses to gluten.

Cellular mechanisms

There are now several reports (from *in-vitro* lymphocyte cultures and leucocyte-inhibition studies) suggesting a significant proportion of patients with coeliac disease exhibit cellular reactivity to gluten. Regarding the specificity of the responses to gluten, both with respect to 'antigen' and 'disease', then on the basis of the above two tests positive results seem to occur only in coeliacs (Haeney and Asquith, 1978). The varying proportion of seemingly non-responding coeliacs could be due to insensitive techniques or the dietary status of the individual. Thus it appears that positive reactions to gluten are likely to be recordable using blood taken from coeliacs whilst on a gluten-free diet; there are other factors also (Haeney and Asquith, 1976).

Furthermore, on the basis of certain data (reviewed above) a proportion of coeliacs are anergic and show evidence of non-specific T-cell impairment. Currently this does not look impressive enough to suggest it is relevant to the mechanism of gluten toxicity. However, more information is needed as it is still possible that tests of non-specific T-cell function in the mucosa would show a sufficient degree of abnormality to be relevant to the initial processing of ingested antigen. It is known that certain antigens are T-cell independent and this may apply to gluten. One possibility therefore is that a major local T-cell defect primarily involving a suppressor T-cell population could lead to anomalous immunization with gluten and hence be a fundamental mechanism explaining coeliac disease.

Hyposplenism

An interesting side issue is the relevance of the anatomical and functional hyposplenism found in many coeliacs, apparently correlating with peripheral T-lymphocyte counts (Bullen and Losowsky, 1977). In animals the spleen appears to have an effect on the fate of orally administered antigen (Rothberg, Kraft, Asquith and Michalek, 1972). Primary hyposplenism in coeliacs could modify the numbers of circulating lymphocytes primed at the intestinal mucosa. Alternatively at its lowest value, i.e. if the hyposplenism was secondary to the coeliac process, then it could aggravate an existing immune abnormality.

This then is the evidence suggesting that the humoral and cellular components of the affector arm in coeliacs is altered with respect to gluten reactivity.

EFFECTOR ARM

Allowing the concept that the affector arm is 'primed', what are the possible mechanisms by which tissue damage could be effected? The most relevant tissue is, of course, the intestine and one assumes on the basis of the elegant studies of Shiner (1973) that it is the epithelial cell and supporting basement membrane that are the first targets of the effector mechanisms. However, other tissues are also damaged, for example the skin in dermatitis herpetiformis and the lung in the allergic alveolitis associated with coeliac disease (Berrill *et al.*, 1975). It is reasonable to assume that several effector mechanisms could be involved, some related to local intestinal damage and others related to peripheral damage. Effector mechanisms could include: (1) K-cell binding, via its Fc receptor, to target cells sensitized with antigluten antibody (Ezoeke *et al.*, 1974), (2) complement-mediated cytolysis, (3) lymphokines released from activated T-cells, (4) other agents released from immune-dependent or independent mechanisms, for example vasoactive amines and prostaglandins (Ch. 3). This is an area needing further study.

PRIMARY OR SECONDARY?

Taking an overview of the evidence regarding affector and effector involvement, one additional approach is still badly needed. So far few studies provide results on more than one immunological parameter. Tests of multiple parameters are required on groups of patients studied sequentially, first on a normal diet, then following gluten withdrawal and subsequent gluten re-challenge with a reasonably well-defined component of gluten, for example α gliadin. Even if we do have a Type I, II, III or IV reaction occurring singly, together or sequentially (Asquith, 1974b), then it still would not be clear whether such reactions are primary, i.e. the basic defect in coeliac disease, or secondary to non-immunologically determined intestinal damage.

MODIFYING INFLUENCES

The nature of the damaging material has not been considered in a pathogenic sense, yet this is central to the issue. Consideration must be given to the chemical characteristics of native wheat (for example, its α-gliadin content) and its processing, including the milling and the baking of the resultant flour. Chemical or other additives could increase gluten's toxicity or potentially destroy it. On the basis of the evidence from Galway (Phelan *et al.*, 1974) it may be that addition of specific carbohydrases to bread could make it non-toxic. Possibly this is why Americans of Irish descent appear to have a lower incidence of coeliac disease than the inhabitants of Ireland. Bread baked in America or Ireland is different.

Additional factors influencing toxicity could include the amount of wheat-containing foods ingested and the rate of presentation of gluten to the small intestine. Thus villous abnormalities can follow partial gastrectomy, while coeliac disease has presented for the first time following peptic ulcer surgery (Franklin, 1970). Although it has been suggested that this latter observation is due to chance, the possibility remains that the two are more fundamentally related. Following gastric surgery, the physical characteristics of the gluten load presented to the proximal small intestine may have changed enough to make it toxic in a susceptible individual.

Finally, although genetic data, as currently presented, suggest that a disease-specific set of genetic markers might emerge, this is not necessarily so. It becomes more likely if we assume that coeliac disease is homogeneous with a possible single mechanism of toxicity. Judging by the total available clinical, haematological, biochemical, morphological, enzymatic, immunological and genetic data, this seems unlikely.

CONCLUSION

Results of numerous studies of humoral and cellular immunity in coeliac disease reveal impressive changes in immune reactivity, suggesting that patients are immunized with gluten. However, as judged on certain parameters, for example the results of serum antibody tests, healthy individuals also appear immunized. It is still not clear whether any important differences in the immunological status (with respect to gluten) of these two groups of individuals are quantitative or qualitative. Assuming an essential difference, it seems reasonable to conclude that the characteristic flat mucosa could result from an immunological reaction to gluten; or put simply, 'a coeliac may be a coeliac because he is immunized' (Asquith, 1974b). If that is so then it seems unlikely, if not incredible, that only one type of immunological

reaction to gluten will be operating in a given coeliac at any one moment in time.

The difficulty with the immunological hypothesis is the initial assumption of an essential difference. It is suggested that the explanation of this difference is likely to be relevant to the basic aetiology. This essential difference could be unrelated to immune mechanisms; for example, a specific enzyme defect may be the primary abnormality. The current genetic studies are exciting and should soon unravel at least the inheritance of this fascinating condition.

EPILOGUE

Coeliac disease has been given various names, some of them formulated on the basic assumption that it is gluten-induced, for example 'gluten-sensitive enteropathy', yet no universal agreement has been reached on nomenclature. The mechanism of gluten toxicity is also still in dispute. These two basic points, and four subsidiary ones, suggest that the concept with respect to name and the further problem of elucidating the mechanism of gluten toxicity could be investigated differently. The four subsidiary points are (1) gluten-sensitive intestinal lesions are well recognized, (2) gluten-sensitive non-intestinal lesions, for example dermatitis herpetiformis, are now accepted, (3) there are recent reports of asymptomatic coeliacs who are gluten-sensitive, particularly first-degree relatives diagnosed as part of prospective family studies, and (4) there are a few cases of coeliacs who initially were gluten-sensitive but subsequently became unresponsive. It is postulated (Asquith, 1977) that multifactorial cluster analysis of commonly available tests done both before and after gluten withdrawal, with appropriate 'numerical loading' for the important parameters, could overcome these various difficulties, particularly with respect to definition. However, it was additionally suggested that such a proposal could allow a rational approach to the solving of gluten toxicity, including its inheritance.

REFERENCES

Alarcon-Segovia, D., Herskovic, T., Wakim, K. G., Green, P. A. & Scudamore, H. H. (1964) Presence of circulating antibodies to gluten and milk fractions in patients with non-tropical sprue. *American Journal of Medicine*, **36**, 485–499.

Albert, E. D. (1976) The HLA system: serologically defined antigens. In *Clinical Immunobiology*, ed. Bach, F. H. & Good, R. A. Vol. 3, pp. 237–271. New York: Academic Press.

Aldersberg, D., Colcher, H. & Drachman, S. R. (1951) Studies on the effects of cortisone and pituitory adreno-corticotropic hormone (ACTH) in the sprue syndrome. *Gastroenterology*, **19**, 674–697.

Allardyce, R. A. & Shearman, D. J. C. (1975) Leukocyte

reactivity to α gliadin in dermatitis herpetiformis and adult coeliac disease. *International Archives of Allergy and Applied Immunology*, **48**, 395–400.

Alp, M. H. & Wright, R. (1971) Autoantibodies to reticulin in patients with idiopathic steatorrhoea, coeliac disease, and Crohn's disease, and their relation to immunoglobulins and dietary antibodies. *Lancet*, **ii**, 682–685.

Alvey, C., Anderson, C. M. & Freeman, M. (1957) Wheat gluten and coeliac disease. *Archives of Disease in Childhood*, **32**, 434–437.

Ammann, A. J. & Hong, R. (1971) Unique antibody to basement membrane in patients with selective IgA deficiency and coeliac disease. *Lancet*, **i**, 1264–1266.

Anand, B. S., Piris, J., Offord, R. E. & Truelove, S. C.

(1976) Unpublished observations, quoted by Sikora, K.,
Anand, B. S., Truelove, S. C., Ciclitira, P. J. & Offord,
R. E. *Lancet*, **ii**, 389–391.

Anand, B. S., Truelove, S. C. & Offord, R. E. (1977a) Skin
test for coeliac disease using a subfraction of gluten.
Lancet, **i**, 118–120.

Anand, B. S., Offord, R. E., Piris, J. & Truelove, S. C.
(1977b) Isolating the component of gluten which causes
the mucosal damage in coeliac disease. *Gut*, **18**, A408.

Anderson, C. M. (1960) Histological changes in the duodenal
mucosa in coeliac disease. Reversibility during treatment
with a wheat gluten-free diet. *Archives of Disease in
Childhood*, **35**, 419–427.

Ansaldi, N., de Sanctis, C., Fabris, C. & Ponzone, A. (1970)
Lymphocyte blast formation induced *in vitro* by PHA and
gluten in children with coeliac disease. *Minerva Pediatrica*,
22, 1907–1912.

Asquith, P. (1970) Adult coeliac disease. A clinical,
morphological and immunological study. MD Thesis,
Birmingham.

Asquith, P. (1974a) Adult coeliac disease and malignancy.
Journal of the Irish Medical Association, **67**, 417–425.

Asquith, P. (1974b) Immunology. In *Clinics in
Gastroenterology*, ed. Cooke, W. T. & Asquith, P. Vol. 3,
No. 1, Ch. 14, pp. 213–234. London: Saunders.

Asquith, P. (1974c) In *Coeliac Disease. Proceedings of the
Second International Coeliac Symposium*, ed. Hekkens,
W. Th. J. M. & Peña, A. S., p. 213. Leiden: Stenfert
Kroese.

Asquith, P. (1974d) In discussion. In *Coeliac Disease.
Proceedings of the Second International Coeliac Symposium*,
ed. Hekkens, W. Th. J. M. & Peña, A. S., p. 24. Leiden:
Stenfert Kroese.

Asquith, P. (1975) Coeliac Disease. In *Topics in
Gastroenterology*, 3rd edn, ed. Truelove, S. C. &
Goodman, M. J., Ch. 18, pp. 273–285. Oxford:
Blackwell.

Asquith, P. (1977) The definition of coeliac disease. In
preparation.

Asquith, P., Housley, J. & Cooke, W. T. (1969). Cell-
mediated immune response to dietary antigens in adult
coeliac disease. In *Coeliac Disease*, ed. Booth, C. C. &
Dowling, R. H., pp. 144–149. Edinburgh: Churchill
Livingstone.

Asquith, P., Thompson, R. A. & Cooke, W. T. (1969)
Serum-immunoglobulins in adult coeliac disease. *Lancet*,
ii, 129–131.

Asquith, P., Thompson, R. A. & Cooke, W. T. (1970a)
Serum and intestinal immunoglobulins in adult coeliac
disease. In *Coeliac Disease*, ed. Booth, C. C. & Dowling,
R. H., pp. 151–161. Edinburgh: Churchill Livingstone.

Asquith, P., Thompson, R. A. & Cooke, W. T. (1970b)
Quantitation of secretory IgA in the serum of patients
with gastrointestinal disease. *Gut*, **11**, 368.

Asquith, P., Thompson, R. A. & Cooke, W. T. (1971)
Quantitation of serum secretory IgA in gastrointestinal
disease. *Clinical Research*, **19**, 562.

Austad, W. I., Cornes, J. S., Gough, K. R., McCarthy,
C. F. & Read, A. E. (1967) Steatorrhoea and malignant
lymphoma. The relationship of malignant tumours of the
lymphoid tissue and coeliac disease. *Americal Journal of
Digestive Diseases*, **12**, 475–490.

Baker, P. G. & Read, A. E. (1976) Positive skin reactions to
gluten in coeliac disease. *Quarterly Journal of Medicine*,
45, 603–610.

Baker, P. G., Verrier Jones, J., Peacock, D. B. & Read,
A. E. (1975) The immune response to ØX174 in man.

III. Evidence for an association between hyposplenism
and immunodeficiency in patients with coeliac disease.
Gut, **16**, 538–542.

Baklien, K., Brandtzaeg, P. & Fausa, O. (1977)
Immunoglobulins in jejunal mucosa and serum from
patients with adult coeliac disease. *Scandinavian Journal
of Gastroenterology*, **12**, 149–159.

Barry, R. E. & Read, A. E. (1973) Coeliac disease and
malignancy. *Quarterly Journal of Medicine*, **42**, 665–675.

Bayless, T. M., Yardley, J. H. & Hendrix, T. R. (1974)
Coeliac disease and possible disease relationships. In
*Coeliac Disease. Proceedings of the Second International
Coeliac Symposium*, ed. Hekkens, W. Th. J. M. & Peña,
A. S., pp. 351–359. Leiden: Stenfert Kroese.

Beale, A. J., Parish, W. E., Douglas, A. P. & Hobbs, J. R.
(1971) Impaired IgA responses in coeliac disease. *Lancet*,
i, 1198–1220.

Bendixen, G. & Søborg, M. (1970) Comments on the
leucocyte migration technique as an *in vitro* method for
demonstrating cellular hypersensitivity in man. *Journal of
Immunology*, **104**, 1551–1552.

Berrill, W. T., Eade, O. E., Fitzpatrick, P. F., Hyde, I.,
Macleod, W. M. & Wright, R. (1975) Birdfancier's lung
and jejunal villous atrophy. *Lancet*, **ii**, 1006–1007.

Blecher, T. E., Brzechwa-Ajdukiewicz, A., McCarthy,
C. F. & Read, A. E. (1969) Serum immunoglobulins
and lymphocyte transformation studies in coeliac disease.
Gut, **10**, 57–62.

Blumgart, H. L. (1923) Three fatal adult cases of
malabsorption of fat with emaciation and anaemia, and in
two acidosis and tetany. *Archives of Internal Medicine*,
32, 113–128.

Booth, C. C. (1974) Definition of adult coeliac disease. In
*Coeliac Disease. Proceedings of the Second International
Coeliac Symposium*, ed. Hekkens, W. Th. J. M. & Peña,
A. S., pp. 17–22. Leiden: Stenfert Kroese.

Borek, F., Stupp, Y. & Sela, M. (1965) Immunogenicity
and the role of size; response of guinea-pigs to
oligotyrosine and tyrosine derivatives. *Science*, **150**, 1177–
1178.

Brandt, L. & Stenstam, M. (1975) Subnormal lymphocyte-
counts in adult coeliac disease. *Lancet*, **i**, 978–979.

Brandtzaeg, P. & Baklien, K. (1976) Immunohistochemical
studies of the formation and epithelial transport of
immunoglobulins in normal and diseased human intestinal
mucosa. *Scandinavian Journal of Gastroenterology*, **2**,
Suppl. 36, 5–45.

Breton, A., Vandendorp, F. & Dubois, O. (1959) L'effet
pathogène du gluten au cours de la maladie coeliaque:
déficit enzymatique ou réaction allergique? *Pediatrie*, **14**,
5–20.

Brostoff, J. (1976) Assessment of immunological
responsiveness in man. In *Twelfth Symposium on
Advanced Medicine*, ed. Peters, D. K., pp. 13–22.
Tunbridge Wells: Pitman Medical.

Brow, J. R., Parker, E., Weinstein, W. M. & Rubin, C. E.
(1971) The small intestinal mucosa in dermatitis
herpetiformis. I. Severity and distribution of the small
intestinal lesion and associated malabsorption.
Gastroenterology, **60**, 355–361.

Brown, D. L., Cooper, A. G. & Hepner, G. W. (1969) IgM
metabolism in coeliac disease. *Lancet*, **i**, 858–861.

Brown, I. L., Ferguson, A., Carswell, F., Horne, C. H. W.
& MacSween, R. N. M. (1973) Autoantibodies in children
with coeliac disease. *Clinical and Experimental
Immunology*, **13**, 373–382.

Bucknall, R. C., Verrier Jones, J. & Peacock, D. B. (1975)

The immune response to ØX174 in man. II. Primary and secondary antibody production in patients with Crohn's disease. *American Journal of Digestive Diseases*, **20**, 430–436.

Bullen, A. W. & Losowsky, M. S. (1976) Cell-mediated immunity (CMI) to gluten fraction III (GFIII) in adult coeliac disease (ACD). *Gut*, **17**, 813.

Bullen, A. W. & Losowsky, M. S. (1977) Peripheral blood lymphocyte subpopulations in adult coeliac disease (CD). *Gut*, **18**, A408–A409.

Burnet, F. M. (1970) The concept of immunological surveillance. *Progress in Experimental Tumor Research*, **13**, 1–27.

Clausen, J. E. (1973) Comparison between capillary tube and agarose migration technique in the study of human peripheral blood leucocytes. *Acta Allergologica*, **28**, 145–158.

Cooke, K. B. (1969) Essential paraproteinaemia. *Proceedings of the Royal Society of Medicine*, **62**, 777–778.

Cooke, W. T. (1968) Adult coeliac disease. In *Progress in Gastroenterology*, ed. Jerzy Glass, G. B. Vol. 1. New York: Grune and Stratton.

Cooke, W. T. & Asquith, P. (1974) In *Coeliac Disease*, ed. Cooke, W. T. & Asquith, P. Clinics in gastroenterology, Vol. 3, No. 1, Ch. 1, pp. 3–10. London: Saunders.

Coombs, R. R. A. & Gell, P. G. H. (1976) Classification of allergic reactions responsible for clinical hypersensitivity and disease. In *Clinical Aspects of Immunology*, 3rd edn, ed. Gell, P. G. H., Coombs, R. R. A. & Lachmann, P. J., pp. 761–782. London: Blackwell.

Cordone, G., Gemme, G., Comelli, A., Vianello, M. G. & Caladoni, S. (1975) Peptidase and coeliac disease. *Lancet*, **i**, 807–808.

Cornell, H. J. (1974) Gliadin degradation and fractionation. In *Coeliac Disease. Proceedings of the Second International Coeliac Symposium*, ed. Hekkens, W. Th. J. M. & Peña, A. S., pp. 74–75. Leiden: Stenfert Kroese.

Crabbé, P. A. (1967) In *Signification du Tissu Lymphoide des musques 'digestives'*. Bruxelles: Editions Arscia SA.

Crabbé, P. A. & Heremans, J. F. (1966) The distribution of immunoglobulin-containing cells along the human gastrointestinal tract. *Gastroenterology*, **51**, 305–316.

David, J. R. & David, R. R. (1972) Cellular hypersensitivity and immunity. Inhibition of macrophage migration and the lymphocyte mediators. *Progress in Allergy*, **16**, 300–449.

Dicke, W. K. (1950) Coeliakie. MD Thesis, Utrecht.

Dissanayake, A. S., Jerrome, D. W., Offord, R. E., Truelove, S. C. & Whitehead, R. (1974) Identifying toxic fractions of wheat gluten and their effect on the jejunal mucosa in coeliac disease. *Gut*, **15**, 931–946.

Doe, W. F., Booth, C. C. & Brown, D. L. (1973). Evidence for complement binding immune complexes in adult coeliac disease, Crohn's disease and ulcerative colitis. *Lancet*, **i**, 402–403.

Doe, W. F., Evans, D., Hobbs, J. R. & Booth, C. C. (1972) Coeliac disease, vasculitis and cryoglobulinaemia. *Gut*, **13**, 112–123.

Doe, W. F., Henry, K. & Booth, C. C. (1974) Complement in coeliac disease. In *Coeliac Disease. Proceedings of the Second International Coeliac Symposium*, ed. Hekkens, W. Th. J. M. & Peña, A. S., pp. 189–196. Leiden: Stenfert Kroese.

Doe, W. F., Henry, K., Holt, L. & Booth, C. C. (1972) An immunological study of adult coeliac disease. *Gut*, **13**, 325–325.

Douglas, A. P. & Weetman, A. P. (1975). Lymphocytes and the gut. *Digestion*, **13**, 344–371.

Douglas, A. P., Crabbé, P. A. & Hobbs, J. R. (1970) Immunochemical studies of the serum, intestinal secretions and intestinal mucosa in patients with adult coeliac disease and other forms of the coeliac syndrome. *Gastroenterology*, **59**, 414–425.

Douglas, A. P., Weetman, A. P. & Haggith, J. W. (1976) The distribution and enteric loss of ^{51}Cr-labelled lymphocytes in normal subjects and in patients with coeliac disease and other disorders of the small intestine. *Digestion*, **14**, 29–43.

Douwes, F. R. (1976) Gluten and lymphocyte sensitization in coeliac disease. *Lancet*, **ii**, 1353.

Dumonde, D. C., Wolstencroft, R. A., Panayi, G. S., Matthew, M., Morley, J. & Howson, W. T. (1969) 'Lymphokines': non-antibody mediators of cellular immunity generated by lymphocyte activation. *Nature (London)*, **224**, 38–42.

Eidelman, S., Davis, S. D., Lagunoff, D. & Rubin, C. E. (1966) The relationship between intestinal plasma cells and serum immunoglobulin A (IgA) in man. *Journal of Clinical Investigation*, **45**, 1003–1004.

Ezeoke, A., Ferguson, N., Fakhri, O., Hekkens, W. Th. J. M. & Hobbs, J. R. (1974) Antibodies in the sera of coeliac patients which can co-opt K-cells to attack gluten-labelled targets. In *Coeliac Disease. Proceedings of the Second International Coeliac Symposium*, ed. Hekkens, W. Th. J. M. & Peña, A. S., pp. 176–186. Leiden: Stenfort Kroese.

Falchuk, Z. M., Gebhard, R. L. & Strober, W. (1974) The pathogenesis of gluten sensitive enteropathy (celiac sprue): organ culture studies. In *Coeliac Disease. Proceedings of the Second International Coeliac Symposium*, ed. Hekkens, W. Th. J. M. & Peña, A. S., pp. 107–117. Leiden: Stenfert Kroese.

Falchuk, Z. M., Laster, L. & Strober, W. (1971) Gluten sensitive enteropathy: intestinal synthesis of antigluten antibody *in vitro*. *Clinical Research*, **19**, 390.

Falchuk, Z. M., Rogentine, G. N. & Strober, W. (1972) Predominance of histocompatibility antigen HL-A8 in patients with gluten-sensitive enteropathy. *Journal of Clinical Investigation*, **15**, 1602–1605.

Falchuk, Z. M., Sessons, C. & Strober, W. (1972) An *in-vitro* model of gluten-sensitive enteropathy (GSE): evidence that gluten is not directly toxic to gastrointestinal (GI) epithelium. *Journal of Clinical Investigation*, **51**, 28a.

Falchuk, Z. M., Gebhard, R. L., Sessoms, C. & Strober, W. (1974) An *in-vitro* model of gluten-sensitive enteropathy. Effect of gliadin on intestinal epithelial cells of patients with gluten-sensitive enteropathy in organ culture. *Journal of Clinical Investigation*, **53**, 487–500.

Ferguson, A. (1974) Lymphocytes in coeliac disease. In *Coeliac Disease. Proceedings of the Second International Coeliac Symposium*, ed. Hekkens, W. Th. J. M. & Peña, A. S., pp. 265–276. Leiden: Stenfert Kroese.

Ferguson, A. & Carswell, F. (1972) Precipitins to dietary proteins in serum and upper intestinal secretions of coeliac children. *British Medical Journal*, **i**, 75–77.

Ferguson, A. & Murray, D. (1971) Quantitation of intraepithelial lymphocytes in human jejunum. *Gut*, **12**, 988–994.

Ferguson, A., Maxwell, J. D. & Hutton, M. M. (1969) Splenic function in adult coeliac disease. *Scottish Medical Journal*, **14**, 261.

Ferguson, A., MacDonald, T. T., McClure, J. P. and Holden, R. J. (1975) Cell-mediated immunity to gliadin within the small intestinal mucosa in coeliac disease. *Lancet*, **i,** 895–897.

Ferguson, R., Asquith, P. & Cooke, W. T. (1974a) Histocompatibility antigens in coeliac disease. *Gut*, **15,** 834.

Ferguson, R., Asquith, P. & Cooke, W. T. (1974b) The jejunal cellular infiltrate in coeliac disease complicated by lymphoma. *Gut*, **15,** 458–461.

Franklin, R. H. (1970) Post-vagotomy diarrhoea? *British Medical Journal*, **i,** 412.

Frazer, A. C. (1956) Discussion on some problems of steatorrhoea and reduced stature. *Proceedings of the Royal Society of Medicine*, **49,** 1009–1013.

Frazer, A. C., Fletcher, R. F., Ross, C. A. C., Shaw, B. Sammons, H. G. & Schneider, R. (1959) Gluten-induced enteropathy. The effect of partially digested gluten. *Lancet*, **ii,** 252–255.

Fry, L., Seah, P. P. & Hoffbrand, A. V. (1974) Dermatitis herpetiformis. In *Clinics in Gastroenterology*, ed. Cooke, W. T. & Asquith, P., Vol 3, No. 1, Ch. 9, pp. 145–157. London: Saunders.

Fry, L., Seah, P. P., McMinn, R. M. H. & Hoffbrand, A. V. (1972) Lymphocytic infiltration of epithelium in diagnosis of gluten-sensitive enteropathy. *British Medical Journal*, **iii,** 371–374.

Fry, L., Seah, P. P., Riches, D. J. & Hoffbrand, A. V. (1973) Clearance of skin lesions in dermatitis herpetiformis after gluten withdrawal. *Lancet*, **i,** 288–291.

Gasbarrini, G., Miglio, F., Serra, M. A. & Bernardi, M. (1974) Immunological studies of the jejunal mucosa in normal subjects and adult celiac patients. *Digestion*, **10,** 122–128.

Gebhard, R. L., Falchuk, Z. M., Katz, I., Sessoms, C., Rogentine, G. N. & Strober, W. (1974) Dermatitis herpetiformis: immunologic concomitants of small intestinal disease and relationship to histocompatibility antigen HL-A8. *Journal of Clinical Investigation*, **54,** 98–103.

Gee, S. (1888) On the coeliac affection. *St. Bartholomew's Hospital Reports*, **24,** 17–20.

Geha, R. S. (1977) Origin of the antibody-dependent cytotoxic cell in man. *Clinical Immunology and Immunopathology*, **7,** 253–261.

Gough, K. R., Read, A. E. & Naish, J. M. (1962) Intestinal reticulosis as a complication of idiopathic steatorrhoea. *Gut*, **3,** 232–239.

Greenberg, A. H., Shen, L. & Roitt, I. M. (1973) Characterization of the antibody-dependent cytotoxic cell. A non-phagocytic monocyte? *Clinical and Experimental Immunology*, **15,** 251–259.

Haeney, M. R. & Asquith, P. (1976) Stimulation of lymphocytes from patients with coeliac disease by a subfraction of gluten. *Lancet*, **ii,** 629–630.

Haeney, M. R. & Asquith P. (1978) Inhibition of leucocyte migration by α gliadin in patients with gastrointestinal disease: its specificity with respect to α gliadin and coeliac disease. In *Perspectives in Coeliac Disease*. ed. McNicholl, B., McCarthy, C. F. & Fottrell, P. F. pp. 229–241. Lancaster: MTP Press.

Halliday, W. J., Maluish, A. & Isbister, W. H. (1974) Detection of antitumour cell mediated immunity and serum blocking factors in cancer patients by the leucocyte adherence inhibition test. *British Journal of Cancer*, **29,** 31–35.

Hardy, D. A. & Ling, N. R. (1969) Effects of some cellular antigens on lymphocytes and the nature of the mixed lymphocyte reaction. *Nature (London)*, **221,** 545–548.

Hardy, D. A., Knight, S. & Ling, N. R. (1970) The interaction of normal lymphocytes and cells from lymphoid cell lines. I. The nature of the activation process. *Immunology*, **19,** 329–342.

Hardy, D. A., Ling, N. R., Wallin, J. & Aviet, T. (1970) Destruction of lymphoid cells by activated human lymphocytes. *Nature (London)*, **227,** 723–725.

Harms, K., Granditsch, G., Rossipal, E., Ludwig, H., Polymenidis, Z., Scholz, S., Wank, R. & Albert, E. D. (1974) HL-A in patients with coeliac disease and their families. In *Coeliac Disease. Proceedings of the Second International Coeliac Symposium*, ed. Hekkens, W. Th. J. M. and Peña, A. S., pp. 215–226. Leiden: Stenfert Kroese.

Harrington, C. I. & Read, N. W. (1977) Dermatitis herpetiformis: effect of gluten-free diet on skin IgA and jejunal structure and function. *British Medical Journal*, **i,** 872–875.

Harris, O. D., Cooke, W. T., Thompson, H. & Waterhouse, J. A. H. (1967) Malignancy in adult coeliac disease and idiopathic steatorrhoea. *American Journal of Medicine*, **42,** 899–912.

Hekkens, W. Th. J. M., van den Aarsen, J., Gilliams, J. P. Lems-van Kan, Ph., Bouma-Frölich, G. (1974) α gliadin structure and degradation. In *Coeliac Disease. Proceedings of the Second International Coeliac Symposium*, ed. Hekkens, W. Th. J. M. & Peña, A. S., pp. 39–45. Leiden: Stenfert Kroese.

Hobart, M. J. & McConnell, I. (1975) *The Immune System: A course on the molecular and cellular basis of immunity*, p. 184. Oxford: Blackwell Scientific Publications.

Hobbs, J. R. & Hepner, G. W. (1968) Deficiency of IgM-globulin in coeliac disease. *Lancet*, **i,** 217–220.

Hobbs, J. R., Hepner, E. W., Douglas, A. P., Crabbé, P. A. & Johannsson, S. G. O. (1969) Immunological mystery of coeliac disease. *Lancet*, **ii,** 649–650.

Hoffman, H. N., Wollaeger, E. E. & Greenberg, E. (1966) Discordance for non-tropical sprue (adult coeliac disease) in a monozygotic twin pair. *Gastroenterology*, **51,** 36–42.

Holmes, G. K. T. (1974) Studies in adult coeliac disease. MD Thesis, Birmingham.

Holmes, G. K. T., Asquith, P. & Cooke, W. T. (1976) Cell-mediated immunity to gluten faction III in adult coeliac disease. *Clinical and Experimental Immunology*, **24,** 259–265.

Holmes, G. K. T., Asquith, P., Stokes, P. L. & Cooke, W. T. (1974) Cellular infiltrate of jejunal biopsies in adult coeliac disease in relation to gluten withdrawal. *Gut*, **15,** 278–283.

Holmes, G. K. T., Stokes, P. L., Sorahan, T. M., Prior, P., Waterhouse, J. A. H. & Cooke, W. T. (1976) Coeliac disease, gluten-free diet and malignancy. *Gut*, **17,** 612–619.

Holt, P. L. J. (1969) In discussion. In *Coeliac Disease*, ed. Booth, C. C. & Dowling, R. H., p. 150. Edinburgh: Churchill Livingstone.

Hood, J. & Mason, A. M. S. (1970) Diffuse pulmonary disease with transfer defect occurring with coeliac disease. *Lancet*, **i,** 445–448.

Housley, J., Asquith, P. & Cooke, W. T. (1969) Immune response to gluten in adult coeliac disease. *British Medical Journal*, **ii,** 159–161.

Immonen, P. (1967) Levels of serum immunoglobulins IgA, IgG and IgM in the malabsorption syndrome in children. *Annales Paediatriae Fenniae*, **13,** 115–153.

Jarnum, S., Jensen, K. B., Søltoft, J. & Westergaardh, (1970) Protein loss and turnover of albumin IgG and IgM in adult coeliac disease. In *Coeliac Disease*, ed. Booth,

C. C. & Dowling, R. H., pp. 163–172. Edinburgh: Churchill Livingstone.

Jondal, M., Holm, G. & Wigzell, H. (1972) Surface markers on human T and B lymphocytes. I. A large population of lymphocytes forming non-immune rosettes with sheep red blood cells. *Journal of Experimental Medicine*, **136**, 207–215.

Jos, J. (1974) In discussion. In *Coeliac Disease. Proceedings of the Second International Coeliac Symposium*, ed. Hekkens, W. Th. J. M. & Peña, A. S., p. 106. Leiden: Stenfert Kroese.

Jos, J., Rey, J. & Frézal, J. (1972) Étude immunohistochimique de la muqueuse intestinale chez l'enfant. *Archives Françaises de Pédiatrie*, **29**, 681–698.

Jos, J., Lenoir, G., de Ritis, G. & Rey, J. (1974). *In-vitro* culturing of biopsies from children. In *Coeliac Disease. Proceedings of the Second International Coeliac Symposium*, ed. Hekkens, W. Th. J. M. & Peña, A. S., pp. 91–105. Leiden: Stenfert Kroese.

Kasarda, D. D., Nimmo, C. C. & Bernardin, J. E. (1974) Structural aspects and genetic relationships of gliadins. In *Coeliac Disease. Proceedings of the Second International Coeliac Symposium*, ed. Hekkens, W. Th. J. M. & Peña, A. S., pp. 25–36. Leiden: Stenfert Kroese.

Katz, J., Kantor, F. S. & Herskovic, T. (1968) Intestinal antibodies to wheat fractions in celiac disease. *Annals of Internal Medicine*, **69**, 1149–1153.

Katz, S. I., Falchuk, Z. M., Dahl, M. V., Rogentine, G. H. & Strober, W. (1972) HL-A8: a genetic link between dermatitis herpetiformis and gluten sensitive enteropathy. *Journal of Clinical Investigation*, **51**, 2977–2979.

Kenrick, K. G. & Walker-Smith, J. A. (1970) Immunoglobulins and dietary protein antibodies in childhood coeliac disease. *Gut*, **11**, 635–640.

Keunning, J. J., Peña, A. S., Van Leewen, A., Van Hooff, J. P. & Van Rood, J. J. (1976) HLA-DW-3 associated with coeliac disease. *Lancet*, **i**, 506–508.

Kowlessar, O. D. (1967) Effect of wheat proteins in celiac disease. *Gastroenterology*, **52**, 893–895.

Krainick, H. G., Debantin, F., Gautier, E., Tobler, R. & Velasco, J. A. (1958) Additional research on the injurious effect of wheat flour in coeliac disease. 1. Acute gliadin reactions (gliadin shock). *Helvetica Pediatrica Acta*, **13**, 432–454.

Krueger, G. R. F. (1972) Chronic immunosuppression and lymphomagenesis in man and mice. *National Cancer Institute Monograph*, **35**, 183–190.

Kumar, P. J., Ferguson, A., Lancaster-Smith, M. & Clark, M. L. (1976) Food antibodies in patients with dermatitis herpetiformis and adult coeliac disease – relationship to jejunal morphology. *Scandinavian Journal of Gastroenterology*, **11**, 5–9.

Kumar, P. J., Silk, D. B. A., Marks, R., Clark, M. L. & Dawson, A. M. (1973) Treatment of dermatitis herpetiformis with corticosteroids and a gluten-free diet: a study of jejunal morphology and function. *Gut*, **14**, 280–283.

Lancaster-Smith, M. J., Benson, M. K. & Strickland, I. D. (1971) Coeliac disease and diffuse interstitial lung disease. *Lancet*, **i**, 473–476.

Lancaster-Smith, M., Packer, S., Kumar, P. J. & Harries, J. T. (1976a) Cellular infiltrate of the jejunum after reintroduction of dietary gluten in children with treated coeliac disease. *Journal of Clinical Pathology*, **29**, 587–591.

Lancaster-Smith, M., Packer, S., Kumar, P. J. & Harries, J. T. (1976b) Immunological phenomena in the jejunum and serum after reintroduction of dietary gluten in children with treated coeliac disease. *Journal of Clinical Pathology*, **29**, 592–597.

Lancaster-Smith, M. J., Perrin, J., Swarbrick, E. T. & Wright, J. T. (1974b) Coeliac disease and autoimmunity. *Postgraduate Medical Journal*, **50**, 45–48.

Lancaster-Smith, M., Kumar, P., Marks, R., Clark, M. L. & Dawson, A. M. (1974a) Jejunal mucosal immunoglobulin-containing cells and jejunal fluid immunoglobulins in adult coeliac disease and dermatitis herpetiformis. *Gut*, **15**, 371–376.

Ling, N. R. (1973) Immune surveillance of lymphoid tissue. A biological role for the mixed lymphocyte reaction. *Immunological Communications*, **2**, 119–127.

Ling, N. R. & Kay, J. E. (1975) *Lymphocyte Stimulation*, 2nd ed. Amsterdam: North-Holland Publishing Co.

Loeb, P. M., Strober, W., Falchuk, Z. M. & Laster, L. (1971) Incorporation of leucine-^{14}C into immunoglobulins by jejunal biopsies of patients with celiac sprue and other gastrointestinal diseases. *Journal of Clinical Investigation*, **50**, 559–569.

McCarthy, C. F., Fraser, I. D., Evans, K. T. & Read, A. E. (1966) Lymphoreticular dysfunction in idiopathic steatorrhoea. *Gut*, **7**, 140–148.

McCarthy, C. F., Mylotte, M., Stevens, F., Egan-Mitchell, B., Fottrell, P. F. & McNicholl, B. (1974) Family studies on coeliac disease in Ireland. In *Coeliac Disease. Proceedings of the Second International Coeliac Symposium*, ed. Hekkens, W. Th. J. M. & Peña, A. S., pp. 311–319. Leiden: Stenfert Kroese.

McDevitt, H. O. & Bodmer, W. F. (1972) Histocompatibility antigens, immune responsiveness and susceptibility to disease. *American Journal of Medicine*, **52**, 1–8.

Maclaurin, B. P., Cooke, W. T. & Ling, N. R. (1971) Impaired lymphocyte reactivity against tumour cells in patients with coeliac disease. *Gut*, **12**, 794–800.

Maclennan, I. C. M. & Harding, B. (1970) Failure of certain cytotoxic lymphocytes to respond mitotically to phytohaemagglutinin. *Nature (London)*, **227**, 1246–1248.

Maclennan, I. C. M. & Harding, B. (1974) Non-T cytotoxicity *in vitro*. In *Progress in Immunology II*. ed. Brent, L. & Holborow, J., Vol. 3, pp. 347–350. Amsterdam: North-Holland Publishing Co.

McNeish, A. S., Rolles, C. J. & Thompson, R. A. (1974) Complement and its degradation products after challenge with gluten in children with coeliac disease. In *Coeliac Disease. Proceedings of the Second International Coeliac Symposium*, ed. Hekkens, W. Th. J. M. & Peña, A. S., pp. 197–199. Leiden: Stenfert Kroese.

Magalhaes, A. F. N., Peters, T. J. & Doe, W. F. (1974) Studies on the nature and significance of connective tissue antibodies in adult coeliac disease and Crohn's disease. *Gut*, **15**, 284–288.

Major, R. H. (1945) *Classic Descriptions of Disease*. Springfield: Thomas, C. C.

Mann, D. L., Katz, S. I., Nelson, D. L., Abelson, L. D. & Strober, W. (1976) Specific B-cell antigen associated with gluten-sensitive enteropathy and dermatitis herpetiformis. *Lancet*, **i**, 110–111.

Marks, J., Shuster, S. & Watson, A. J. (1966) Small bowel changes in dermatitis herpetiformis. *Lancet*, **ii**, 1280.

Martinez, C. (1964) Effect of early thymectomy on development of mammary tumours in mice. *Nature*, **203**, 1188.

Mavromichalis, J., Brueton, M. J., McNeish, A. S. & Anderson, C. M. (1976) Evaluation of the intraepithelial lymphocyte count in the jejunum in childhood enteropathies. *Gut*, **17**, 600–603.

Mawhinney, H. & Love, A. H. G. (1975) The immunoglobulin class response to oral poliovaccine in coeliac disease. *Clinical and Experimental Immunology*, 21, 399–406.

Meeuwisse, G. W. (1970) Diagnostic criteria in coeliac disease. *Acta Paediatrica Scandinavica*, 59, 461–463.

Mietens, C. (1967) Antikörperbildunggegen gliadin und milch proteine II. *Zeitschrift für Kinderheilkunde*, 99, 130–139.

Miller, J. F. A. P. (1962) Effect of neonatal thymectomy on the immunological responsiveness of the mouse. *Proceedings of the Royal Society of London, Series B*, 156, 415–428.

Montgomery, R. D. & Shearer, A. C. I. (1974) The cell population of the upper jejunal mucosa in tropical sprue and post-infective malabsorption. *Gut*, 15, 387–391.

Morganroth, J., Watson, D. W. & French, A. B. (1972) Cellular and humoral sensitivity to gluten fractions in patients with treated non-tropical sprue. *American Journal of Digestive Diseases*, 17, 205–212.

Morris, J. S., Read, A. E., Jones, B., Cotes, J. E. & Edwards, J. H. (1971) Coeliac disease and lung disease. *Lancet*, i, 754.

Morris, P. J. (1975) The major histocompatibility system (HL-A) and disease in man. In *Topics in Gastroenterology*, 3rd edn., ed. Truelove, S. C. & Goodman, M. J., Ch. 13, pp. 197–208. Oxford: Blackwell.

Moticka, E. J. (1974) The non-specific stimulation of immunoglobulin secretion following specific stimulation of the immune system. *Immunology*, 27, 401–412.

Mowbray, J. F., Hoffbrand, A. V., Holborow, E. J., Seah, P. P. & Fry, L. (1973) Circulating immune complexes in dermatitis herpetiformis. *Lancet*, i, 400–402.

Nelson, D. L. & Strober, W. (1974) Quoted by Strober, W., Falchuk, Z. M., Nelson, D. L. & Gebhard, R. M. The Pathogenesis of gluten-sensitive enteropathy. In *Progress in Immunology II*, ed. Brent, L. & Holborow, J., Vol. 4, pp. 221–229. Amsterdam: North Holland Publishing Co.

Nelson, D. L., Falchuk, Z. M., Kasarda, D. & Strober, W. (1975) Gluten-sensitive enteropathy; correlation of organ culture behaviour with HL-A status. *Clinical Research*, 23, 254.

O'Donoghue, D. P., Lancaster-Smith, M., Laviniere, P. & Kumar, P. J. (1976) T-cell depletion in untreated adult coeliac disease. *Gut*, 17, 328–331.

Parrott, D. M. V. (1976) The gut-associated lymphoid tissues and gastrointestinal immunity. In *Immunological Aspects of the Liver and Gastrointestinal Tract*, ed. Ferguson, A. & MacSween, R. N. M., pp. 1–32. Lancaster: MTP Press.

Paulley, J. W. (1954) Observations on the aetiology of idiopathic steatorrhoea. Jejunal and lymph node biopsies. *British Medical Journal*, ii, 1318–1321.

Peacock, D. B., Verrier Jones, J. & Gough, M. (1973) The immune response to ØX174 in man. I. Primary and secondary antibody production in normal adults. *Clinical and Experimental Immunology*, 13, 497–513.

Peña, A. S., Nieuwkoop, J. V., Schuit, H. R. E., Hekkens, W. Th. J. M. & Haek, A. J. Ch. (1976) Transient paraproteinaemia in a patient with coeliac disease. *Gut*, 17, 735–739.

Peña, A. S., Mann, D. L., Hague, M. E., Heck, J., Van Leeuwen, A., Van Rood, J. J. & Strober, W. (1977) B-cell antigens in coeliac disease (gluten-sensitive enteropathy). *Gut*, 18, A409.

Perlmann, P. (1976) Cellular immunity: antibody-dependent cytotoxicity (K-cell activity). In *Clinical Immunobiology*, ed. Bach, F. H. & Good, R. A. Vol. 3, pp. 107–132. New York: Academic Press.

Perlmann, P. & Holm, G. (1969) Cytotoxic effects of lymphoid cells *in vitro*. *Advances in Immunology*, 11, 117–193.

Petreshock, E. P., Pessah, M. & Menachemi, E. (1975) Adenocarcinoma of the jejunum associated with non-tropical sprue. *American Journal of Digestive Diseases*, 20, 796–802.

Pettingale, K. W. (1970) Immunoglobulin and specific antibody responses to antigenic stimulation in adult coeliac disease. *Clinical Science*, 38, 16P.

Phelan, J. J., McCarthy, C. F., Stevens, F. M., McNichol, B. & Fottrell, P. E. (1974) The nature of gliadin toxicity in coeliac disease: a new concept. In *Coeliac Disease. Proceedings of the Second International Coeliac Symposium*, ed. Hekkens, W. Th. J. M. & Peña, A. S., pp. 60–70. Leiden: Stenfert Kroese.

Pink, I. J. & Creamer, B. (1967) Response to a gluten-free diet of patients with coeliac syndrome. *Lancet*, i, 300–304.

Popović, O., Andrejevic, M., Pendić, B., Lovrić, L. & Djordjević, V. (1970) Lymphocyte transformation in coeliac disease. *Lancet*, ii, 725.

Remold, H. G., Katz, A. B., Haber, E. & David, J. R. (1970) Studies on migration inhibitory factor (MIF): recovery of MIF activity after purification by gel filtration and disc electrophoresis. *Cellular Immunology*, 1, 133–145.

Rizzetto, M. & Doniach, D. (1973) Types of 'reticulin' antibodies detected in human sera by immunofluorescence. *Journal of Clinical Pathology*, 26, 841–851.

Robinson, T. J. (1976) Coeliac disease with farmers' lung. *British Medical Journal*, i, 745–746.

Rocklin, R. E. (1974) Products of activated lymphocytes. Leukocyte inhibitory factor (LIF) distinct from migration inhibitory factor (MIF). *Journal of Immunology*, 112, 1461–1466.

Rocklin, R. E., MacDermott, R. P., Chess, L., Schlossman, S. F. & David, J. R. (1974) Studies on mediator production by highly purified human T and B lymphocytes. *Journal of Experimental Medicine*, 140, 1303–1316.

Rossipal, E. (1974) Precipitating antibodies and complement in coeliac children. In *Coeliac Disease. Proceedings of the Second International Coeliac Symposium*, ed. Hekkens, W. Th. J. M. & Peña, A. S., pp. 200–202. Leiden: Stenfert Kroese.

Rothberg, R. M., Kraft, S. C., Asquith, P. & Michalek, S. M. (1972) The effect of splenectomy on the immune response of rabbits to a soluble protein antigen given parenterally or orally. *Cellular Immunology*, 7, 124–131.

Rubin, C. E., Eidelman, S. & Weinstein, W. M. (1970) Sprue by any other name. *Gastroenterology*, 58, 409–413.

Rubin, C. E., Brandborg, L. L., Phelps, P. C. & Taylor, H. C. Jr. (1960) Studies of coeliac disease. 1. The apparent identical and specific nature of the duodenal and proximal jejunal lesion in coeliac disease and idiopathic steatorrhoea. *Gastroenterology*, 38, 28–49.

Rubin, W., Fauci, A. S., Sleisenger, M. H. & Jeffries, G. H. (1965) Immunofluorescent studies in adult celiac disease. *Journal of Clinical Investigation*, 44, 475–485.

Ryan, F. P., Holdsworth, C. D. & Verrier Jones, J. (1977) Impaired immunity in ulcerative colitis with hyposplenism: the response to the intravenous antigen ØX174. *Gut*, 18, A424.

Sampson, R. R., McClelland, D. B. L. & Shearman, D. J. C. (1973) Studies on the quantitation of immunoglobulin in human intestinal secretions. *Gut*, **14**, 616–626.

Savilahti, E. (1972a) Immunoglobulin-containing cells in the intestinal mucosa and immunoglobulins in the intestinal juice in children. *Clinical and Experimental Immunology*, **11**, 415–425.

Savilahti, E. (1972b) Intestinal immunoglobulins in children with coeliac disease. *Gut*, **13**, 958–964.

Scadding, J. G. (1970) Lung biopsy in the diagnosis of diffuse lung disease. *British Medical Journal*, **ii**, 557–564.

Schmerling, D. H. & Shiner, M. (1970) The response of the intestinal mucosa to the intraduodenal instillation of gluten in patients with coeliac disease during remission. In *Coeliac Disease*, ed. Booth, C. C. & Dowling, R. H., pp. 64–75. Edinburgh: Churchill Livingstone.

Schneider, R., Kendall, M. J., Hawkins, C. F. (1974) Gliadin subfractionation. In *Coeliac Disease. Proceedings of the Second International Coeliac Symposium*, ed. Hekkens, W. Th. J. M. & Peña, A. S., pp. 72–73. Leiden: Stenfert Kroese.

Schwartz, R. S. (1974) Immunosuppression and neoplasia. In *Progress in Immunology II*, ed. Brent, L. & Holborow, J. Vol. 5, Clinical Aspects II, pp. 229–232. Amsterdam: North Holland Publishing Co.

Scott, B. B. (1975) Personal communication.

Scott, B. B. & Losowsky, M. S. (1975) Coeliac disease: a cause of various associated diseases? *Lancet*, **ii**, 956–957.

Scott, B. B. & Losowsky, M. S. (1976a) Depressed cell-mediated immunity in coeliac disease. *Gut*, **17**, 900–905.

Scott, B. B. & Losowsky, M. S. (1976b) Cell-mediated autoimmunity in coeliac disease. *Clinical and Experimental Immunology*, **26**, 243–246.

Scott, B. B., Losowsky, M. S. & Rajah, S. M. (1974) HL-A8 and HL-A12 in coeliac disease. *Lancet*, **ii**, 171.

Scott, B. B., Scott, D. G. & Losowsky, M. S. (1977) Evidence for mucosal immune complexes in untreated coeliac disease. *Gut*, **18**, A409.

Seah, P. P., Fry, L., Hoffbrand, A. V. & Holborow, E. J. (1971a) Tissue antibodies in dermatitis herpetiformis and adult coeliac disease. *Lancet*, **i**, 834–836.

Seah, P. P., Fry, L., Rossiter, M. A., Hoffbrand, A. V., & Holborow, E. J. (1971b) Anti-reticulin antibodies in childhood coeliac disease. *Lancet*, **ii**, 681–682.

Seah, P. P., Fry, L., Mazaheri, M. R., Mowbray, J. F., Hoffbrand, A. V. & Holborow, E. J. (1973b) Alternative pathway complement fixation by IgA in the skin in dermatitis herpetiformis. *Lancet*, **ii**, 175.

Seah, P. P., Fry, L., Stewart, J. S., Chapman, B. L., Hoffbrand, A. V. & Holborow, E. J. (1972) Immunoglobulins in the skin in dermatitis herpetiformis and coeliac disease. *Lancet*, **i**, 611–614.

Seah, P. P., Fry, L., Holborow, E. J., Rossiter, M. A., Doe, W. F., Magalhaes, A. F. & Hoffbrand, A. V. (1973a) Antireticulin antibody: incidence and diagnostic significance. *Gut*, **14**, 311–315.

Shiner, M. (1956) Duodenal biopsy. *Lancet*, **i**, 17–19.

Shiner, M. (1973) Ultrastructural changes suggestive of immune reactions in the jejunal mucosa of coeliac children following gluten challenge. *Gut*, **14**, 1–12.

Shiner, M. & Ballard, J. (1972) Antigen–antibody reactions in jejunal mucosa in childhood coeliac disease after gluten challenge. *Lancet*, **i**, 1202–1205.

Sikora, K., Anand, B. S., Truelove, S. C., Ciclitira, P. J. & Offord, R. E. (1976) Stimulation of lymphocytes from patients with coeliac disease by a subfraction of gluten. *Lancet*, **ii**, 389–391.

Söltoft, J. (1969) Immunoglobulin-containing cells in normal jejunal mucosa in ulcerative colitis and regional enteritis. *Scandinavian Journal of Gastroenterology*, **4**, 353–360.

Søltoft, J. (1970) Immunoglobulin-containing cells in non-tropical sprue. *Clinical and Experimental Immunology*, **6**, 413–420.

Søltoft, J. & Søeberg, B. (1972) Immunoglobulin-containing cells in the small intestine in viral hepatitis. *Acta Pathologica et Microbiologica Scandinavica*, Section B, **80**, 379–387.

Søltoft, J. & Weeke, B. (1969) Immunoglobulins in serum and jejunal biopsies in non-tropical sprue. *Acta Medica Scandinavica*, **186**, 459–464.

Spitler, L., Huber, H. & Fudenberg, H. H. (1969) Inhibition of capillary migration by antigen–antibody complexes. *Journal of Immunology*, **102**, 404–411.

Stokes, P. L. & Holmes, G. K. T. (1974) Malignancy. In *Clinics in Gastroenterology*, ed. Cooke, W. T. & Asquith, P., Vol. 3, No. 1, pp. 159–170. London: Saunders.

Stokes, P. L., Asquith, P. & Cooke, W. T. (1973) Genetics of coeliac disease. In *Clinics in Gastroenterology*, ed. McConnell, R. B., 2, No. 3, pp. 547–556. London: Saunders.

Stokes, P. L., Asquith, P., Holmes, G. K. T., Mackintosh, P. & Cooke, W. T. (1972) Histocompatibility antigens associated with adult coeliac disease. *Lancet*, **ii**, 162–164.

Stutman, O. (1974) Tumor development after 3-methyl cholanthrene in immunologically deficient athymic nude mice. *Science*, **183**, 534–536.

Taylor, K. B., Thompson, D. L., Truelove, S. C. & Wright, R. (1961) An immunological study of coeliac disease and idiopathic steatorrhoea. Serological reactions to gluten and milk proteins. *British Medical Journal*, **ii**, 1727–1731.

Thomas, L. (1959) Discussion in *Cellular and Humoral Aspects of the Hypersensitive States*, ed. Lawrence, H. S., pp. 529–532. New York: Hoeber-Harper.

Thompson, R. A. (1974) Anticomplementary activity of serum and immune complexes. *British Medical Journal*, **ii**, 60.

Townley, R. R. W., Bhathal, P. S., Cornell, H. J. & Mitchell, J. D. (1973) Toxicity of wheat gliadin fractions in coeliac disease. *Lancet*, **i**, 1362–1364.

Tubergen, D. G., Feldman, J. D., Pollock, E. M. & Lerner, R. A. (1972) Production of macrophage migration inhibition factor by continous cell lines. *Journal of Experimental Medicine*, **135**, 255–266.

Van Boxel, J. A., Stobo, J. D., Paul, W. E. & Green, I. (1972) Antibody-dependent lymphoid cell-mediated cytotoxicity: no requirement for thymus-derived lymphocytes. *Science*, **175**, 194–196.

Verrier Jones, J. & Cumming, R. H. (1977) Tests for circulating immune complexes. In *Techniques in Clinical Immunology*, ed. Thompson, R. A., Ch. 7, pp. 136–156. Oxford: Blackwell.

Von Büllow, H., Grüttner, R., Lücking, Th., Schulz, K. H. & Tripcke, B. (1974) Cell-mediated immunity in coeliac disease. In *Coeliac Disease. Proceedings of the Second International Coeliac Symposium*, ed. Hekkens, W. Th. J. M. & Peña, A. S., pp. 240–241. Leiden: Stenfert Kroese.

Von Essen, R., Savilahti, E. & Pelkonen, P. (1972) Reticulin antibody in children with malabsorption. *Lancet*, **i**, 1157–1159.

Walker-Smith, J. A. (1973) Discordance for childhood coeliac disease in monozygotic twins. *Gut*, **14**, 374–375.

Wall, A. J., Douglas, A. D., Booth, C. C. & Pearse, A. G. E. (1970) Response of the jejunal mucosa in adult coeliac disease to oral prednisolone. *Gut*, **11**, 7–14.

Watson, D. W. (1969) Immune responses and the gut. *Gastroenterology*, **56**, 944–965.

Weiser, M. M. & Douglas, A. P. (1976) An alternative mechanism for gluten toxicity in coeliac disease. *Lancet*, **i**, 567–569.

WHO (1975) Histocompatibility testing 1975, ed. Kissmeyer-Hielsen, F. Copenhagen: Munksgaard.

Williamson, N., Asquith, P., Stokes, P. L., Jowett, A. W. & Cooke, W. T. (1976) Anticonnective tissue and other antitissue 'antibodies' in the sera of patients with coeliac disease compared with the findings in a mixed hospital population. *Journal of Clinical Pathology*, **29**, 484–494.

Winter, G. C. B., McCarthy, C. F., Read, A. E. & Yoffey, J. M. (1967) Development of macrophages in phytohaemagglutinin in cultures of blood from patients with idiopathic steatorrhoea and with cirrhosis. *British Journal of Experimental Pathology*, **48**, 66–80.

Yeomans, N. D. (1974) Pathogenesis of coeliac sprue. *Lancet*, **ii**, 843–844.

Young, V. H. (1969) Transient paraproteins. *Proceedings of the Royal Society of Medicine*, **62**, 778–780.

7. Inflammatory bowel disease (ulcerative colitis and Crohn's disease)

Sumner C. Kraft

INTRODUCTION

Ulcerative colitis and Crohn's disease are inflammatory bowel disorders of unknown aetiology which must be diagnosed by the exclusion of numerous *specific* diseases. While Crohn's disease may involve any portion of the alimentary canal from the lips to the anus, often in a discontinuous distribution, the symptomatic intestinal manifestations of ulcerative colitis are limited to the colon. Both may be accompanied by similar extraintestinal lesions; the frequency and temporal relations of these complications have led to an increasing acceptance of the likelihood that these conditions represent interrelated systemic disorders. Furthermore, both intestinal diseases generally respond favourably to similar or identical medical therapy (Kirsner, 1970; Thayer, 1970).

Ulcerative colitis is an acute and chronic inflammatory process which diffusely involves the colonic mucosa, although ulceration is not always a prominent feature. In acute disease, the patient may be seriously ill with 20 or more watery, bloody stools per day, dehydration, anaemia, hypoproteinaemia and fever. Many patients follow a chronic course with frequent exacerbations, but this may vary considerably and prolonged remissions are not uncommon. Proctosigmoidoscopy classically reveals evidence of diffuse mucosal abnormalities, including oedema, hyperaemia, fine granularity, petechial haemorrhages, ulceration, friability on cotton wiping, and a mucopurulent, sanguineous exudate. *Crohn's disease* is a persistent or relapsing, transmural, granulomatous inflammatory process resulting in strictures, fissured ulcers, sinuses and fistulas. Clinical accompaniments may include abdominal pain, diarrhoea, malnutrition, inflammatory masses, and severe anal disease. Although confined to the small intestine in half the cases (regional enteritis), ileal and colonic disease often occur together (ileocolitis), or the process may be confined to the colon (Crohn's colitis) and mimic ulcerative colitis. Proctosigmoidoscopy in Crohn's colitis may show patchy, fine or coarse granularity or shallow aphthoid ulceration, with biopsy evidence of sarcoid-type granulomas in about one-third of the cases (Kraft and Kirsner, 1971a; Kraft and Wall, 1976; Wall and Kraft, 1976).

In dealing with disease limited to the colon, the distinction between ulcerative colitis and Crohn's disease is often difficult clinically, radiologically and pathologically, even with the availability of a total proctocolectomy specimen (Schachter, Goldstein, Rappaport, Fennessy and Kirsner, 1970). The pathological diagnosis must rest upon cumulative gross and microscopic features (Schachter and Kirsner, 1975), but a small percentage of patients with nonspecific inflammatory disease of the colon may have to be given the deferred diagnosis of 'indeterminate' colitis. Hypotheses to explain the aetiology of inflammatory bowel disease have attempted to implicate infectious agents, endotoxins, destructive enzymes, various deficiency states, colonic motor changes, vascular disturbances, an autonomic nerve imbalance, psychogenic mechanisms, metabolic defects, connective tissue disorders, defective mucosal regeneration, and immunological phenomena (Kirsner and Palmer, 1954; Kraft, 1976). While this chapter will primarily emphasize the last of this list, several of these categories must interact pathogenetically. Furthermore, many colonic disorders present with similar clinical and radiographic findings and the possibility exists that ulcerative colitis and Crohn's disease each may consist of aetiologically heterogeneous subgroups (Kirsner, 1971).

Indirect evidence implicating immunological mechanisms in the aetiology of inflammatory bowel disease includes the not unusual personal and family histories of allergic disorders; the occasional association of ulcerative colitis with other disorders often linked with immunological mechanisms; the frequency of the disease among young people; the multiplicity of connective tissue-type diseases in occasional patients with ulcerative colitis; increasingly reported numbers of family occurrences of inflammatory bowel disease; and the beneficial response to ACTH and adrenal corticosteriod therapy and, in selected instances, to azathioprine and other potentially immunosuppressive drugs (Kraft and Kirsner, 1975). Progress over the past two decades has been impressive and forms the basis for many detailed discussions (Kraft, Bregman and Kirsner, 1962; Kraft and Kirsner, 1966, 1968, 1971a, b; Watson, 1969; Wright, 1970; Kirsner, 1970). This chapter will highlight the major studies of humoral and cellular immune phenomena in inflammatory bowel disease, with special emphasis on publications appearing since a previous review (Kraft and Kirsner, 1971b). However, some earlier work will be included since more recent observations have possibly served to put hitherto unexplained observations into better perspective.

ULCERATIVE COLITIS

HUMORAL IMMUNE PHENOMENA AND ULCERATIVE COLITIS

The presence of lymphocytes, plasma cells, eosinophils and mast cells in colonic tissues from patients with ulcerative colitis is consistent with the participation of immunological mechanisms in this disease. Since macrophages are known to play an important role in the sequence of events leading to humoral antibody production, their additional presence sets the stage for the potential induction, perpetuation and termination of local antigen–antibody reactions (Kraft and Kirsner, 1966). Increasing attention is also being directed to lymphocytes within the epithelial cell layer of the intestines of patients with inflammatory bowel disease; many of these heterogeneous theliolymphocytes (Fichtelius, 1968) appear to be transformed or in mitosis, suggesting that they too are capable of responding to antigens and may have an active immunological function (Otto, 1973).

Although ulcerative colitis-like syndromes have been described in rare patients with major defects of the humoral or cellular immune systems (Kirk and Freedman, 1967; Rothberg and ten Bensel, 1967), these are not a frequent manifestation of the recognized isolated or combined immunodeficiency disorders. Indeed, it is doubtful whether such patients should be categorized as cases of non-specific inflammatory bowel disease. The integrity of the humoral immune system in most patients with ulcerative colitis is evidenced by normal or elevated serum gamma-globulin concentrations (Bicks, Kirsner and Palmer, 1959a; de Dombal, 1969), apparently normal antibody responses to standard bacterial immunizations and to common upper-respiratory viral agents and enteropathogens (Lo Grippo, Anselm, Hayashi and Priest, 1970), and studies of mesenteric lymph node morphology from the colectomy specimens of patients with ulcerative colitis (Skinner and Whitehead, 1974a).

Occasional laboratory observations suggesting the involvement of humoral immune mechanisms in ulcerative colitis have included Coombs-positive haemolytic anaemias (Lorber, Schwartz and Wasserman, 1955), hypergammaglobulinaemia, and other serum and tissue immunoglobulin abnormalities to be discussed below. It is well known that the intestine has important homeostatic regulating functions in relation to albumin and other plasma proteins and that changes in these components occur in patients with inflammatory bowel disease (Steinfeld, Davidson, Jordon and Greene, 1960; Bendixen, 1970; Jarnum and Jensen, 1975). Unfor-

tunately, changes secondary to the intestinal disease process have not always been given enough consideration in evaluating assumed immunological phenomena. Obviously, the immunological 'building blocks' of both the humoral and cell-mediated immune systems may be depleted in a variety of exudative enteropathies, resulting in immunological observations which are primarily epiphenomena and often reversible with control of the disease process (Strober, Wochner, Carbone and Waldmann, 1967; Weiden, Blaese, Strober, Block and Waldmann, 1972). These types of protein loss, including the removal of albumin and other large molecules from the interstitial space, involve very specific reactions by intestinal vascular and lymphatic capillaries; and the colon may function less effectively and more slowly than the small bowel in this clearance of interstitial macromolecules (Sterns and Sheppard, 1974a,b).

Serum immunoglobulins

Serum concentrations of the major immunoglobulin classes follow no predictable pattern among patients with ulcerative colitis, and show no consistent relationship to the state of activity, extent or severity of the disease (Kraft and Kirsner, 1971b; Weeke and Jarnum, 1971; Hardy Smith and Macphee, 1971; Loygue et al., 1972; Marner, Friborg and Simonsen, 1975). Serial studies of immunoglobulins in individual patients may be more rewarding than an assessment at a single point in time. In one early study (Bicks, Kirsner and Palmer, 1959b), steroid therapy was most effective in patients with ulcerative colitis and hypergammaglobulinaemia; while Weeke and Jarnum (1971) found that patients with active ulcerative colitis who responded favourably to medical treatment tended to have higher serum levels of IgG than those who did not improve. The prognostic value of other serum protein determinations in severe attacks of ulcerative colitis was emphasized earlier by de Dombal (1967); for example, a rise in the serum alpha$_2$-globulin value was found in longitudinal studies to precede clinical relapses by a few months. While the serum IgA concentration may be elevated when symptoms of ulcerative colitis have been present for longer than 10 years (Kraft, Ford, McCleery and Kirsner, 1968; Weeke and Jarnum, 1971), some of these patients continue to increase their serum IgA concentrations following total proctocolectomy (Hardy Smith and Macphee, 1971; Sandor et al., 1975). Although serum IgG and IgM values may be increased, Bendixen et al. (1970) noted that a few patients with active ulcerative colitis had elevated fractional catabolic rates for these two immunoglobulins on isotopic turnover studies.

Gelernt, Present and Janowitz (1972) reported transient elevations of serum IgM concentrations following bowel resection for either ulcerative colitis or Crohn's disease; no significant changes were noted in the serum

IgA or IgG values pre- and post-operatively. This suggested the possibility that severe disease activity might be associated with increased IgM production, leading to the higher serum concentrations when postulated intestinal binding sites for IgM were removed. Although a subsequent study (Soltis and Wilson, 1975) confirmed the rise in serum IgM concentrations following bowel resection, the changes were not specific for patients with chronic inflammatory bowel disease, and detailed serological studies indicated that the IgM rise did not represent antibody directed against colon antigens. Studies of this type emphasize the need to compare serum and mucosal immunoglobulins concomitantly whenever possible. However, immunoglobulin measurements in intestinal secretions and faeces provide only semi-quantitative results, because of the uncertain effects of enzymatic digestion and the general non-availability of satisfactory standard preparations of secretory immunoglobulins (Samson, McClelland and Shearman, 1973).

Patients with ulcerative colitis have been reported to have greater than normal proportions and absolute numbers of peripheral blood B-lymphocytes, especially of those bearing surface IgA or IgM (Strickland, Korsmeyer, Soltis, Wilson and Williams, 1974; Ramachandar et al., 1974; Sachar et al., 1976). In contrast, Thayer, Charland and Field (1976) and Hoj and Sorensen (1976) found no differences in the number of immunoglobulin-bearing circulating B-cells between patients with ulcerative colitis and healthy controls. Furthermore, the patients studied by Thayer et al. (1976) had markedly decreased proportions and absolute numbers of B-cells capable of forming rosettes with antibody–complement-coated sheep erythrocytes (complement-receptor lymphocytes). While the meaning of these observations is uncertain, it is known that such B-cell data may be quite unrelated to circulating and secretory immunoglobulin measurements in the same individuals (Lawton, Royal, Self and Cooper, 1972).

Tomasi (1972) speculated that secretory IgA deficiency, perhaps related to abnormalities in the epithelial synthesis of secretory component, could allow ingested or bacterial antigens to penetrate deeper into the intestinal mucosa where humoral or cellular immune reactions could lead to a disease such as ulcerative colitis. In one immunofluorescent study (Das, Erber and Rubinstein, 1975), decreased secretory component was noted in colonoscopic biopsies from patients with idiopathic proctitis in contrast to control subjects with radiologically suspected polyps. However, Skinner and Whitehead (1974b) reported that the distribution of secretory component in colectomy specimens from patients with ulcerative colitis seemed unremarkable. While elevated levels of serum secretory 11S IgA have been detected in both types of inflammatory bowel

disease (Thompson, Asquith and Cooke, 1969; Asquith, Thompson and Cooke, 1971), there need not be a direct relationship between the respective concentrations of secretory IgA in the serum and external secretions. In addition, quantitative differences may be less important than are the structural and functional characteristics of the secretory immunoglobulins of the IgG, IgM and IgE classes (Tomasi and Bienenstock, 1968; Tomasi and Grey, 1972). For example, there is no information available as yet regarding the subclass and allotypic characteristics of circulating secretory IgA. Both IgE immunocytes in the lamina propria and IgE in intestinal fluids are available to participate in immediate-type immunological reactions in the human intestinal mucosa, in spite of very low serum concentrations of IgE (Tada and Ishizaka, 1970; Brown, Borthistle and Chen, 1975). Serum IgE levels are not raised in most patients with ulcerative colitis (Brown, Lansford and Hornbrook, 1973).

Tissue immunoglobulins

There have been several immunohistochemical studies of the distribution of immunoglobulins and immunoglobulin-containing lymphoid cells in the colonic mucosa in the past few years. Gelzayd, Kraft, Fitch and Kirsner (1968) studied rectal biopsies from adults with proctoscopically quiescent or mildly active ulcerative colitis. A reduced number of discrete IgA cells in 6 of 9 subjects was considered more apparent than real because IgA was often present in the extracellular interstitium and only IgA-containing cells with a distinct cytoplasm or nucleus could be counted. All ulcerative colitis tissues showed a normal distribution of IgA within the apical portion of the cytoplasm of epithelial cells (Gelzayd, Kraft and Fitch, 1967). The number of IgG cells per unit area of superficial mucosal interstitium also appeared reduced; but the unusual observation (Crabbé and Heremans, 1966) of large numbers of IgD-containing lymphoid cells in the rectal mucosa in ulcerative colitis was not confirmed.

In a more recent study of patients with active ulcerative colitis, characterized by a dense mucosal–submucosal infiltration of lymphocytes and plasma cells, Brandtzaeg, Baklien, Fausa and Hoel (1974) reported somewhat different results. Using directly ethanol-fixed tissues, much specific background staining of the connective tissue ground substance and interstitial fluid for IgG, and to a lesser extent for IgA, obscured the ability to clearly identify IgG and IgA cells. Portions of the same tissue sections were then extracted for 48 hours by controlled washing in saline to remove the diffusible extracellular components prior to fixation (Brandtzaeg, 1974). In comparison to control subjects without overt inflammation, the colonic tissue specimens from the patients with ulcerative colitis showed increased numbers of IgA-, IgM- and IgG-containing plasma cells, and with respect to IgG cells the increase was especially noticeable deeper in the submucosa. These studies have since been extended with similar results (Baklien and Brandtzaeg, 1975; Brandtzaeg and Baklien, 1976).

Other workers (Söltoft, Binder and Gudmand-Höyer, 1973; Ballard and Shiner, 1974) have also reported an elevated number of rectal IgG- and IgA-containing immunocytes in active ulcerative colitis, with the IgG cells even persisting in the inactive stages of the disease in a few serial follow-up studies (Söltoft et al., 1973). Skinner and Whitehead (1974b) quantitated immuno-globulin-containing cells in the mucosa of 46 colectomy specimens from patients with active ulcerative colitis and found statistically increased numbers of IgA, IgG and IgM cells, but a comparison of control and inactive ulcerative colitis tissues showed no such differences. Furthermore, Fodor, Dumitrasku, Radu, Dejica and Grigorescu (1974) noted a decreased density of IgA-containing plasma cells in the rectal mucosa of patients with ulcerative colitis in remission. The distribution of IgE cells in the colonic mucosa in ulcerative colitis also requires additional correlation with disease activity since findings of large numbers of such cells in some patients (Fodor et al., 1974; Brown et al., 1975; Heatley et al., 1975b; Rimpila, O'Neal, Diab, Roth and Kraft, 1976) have not been noted by other workers (Söltoft et al., 1973; Skinner and Whitehead, 1974b; Baklien and Brandtzaeg, 1975; Lloyd, Green, Fox, Mani and Turn-berg, 1975).

Whereas interstitial immunoglobulin deposition in ulcerative colitis may merely reflect a non-specific mani-festation of inflammation, the presence of both increased numbers of immunocytes and a pronounced local IgG-cell response certainly is consistent with the participa-tion of local immunological mechanisms. It is thus of interest that immunofluorescent tests by Monteiro, Fossey, Shiner, Drasar and Allison (1971) demonstrated colorectal mucosal antibodies against anaerobic bacteria in 11 patients with ulcerative colitis, in contrast to non-colitic patients. Although the mucosal antibody was predominantly of the IgG class, it was not thought to be derived from serum, since serum antibodies did not react with the anaerobic faecal bacteria.

Another approach to the study of tissue immuno-globulins is to examine the kinetics of immunoglobulin secretion in the intestine using in-vitro techniques. Employing tissue cultures and radioactively labelled amino acids, Aiuti and Garofalo (1972) and Fiorilli, Luzi and Aiuti (1975) found a definite increase in IgA and IgG synthesis in rectal mucosal biopsies from un-treated patients with ulcerative colitis in comparison with normal control subjects and patients with bacterial enterocolitis. Others have devised intestinal mucosal organ-culture techniques which will allow human biopsy

specimens to remain viable for at least 24 hours and will permit simultaneous in-vitro studies of protein bio-synthesis and secretion, as well as epithelial cell renewal and migration (Eastwood and Trier, 1973a, b; Mac-Dermott, Donaldson and Trier, 1974).

Circulating antibodies

In contrast to the sparsity of information about specific antibody activities associated with immunoglobulins in intestinal tissues in ulcerative colitis, much evidence has accumulated about serum antibodies in such patients, leading to theories of the possible isolated or combined roles of colonic mucosal epithelial cells, intestinal micro-organisms, dietary proteins and other factors in the immunopathogenesis of this disorder. The greatest handicap we face in a discussion of the immunology of inflammatory bowel disease is uncertainty regarding the nature of the antigen(s) involved. Regardless of whether we are concerned with humoral or cell-mediated immune mechanisms, a proper understanding of any type of immunological tissue damage still requires adequate antigenic identification (Taylor and Truelove, 1962; Kraft and Kirsner, 1966, 1971b).

Anticolon antibodies

Much effort has been given to identifying specific colon antigens and anticolon antibodies in patients with ulcera-tive colitis, stemming from the finding of an increased frequency of haemagglutinating antibodies directed against colon mucosa in the sera of patients with ulcera-tive colitis, in contrast to sera from control subjects (Cornelis, 1958; Broberger and Perlmann, 1959). Bro-berger and Perlmann (1959) used normal human foetal colon extracted with phenol-water at 65°C and indicated that the colonic antigenic determinants were carbohy-drate in nature, probably involving a gastrointestinal mucopolysaccharide as found in mucin and which was most likely to be immunologically heterogeneous. Other data (Broberger and Perlmann, 1962; Koffler, Minko-witz, Rothman and Garlock, 1962), based on immuno-fluorescent staining of the cytoplasm of colonic epithelial cells, also suggested a predominantly polysaccharide antigenic composition.

In the search for a more available source of antigen, Perlmann, Hammarström, Lagercrantz and Gustafsson (1965) observed that phenol–water extracts of germ-free rat colon and faeces also reacted with sera from certain patients with ulcerative colitis. This antigen was immunologically related to the human colonic antigen (Lagercrantz, Hammarström, Perlmann and Gustafsson, 1966), and additionally shared antigenic determinants with a lipopolysaccharide extractable from E. coli 014 (Perlmann et al., 1965). Further experiments (Lager-crantz, Hammarström, Perlmann and Gustafsson, 1968; Hammarström, Carlsson, Perlmann and Svensson, 1971) indicated that a heterogenetic antigen which is a constituent of most *Enterobacteriaceae* strains, the so-called common antigen of Kunin (Kunin, 1963), was the component in *E. coli* 014 which cross-reacted with the colon antigen.

The complexity of this problem is illustrated by the production of anticolon antibodies in rabbits after immunization with *E. coli* 014 (Asherson and Holborow, 1966) or strains of *E. coli* isolated from the faeces of patients with ulcerative colitis (Cooke, Filipe and Dawson, 1968), the inhibition of the detection of anti-rat colon antibodies in ulcerative colitis sera by absorption with extracts of *E. coli* 014 (Perlmann *et al.*, 1965; Perlmann, Hammarström, Lagercrantz and Campbell, 1967), and the demonstration of anticolon antibodies in germ-free rats monocontaminated with certain *Clostridia* strains (Hammarström, Perlmann, Gustafsson and Lagercrantz, 1969). In view of its inherent contamination with dietary constituents and microbial antigens, colonic tissue represents a difficult material for immunological study and the results of many of the early studies using crude colonic mucosal extracts have to be interpreted with caution. Available sources of germ-free human faeces (Barnes *et al.*, 1969) might enhance the search for colon-specific antigens and antibodies; but even the normal human foetal colon may have the capacity to absorb materials contained within swallowed amniotic fluid (Lev and Orlic, 1974).

There has been much additional heterogeneity among the various anticolon antibody populations described to date. This is perhaps not surprising in view of the multitude of colonic antigens which have been described and which possess varying degrees of digestive tract, organ and species specificity (Nairn, Fothergill, McEntegart and Porteous, 1962; Nairn and de Boer, 1966; Zweibaum, Oudea, Halpern and Veyre, 1966; Henry, Bernard and Depieds, 1968; Zweibaum and Bouhou, 1970; Martin and Martin, 1970; Remacle-Bonnet and Depieds, 1974). Human sera have reacted differently when immunofluorescently tested against both rat and human colonic tissues, and there has not been a close correlation between the anticolon antibody results obtained using immunofluorescence and passive haemagglutination (Lagercrantz *et al.*, 1966; McGiven, Ghose and Nairn, 1967; Zeromski, Perlmann, Lagercrantz, Hammarström and Gustafsson, 1970b). Thus, Zeromski *et al.* (1970b) studied 10 human sera which gave positive immunofluorescent tests for anti-rat colon or antibacterial antibodies and demonstrated this antibody activity in almost equal association with IgG, IgM and IgA. In one patient, circulating anticolon antibody was associated with secretory IgA; none had anticolon antibodies belonging to the IgD or IgE classes. On the other hand, haemagglutinating antibodies to phenol–water extracts of germ-free rat colon have been primarily

of the IgM class (Perlmann *et al.*, 1965), as are the haemagglutinating antibodies against enteric bacteria which are demonstrable in most human sera (Kunin, 1962; Michael and Rosen, 1963). Benedict (1965) has pointed out that the passive haemagglutination technique is much more efficient at detecting IgM antibody. Indeed, immunofluorescent studies (Cohen and Norins, 1968) showed serum antibodies to Gram-negative bacteria to be associated with IgG and IgA, as well as IgM.

The significance of anticolon antibodies in the pathogenesis of ulcerative colitis is unclear (Lagercrantz, Perlmann and Hammarström, 1971) although they have been used to inhibit DNA synthesis in colonic mucosal epithelial cells in guinea-pigs and rats (Hausamen, Halcrow and Taylor, 1969). Nevertheless, serum containing anticolon antibodies has not been cytotoxic to human foetal colon cells in tissue culture (Broberger and Perlmann, 1963); specific anticolon antibodies have not been demonstrated in colonic tissues in ulcerative colitis; and the presence of circulating anticolon antibodies in patients with ulcerative colitis has not correlated with the severity, duration, course and extent of the disease, the presence or absence of extra-colonic manifestations, or treatment with adrenal corticosteroids (Harrison, 1965; Wright and Truelove, 1966; Lagercrantz *et al.*, 1966; Deodhar, Michener and Farmer, 1969; Marcussen, 1974). While several investigators have been unable to detect circulating antibodies to colonic mucosa in patients with ulcerative colitis, such divergent results could represent different methods of antibody assay, variability of the antigenic source, composition and extraction procedures, or the heterogeneity of the ulcerative colitis population (Kraft, Rimpila, Fitch and Kirsner, 1966). The finding (Gibbs and French, 1971) of circulating antibody to human colon mucus in patients with thyroid disease or chronic asthma, and the observation that this antibody tends to be short-lived in serial studies on individual patients, again raises doubts as to whether the presence of the various anticolon antibodies has any causative or prognostic significance in patients with inflammatory bowel disease.

In all immunological states involving antibodies detectable in the serum, antibodies are necessary but not alone sufficient to cause symptoms (Farr, 1963). The demonstration of circulating antitissue antibodies does not necessarily indicate an immunological basis for any disease, but may rather be an epiphenomenon secondary to tissue damage, similar to reports of circulating antibodies to heart antigens in some patients after an uncomplicated myocardial infarction (Ehrenfeld, Gery and Davies, 1961; Hess, Fink, Taranta and Ziff, 1964). A further possibility, that anticolon antibody may have a protective action against damage, was suggested by Thomas (1964) over a decade ago, and has recently been applied by Shorter, Huizenga and Spencer (1972a) in a working hypothesis for the aetiology and pathogenesis of non-specific inflammatory bowel disease which will be discussed below. Thomas (1964) also stressed that antibodies to tissue elements may be of value in the recovery from damage, facilitating the removal of debris by immunological mechanisms, perhaps involving complement and leucocytes. The use of newer methodology may clarify some of these issues. For example, horseradish peroxidase-conjugated antibodies may constitute a valuable tool for studies of colonic antigen localization at the ultrastructural level (Zeromski, Perlmann, Lagercrantz and Gustafsson, 1970a).

An additional caution in studies of anticolon antibodies has concerned differentiating blood-group antigens which are extractable with phenol–water and which mutually share antigenic determinants with both Gram-negative enteric bacteria (Drach, Reed and Williams, 1972) and mucosal epithelial-cell antigens (Hammarström, Lagercrantz, Perlmann and Gustafsson, 1965). While extracts of germ-free rat caecum contained antigens similar to blood group A and H antigens, absorption studies by Hammerström et al. (1965) indicated that the anticolon antibodies in patients with ulcerative colitis were not reacting with blood-group antigens. Similar absorption studies have been used by Holmgren et al. (1972) to argue against a role for blood-group antigens in the observed antigenic relationship between human kidney, germ-free rat colon, and the common antigen of Enterobacteriaceae extracted from E. coli 014.

Antibacterial antibodies

In addition to the possible consequences of sharing antigenic determinants, bacteria could affect the colonic epithelium by directly damaging mucosal cells, by altering the configuration of colonic antigens, or by attaching as in a hapten combination (Kirsner, 1965). For example, Bregman and Kirsner (1965) considered that alpha-epsilon-diaminopimelic acid, a component of the cell walls of intestinal bacteria, or other metabolic products of enteric microorganisms, may contribute to the antigenic potential of the colon in ulcerative colitis. Also, Gram-negative bacteria are good sources of endotoxins, known to be effective both as antigens and adjuvants (Thomas, 1961). A local Schwartzman phenomenon related to bacterial endotoxins still may be one of the immunologically non-specific factors involved in the tissue reaction in ulcerative colitis (Pardo Gilbert and Zamacoma Ravelo, 1968).

The demonstration by Monteiro et al. (1971) of antibodies to certain faecal anaerobic bacteria in the colorectal mucosa of patients with ulcerative colitis whose sera were reactive only with aerobes makes it reasonable to ask if certain serum antibacterial antibodies tend to be more prominent in this disease. As mentioned already, most human sera do contain antibodies to Gram-negative intestinal bacteria. Conflicting reports exist as to whether (Perlmann et al., 1965; Lagercrantz et al., 1968; Thayer, Brown, Sangree, Katz and Hersh, 1969; Lagercrantz et al., 1971) or not (Fink, Mais, Locke and Hall, 1967b; Kovács, 1974) antibodies to E. coli 014 are detectable more frequently and in higher titres in sera from patients with ulcerative colitis than in sera from control subjects. While the occurrence of positive antibody titres to E. coli 014 seems to bear no relationship to the site or extent of disease, or to age, sex or race, these antibodies also have been demonstrated with greater than expected frequency in sera from healthy female relatives of patients with ulcerative colitis (Lagercrantz et al., 1971). Serum antibody titres to E. coli 0119, Proteus mirabilis and Pseudomonas aeruginosa generally have not differed between ulcerative colitis and control subjects (Fink et al., 1967b; Thayer et al., 1969; LoGrippo et al., 1970; Lagercrantz et al., 1971).

Brown and Lee (1973) performed radioimmunological measurements of serum antibodies reactive with nonpathogenic strains of E. coli and found that mean antibody concentrations in 8 patients with ulcerative colitis were not significantly different from normal subjects. However, there was a tendency towards lower concentrations of IgG and IgA antibodies in these patients and 3 had no detectable circulating IgG anti-E. coli antibodies, the only patients except for those with hypogammaglobulinaemia in whom this was observed. Subsequently (Brown and Lee, 1974), concentrations of serum IgG, IgA and IgM antibodies to Bacteroides fragilis were found to be increased in patients with ulcerative colitis; but serum levels of antibody to Enterococcus species were only moderately elevated. Similar methods have been adapted for studying the antibacterial antibodies associated with immunoglobulins in external secretions (Ste-Marie, Lee and Brown, 1974). Since serum isohaemagglutinins appear after oral immunization to Gram-negative bacteria which contain blood-group-active antigens (Springer and Horton, 1969), apparent differences (Arend and Fehlhaber, 1969; Arend, 1970) in the reactivity of patients with blood group O and ulcerative colitis to immunization with blood-group B antigen also merit further study.

Antiviral antibodies

The possibility of a viral aetiology for inflammatory bowel disease has been under intermittent investigation for over 25 years (Victor, Kirsner and Palmer, 1950; Sloan, Bargen and Gage, 1950) and continues to be considered. In a serological survey for antibodies against 12 viral antigens, Farmer et al. (1973) found that only antibodies to cytomegalovirus were present more frequently and in significantly higher titres in patients with ulcerative colitis than in matched control subjects. While these and other data suggested an unusually high prevalence of cytomegalovirus among the particular patients studied, there is no current evidence to support a role for this virus in the pathogenesis of ulcerative colitis. However, there are a number of case reports (Powell, Warner, Levine and Kirsner, 1961; Levine, Warner and Johnson, 1964; Tamura, 1973; Keren, Milligan, Strandberg and Yardley, 1975) of patients with cytomegalovirus infection and clinical ulcerative colitis and it is possible that in some cases this organism or other viruses may be involved in exacerbating or prolonging the disease (Farmer et al., 1973). LoGrippo et al. (1970) found normal neutralizing antibody levels to cytomegalovirus, as well as to 12 enteroviruses, herpes simplex and herpes zoster in the vast majority of 86 consecutively studied patients with ulcerative colitis. Grotsky, Glade, Hirshaut, Sachar and Janowitz (1970) reported no differences in the incidence of circulating antibodies to the herpes-like Epstein–Barr virus among patients with ulcerative colitis and normal control subjects. Serum antibodies to synthetic double-stranded RNA have not been detected (Korsmeyer, Williams, Wilson and Strickland, 1976) in patients with ulcerative colitis, in contrast to the findings in Crohn's disease to be discussed below.

Anti-milk antibodies

While a number of reports have appeared of milk-induced gastrointestinal diseases, including ulcerative colitis, immunization to ingested proteins is a naturally occurring phenomenon (Rothberg, Kraft, Farr, Kriebel and Goldberg, 1971) and it has been difficult to distinguish between the roles of immunological and non-immunological factors in these conditions. Certainly the efficacy of elimination diets in the control of symptoms does not constitute convincing evidence of an immunological basis for a disease, and the mechanism of milk intolerance in certain patients with ulcerative colitis remains to be established. Non-immunological mechanisms involving chemical, metabolic or mechanical causes might alternatively be implicated (Kraft and Kirsner, 1966).

Among studies of patients with ulcerative colitis, there have been conflicting reports of the incidence of serological reactions of high titre to one or more of the cow's milk antigens, possibly related to differences in the antibody tests and the antigens which were used. Thus, a relative excess of high-titre haemagglutinating antibodies against casein or beta-lactoglobulin was observed (Taylor and Truelove, 1961; Taylor, Truelove and Wright, 1964) in sera from adult patients with ulcerative colitis, in comparison with sera from healthy control subjects or adults with regional enteritis. Others (Sewell, Cooke, Cox and Meynell, 1963; Dudek, Spiro and

Thayer, 1965) used comparable serological tests and antigens but did not confirm the above findings. Recent studies have reinvestigated this problem, employing both primary and secondary antibody assay techniques and multiple cow's milk antigens. In our laboratory (McCaffery, Kraft and Rothberg, 1972), only in studies employing the passive haemagglutination of raw skimmed milk-coated erythrocytes were high titres found more frequently in sera from patients with inflammatory bowel disease than in sera from a heterogeneous group of control subjects. These findings suggested either that antibodies to milk play no pathogenetic role in these diseases or, at most, that certain of these patients may demonstrate an increased permeability and reactivity of the intestinal mucosa to some dietary antigens. Jewell and Truelove (1972a) reached similar conclusions using casein, alpha-lactalbumin and beta-lactoglobulin as antigens, as did Falchuk and Isselbacher (1976) using bovine serum albumin.

In view of the association of IgE with reaginic antibody (Ishizaka, 1970), and the knowledge that increased numbers of mast cells with the capacity to fix IgE (Ishizaka and Ishizaka, 1968) may be part of the tissue reaction in ulcerative colitis (Sommers, 1966; Korelitz and Sommers, 1974; Dobbins, 1975), it should now be possible to design experiments to study the role of reaginic mechanisms in this and other diseases sometimes attributed to so-called food allergy (Kraft and Kirsner, 1976). Jewell and Truelove (1972b) investigated the possibility that milk sensitivity in ulcerative colitis might be mediated by reaginic antibodies, using intradermal testing and by measuring IgE-specific antibodies in the serum. No circulating IgE anti-milk antibodies were found. Intradermal tests, especially using casein, were frequently positive in patients with ulcerative colitis, but the results did not differ from those found in healthy subjects and in patients with Crohn's disease. Skin testing to foods is generally considered unreliable and reagins to a variety of antigens may be demonstrable in a given individual without clinical evidence of sensitivity (Lindblad and Farr, 1961).

Antireticulin antibodies

As discussed in Chapter 6, both serum antibodies to reticulin and high-titre serum antibodies to gluten fraction III have been detected more frequently in patients with coeliac disease than in control subjects (Alp and Wright, 1971). While circulating antibodies to reticulin and/or basement membrane were also found in approximately 10 per cent of patients with ulcerative colitis, in inflammatory bowel disease there was no correlation between positive tests and the presence of serum antibodies to gluten. The meaning of demonstrable reticulin antibodies is not clear; they may merely reflect absorption of reticulin antigens in the diet or be secondary to tissue damage, but there is no evidence that they are responsible for the perpetuation of the bowel lesion.

Miscellaneous antibodies

Other circulating reactants which have been inconsistently or occasionally detected in sera from patients with ulcerative colitis include antinuclear factors, rheumatoid factor, antierythrocyte antibodies, antibodies to gastric and small intestinal mucous cells, gastric parietal cell antibodies, antibodies to thyroglobulin, adrenal antibodies, precipitins to pancreatic homogenates, antibodies to bile ductular cells, and antibodies to phenol–water extracts of liver or kidney (Kraft and Kirsner, 1971a). Serum antibodies to secretory IgA have been detected with equal frequency in patients with ulcerative colitis and in normal subjects (Wilson, 1972). Very occasional patients with ulcerative colitis show positive indirect haemagglutination tests for amoebiasis, but the prevalence is no greater than among control subjects (Healy and Kraft, 1972).

Circulating antigens

Increased plasma or serum levels of carcinoembryonic antigen (CEA) have been detected in up to 30 or 40 per cent of patients with inflammatory bowel disease, those patients with active disease seeming to have the higher titres (Moore, Kantrowitz and Zamcheck, 1972; Rule, Goleski-Reilly, Sachar, Vandevoorde and Janowitz, 1973; Booth, King, Leonard and Dykes, 1974). This applies equally to patients with Crohn's disease of the small and/or large bowel. Mitchell, Gill, Orchard and Parkins (1975) have correlated increased plasma CEA levels with the severity of the initial attack of ulcerative colitis. The elevated levels for the most part have been in the equivocally positive range, i.e. between 2·5 and 5·0ng per ml using the zirconyl–phosphate gel technique (Lo Gerfo, Krupey and Hansen, 1971). The source, nature and significance of this antigenaemia remain to be determined, but no correlation between elevated circulating CEA levels and a high risk of bowel cancer has been shown in inflammatory bowel disease. Indeed, some such patients with carcinomatous changes of the colon show levels which are within the normal range (Booth *et al.*, 1974; Dilawari, Lennard-Jones, Mackay, Ritchie and Sturzaker, 1975). Nevertheless, Isaacson (1976) used an immunoperoxidase technique and demonstrated CEA in the malignant or premalignant mucosae of colectomy specimens from a small group of patients with ulcerative colitis, and the methodology is available to measure CEA levels in colonic mucus (Molnar, Vandevoorde and Gitnick, 1976). Although Straus, Rule, Grotsky, Janowitz and Glade (1972) found that some patients with ulcerative colitis and Crohn's disease have circulating lymphocytes which have been sensitized to a meconium antigen which shares deter-

minants with purified CEA, subsequent *in-vitro* studies in such patients failed to demonstrate cell-mediated immunity to purified CEA (Straus, Vernace, Janowitz and Paronetto, 1975). A more general discussion of the use of CEA tests is presented in Chapter 15.

Antigen–antibody complexes

Kohler (1973) has emphasized that skin rashes, arthritis or arthralgia, glomerulonephritis and systemic vasculitis, some of the extraintestinal manifestations of ulcerative colitis, are suggestive evidence of immune complex disease. While Koffler *et al.* (1962) inferred the local formation of cytotoxic antigen–antibody complexes by demonstrating both the C3 component of complement and gamma-globulin in ulcerative colitis colorectal specimens, until recently there had been little to suggest the participation of immune complexes in the pathogenesis of this disease (Kraft and Kirsner, 1966). Nevertheless, the first component of complement is thought (Colten, Gordon, Rapp and Borsos, 1968) to be synthesized primarily in the columnar epithelial cells of the small intestine; and there has been speculation (Pepys, Wansbrough-Jones, Dash and Mirjah, 1975) that complement and complement-receptor lymphocytes play a role in the induction of immunological responses in the intestine.

It has long been known that serum complement levels decrease in active phases of post-streptococcal glomerulonephritis, systemic lupus erythematosus and rheumatoid arthritis (Williams and Law, 1958). In contrast to the low serum complement levels in those conditions, however, patients with active ulcerative colitis have been reported (Thayer and Spiro, 1963a; Law, 1964; Fletcher, 1965; Fogel, Hook and Polish, 1967) to have normal or high serum complement activity. With the availability of improved methodology, renewed effort has been directed at individual complement components to learn whether activation of the complement pathway might play a role in the pathogenesis of ulcerative colitis.

Thus, Ward and Eastwood (1975) recently described significantly elevated serum C4 levels in patients with ulcerative colitis in severe relapse, although this finding even persisted years after total colectomy; a similar, but less exaggerated, disturbance was seen in the serum C3 levels. Hodgson, Potter and Jewell (1975) found normal concentrations of C3 in sera from 5 patients with active, unspecified inflammatory bowel disease, but metabolic data indicated an increased C3 consumption in these patients. Teisberg and Gjone (1975) reported normal levels of C3, C4 and C3 proactivator protein (C3PA) in 25 patients with ulcerative colitis, but activation products of both C3 and C3PA were observed in approximately half of these subjects and correlated with the extent of the disease process. While Feinstein, Kaplan and Thayer (1976) noted an elevated mean C3PA titre in 26 patients with ulcerative colitis, those patients with exacerbation of disease had the highest levels. All four of these studies are consistent with the participation of the complement system in ulcerative colitis, and the authors point out that normal serum levels of complement factors may merely reflect increased synthesis in compensation for increased utilization.

With this background information, it is of interest that several laboratories have provided evidence for the presence of soluble immune complexes in sera from some patients with ulcerative colitis. Doe, Booth and Brown (1973) and Mowbray, Hoffbrand, Holborow, Seah and Fry (1973) detected small, circulating immune complexes in a few patients with ulcerative colitis using the ability of C1q to precipitate soluble complexes in agar gel. Positive reactions were found even more frequently in patient with Crohn's disease, but very rarely in healthy control subjects. Doe et al. (1973) emphasized that further analysis of the components present in these immune complexes was needed to determine their part, if any, in the pathogenesis of these bowel diseases. Clarification of certain technical issues is also necessary since Soltis and Wilson (1976) have reported that heating may increase serum anticomplementary activity as measured by C1q binding.

Another laboratory (Jewell, MacLennan and Truelove, 1972; Jewell and MacLennan, 1973) demonstrated circulating immune complexes in patients with inflammatory bowel disease by showing that such sera produced significantly greater inhibition of antibody-induced, lymphocyte-mediated cytotoxicity (MacLennan, 1972) than did sera from normal subjects. In ulcerative colitis, inhibition of cytotoxicity correlated well with the severity of disease and the degree of proctoscopic inflammation, but not with the length of history, extent of disease, or the use of corticosteroid therapy. The observed inhibition was considered to be due to serum antigen–antibody complexes which contained less than 5 molecules of IgG, and not to aggregated IgG molecules or to monomeric IgG or IgM.

These intriguing data require much follow-up study but suggest that our problems in understanding some of the cellular immune phenomena to be discussed below may ultimately relate to either unexplained or still unavailable humoral immune data (Shorter, Tomasi, Huizenga, Spencer and Stobo, 1976), serving to emphasize the increasingly apparent overlap of humoral and cell-mediated immunological mechanisms in health and disease (Kraft and Kirsner, 1975). This is further evidenced by the reports (Korsmeyer, Strickland, Wilson and Williams, 1974; Strickland, Friedler, Henderson, Wilson and Williams, 1975) of serum lymphocytotoxic activity in up to 40 per cent of patients with ulcerative colitis or Crohn's disease. This phenomenon involves the killing of sensitized lymphocytes by cytotoxic antibody molecules in the presence of complement. An apparent resistance of lymphocytes from patients with inflammatory bowel disease to the lymphocytotoxic activity of such sera was observed and thought to be due either to saturation of the patients' lymphocyte receptors by absorbed or blocking IgG–IgG complexes, or to depletion of a susceptible population of lymphocytes. Further studies (Korsmeyer, Williams, Wilson and Strickland, 1975; Korsmeyer et al., 1976) have also demonstrated these antilymphocyte antibodies in 30–50 per cent of family members and other household contacts of inflammatory bowel disease probands in contrast only 4 per cent of control family members. Such data suggested exposure to a common environmental agent, possibly a virus, but genetic factors were implicated by also finding an increased prevalence of lymphocytotoxic antibody in sera from consanguineous relatives without household contact.

Brandtzaeg et al. (1974) speculated that locally produced IgG antibodies may directly, or in cooperation with lymphocytes, be responsible for the chronicity and recurrences seen in ulcerative colitis. Degradation of IgG in the inflammatory lesions could give rise to a chemotactic product specific for neutrophils; and antigen-complexed IgG antibodies could act as potent complement activators to produce a local immune complex disease. It has also been suggested (Laham, Panesh and Caldwell, 1976) that complement activation may modulate lymphocyte responses and provide a feedback control loop between cellular and humoral immunity. Nevertheless, Baklien and Brandtzaeg (1974a, b) caution against forming premature conclusions based primarily on the immunofluorescent identification of IgG and C3 in cryostat sections of ulcerative colitis tissues (Ballard and Shiner, 1974).

CELLULAR IMMUNE PHENOMENA AND ULCERATIVE COLITIS

Much of the emphasis in the immunology of inflammatory bowel disease over the past decade has involved investigations of cell-mediated immunological reactions. This was encouraged not only by the apparently limited role of the humoral-type mechanisms just described, but also by the possible involvement of microorganisms and the knowledge that cellular immunological responses commonly participate in microbial tissue reactions. This is a rapidly changing area of immunology and much remains to be learned about the steps and mediators involved in the afferent and efferent limbs of the cellular immune responses, i.e. the interactions of antigen, monocytes, macrophages, lymphocytes, antibody, complement, and target cells (Chs. 1–3). In patients with inflammatory bowel disease, cell-mediated immune phenomena have been studied with in-vivo methods, as well as with techniques developed to serve as in-vitro correlates of cellular immunity.

In-vivo studies

Using conventional skin testing with mumps, candida and trichophyton antigens, normal reactions were obtained by Binder, Spiro and Thayer (1966) in patients with ulcerative colitis. The cutaneous basophilia described (Rebuck, Hodson, Priest and Barth, 1963) in patients with inflammatory bowel disease, using the so-called skin window technique (Priest, Rebuck and Harvey, 1960), also may have represented a cellular reaction to diphtheria products which were injected into the dermis as part of the procedure (Wolf-Jurgensen, Anthonisen and Riis, 1965). On the other hand, Sachar et al. (1976) recently reported cutaneous anergy to 2,4-dinitrochorobenzene in 14 of 28 patients with ulcerative colitis.

Positive delayed-type skin responses to injected autologous leucocytes have been produced in patients with ulcerative colitis (Watson, Styler and Bolt, 1965; Stoebner and Patterson, 1965), but the induration was less pronounced than had been observed (Friedman, Bardawil, Merrill and Hanau, 1960) in patients with systemic lupus erythematosus in whom it was considered to represent autosensitization to nucleoprotein. In another study (Barta and Benysek, 1968), 14 of 44 patients with ulcerative colitis gave positive intracutaneous responses to DNA as manifested by a predominantly mononuclear cell infiltration. A local inflammatory response has also been reported (Fink, Donnelly and Jablokow, 1967a) in patients with ulcerative colitis following the intramucosal rectal injection of autologous mixed leucocytes, but not cell-free plasma. Intradermal skin tests using autologous colon did not produce reactions in one small group of patients with ulcerative colitis studied by Fink and Mais (1968); however, positive responses were induced in both the patients and normal control subjects by similarly injecting colon antigen which had been incubated with live E. coli 014 or E. coli 0119:B14.

None of the above studies provides other than morphological evidence that the positive skin responses were due to cell-mediated immune reactions. More recent and reliable methods for studying cell-mediated immunity have involved measurements of T-lymphocytes, and in-vitro techniques such as lymphocyte transformation, leucocyte migration inhibition, and lymphocyte cytotoxicity.

Circulating T-lymphocytes

The normal responsiveness of the cellular immune system in most patients with ulcerative colitis is supported by the observations of Strickland et al. (1974) of normal T-cell proportions in the peripheral blood of such patients; decreased T-cell numbers were noted but could be related to depressed total peripheral blood lymphocyte counts. As has been reported (De Horatius,

Strickland and Williams, 1974) in a variety of chronic liver diseases, a few of their patients with ulcerative colitis and associated liver disease such as sclerosing cholangitis, chronic active hepatitis and cirrhosis, showed significant reductions of both T-cell numbers and proportions, when compared with the remaining ulcerative colitis patients. While Thayer, Charland and Field (1976) found no differences in the means of either the absolute numbers or proportions of T-cells between 18 patients with extensive ulcerative colitis and healthy control subjects, there was a subpopulation of these patients whose T-cells were reduced. Sachar et al. (1976) and Hoj and Sorensen (1976) encountered similar cases. Important unknowns in this type of study include the degree to which circulating T- and B-cells are influenced by lymphocyte sequestration in the diseased intestinal tissues, and the possibility that standard assays may fail to demonstrate receptors on lymphocytes which have been masked either by antilymphocyte antibodies or circulating immune complexes (Editorial, 1975).

Lymphocyte transformation

Circulating lymphocytes from groups of patients with ulcerative colitis have been reported to have normal mean in-vitro responses to non-specific plant mitogens (Hinz, Perlmann and Hammarström, 1967; Stefani and Fink, 1967; Walker and Greaves, 1969; Parent, Barrett and Wilson, 1971; Asquith, Kraft and Rothberg, 1974) and allogeneic lymphocytes (Townsend, Sakai, Fish and Ritzmann, 1973), but occasional patients within these and other studies (Sachar et al., 1973; Hunt and Trotter, 1973) have had impaired lymphocyte responses to phytohaemagglutinin. Since equally low cell-response indices may be observed in healthy individuals, however, no clinical implications should be drawn from such isolated in-vitro data.

Bull (1974) has further emphasized that, at best, plant mitogens may only partly reflect the capacity of lymphocytes to respond to environmental antigens; the mitogenic responses of whole populations of mononuclear cells are not likely to provide helpful pathogenetic clues; and the reactivity of particular lymphoid subpopulations may be more meaningful. We certainly also need to compare the immunobiological activities of circulating lymphocytes with those of populations of gut-associated lymphocytes isolated from the human intestinal wall (Mavligit, Jubert, Gutterman, McBride and Hersh, 1974; Rudzik and Bienenstock, 1974; Clancy, 1976; Bull and Bookman, 1976) and from mesenteric lymph nodes (Hinz et al., 1967; Guillou, Brennan and Giles, 1973; Bird and Britton, 1974). For example, Hinz et al. (1967) showed that lymphocytes separated from lymph nodes draining the diseased colons of patients with ulcerative colitis were stimulated less by extracts of

E. coli 014 and *E. coli* 075 than were peripheral blood lymphocytes from the same individuals. However, circulating and lymph-node lymphocytes from control subjects reacted similarly.

Nasz *et al.* (1973) reported positive lymphocyte transformation tests to adenovirus types 1, 2, 5 and 6 in approximately one-third of patients with ulcerative colitis, in contrast to less than 10 per cent positive results in healthy persons, suggesting again that virus-induced disturbances of the immune reaction might be important in ulcerative colitis. Watson and Pinedo (1971) found that 2 of 10 patients with ulcerative colitis showed relatively high lymphocyte stimulation responses to 1 or more of 4 unidentified antigens prepared from the stool and resected colon of a patient with ulcerative colitis. Circulating lymphocytes from 5 of 8 patients with Crohn's disease, but none of 8 control subjects, showed similar mitogenic responses. More recently, Hunt and Trotter (1973) used viable autologous rectal epithelial cells as the stimulant and noted a significantly greater response of peripheral blood lymphocytes from patients with acute severe ulcerative colitis when compared with findings in normal subjects and patients with quiescent ulcerative colitis. In contrast, using extracts of *E. coli* 0119:B14, Stefani and Fink (1967) described absent or diminished lymphocyte reactions in patients with active ulcerative colitis, in comparison to the responses of circulating lymphocytes from patients with the disease in remission and from normal donors. Despite the use of similar lymphocyte techniques, it is obvious that no meaningful conclusions will result from comparing studies done with such diverse antigenic stimuli and limited numbers of heterogeneous patients. Also, the possible effects of such variables as iron deficiency anaemia (Joynson, Jacobs, Murray Walker and Dolby, 1972; Chandra and Saraya, 1975), the blocking action of serum factors associated with tissue injury or bacterial sepsis (Taguchi, Gordon and MacLean, 1974), aspirin ingestion (Crout, Hepburn and Ritts, 1975), and even chronic cigarette smoking (Silverman, Potvin, Alexander and Chretien, 1975) require consideration.

Leucocyte migration inhibition

Bendixen (1967, 1969, 1970) reported that the *in-vitro* migration of circulating leucocytes (60 per cent mononuclear cells, 40 per cent neutrophils) from most patients with active ulcerative colitis was inhibited by homogenates prepared from lyophilized sterile, foetal, colonic and jejuno-ileal mucosae. This phenomenon has been considered likely to be an *in-vitro* correlate of cellular immunity (Soborg and Bendixen, 1967). While this may or may not be true, the occurrence (Bendixen 1969, 1970) of similar leucocyte migration inhibition in tests of occasional patients with Crohn's disease and

other intestinal disorders speaks somewhat against the disease specificity of the observation. Furthermore, Williams, Richens, Gough and Ancill (1975) used a similar technique and noted migration inhibition when leucocytes from patients with either ulcerative colitis or Crohn's disease were tested in the presence of whole colon homogenates prepared from a patient with Crohn's disease. As originally stressed (Bendixen, 1967), greater purification or isolation of the involved antigen(s) must be achieved before the possible pathogenetic significance of such data becomes apparent.

Using a phenol–water extract of *E. coli* 0119:B14, Watson and Martucci (1974) found no significant differences in the inhibition of peripheral leucocyte migration between tests in 21 patients with chronic non-specific inflammatory bowel disease of unspecified type and in 19 normal control subjects. Thus, as was noted for circulating antibodies, cellular immunity to coliform antigens appears to be a normal phenomenon in man.

Using enterobacterial common antigen isolated from *Salmonella typhimurium*, Bull and Ignaczak (1973) noted that antigen-stimulated lymphocytes from 8 patients with ulcerative colitis caused more marked migration inhibition of guinea-pig macrophages than did lymphocytes from healthy volunteers and those from most patients with other intestinal diseases. It was also of interest that unstimulated lymphocytes from 3 severely ill patients with ulcerative colitis seemed to elaborate macrophage migration-inhibition factor, perhaps reflecting an intense antigenic stimulation as a part of the active inflammatory process. Inhibition of peripheral leucocyte migration with enterobacterial common antigen was also obtained by Bartnik, Swarbrick and Williams (1974) in tests of 11 of 20 patients with ulcerative colitis, in contrast to only 1 of 33 control subjects. The occurrence and the degree of migration inhibition appeared to be related to the activity of the disease. Similar findings were reported by Fixa *et al.* (1975) who tested the effects of a human foetal colon extract and the lipopolysaccharide antigen from *E. coli* 014, both of which are known to share antigenic determinants with the common enterobacterial antigen, on leucocytes from 35 patients with active or inactive ulcerative colitis and 25 control subjects. While lymphocytes sensitized to common enterobacterial antigen could play an important role in the pathogenesis of ulcerative colitis, much more evidence is needed in this regard.

Cytotoxic action of lymphocytes

One of the most sustained areas of investigation has followed the *in-vitro* observations of Perlmann and Broberger (1963) and Watson, Quigley and Bolt (1966) that circulating lymphocytes from patients with inflammatory bowel disease may be cytotoxic to cultures of human foetal and adult colonic epithelial cells.

This phenomenon has since been extensively studied by Shorter and co-workers (Shorter, Spencer, Huizenga and Hallenbeck, 1968; Shorter, Cardoza, Spencer and Huizenga, 1969; Shorter, Cardoza, Huizenga, ReMine and Spencer, 1969; Shorter, Cardoza, ReMine, Spencer and Huizenga, 1970; Shorter, Huizenga, ReMine and Spencer, 1970; Shorter, Huizenga, Spencer, Aas and Guy, 1971; Shorter, Huizenga, Spencer and Guy, 1972b; Shorter, Huizenga, Spencer and Weedon, 1973). They have repeatedly observed that peripheral blood mononuclear cells from patients with either ulcerative colitis or Crohn's disease can lyse isologous or allogeneic colonic epithelial cells in tissue culture. It appears to be a rapid, non-complement-dependent effect of lymphocytes and their cell-free filtrates, and was not detected 10 days following colectomy. It was abolished or reduced by preincubation of the test lymphocytes variously with horse antihuman thymus serum, serum from another patient with inflammatory bowel disease, or a lipopolysaccharide extract of *E. coli* 0119:B14. The cytotoxic capacity was also induced in circulating lymphocytes obtained from normal adults by prior incubation in a medium containing either the same lipopolysaccharide extract or serum from a patient with inflammatory bowel disease. In the latter situation, the induction was thought to require the presence of a cytophilic antibody of the IgM class. The cytotoxic phenomenon is thought to involve a non-specific target cell destruction effected via the specific release of lymphotoxin by sensitized lymphocytes. More recently it was learned (Stobo, Tomasi, Huizenga, Spencer and Shorter, 1976) that the cytotoxic cell is not included with the majority of either the T- or B-lymphocytes and may thus belong to the null or 'K' subpopulation of lymphoid cells. However, this non-phagocytic cell bore a surface receptor capable of combining to the Fc portion of immunoglobulin. An increased number of circulating null cells has been noted in patients with ulcerative colitis, but not in Crohn's disease (Hoj and Sorensen, 1976). Other laboratories (Carlsson, Hammarström, Lanteli and Perlmann, 1971; Hunt, 1972; Hunt and Trotter, 1975; Kovács, Onody and Petranyi, 1975) also appear to be studying this cytotoxicity phenomenon in patients with inflammatory bowel disease.

Hopefully, continued work will clarify the meaning of these interesting observations and answer several existing questions. What is the origin of the cytotoxic lymphocyte population(s)? Do these effector cells bear complement receptors? Is this a primary or secondary phenomenon? Does it involve mechanisms other than lymphotoxin production and release? Does it represent antibody-dependent cell-mediated cytotoxicity? As already indicated, serum from patients with inflammatory bowel disease is not cytotoxic to colonic epithelial cells *in vitro* (Broberger and Perlmann, 1963); but

locally produced antibodies or immune complexes in the inflammatory lesion may direct lymphocytes toward cytotoxic reactions (Brandtzaeg and Baklien, 1974).

Perhaps the most immediate impact of all these fascinating cellular immune observations is to increase interest in the role of enteric bacteria, in conjunction with both humoral and cellular immune mechanisms, in the pathogenesis of ulcerative colitis and Crohn's disease. A search for sensitized lymphocytes at the site of the tissue reaction remains important. However, just as tests developed for the assessment of serum antibodies may not be ideal for evaluating antibodies and immunoglobulins in external secretions, *in-vitro* tests based on lymphocyte transformation, migration inhibition, and cytotoxicity may be somewhat difficult to apply to studies of lymphocytes isolated from different gut compartments. Thus, propriolymphocytes, theliolymphocytes, and lymphocytes from Peyer's patches and mesenteric nodes each may be more heterogeneous than is apparent by currently available isolation and identification techniques (Kraft and Kirsner, 1976).

CROHN'S DISEASE

Many of the clinical-type observations which suggested the possibility of immune involvement in the pathogenesis of ulcerative colitis also have been recorded in patients with Crohn's disease. For example, polyarthritis, eczema and hay fever are found with increased prevalence both in patients with Crohn's disease and their first-degree relatives (Hammar, Ashurst and Naish, 1968; Haslock, 1973). The immunogenetic implications of several observations of the prevalence of certain histocompatibility antigens in inflammatory bowel disease, especially in association with ankylosing spondylitis, will be discussed below under the heading 'Immunological Hypotheses'.

Morphologically, one of the earliest tissue changes detectable (Aluwihare, 1971) with the electron microscope in Crohn's disease is an increase in the proportion of lymphocytes and plasma cells in the lamina propria, and these lymphocytes not infrequently have prominent and unusual nucleoli. Aluwihare (1971) emphasized that the ultrastructural relationships between lymphocytes, macrophages, epithelial cells and intramural bacteria suggested the need for further immunological study. This view was supported by the electron microscopic studies of Ranlöv, Nielsen and Wanstrup (1972), using terminal ileal tissues and regional lymph nodes resected from two patients with advanced Crohn's disease. Large, activated, polyribosome-rich lymphocytes frequently were seen in association with small lymphocytes, plasma cells and mast cells. Increased numbers of theliolymphocytes (Otto, 1973), lamina propria plasma cell:lymphocyte ratios greater than unity (Ferguson, Allan and Cooke, 1975), hypertrophied plasma cells (Rippey and Sommers, 1967), and increased numbers of macrophages (Korelitz and Sommers, 1974) and mast cells (Hiatt and Katz, 1962; Rao, 1973) have also been described in Crohn's disease tissues.

HUMORAL IMMUNE PHENOMENA AND CROHN'S DISEASE

Most patients with Crohn's disease show no impairment in the capacity to produce circulating antibodies (Bucknall, Verrier Jones and Peacock, 1975); although a few cases have been reported (Eggert, Wilson and Good, 1969; Söltoft, Petersen and Kruse, 1972) with coexistent severe hypogammaglobulinaemia, perhaps arguing against an important pathogenetic role for humoral-type immune processes in the production of the intestinal lesion. Rare patients with Crohn's disease also have had an associated selective IgA deficiency (Jensen, Goltermann, Jarnum, Weeke and Westergaard, 1970; Tomasi, Bull, Tourville, Montes and Yurchak, 1971; Söltoft et al., 1972; Bergman, Johansson and Krause, 1973), but more have had high serum IgA levels, especially patients with extensive or untreated disease involving the small intestine (Kraft et al., 1968; Hobbs and Hepner, 1968; Poen et al., 1969; Deodhar et al., 1969; Bolton, James, Newcombe, Whitehead and Hughes, 1974; Sandor et al., 1975). In contrast, serum IgG and IgM levels usually have been normal or reduced in chronic cases (Kraft et al., 1968; Poen et al., 1969; Weeke and Jarnum, 1971), perhaps as a result of increased catabolic rates (Bendixen et al., 1968; Jensen et al., 1970) which seems only partly dependent on intestinal protein loss (Beeken, Busch and Sylwester, 1972). There is evidence (Jarnum and Jensen, 1975) of a greater faecal loss of IgG than albumin in patients with Crohn's disease involving the small intestine. Serum IgE concentrations are only occasionally elevated in patients with Crohn's disease and do not differ significantly from those of normal control subjects or patients with ulcerative colitis (Brown et al., 1973; Bergman et al., 1973). Concentrations of IgA and IgE in intestinal fluids (Bergman et al., 1973; Jones, Beeken, Roessner and Brown, 1976) and IgA synthesis by jejunal organ cultures (Jones et al., 1976) have also been normal in Crohn's disease.

As might be expected, more immunoglobulin-containing lymphoid cells and larger concentrations of immunoglobulins have been observed (Persson and Danielsson, 1973; Persson, 1974) in the terminal ileum in Crohn's disease than in specimens from control subjects without ileal inflammation. There appeared to be a relative decrease of IgA-containing cells and a relative increase of IgG and IgM cells in the diseased ileal tissues. These results were confirmed and extended to include cases with involvement of the colon (Baklien and Brandtzaeg, 1975; Brandtzaeg and Baklien, 1976); IgG cells were dramatically increased in areas of severe inflammation. In areas with intact mucosa, IgA cells still predominated and the glandular distribution of secretory component appeared normal. Meuwissen, Felkamp-Vroom, Brutel de la Riviere and Tytgat (1976) also noted significantly reduced ratios of IgA:IgM plasma cells within the lamina propria of intestinal tissues from patients with Crohn's disease, compared to normal controls and patients with ulcerative colitis. Green and Fox (1975) similarly observed reduced numbers of IgA cells and increased numbers of IgM cells in non-ulcerated affected areas of bowel resected from patients with Crohn's disease, but the distribution of IgA in unaffected areas of bowel was normal. In an earlier study, Söltoft (1969) had found increased numbers of immunocytes in the virtually normal jejunal mucosa of 9 patients with Crohn's disease of the distal ileum and colon, but the distribution of IgA, IgG and IgM cells did not differ from control tissues. Mul, de Boer, Taminiau and Ballieux (1975) reported similar findings in jejunal biopsies from 6 patients with Crohn's disease and further noted that the ratio between IgA (kappa)-producing and IgA (lambda)-producing lymphoid cells was approximately 63:37, no different than observed in other patients with and without local inflammation in the biopsy specimens. Some (Brown et al., 1975), but not others (Skinner and Whitehead, 1974b; Green and Fox, 1975; Baklien and Brandtzaeg, 1975), have noted increased numbers of IgE cells in the intestinal mucosa in Crohn's disease.

Proportions and absolute numbers of peripheral blood B-cells bearing surface IgA or IgM have been noted to be increased significantly in Crohn's disease, as in ulcerative colitis, a finding which was unrelated to the activity, site or duration of disease, or to mode of treatment (Strickland et al., 1974; Ramachandar et al., 1974). Thayer et al. (1976) and Hoj and Sorensen (1976) found no such increase in immunoglobulin-bearing B-cells, but circulating complement-receptor B-cells were decreased (Thayer et al., 1976), as was also noted in patients with ulcerative colitis. These and the above immunofluorescent observations, coupled with the elevation of serum secretory IgA levels (Thompson et al., 1969; Asquith et al., 1971) and apparent changes in salivary IgA production in some patients with Crohn's disease (Basu, Asquith, Thompson and Cooke, 1975), indicate the importance of continued investigations of both cell-bound and diffusible immunoglobulins and their associated antibody activities at the tissue level

Although earlier immunofluorescent studies (Harrison, 1965; Wright and Truelove, 1966) had not detected circulating antihuman colon antibodies in patients with Crohn's disease, subsequent work (Lagercrantz et al.,

1966; Deodhar *et al.*, 1969; Thayer *et al.*, 1969) has shown serum antibodies to germ-free rat colon or faeces, and to *E. coli* 014, as frequently as was noted in ulcerative colitis. Recent studies (McCaffery *et al.*, 1972; Jewell and Truelove, 1972a; Falchuk and Isselbacher, 1976) have been unable to differentiate patients with Crohn's disease from those with ulcerative colitis on the basis of the incidence or amount of antibodies detectable against skimmed milk antigens, bovine serum albumin, casein, beta-lactoglobulin or alpha-lactalbumin. Serum antibodies to reticulin appear to be more prevalent among patients with Crohn's disease than in patients with ulcerative colitis, but less frequent than among those with coeliac disease (Alp and Wright, 1971; Magalhaes, Peters and Doe, 1974). Circulating thyroid, gastric parietal cell and antinuclear antibodies (Deodhar *et al.*, 1969; Perrett *et al.*, 1971), as well as serum antibodies to the Epstein–Barr virus (Grotsky *et al.*, 1970, 1971), are not found more frequently in patients with Crohn's disease than in control subjects. However, serum antibodies to synthetic double-stranded RNA are found (Korsmeyer *et al.*, 1976) more frequently in patients with Crohn's disease (23 per cent) and in their relatives (19 per cent) than in control families (3 per cent).

The reports (Jewell *et al.*, 1972; Jewell and Mac-Lennan, 1973; Doe *et al.*, 1973; Mowbray *et al.*, 1973) of circulating small antigen–antibody complexes in sera from some patients with ulcerative colitis also described identical serological phenomena in patients with Crohn's disease. In a recent confirmatory report (Lurhuma, Cambiaso, Masson and Heremans, 1976), circulating antigen–antibody complexes were described in 58 of 66 patients with Crohn's ileitis; while Ezer and Hayward (1974) demonstrated apparent immune complexes in sera from 12 of 24 patients with Crohn's disease by the inhibition of complement-dependent lymphocyte rosette formation. Korsmeyer *et al.* (1974, 1976) demonstrated possible IgG–IgG complexes containing complement-dependent lymphocytotoxic antibody in sera from patients with Crohn's disease, as in ulcerative colitis. Significantly elevated serum concentrations of the C4 component of complement have recently been described (Ward and Eastwood, 1975) in patients with Crohn's disease even when in remission; in non-operated patients with ulcerative colitis, an increased C4 level was found only in active cases, suggesting possible differences in complement metabolism or tissue repair processes during inactive phases of the two diseases. The previously mentioned complement studies of Teisberg and Gjone (1975) and Feinstein *et al.*, (1976) did not vary appreciably when applied to sera from patients with Crohn's disease instead of ulcerative colitis. In the former study, the presence of complement activation was correlated with disease activity in both groups of patients.

CELLULAR IMMUNE PHENOMENA AND CROHN'S DISEASE

Special attention is being directed to the integrity and reactivity of the cell-mediated immune system in patients with Crohn's disease. This is not unreasonable (Kraft, 1971a) in view of (a) the hyperplastic lymphoid reaction in the involved bowel, with or without sarcoid-like granulomas; (b) the known impaired expression of cellular immunity in patients with sarcoidosis, a condition which conceivably could be caused by a common or closely related agent (Mitchell, Cannon, Dyer, Hinson and Willoughby, 1970); (c) observations of an increased enteric loss of lymphocytes (Weetman, Haggith and Douglas, 1974) and an absolute lymphopenia (Strober *et al.*, 1967; Grotsky *et al.*, 1971; Hoj and Sorensen, 1976) in some patients with Crohn's disease; (d) the finding of high rates of DNA synthesis in 72-hour cultures of Crohn's disease mucosal lymphocytes (Clancy, 1976); (e) the possibility that Crohn's disease may be an infectious disease, perhaps analogous to the tuberculoid form of leprosy (Golde, 1968), in which there is a high degree of cell-mediated immunological reactivity (Turk, 1969); (f) the rare association of the disease with severe immunoglobulin deficiency but intact cellular immunity; and (g) the inability to differentiate ulcerative colitis and Crohn's disease on the basis of the prevalence of innumerable humoral antibodies or apparent circulating immune complexes. What can one say about the current status of cellular immunity in patients with Crohn's disease?

Using a combination of morphological features, Skinner and Whitehead (1974a) found no evidence of diminished immunoreactivity in mesenteric lymph nodes from patients with Crohn's colitis, although conceding that this did not preclude differences in the reactivity of lymphoid tissue within the intestinal wall. The *in-vitro* proliferative responses of lymphocytes separated from the mesenteric lymph nodes of patients with Crohn's disease have been either normal (Bird and Britton, 1974) or impaired (Guillou *et al.*, 1973). Limited studies (Strickland, Husby, Black and Williams, 1975; Meuwissen *et al.*, 1976) of resected intestinal tissues from patients with Crohn's disease have shown large numbers of T-lymphocytes, especially in the deeper layers of the inflamed bowel and surrounding epithelioid cell granulomas.

Conventional skin test reactivity has been reported to be normal (Binder *et al.*, 1966) or depressed (Meuwissen, Schellekens, Huismans and Tytgat, 1975) in Crohn's disease, and either normal (Fletcher and Hinton, 1967; Ropke, 1972; Bolton *et al.*, 1974) or depressed (Phear, 1958; Jones Williams, 1965) skin responses to tuberculoprotein have been described. Bird and Britton (1974) obtained negative skin reactivity to purified protein derivative in 7 of 12 patients with Crohn's disease, in contrast to positive tests in each of 9 healthy control subjects. On the other hand, the *in-vitro* lymphocyte responses to tuberculin did not differ significantly between the two groups. Patients with positive *in-vitro* and negative *in-vivo* tests of tuberculin sensitivity have been observed by others (Caspary and Field, 1971; Nilsson, 1971). Interestingly, there are two preliminary reports (Asquith *et al.*, 1975; Ng and Vicary, 1976) of the apparent conversion to positive tuberculin and other skin test reactivity in patients with Crohn's disease after treatment with transfer factor. The frequent finding (Verrier Jones, Housley, Ashurst and Hawkins, 1969) of absent skin reactivity to 2,4-dinitrochlorobenzene suggested a relative depression of cellular immunity, but Bolton *et al.* (1974) and MacPherson, Albertini and Beeken (1976) found such reactions to be normal in Crohn's disease patients who were not on immunosuppressive therapy.

Peripheral blood T-cell proportions and numbers in Crohn's disease have (Strickland *et al.*, 1974; Strickland and Williams, 1975; Sachar *et al.*, 1976) or have not (Bird and Britton, 1974; Thayer *et al.*, 1976) been significantly decreased, perhaps related to different ways of recording such data, the variable loss of these lymphocytes into the intestinal lumen and other factors. Possible roles for qualitative defects in T-cells and the loss of select subpopulations of T-cells have not been excluded. For example, some patients with Crohn's disease have shown depressed responses to allogeneic lymphocytes (Townsend *et al.*, 1973; Richens, Williams, Gough and Ancill, 1974b), and Cave and Brooke (1973) found reduced colchicine-induced mitotic indices using lymphocytes from patients with Crohn's disease in contrast to control lymphocytes.

Using lymphocyte transformation, some have described a variable impairment of the responses of circulating lymphocytes to phytohaemagglutinin (Walker and Greaves, 1969; Brown, Taub, Present and Janowitz, 1970; Parent *et al.*, 1971; Maclaurin, Cooke and Ling, 1972; Sachar *et al.*, 1973; Guillou *et al.*, 1973) and concanavalin (Brown *et al.*, 1970) in Crohn's disease. However, many workers have been unable to confirm such observations (McHattie, Magil, Jeejeebhoy and Falk, 1971; Aas, Huizenga, Newcomer and Shorter, 1972; Ropke, 1972; Townsend *et al.*, 1973; Asquith *et al.*, 1973; Richens *et al.*, 1974; Bolton *et al.*, 1974; Bird and Britton, 1974; Meuwissen *et al.*, 1975; MacPherson *et al.*, 1976). The results in our laboratory (Asquith *et al.*, 1973) showed considerable overlap among inflammatory bowel disease and control subjects and considerable variability in the optimal dose of a mitogen needed to elicit a maximal response in a given subject. There was a trend towards poorer lymphocyte responsiveness in patients with Crohn's disease of moderate to severe clinical activity. While medications may represent potential variables, negative *in-vitro* studies of the in-

fluence of sulphasalazine therapy on lymphocyte responses have been described (Sachar *et al.*, 1973). On the other hand, corticosteroid administration has been shown (Claman, 1972; Helms, Miller, Grendell and Bull, 1974) to suppress *in-vitro* lymphocyte responsiveness and to reduce the number of circulating T-cells; the possibility of depressed *in-vitro* lymphocyte responses related to acute and chronic starvation must also be considered (Holm and Palmblad, 1976; Bird and Britton, 1974).

Utilizing a migration-inhibition technique, Bendixen (1967) originally suggested that the migration or peripheral blood leucocytes from patients with Crohn's disease was not inhibited following exposure to homogenates of sterile foetal, colonic or jejunoileal mucosa. This no longer appears to be strictly so (Bendixen, 1969, 1970) and circulating leucocytes from a high proportion of patients with Crohn's disease have shown distinct migration-inhibition responses to crude extracts of faeces (Dykes, 1970, 1972) or to preparations of diseased colonic mucosa from a patient with Crohn's disease (Richens, Williams, Gough and Ancill, 1974a; Williams *et al.*, 1975). Bull and Ignaczak (1973) and Bartnik *et al.* (1974) also found that lymphocyte cultures from patients with regional enteritis caused migration inhibition in response to enterobacterial common antigen, but to a lesser extent than was observed in similar tests of patients with ulcerative colitis.

The cumulative data discussed to this point do not provide evidence of decisive differences in immunological mechanisms, either cellular or humoral, between patients with these two types of inflammatory bowel disease. In addition, the extensive data pertaining to the *in-vitro* colonic cell toxicity, shown by circulating lymphocytes from patients with ulcerative colitis, apply equally to lymphocytes from patients with Crohn's disease of the small or large intestine, or of both sites (Shorter *et al.*, 1976).

CROHN'S DISEASE, SARCOIDOSIS AND CHRONIC GRANULOMATOUS DISEASE

There has been renewed interest in a possible pathogenetic link between Crohn's disease and sarcoidosis (Kraft, 1971b; Janowitz and Sachar, 1976), especially since the sarcoid-like reaction in Crohn's disease remains one of the most reliable diagnostic features, and may even have prognostic value (Glass and Baker, 1976). In addition to sharing non-caseating epithelioid cell granulomas and Langhans-type giant cells, these two conditions may be associated with uveitis, erythema nodosum, arthritis and circulating immune complexes (Verrier Jones, Cumming, Asplin, Laszlo and White, 1976), while both conditions generally show favourable therapeutic responses to corticosteroids. Crohn's disease may even appear in a miliary form (Heaton, McCarthy,

Horton, Cornes and Read, 1967; Manns, 1972; Daum, Boley and Cohen, 1974), and elevated serum lysozyme levels are frequent in sarcoidosis (Pascual, Gee and Finch, 1973). Early attempts (Sanders, 1964; Jones Williams, 1965) to devise a skin test for regional enteritis, analogous to the controversial (Israel and Goldstein, 1971; Thomas, 1971; Scadding, 1971; Hurley and Lane, 1971; Hurley, Sullivan and Hurley, 1975) Kviem test, were unsuccessful. Although many (Jones Williams, 1965, 1971; Siltzbach, Vieira, Topilsky and Janowitz, 1971; Hannuksela, Alkio and Selroos, 1971; Chapman, Gleeson and Taylor, 1971) disagree, at least three groups (Mitchell et al., 1970; Bartnik and Zych, 1972; Karlish, Cox, Hampson and Hemsted, 1972) reported microscopically positive Kviem tests in about 50 per cent of patients with Crohn's disease. Batch differences have since been considered the most likely explanation for this controversy (James, 1975; Siltzbach, 1976; Douglas et al., 1976).

Mitchell and Rees (1969, 1970) produced sarcoid-like granulomas in the footpads of mice injected with either lymph nodes or homogenates of small intestine from patients with Crohn's disease. Subsequent studies (Mitchell, Rees and Goswami, 1976) have confirmed retention of the ability to produce granulomas following passage of the homogenized, ultrafiltered mouse tissues; have shown different patterns of systemic dissemination of granulomas when using either sarcoid or Crohn's disease homogenates as the starting inoculum; and have noted failure to induce granulomas if the original human tissues had been autoclaved. Further suggestions of a transmissible agent in Crohn's disease come from observations in rabbits inoculated intra-ileally with Crohn's tissue homogenates (Cave, Mitchell, Kane and Brooke, 1973; Cave, Mitchell and Brooke, 1975), and in mice receiving footpad injections of similar intestinal granulomas and lymph nodes (Taub, Sachar, Siltzbach and Janowitz, 1975; Taub, Sachar, Janowitz and Siltzbach, 1976). In the latter laboratory, granulomas also were induced in mice receiving footpad injections of affected intestinal tissues obtained from patients with ulcerative colitis or from patients undergoing bowel resection for unrelated intra-abdominal conditions. Others (Bolton, Owen, Heatley, Jones Williams and Hughes, 1973; Heatley, Bolton, Owen, Jones Williams and Hughes, 1975a) have been unsuccessful in inducing sarcoid-like granulomas in rats, guinea-pigs and mice; but techniques, reagents and the character of the tissue reaction (Simonowitz, Block, Riddell, Kraft and Kirsner, 1977) vary widely among laboratories, and care must be taken to avoid bowel contact with antiseptic skin preparations (Orr et al., 1975).

The potential importance of the studies of Mitchell, Rees, Cave and co-workers is augmented by in-vitro observations of positive migration-inhibition phenomena using sarcoid spleen cells and peripheral lymphocytes from patients with either Crohn's disease (Willoughby and Mitchell, 1971; Brostoff and Walker, 1971; Richens, Gough and Williams, 1973) or sarcoidosis (Caspary and Field, 1971). The possibility of interrelationships between Crohn's disease and sarcoidosis becomes even stronger if one considers that Crohn's disease has been reported (Willoughby, Mitchell and Wilson, 1971) in a sibship having multiple cases of sarcoidosis, and that the two conditions may occur in the same individual (Dines, DeRemee and Green, 1971; Padilla and Sparberg, 1972). While the ultrastructural demonstration of bacteria within the lesions of Crohn's disease (Aluwihare, 1971) and sarcoidosis (Greenberg, Gyorkey, Weg, Jenkins and Gyorkey, 1970), and the recovery of bacterial variants from Crohn's disease tissues (Parent and Mitchell, 1976), raise the hope that the suggested transmissible agents might be identifiable with continued study, the overlapping infectious, genetic and immunological aspects of these conditions will have to be delineated with great care.

Nonetheless, there is mounting evidence (Aronson, Phillips, Beeken and Forsyth, 1975; Cave et al., 1975; Gitnick, Arthur and Shibata, 1976; Gitnick and Rosen, 1976) for the presence of viral agents in intestinal tissues from some patients with Crohn's disease. Although evidence of pathogenicity has not been established, identification and characterization remains incomplete, and distinctions must be made with respect to the many viruses normally present in the alimentary tract (Flewett and Boxall, 1976), this is intriguing information in view of the possible role of viruses in the induction of serum antibodies directed against lymphocytes or RNA in the majority of patients with Crohn's disease (Korsmeyer et al., 1976). Negative studies (Cook and Turnbull, 1975; Whorwell, Baldwin and Wright, 1976) do not exclude the presence and participation of a virus in this disease.

Finally, there has been speculation (Kraft, 1967; Yogman, Touloukian and Gallagher, 1974), based on histological and clinical overlapping, that there might be a relationship between Crohn's disease and the syndrome of chronic granulomatous disease of childhood. Gastrointestinal studies (Ament and Ochs, 1973) in patients with the latter condition, an inborn defect of the bactericidal capacity of neutrophils (Quie, White, Holmes and Good, 1967; Schlegel, 1975), showed that 4 of 9 cases had digestive symptoms and that the granulomas and giant cells found in the rectal mucosa could not be morphologically differentiated from those seen in Crohn's disease. Chronic granulomatous disease may also produce diffuse histological changes of the gastric antrum (Griscom et al., 1974) or small intestine (Yogman et al., 1974), which appear similar or identical to those seen in Crohn's disease and which may cause problems in differential diagnosis. Interestingly, a sister of at least one child with chronic granulomatous disease is said (Quie *et al.*, 1967) to have had ulcerative colitis. In spite of these intriguing suggestions, Ament (1974) found that the *in-vitro* bactericidal activities of leucocytes from 20 patients with Crohn's disease were normal, and two groups (Ward and Eastwood, 1976; Segal and Loewi, 1976) found no evidence of defective neutrophilic function in patients with Crohn's disease as measured by the capacity to reduce nitroblue tetrazolium dye, leading to the conclusion that quite different pathogenetic mechanisms are probably involved in the two disorders. While much remains to be learned about granuloma formation (Epstein, 1967; Adams, 1976), the deposition of antigen–antibody complexes may cause granulomatous disease in laboratory animals (Spector and Heesom, 1969), cell-mediated immunologic granulomas have been well documented (Warren, Domingo and Cowan, 1967), and a functional classification of immunologic and non-immunologic granulomas (Warren, 1976) does appear to be a worthwhile approach to a better understanding of the aetiopathogenesis of conditions such as sarcoidosis and Crohn's disease.

IMMUNOSUPPRESSIVE DRUG THERAPY

Potentially immunosuppressive drugs such as adrenal corticosteroids and sulphasalazine have long been used with good results in the treatment of inflammatory bowel disease. Nevertheless, a 14-centre cooperative controlled trial (Best, Becktel, Singleton and Kern, 1976; Singleton, 1976) is in progress to determine the efficacy of these two agents, as well as azathioprine, in both active and quiescent Crohn's disease. The investigators hope to have randomized over 600 patients into this study by 1977. Another controlled, double-blind, multicentre trial is under way using sulphasalazine in primarily resected patients with Crohn's disease (Wenckert *et al.*, 1976); while there is a preliminary report (Blichfeldt, Blomhoff, Myhre and Gjone, 1976) of a controlled study of the efficacy and safety of metronidazole in Crohn's disease (Ursing and Kamme, 1975; Mitelman, Hartley-Asp and Ursing, 1976). Metronidazole and related agents have been shown capable of suppressing cell-mediated immunologic granuloma formation (Grove, Mahmond and Warren, 1976; Webster, Butterworth, Mahmoud, Mngola and Warren, 1975). Can we gain further insight into the complex, multifactorial pathogenesis of ulcerative colitis and Crohn's disease by studying the results of well-designed trials of immunosuppressive drug therapy?

Since an encouraging case report by Bean in 1962, many patients with these diseases have been treated with immunosuppressive agents, including 6-mercapto-purine, nitrogen mustard, chlorambucil and azathioprine. Although azathioprine seems to be under increasing usage, several problems impede a meaningful interpretation of any apparently beneficial effects (Wright 1970; Kraft and Kirsner, 1971b). These include the difficulties in differentiating ulcerative colitis from Crohn's disease, deficient knowledge of the specific antigens and immunological phenomena involved, natural variations in the clinical course of these conditions, limited objective evidence of immunosuppression, and uncertainties related to the many potential modes of action of the drug and its varying effects on different lymphocyte subpopulations and on macrophages.

In anecdotal studies, 60–70 per cent of patients with either ulcerative colitis or Crohn's disease seem to have derived benefits from azathioprine, as judged by clinical and radiological improvement for varying periods of time. However, only 6 double-blind, controlled studies have been recorded, 2 in ulcerative colitis (Jewell and Truelove, 1972c, 1974; Rosenberg, Wall, Levin, Binder and Kirsner, 1975b) and 4 in patients with Crohn's disease (Rhodes, Bainton, Beck and Campbell 1971; Willoughby, Kumar, Beckett and Dawson, 1971; Rosenberg, Levin, Wall and Kirsner, 1975a; Klein, Binder, Mitchell, Aaronson and Spiro, 1974). The details and results of these 6 studies were recently summarized (Kraft, 1974). The consensus was that clinical signs and symptoms were not strikingly improved in patients with ulcerative colitis, but that less prednisone was required in managing the azathioprine-treated groups. Since azathioprine may suppress host defences and cause several long-term complications (Schein and Winokur, 1975), caution has been urged (Bowen, Irons, Rhodes and Kirsner, 1966; Cooke, 1970) in considering such adjunctive therapy in patients with ulcerative colitis who are already vulnerable to many systemic and local problems, including infections, hepatic damage and colonic neoplasms. In the four controlled trials in patients with Crohn's disease, relapses were less frequent with azathioprine treatment, but the results were far from convincing; for example, fistulas and other complications were not affected or prevented in some cases. Certain subgroups of Crohn's disease may be especially responsive to azathioprine (Klein *et al.*, 1974); immunological studies in these patients could be very rewarding.

There have been few attempts to correlate azathioprine therapy in inflammatory bowel disease with objective evidence of immunosuppression. Campbell *et al.* (1974) serially measured plasma cells in the lamina propria of the rectum, and tested circulating lymphocytes with regard to surface immunoglobulins, phytohaemagglutinin responsiveness and antibody-mediated cytotoxicity. Only the lamina propria plasma cells and the circulating cytotoxic lymphocytes were found to be depressed after prolonged azathioprine treatment. Upon discontinuing the drug, these two lymphoid subpopulations rapidly returned towards normal levels, usually within 3–5 weeks. Their data involved 6 patients who had received azathioprine for several years and did not permit a correlation of the immunological findings with disease activity. There have been unsuccessful efforts to show such a correlation in Crohn's disease by testing the ability of peripheral blood lymphocytes to form spontaneous rosettes with sheep erythrocytes (Clarke, Richens, Williams, Gough and Ancil, 1974). These two reports point out that a study limited to peripheral blood lymphocytes is likely to give an incomplete representation of one's humoral and cellular immunological status at the tissue level. In a broader sense, they illustrate that meaningful therapeutic advances must be dependent upon a better understanding of immunological and other pathogenetic mechanisms in inflammatory bowel disease. This applies not only to azathioprine and metronidazole, but also to the use of BCG vaccine (Geffroy, Colin, Hecketsweiler and Segrestin, 1971; Rachail, Pellet, Bruttmann, Coulomb and Faure, 1973), transfer factor (Asquith *et al.*, 1975; Ng and Vicary, 1976), levamisole (Lehner, Wilton and Ivanyi, 1976), thymectomy (Cesnik, 1968; Cesnik and Schmid, 1971), epsilon-aminocaproic acid (Salter and Read, 1970; Mowat *et al.*, 1973), sodium cromoglycate (Heatley, Calcraft, Rhodes, Owen and Evans, 1974; Mani, Lloyd, Green, Fox and Turnberg, 1976), and other experimental treatments whose modes of action remain uncertain.

AETIOPATHOGENESIS OF INFLAMMATORY BOWEL DISEASE: IMMUNOLOGICAL HYPOTHESES

Since there are many clinical, epidemiological, familial and immunological similarities between ulcerative colitis and Crohn's disease, no clear-cut separation between the two conditions will be attempted in summarizing the major hypotheses of the aetiopathogenetic roles of humoral and cellular immune mechanisms. These hypotheses have included efforts to implicate autoimmunity, lymphocyte sensitization, immunogenetic factors, immune complexes, and combinations thereof, with the involvement of bacteria being germane to most of these views.

Some (Perlmann *et al.*, 1967; Lagercrantz *et al.*, 1968; Perlmann and Broberger, 1969) consider the occurrence of autoimmunity already to be well established in ulcerative colitis, although conceding that it is not known whether autoimmunity causes the tissue damage or contributes to its maintenance in a secondary manner. The heterogenetic antigen (Kunin, 1963) in most enteric bacteria which shares antigenic determinants with human colonic mucosa is hypothesized to give rise to

anticolon antibody formation through disruption of natural tolerance. Since the heterogenetic antigen also is present in healthy individuals, additional factors are required to explain the induction of anticolon autoimmunity in patients with inflammatory bowel disease. Perlmann and Broberger (1969) speculated that this could be on a genetic basis, perhaps reflecting a hereditary abnormality in the absorption of macromolecules through the intestinal wall. Furthermore, the *in-vitro* cytotoxic anticolon effect of lymphocytes from patients with inflammatory bowel disease was considered circumstantial evidence that cell-mediated autoimmune reactions also may contribute to the tissue damage in such patients.

The working hypothesis of Shorter *et al.* (1972a, 1976) is also based on the concept of hypersensitivity to bacterial antigens which are normally present in the gastrointestinal tract. Basically, they speculate that gut-associated lymphoid tissues become sensitized to common enterobacterial antigen as a result of increased mucosal permeability. Since shared antigenic determinants exist between this bacterial lipopolysaccharide and colonic epithelial cells, the stage is then set for a self-perpetuating, predominantly cell-mediated, possibly antibody-dependent immunological reaction directed against the bowel wall in perhaps genetically predisposed individuals. It is suggested that either antigen–antibody complexes or IgM antibody are responsible for the *in-vivo* arming of the Fc-receptor-bearing null (K-) lymphocytes for cytotoxicity. Several ideas are presented to explain why hypersensitivity to the ubiquitous enterobacterial antigen does not lead to immediate bowel injury, why all people need not react adversely, what predisposing factors are involved, and why the intestinal lesion often becomes chronic. It is also speculated that ulcerative colitis and Crohn's disease represent parts of a spectrum of a single pathogenetic process, with the different tissue manifestations being dependent in part on the site of interaction of antigen and lymphocytes. To explain how many patients may have long periods of remission, some type of selective immunosuppression is considered, either as a result of the suppression of lymphocyte-mediated immune reactions by antibacterial or anticolon antibodies, or due to the development of a form of tolerance. It is known that B-cells and suppressor T-cells are involved to varying degrees in different forms of tolerance (Grabar, 1975), but suppressor T-cells may also be involved as intermediaries in antibody-induced immunosuppression (Mitchell, 1976).

An earlier hypothesis (Burch, de Dombal and Watkinson, 1969) argued that ulcerative colitis is an 'auto-aggressive' process which develops only in those individuals having a predisposition for the disease based on polygenic factors. Thus, specific somatic gene mutations in mesenchymal stem cells were thought to initiate the disease process and lead to the activation of endogenous defences mediated through alpha$_2$-globulins, mast cells and other immunological mechanisms. Burch *et al.* (1969) pointed out that one or more of the genes predisposing to ulcerative colitis might also predispose the patient to associated conditions such as sacroiliitis, ankylosing spondylitis and uveitis. Genes encoding for histocompatibility antigens, common to the colonic mucosa and to these other tissues, were considered likely to be responsible for such pleiotropic effects. The subsequent tissue typing studies discussed below lend support to this view. No unusual ABO blood-group frequencies have been detected in inflammatory bowel disease (Winstone, Henderson and Brooke, 1960); while a reported (Sheehan, Necheles, Lindeman, Meyer and Patterson, 1967) 10 per cent association between the X-linked trait of erythrocyte glucose-6-phosphate dehydrogenase deficiency and Crohn's disease, but not ulcerative colitis, was followed by a study (Katsaros and Truelove, 1969) in which no examples of this trait were found in either disorder.

Specific antigens of the HLA histocompatibility system have been identified (Morris, 1974) to occur with increased frequencies in diseases with immunological features, such as systemic lupus erythematosus, ragweed pollenosis, chronic active hepatitis, pernicious anaemia and adult coeliac disease; in diseases with a strong genetic influence, such as diabetes mellitus and psoriasis; and in certain malignancies. Also, the strong association of HLA B27 in patients with ankylosing spondylitis (Schlosstein, Terasaki, Bluestone and Pearson, 1973; Brewerton *et al.*, 1973a; Dick, Sturrock, Dick and Buchanan, 1974; Russell, Schlaut, Percy and Dossetor, 1974) or acute anterior uveitis (Brewerton, Caffrey, Nicholls, Walters and James, 1973b) has been recognized.

It is not surprising, therefore, that similar HLA associations have been sought in groups of patients with inflammatory bowel disease. For example, (a) ankylosing spondylitis, iritis and other immune-associated diseases are not uncommon in such patients; (b) familial occurrences (Singer, Anderson, Frischer and Kirsner, 1971) are being recognized with increasing frequency, including multiple instances (Kirsner, 1973) of ulcerative colitis or Crohn's disease among sets of identical twins, and the occurrence of these conditions in all three members of one family (Rosenberg, Kraft and Kirsner, 1976); (c) humoral immunological abnormalities have long been recognized (Thayer and Spiro, 1963b; Polcak, Vokurka and Skalova, 1967; Polcak and Skalova, 1968; Lagercrantz *et al.*, 1971) in some of the apparently healthy relatives of patients with inflammatory bowel disease; and (d) various chromosomal abnormalities have been detected on rectal tissue karyotyping in

patients with chronic ulcerative colitis (Xavier, Prolla, Bemvenuti and Kirsner, 1974). The cumulative results of numerous studies (Thorsby and Lie, 1971; Gleeson, Walker, Wentzel, Chapman and Harris, 1972; Asquith, Mackintosh, Stokes, Holmes and Cooke, 1974; Lewkonia, Woodrow, McConnell and Evans, 1974; Brewerton, Caffrey, Nicholls, Walters and James, 1974; Morris, Metzger, Bluestone and Terasaki, 1974; Russell *et al.*, 1974, 1975; Jacoby and Jayson, 1974; Nahir, Gideoni, Eidelman and Barzilai, 1976) provide no evidence of a consistent association between specific HLA antigens and either ulcerative colitis or Crohn's disease, except for a positive correlation with HLA B27 in patients also having ankylosing spondylitis (Asquith *et al.*, 1974; Brewerton *et al.*, 1974; Morris *et al.*, 1974; Russell *et al.*, 1974; Russell *et al.*, 1975) or iritis (Morris *et al.*, 1974).

The association of particular HLA antigens with certain diseases suggests that these cell surface antigens could genetically predispose one to that disease by virtue of shared determinants with microbial, food or other environmental factors. This might enhance mucosal penetration by providing a receptor site or by preventing a protective response due to a form of immune tolerance (Morris, 1974). It has also been postulated (Svejgaard and Ryder, 1976) that HLA antigens may lead to disease by interfering with the interaction between nonimmunological ligands, such as hormones, and their receptors on cell surfaces. Finally, histocompatibility antigens have been shown to be linked closely to immune response genes in laboratory animals, and there have been increasing data linking such a mechanism to the association between HLA and diseases in man (McDevitt and Bodmer, 1974; Boettcher, 1975). Thus, in adult coeliac disease the presence of HLA B8 has now been associated with increased serum globulin levels (Ferguson, Asquith and Cooke, 1974), higher titres of serum antibodies to gluten (Scott, Swinburne, Rajah and Losowsky, 1974), and a decreased lymphocyte population in the lamina propria of the jejunum (Ferguson *et al.*, 1974) when receiving gluten, as well as with differences in the reactivity of the jejunal mucosa in organ culture (Nelson, Falchuk, Kasarda and Strober, 1974). Further studies (Katz, Mann, Nelson, Abelson and Strober, 1976) have shown that adult coeliac disease is associated with the simultaneous presence of an HLA gene, in linkage disequilibrium with HLA B8, and a disease specific non-HLA gene coding for antigen(s) on the surface of B-cells. The latter gene may represent an abnormal human immune response gene (Katz *et al.*, 1976). Such data support the concept (Nelson *et al.*, 1974; Strober, Falchuk, Rogentine, Nelson and Klaeveman, 1975) that such genes are not merely markers, but may play an important role in the pathogenesis of a disease; comparable immunogenetic studies would be of interest in inflammatory bowel disease (Lewkonia and McConnell, 1976).

It would also be important to analyse the components of the circulating, complement-binding, antigen–antibody complexes which have been identified in some patients with these same conditions. While such serological observations may merely reflect the uptake and transport of highly antigenic material from the intestinal lumen (Walker and Isselbacher, 1974), perhaps immune complexes are being formed in the intestinal mucosa in inflammatory bowel disease, as was suggested by the early immunofluorescent studies of Koffler *et al.* (1962) and the more recent findings of Monteiro *et al.* (1971). Erythema nodosum, uveitis, arthritis and other extra-intestinal manifestations could also reflect localization of soluble complexes at these sites (Doe *et al.*, 1973). Antigen–antibody complexes thus may trigger or perpetuate inflammatory responses and, under certain circumstances, antibody may combine with target cell antigens and render the cells susceptible to damage by non-immune lymphocytes (Brandtzaeg *et al.*, 1974). The finding (Korsmeyer *et al.*, 1974, 1976) of non-HLA-related serum lymphocytotoxic activity in patients with inflammatory bowel disease and their families also may reflect the presence of high-molecular-weight complexes of IgG; certainly, antilymphocyte antibodies may interfere with normal immune responses and contribute to disease chronicity. The finding by Sion and Friedell (1974) of serum lymphocytotoxins in patients with ulcerative colitis led to additional speculation about the role of tolerance in this disease.

There is still the additional hypothesis that pathogenic strains of *E. coli* (Cooke, 1968) or other organisms are responsible for ulcerative colitis and Crohn's disease, or that enteric organisms which ordinarily are classified as non-pathogens may proliferate and even become invasive in these diseases (Aluwihare, 1971; Vince, Dyer, O'Grady and Dawson, 1972; Cooke, Evans, Hywel-Jones and Lennard-Jones, 1974). *E. coli* has been the most frequently isolated organism associated with portal bacteraemia at the time of colectomy for ulcerative colitis (Eade and Brooke, 1969). Reports of coincident salmonellosis and ulcerative colitis continue to appear (Dronfield, Fletcher and Langman, 1974; Happel and Hershfield, 1974), creating problems of both recognition and management, but also suggesting more than a chance association between the two conditions. For example, the heterogenetic antigen of Kunin (1963) is present on the surface of *Salmonella*, *Shigella* and *Proteus* species, just as with *E. coli* 014.

Golde (1968) suggested that Crohn's disease was caused by a mycobacteria-related organism which defied culture and conventional tissue identification. It is thus of interest that Watson and Martucci (1975) have reported significant sensitivity to several mycobacterial antigens in patients with Crohn's disease on the basis of peripheral leucocyte migration-inhibition studies, although earlier (Morganroth and Watson, 1970) serum precipitin and delayed skin reactions to some of the same mycobacterial antigens had been negative in such patients. Electron-microscopic studies of the colon in inflammatory bowel disease by Dobbins and Siemers (1972) provided some presumptive support for viral involvement, but Gonzalez-Licea and Yardley (1966) and Nagle and Kurtz (1967) did not observe viral invasion of the colon in ulcerative colitis. The more recent evidence for the presence of viral agents in intestinal tissues from some patients with Crohn's disease was discussed above.

EPILOGUE

A clearer understanding is needed of the possible *in-vivo* relationships between bacterial and colonic antigens in inflammatory bowel disease, and further efforts should strive to document specific antigens and antibodies in the diseased intestinal tissues. In view of the ubiquitousness of the common enterobacterial antigen of Kunin and its cross-reactivity with cellular antigens of diverse origin (e.g. colonic and renal epithelium), why do only certain individuals develop inflammatory bowel disease? In this regard, the studies pursuing a genetic predisposition seem worthy. Also, the documentation of antigen–antibody complexes in the serum provides an exciting opportunity for antigen identification. Any type of immunological tissue damage requires the participation of antigen(s), although circulating immune complexes generally require some sort of tissue abnormality or co-factor before localizing at a given site. The recent viral studies certainly merit continuation.

There is much heterogeneity among populations of patients with ulcerative colitis and Crohn's disease, and a need exists to study subgroups with similarities based on abnormal serological features, common HLA antigens, positive family histories of inflammatory bowel disease and personal histories of multiple, extraintestinal disease manifestations. While there seems to have been much emphasis in recent years on cell-mediated immune phenomena, some of the unexplained earlier observations in the area of humoral immunity must be re-examined in the light of newer information (Spiegelberg, 1974; Rosenthal, Lipsky and Shevach, 1975), improved and more sensitive methods, and the knowledge that the humoral and cellular limbs of the immune system closely interact by virtue of several different subpopulations of immunoregulatory cells (Waldmann *et al.*, 1974; Dannenberg, 1975). Continuing studies of the role of the classical and alternate pathways of complement activation appear important in this respect. Another deficient area of knowledge is the functional status of the reticuloendothelial system in inflammatory bowel disease, an important part of the afferent limb of the immune response (Saba, 1970). Additional considerations suggest the need to reinvestigate the interaction of IgE (Heatley et al., 1975a; Lloyd et al., 1975) and mast cells (Kraft and Kirsner, 1960; Sommers, 1966; Rao 1973), and the release of kinins (Erdos, 1966; Kellermeyer and Graham, 1968) and other soluble mediators in the tissue reactions in these diseases.

The possible role of local immune mechanisms in protecting the intestinal mucosa from pathogenic bacteria and other environmental antigens remains uncertain. Much of this type of work has concerned so-called coproantibodies which appear in the intestinal lumen following either local synthesis or serum transudation. In addition to these antibodies of diverse origin and immunoglobulin class, cell-mediated immune mechanisms undoubtedly play a role in preventing untoward local antigen effects. Brandtzaeg (1973) has proposed two lines of defence with respect to local immune responses. The first is represented by the classical IgA response and supplies the mucosa with protective antibodies associated with the secretory IgA and IgM classes. Secondary local defence stems from complement-fixing IgG antibodies which are derived both from serum transudation and synthesis in local immunocytes, which are themselves the descendants of circulating lymphocytes. Undoubtedly these various defence mechanisms function concomitantly, coupled with non-immunological host defences (Apffel, 1976), and may vary with the nature of the antigen and other local tissue factors.

Observations (Bellamy and Nielsen, 1974) of the immune-mediated emigration of neutrophils into the lumen of the intestine have further emphasized the diversity of the potential protective mechanisms at mucosal surfaces. To take this a step further, the presence of gamma-globulin in the inflammatory bowel lesion may stimulate the phagocytic activity of polymorphonuclear neutrophils or lead to other physiological roles of this protein (Najjar, 1974). Recently (Segal and Loewi, 1976), the migration of neutrophils into skin windows has been found to be abnormally reduced in patients with Crohn's disease, but various in-vitro parameters of neutrophil function have consistently been normal in such patients (Ward and Eastwood, 1976; Segal and Loewi, 1976; Renz, Ward, Eastwood and Harkness, 1976; Binder and Riis, 1976).

We seem to be coming closer to an understanding of the role of the immunological apparatus of the intestine in both health and disease. Combinations of humoral and cellular immune phenomena, involving both induction and paralysis (Kagnoff, 1974), must occur in response to ingested and other luminal antigens. It is difficult to disregard any of the immunological hypotheses of the pathogenesis of inflammatory bowel disease, based upon data showing interactions among intestinal plasma cells, various subpopulations of B- and T-lymphocytes, eosinophils, neutrophils, macrophages, mast cells and plasma proteins, in close approximation with epithelial cells, and in constant exposure to the ubiquitous antigens which share determinants with colonic mucosal constituents, histocompatibility antigens and other normal body components. Which of the immunological observations reviewed herein are of aetiopathogenetic importance, and which are better considered as epiphenomena, remains to be established.

REFERENCES

Aas, J., Huizenga, K. A., Newcomer, A. D. & Shorter, R. G. (1972) Inflammatory bowel disease: lymphocytic responses to nonspecific stimulation in vitro. Scandinavian Journal of Gastroenterology, 7, 299–303.

Adams, D. O. (1976) The granulomatous inflammatory response: a review. American Journal of Pathology, 84, 164–192.

Aiuti, F. & Garofalo, J. A. (1972) Rectal immunoglobulin synthesis in ulcerative colitis. New England Journal of Medicine, 287, 1151.

Alp, M. H. & Wright, R. (1971) Autoantibodies to reticulin in patients with idiopathic steatorrhoea, coeliac disease, and Crohn's disease, and their relation to immunoglobulins and dietary antibodies. Lancet, ii, 682–685.

Aluwihare, A. P. R. (1971) Electron microscopy in Crohn's disease. Gut, 12, 509–518.

Ament, M. E. (1974) Intestinal granulomatosis in chronic granulomatous disease and in Crohn's disease. New England Journal of Medicine, 290, 228.

Ament, M. E. & Ochs, H. D. (1972) Gastrointestinal pathology in chronic granulomatous disease (CGD) of children: a clue to the etiology of Crohn's disease? Gastroenterology, 62, 836.

Ament, M. E. & Ochs, H. D. (1973) Gastrointestinal manifestations of chronic granulomatous disease. New England Journal of Medicine, 288, 382–387.

Apffel, C. A. (1976) Nonimmunological host defenses: a review. Cancer Research, 36, 1527–1537.

Arend, P. (1970) Alterations in the formation of 'natural' isoantibodies during the course of non-specific chronic ulcerative colitis. Gastroenterology, 58, 924.

Arend, P. & Fehlhaber, G. (1969) Der unterschiedliche Einfluss einer erhöhten enteralen Antigenresorption auf das Verhalten der 'natürlichen' Antikörper bei Personen der Blutgruppen O und A. Vergleichende blutgruppenserologische Untersuchungen an Patienten mit ulcerierender Colitis und Gesunden. Klinische Wochenschrift, 47, 535–541.

Aronson, M. D., Phillips, C. A., Beeken, W. L. & Forsyth, B. R. (1975) Isolation and characterization of a viral agent from intestinal tissue of patients with Crohn's disease and other intestinal disorders. Progress in Medical Virology, 21, 165–176.

Asherson, G. L. & Holborow, E. J. (1966) Autoantibody production in rabbits. VII. Autoantibodies to gut produced by the injection of bacteria. Immunology, 10, 161–167.

Asquith, P., Kraft, S. C. & Rothberg, R. M. (1973) Lymphocyte responses to nonspecific mitogens in inflammatory bowel disease. *Gastroenterology*, **65**, 1–7.

Asquith, P., Thompson, R. A. & Cooke, W. T. (1971) Quantitation of serum secretory IgA in gastrointestinal disease. *Clinical Research*, **19**, 562.

Asquith, P., Mackintosh, P., Stokes, P. L., Holmes, G. K. T. & Cooke, W. T. (1974) Histocompatibility antigens in patients with inflammatory-bowel disease. *Lancet*, **i**, 113–115.

Asquith, P., Mallas, E., Ross, I., Montgomery, R. D., Cooke, W. T. & Thompson, R. A. (1975) Transfer factor in the treatment of Crohn's disease. *Gut*, **16**, 832.

Baklien, K. & Brandtzaeg, P. (1974a) Local immunity and ulcerative colitis. *Lancet*, **ii**, 411–412.

Baklien, K. & Brandtzaeg, P. (1974b) Immunohistochemical localisation of complement in intestinal mucosa. *Lancet*, **ii**, 1087–1088.

Baklien, K. & Brandtzaeg, P. (1975) Comparative mapping of the local distribution of immunoglobulin-containing cells in ulcerative colitis and Crohn's disease of the colon. *Clinical and Experimental Immunology*, **22**, 197–209.

Ballard, J. & Shiner, M. (1974) Evidence of cytotoxicity in ulcerative colitis from immunofluorescent staining of the rectal mucosa. *Lancet*, **i**, 1014–1017.

Barnes, R. D., Fairweather, D. V. I., Holliday, J., Keane, C., Piesowicz, A., Soothill, J. F. & Tuffrey, M. (1969) A germfree infant. *Lancet*, **i**, 168–171.

Bárta, K. & Benýšek, L. (1968) Cutaneous hypersensitivity to deoxyribonucleic acid (DNA) in patients with ulcerative colitis. *Digestion*, **1**, 107–114.

Bartnik, W. & Zych, D. (1972) The Kviem controversy. *Lancet*, **i**, 154.

Bartnik, W., Swarbrick, E. T. & Williams, C. (1974) A study of peripheral leucocyte migration in agarose medium in inflammatory bowel disease. *Gut*, **15**, 294–300.

Basu, M. K., Asquith, P., Thompson, R. A. & Cooke, W. T. (1975) Oral manifestations of Crohn's disease. *Gut*, **16**, 249–254.

Bean, R. H. D. (1962) The treatment of chronic ulcerative colitis with 6-mercaptopurine. *Medical Journal of Australia*, **2**, 592–593.

Beeken, W. L., Busch, H. J. & Sylwester, D. L. (1972) Intestinal protein loss in Crohn's disease. *Gastroenterology*, **62**, 207–215.

Bellamy, J. E. C. & Nielsen, N. O. (1974) Immune-mediated emigration of neutrophils into the lumen of the small intestine. *Infection and Immunity*, **9**, 615–619.

Bendixen, G. (1967) Specific inhibition of the *in-vitro* migration of leucocytes in ulcerative colitis and Crohn's disease. *Scandinavian Journal of Gastroenterology*, **2**, 214–221.

Bendixen, G. (1969) Cellular hypersensitivity to components of intestinal mucosa in ulcerative colitis and Crohn's disease. *Gut*, **10**, 631–636.

Bendixen, G. (1970) Cellular hypersensitivity to intestinal mucosa components in ulcerative colitis and Crohn's disease. *Tijdschrift voor Gastroenterologie*, **13**, 459–466.

Bendixen, G., Goltermann, N., Jarnum, S., Jensen, K. B., Weeke, B. & Westergaard, H. (1970) Immunoglobulin and albumin turnover in ulcerative colitis. *Scandinavian Journal of Gastroenterology*, **5**, 433–441.

Bendixen, G., Jarnum, S., Söltoft, J., Westergaard, H., Weeke, B. & Yssing, M. (1968) IgG and albumin turnover in Crohn's disease. *Scandinavian Journal of Gastroenterology*, **3**, 481–489.

Benedict, A. A. (1965) Sensitivity of passive haemagglutination for assay of 7S and 19S antibodies in primary rabbit anti-bovine serum albumin sera. *Nature (London)*, **206**, 1368–1369.

Bergman, L., Johansson, S. G. O. & Krause, U. (1973) The immunoglobulin concentrations in serum and bowel secretion in patients with Crohn's disease. *Scandinavian Journal of Gastroenterology*, **8**, 401–406.

Best, W. R., Becktel, J. M., Singleton, J. W. & Kern, F. (1976) Development of a Crohn's disease activity index: National Cooperative Crohn's Disease Study. *Gastroenterology*, **70**, 439–444.

Bicks, R. O., Kirsner, J. B. & Palmer, W. L. (1959a) Serum proteins in ulcerative colitis. I. Electrophoretic patterns in active disease. *Gastroenterology*, **37**, 256–262.

Bicks, R. O., Kirsner, J. B. & Palmer, W. L. (1959b) Serum proteins in ulcerative colitis. II. The effects of therapy correlated with electrophoretic patterns. *Gastroenterology*, **37**, 263–267.

Binder, H. J., Spiro, H. M. & Thayer, W. R., Jr (1966) Delayed hypersensitivity in regional enteritis and ulcerative colitis. *American Journal of Digestive Diseases*, **11**, 572–574.

Binder, V. & Riis, P. (1976) The leucocyte chemotactic function in patients with Crohn's disease. *Scandinavian Journal of Gastroenterology*, **11**, Suppl. 38, 89.

Bird, A. G. & Britton, S. (1974) No evidence for decreased lymphocyte reactivity in Crohn's disease. *Gastroenterology*, **67**, 926–932.

Blichfeldt, P., Blomhoff, J. P., Myhre, E. & Gjone, E. (1976) Metronidazole in Crohn's disease – a preliminary report of a double blind cross over study. *Scandinavian Journal of Gastroenterology*, **11**, Suppl. 38, 100.

Bolton, P. M., James, S. L., Newcombe, R. G., Whitehead, R. H. & Hughes, L. E. (1974) The immune competence of patients with inflammatory bowel disease. *Gut*, **15**, 213–219.

Bolton, P. M., Owen, E., Heatley, R. V., Jones Williams, W. & Hughes, L. E. (1973) Negative findings in laboratory animals for a transmissible agent in Crohn's disease. *Lancet*, **ii**, 1122–1124.

Booth, S. N., King, J. P. G., Leonard, J. C. & Dykes, P. W. (1974) The significance of elevation of serum carcinoembryonic antigen (CEA) levels in inflammatory diseases of the intestine. *Scandinavian Journal of Gastroenterology*, **9**, 651–656.

Bowen, G. E., Irons, G. V., Jr, Rhodes, J. B. Kirsner, J. B. (1966) Early experiences with azathioprine in ulcerative colitis. A note of caution. *Journal of the American Medical Association*, **195**, 460–464.

Brandtzaeg, P. (1973) Structure, synthesis and external transfer of mucosal immunoglobulins. *Annales d'Immunologie*, **124C**, 417–438.

Brandtzaeg, P. (1974) Mucosal and glandular distribution of immunoglobulin components. Immunohistochemistry with a cold ethanol-fixation technique. *Immunology*, **26**, 1101–1114.

Brandtzaeg, P. & Baklien, K. (1974) Bowel diseases involving local immunoglobulin systems. *Acta Pathologica et Microbiologica Scandinavica*, Section A, Suppl. 248, 43–60.

Brandtzaeg, P. & Baklien, K. (1976) Immunohistochemical studies of the formation and epithelial transport of immunoglobulins in normal and diseased human intestinal mucosa. *Scandinavian Journal of Gastroenterology*, **11**, Suppl. 36, 1–45.

Brandtzaeg, P., Baklien, K., Fausa, O. & Hoel, P. S. (1974) Immunohistochemical characterization of local immunoglobulin formation in ulcerative colitis. *Gastroenterology*, **66**, 1123–1136.

Bregman, E. & Kirsner, J. B. (1965) Amino acids of colon and rectum. Possible involvement of diaminopimelic acid of intestinal bacteria in antigenicity of ulcerative colitis colon. *Proceedings of the Society for Experimental Biology and Medicine*, **118**, 727–731.

Brewerton, D. A., Caffrey, M., Nicholls, A., Walters, D. & James, D. C. O. (1973b) Acute anterior uveitis and HL-A 27. *Lancet*, **ii**, 994–996.

Brewerton, D. A., Caffrey, M., Nicholls, A., Walters, D. & James, D. C. O. (1974) HL-A 27 and arthropathies associated with ulcerative colitis and psoriasis. *Lancet*, **i**, 956–958.

Brewerton, D. A., Caffrey, M., Hart, F. D., James, D. C. O., Nicholls, A. & Sturrock, R. D. (1973a) Ankylosing spondylitis and HL-A 27. *Lancet*, **i**, 904–907.

Broberger, O. & Perlmann, P. (1959) Autoantibodies in human ulcerative colitis. *Journal of Experimental Medicine*, **110**, 657–674.

Broberger, O. & Perlmann, P. (1962) Demonstration of an epithelial antigen in colon by means of fluorescent antibodies from children with ulcerative colitis. *Journal of Experimental Medicine*, **115**, 13–26.

Broberger, O. & Perlmann, P. (1963) *In-vitro* studies of ulcerative colitis. I. Reactions of patients' serum with human fetal colon cells in tissue cultures. *Journal of Experimental Medicine*, **117**, 705–716.

Brostoff, J. & Walker, J. G. (1971) Leucocyte migration inhibition with Kveim antigen in Crohn's disease. *Clinical and Experimental Immunology*, **9**, 707–711.

Brown, S. M., Taub, R. N., Present, D. H. & Janowitz, H. D. (1970) Short-term lymphocyte cultures in regional enteritis. *Lancet*, **i**, 1112.

Brown, W. R. & Lee, E. M. (1973) Radioimmunologic measurements of naturally occurring bacterial antibodies. I. Human serum antibodies reactive with *Escherichia coli* in gastrointestinal and immunologic disorders. *Journal of Laboratory and Clinical Medicine*, **82**, 125–136.

Brown, W. R. & Lee, E. M. (1974) Radioimmunological measurements of bacterial antibodies. II. Human serum antibodies reactive with *Bacteroides fragilis* and *Enterococcus* in gastrointestinal and immunological disorders. *Gastroenterology*, **66**, 1145–1153.

Brown, W. R., Borthistle, B. K. & Chen, S.-T. (1975) Immunoglobulin E (IgE) and IgE-containing cells in human gastrointestinal fluids and tissues. *Clinical and Experimental Immunology*, **20**, 227–237.

Brown, W. R., Lansford, C. L. & Hornbrook, M. (1973) Serum immunoglobulin E (IgE) concentrations in patients with gastrointestinal disorders. *American Journal of Digestive Diseases*, **18**, 641–645.

Bucknall, R. C., Verrier Jones, J. & Peacock, D. B. (1975) The immune response to ØX 174 in man. II. Primary and secondary antibody production in patients with Crohn's disease. *American Journal of Digestive Diseases*, **20**, 430–436.

Bull, D. M. (1974) Lymphocyte responsiveness to plant mitogens in diseases of unknown cause. *Gastroenterology*, **67**, 1071–1073.

Bull, D. M. & Bookman, M. A. (1976) Isolation and functional characterization of human intestinal submucosal lymphoid cells. *Clinical Research*, **24**, 431A.

Bull, D. M. & Ignaczak, T. F. (1974) Enterobacterial common antigen-induced lymphocyte reactivity in inflammatory bowel disease. *Gastroenterology*, **64**, 43–50.

Burch, P. R. J., de Dombal, F. T. & Watkinson, G. (1969) Aetiology of ulcerative colitis. II. A new hypothesis. *Gut*, **10**, 277–284.

Campbell, A. C., Skinner, J. M., Hersey, P., Roberts-Thomson, P., MacLennan, I. C. M. & Truelove, S. C. (1974) Immunosuppression in the treatment of inflammatory bowel disease. I. Changes in lymphoid sub-populations in the blood and rectal mucosa following cessation of treatment with azathioprine. *Clinical and Experimental Immunology*, **16**, 521–533.

Carlsson, H. E., Hammarström, S., Lanteli, M. & Perlmann, P. (1971) Antibody-induced destruction of colon antigen-coated chicken erythrocytes by normal human lymphocytes. *European Journal of Immunology*, **1**, 281–285.

Caspary, E. A. & Field, E. J. (1971) Lymphocyte sensitization in sarcoidosis. *British Medical Journal*, **ii**, 143–145.

Cave, D. R. & Brooke, B. N. (1973) A study of lymphocyte function in Crohn's disease using the mitotic index. *British Journal of Surgery*, **60**, 319.

Cave, D. R., Mitchell, D. N. & Brooke, B. N. (1975) Experimental animal studies of the etiology and pathogenesis of Crohn's disease. *Gastroenterology*, **69**, 618–624.

Cave, D. R., Mitchell, D. N., Kane, S. P. & Brooke, B. N. (1973) Further animal evidence of a transmissible agent in Crohn's disease. *Lancet*, **ii**, 1120–1122.

Cesnik, H. (1968) Thymektomie bei Colitis ulcerosa. Vorläufiger Bericht über einen Behandlungsversuch bei 7 Patienten. *Langenbecks Archiv fur klinische Chirurgie*, **321**, 86–98.

Cesnik, H. & Schmid, K. O. (1971) Über Lymphfollikel im Thymus bei Colitis ulcerosa. *Langenbecks Archiv fur klinische Chirurgie*, **328**, 128–138.

Chandra, R. K. & Saraya, A. K. (1975) Impaired immunocompetence associated with iron deficiency. *Journal of Pediatrics*, **86**, 899–902.

Chapman, J. A., Gleeson, M. H. & Taylor, G. (1971) Kveim tests in Crohn's disease. *Lancet*, **ii**, 1097.

Claman, H. N. (1972) Corticosteroids and lymphoid cells. *New England Journal of Medicine*, **287**, 388–397.

Clancy, R. (1976) Isolation and kinetic characteristics of mucosal lymphocytes in Crohn's disease. *Gastroenterology*, **70**, 177–180.

Clarke, J. R., Richens, E. R., Williams, M. J., Gough, K. R. & Ancill, R. J. (1974) An evaluation of the rosette-inhibition test in Crohn's disease. *Gut*, **15**, 725–727.

Cohen, I. R. & Norins, L. C. (1968) Antibodies of the IgG, IgM, and IgA classes in newborn and adult sera reactive with gram-negative bacteria. *Journal of Clinical Investigation*, **47**, 1053–1062.

Colten, H. R., Gordon, J. M., Rapp, H. J. & Borsos, T. (1968) Synthesis of the first component of guinea-pig complement by columnar epithelial cells of the small intestine. *Journal of Immunology*, **100**, 788–792.

Cook, M. G. & Turnbull, G. J. (1975) A hypothesis for the pathogenesis of Crohn's disease based on an ultrastructural study. *Virchows Archiv A: Pathological Anatomy and Histology*, **365**, 327–336.

Cooke, E. M. (1968) Properties of strains of *Escherichia coli* isolated from the faeces of patients with ulcerative colitis, patients with acute diarrhoea and normal persons. *Journal of Pathology and Bacteriology*, **95**, 101–113.

Cooke, E. M., Filipe, M. I. & Dawson, I. M. P. (1968) The production of colonic auto-antibodies in rabbits by immunisation with *Escherichia coli*. *Journal of Pathology and Bacteriology*, **96**, 125–130.

Cooke, E. M., Ewins, S. P., Hywel-Jones, J. &

Lennard-Jones, J. E. (1974) Properties of strains of *Escherichia coli* carried in different phases of ulcerative colitis. *Gut*, **15**, 143–146.

Cornelis, W. (1958) *Contribution à l'étude et expérimentale de la rectocolite hémorragique. Mémoires assistant étranger.* Paris: Faculté Médecine.

Crabbé, P. A. & Heremans, J. F. (1966) Presence of large numbers of plasma cells containing IgD in the rectal mucosa of a patient with ulcerative colitis. *Acta Clinica Belgica*, **21**, 73–83.

Crout, J. E., Hepburn, B. & Ritts, R. E., Jr (1975) Suppression of lymphocyte formation after aspirin ingestion. *New England Journal of Medicine*, **292**, 221–223.

Dannenberg, A. M., Jr (1975) Macrophages in inflammation and infection. *New England Journal of Medicine*, **293**, 489–493.

Das, K. M., Erber, W. & Rubinstein, A. (1975) Immunological studies in patients with idiopathic proctitis: changes in systemic immune reactions, secretory component and immunoglobulins in histologically involved and uninvolved colonic mucosa. *Gastroenterology*, **68**, 880.

Daum, F., Boley, S. J. & Cohen, M. I. (1974) Miliary Crohn's disease. *Gastroenterology*, **67**, 527–530.

de Dombal, F. T. (1967) Serum proteins in ulcerative colitis: electrophoretic patterns in the inferior mesenteric artery and vein. *Gut*, **8**, 482–485.

de Dombal, F. T. (1969) Prognostic value of estimating serum proteins in cases of ulcerative colitis in remission. *Gut*, **10**, 491–496.

DeHoratius, R., Strickland, R. G. & Williams, R. C. (1974) T and B lymphocytes in acute and chronic hepatitis. *Clinical Immunology and Immunopathology*, **2**, 353–360.

Deodhar, S. D., Michener, W. M. & Farmer, R. G. (1969) A study of the immunologic aspects of chronic ulcerative colitis and transmural colitis. *American Journal of Clinical Pathology*, **51**, 591–597.

Dick, H. M., Sturrock, R. D., Dick, W. C. & Buchanan, W. W. (1974) Inheritance of ankylosing spondylitis and HL-A antigen W27. *Lancet*, **ii**, 24–25.

Dilawari, J. B., Lennard-Jones, J. E., Mackay, A. M., Ritchie, J. K. & Sturzaker, H. G. (1975) Estimation of carcinoembryonic antigen in ulcerative colitis with special reference to malignant change. *Gut*, **16**, 255–260.

Dines, D. E., DeRemee, R. A. & Green, P. A. (1971) Sarcoidosis associated with regional enteritis (Crohn's disease). Report of two cases. *Minnesota Medicine*, **54**, 617–620.

Dobbins, W. O., III (1975) Colonic epithelial cells and polymorphonuclear leukocytes in ulcerative colitis: an electron microscopic study. *American Journal of Digestive Diseases*, **20**, 236–252.

Dobbins, W. O., III & Siemers, P. T. (1972) A viral etiology for inflammatory bowel disease? *Gastroenterology*, **62**, 742.

Doe, W. F., Booth, C. C. & Brown, D. L. (1973) Evidence for complement-binding immune complexes in adult coeliac disease, Crohn's disease, and ulcerative colitis. *Lancet*, **i**, 402–403.

Douglas, A. C., Wallace, A., Clark, J., Stephens, J. H., Smith, I. E. & Allan, N. C. (1976) The Edinburgh spleen: source of a validated Kveim–Siltzbach test material. *Annals of the New York Academy of Sciences*, **278**, 670–679.

Drach, G. W., Reed, W. P. & Williams, R. C. (1972) Antigens common to human and bacterial cells. II. *E. coli* 014, the common Enterobacteriaceae antigen, blood groups A and B, and *E. coli* 086. *Journal of Laboratory and Clinical Medicine*, **79**, 38–46.

Dronfield, M. W., Fletcher, J. & Langman, M. J. S. (1974) Coincident Salmonella infections and ulcerative colitis: problems of recognition and management. *British Medical Journal*, **i**, 99–100.

Dudek, B., Spiro, H. M. & Thayer, W. R., Jr (1965) A study of ulcerative colitis and circulating antibodies to milk proteins. *Gastroenterology*, **49**, 544–547.

Dykes, P. W. (1970) Delayed hypersensitivity in Crohn's disease. *Proceedings of the Royal Society of Medicine*, **63**, 906–908.

Dykes, P. W. (1972) Immunology of Crohn's disease. *Clinics in Gastroenterology*, **1**, 349–366.

Eade, M. N. & Brooke, B. N. (1969) Portal bacteraemia in cases of ulcerative colitis submitted to colectomy. *Lancet*, **i**, 1008–1009.

Eastwood, G. L. & Trier, J. S. (1973a) Organ culture of human rectal mucosa. *Gastroenterology*, **64**, 375–382.

Eastwood, G. L. & Trier, J. S. (1973b) Epithelial cell renewal in cultured rectal biopsies in ulcerative colitis. *Gastroenterology*, **64**, 383–390.

Editorial (1975) Lymphocyte subpopulations in chronic inflammatory diseases. *British Medical Journal*, **ii**, 1–2.

Eggert, R. C., Wilson, I. D. & Good, R. A. (1969) Agammaglobulinemia and regional enteritis. *Annals of Internal Medicine*, **71**, 581–585.

Ehrenfeld, E. N., Gery, I. & Davies, A. M. (1961) Specific antibodies in heart-disease. *Lancet*, **i**, 1138–1141.

Epstein, W. L. (1967) Granulomatous hypersensitivity. *Progress in Allergy*, **11**, 36–88.

Erdös, E. G. (1966) Release and inactivation of kinins. *Gastroenterology*, **51**, 893–900.

Ezer, G. & Hayward, A. R. (1974) Inhibition of complement-dependent lymphocyte rosette formation: a possible test for activated complement products. *European Journal of Immunology*, **4**, 148–150.

Falchuk, K. R. & Isselbacher, K. J. (1976) Circulating antibodies to bovine albumin in ulcerative colitis and Crohn's disease. Characterization of the antibody response. *Gastroenterology*, **70**, 5–8.

Farmer, G. W., Vincent, M. M., Fuccillo, D. A., Horta-Barbosa, L., Ritman, S., Sever, J. L. & Gitnick, G. L. (1973) Viral investigations in ulcerative colitis and regional enteritis. *Gastroenterology*, **65**, 8–18.

Farr, R. S. (1963) Some comments regarding the allergic state. *Archives of Environmental Health*, **6**, 92–98.

Feinstein, P. A., Kaplan, S. R. & Thayer, W. R., Jr (1976) The alternate complement pathway in inflammatory bowel disease. Quantitation of the C3 proactivator (factor B) protein. *Gastroenterology*, **70**, 181–185.

Ferguson, R., Allan, R. N. & Cooke, W. T. (1975) A study of the cellular infiltrate of the proximal jejunal mucosa in ulcerative colitis and Crohn's disease. *Gut*, **16**, 205–208.

Ferguson, R., Asquith, P. & Cooke, W. T. (1974) Histocompatibility antigens in coeliac disease. *Gut*, **15**, 834.

Fichtelius, K. E. (1968) The gut epithelium – a first level lymphoid organ? *Experimental Cell Research*, **49**, 87–104.

Fink, S. & Mais, R. F. (1968) Cell-mediated immune reaction to colon altered by bacteria. *Gut*, **9**, 629–632.

Fink, S., Donnelly, W. J. & Jablokow, V. R. (1967a) Rectal reaction to injected ulcerative colitis leucocytes and plasma. *Gut*, **8**, 20–23.

Fink, S., Mais, R. F., Locke, R. F. & Hall, A. G. (1967b) *E. coli* agglutinating activity of ulcerative colitis sera. *Proceedings of the Society for Experimental Biology and Medicine*, **125**, 402–404.

Fiorilli, M., Luzi, G. & Aiuti, F. (1975) Immunoglobulin production by the rectal mucosa in subjects with ulcerative colitis. *Rendiconti di Gastro-enterologia*, 7, 1–4.

Fixa, B., Komarkova, O., Skaunic, V., Nerad, M. & Kojecky, Z. (1975) Inhibition of leucocyte migration by antigens from human colon and *E. coli* 014 in patients with ulcerative colitis. *Scandinavian Journal of Gastroenterology*, 10, 491–493.

Fletcher, J. (1965) Serum complement levels in active ulcerative colitis. *Gut*, 6, 172–175.

Fletcher, J. & Hinton, J. M. (1967) Tuberculin sensitivity in Crohn's disease. *Lancet*, ii, 753–754.

Flewett, T. H. & Boxall, E. (1976) The hunt for viruses in infections of the alimentary system: an immunoelectron-microscopical approach. *Clinics in Gastroenterology*, 5, 359–385.

Fodor, O., Dumitrascu, D., Radu, D., Dejica, D. & Grigorescu, M. (1974) Inflammation of the intestinal mucosa and immunoglobulin production. *Annales de Gastroenterologie et d'Hepatologie (Paris)*, 10, 377–387.

Fogel, B. J., Hook, W. A. & Polish, E. (1967) A note on serum complement activity with particular reference to ulcerative colitis. *Military Medicine*, 132, 282–285.

Friedman, E. A., Bardawil, W. A., Merrill, J. P. & Hanau, C. (1960) 'Delayed' cutaneous hypersensitivity to leukocytes in disseminated lupus erythematosus. *New England Journal of Medicine*, 262, 486–491.

Geffroy, Y., Colin, R., Hecketsweiler, P. & Segrestin, M. (1971) Traitment de la maladie de Crohn par le BCG. Données biologiques – essai d'interprétation. *Archives Françaises des Maladies de l'Appareil Digestif*, 60, 299–308.

Gelernt, I. M., Present, D. H. & Janowitz, H. D. (1972) Alterations in serum immunoglobulins after resection of ulcerative and granulomatous disease of the intestine. *Gut*, 13, 21–23.

Gelzayd, E. A., Kraft, S. C. & Fitch, F. W. (1967) Immunoglobulin A: localization in rectal mucosal epithelial cells. *Science*, 157, 930–931.

Gelzayd, E. A., Kraft, S. C., Fitch, F. W. & Kirsner, J. B. (1968) Distribution of immunoglobulins in human rectal mucosa. II. Ulcerative colitis and abnormal mucosal control subjects. *Gastroenterology*, 54, 341–347.

Gibbs, N. M. & French, L. W. (1971) The colon mucus antibody. *Journal of Clinical Pathology*, 24, 867–869.

Gitnick, G. L. & Rosen, V. J. (1976) Electron microscopic studies of viral agents in Crohn's disease. *Lancet*, ii, 217–219.

Gitnick, G. L., Arthur, M. H. & Shibata, I. (1976) Cultivation of viral agents from Crohn's disease. A new sensitive system. *Lancet*, ii, 215–217.

Glass, R. E. & Baker, W. N. W. (1976) Role of the granuloma in recurrent Crohn's disease. *Gut*, 17, 75–77.

Gleeson, M. H., Walker, J. S., Wentzel, J., Chapman, J. A. & Harris, R. (1972) Human leucocyte antigens in Crohn's disease and ulcerative colitis. *Gut*, 13, 438–440.

Golde, D. W. (1968) Aetiology of regional enteritis. *Lancet*, i, 1144–1145.

Gonzalez-Licea, A. & Yardley, J. H. (1966) A comparative ultrastructural study of the mucosa in idiopathic ulcerative colitis, shigellosis and other human colonic diseases. *Bulletin of the Johns Hopkins Hospital*, 118, 444–461.

Grabar, P. (1975) Hypothesis. Auto-antibodies and immunological theories: an analytical review. *Clinical Immunology and Immunopathology*, 4, 453–466.

Green, F. H. Y. & Fox, H. (1975) The distribution of mucosal antibodies in the bowel of patients with Crohn's disease. *Gut*, 16, 125–131.

Greenberg, S. D., Györkey, F., Weg, J. C., Jenkins, D. E. & Györkey, P. (1970) The ultrastructure of the pulmonary granuloma in 'sarcoidosis'. *American Review of Respiratory Disease*, 102, 648–652.

Griscom, N. T., Kirkpatrick, J. A., Jr, Girdany, B. R., Berdon, W. E., Grand, R. J. & Mackie, G. G. (1974) Gastric antral narrowing in chronic granulomatous disease of childhood. *Pediatrics*, 54, 456–460.

Grotsky, H. W., Glade, P. R., Hirshaut, Y., Sachar, D. & Janowitz, H. D. (1970) Herpes-like virus and granulomatous colitis. *Lancet*, ii, 1256–1257.

Grotsky, H. W., Hirshaut, Y., Sorokin, C., Sachar, D., Janowitz, H. D. & Glade, P. R. (1971) Epstein-Barr virus and inflammatory bowel disease. *Experientia*, 27, 1474–1475.

Grove, D. I., Mahmoud, A. A. F. & Warren, K. S. (1976) Suppression of cell-mediated immunity by metronidazole. *Clinical Research*, 24, 285A.

Guillou, P. J., Brennan, T. G. & Giles, G. R. (1973) Lymphocyte transformation in the mesenteric lymph nodes of patients with Crohn's disease. *Gut*, 14, 20–24.

Hammarström, S., Carlsson, H. E., Perlmann, P. & Svensson, S. (1971) Immunochemistry of the common antigen of Enterobacteriaceae (Kunin). *Journal of Experimental Medicine*, 134, 565–576.

Hammarström, S., Lagercrantz, R., Perlmann, P. & Gustafsson, B. E. (1965) Immunological studies in ulcerative colitis. II. 'Colon' antigen and human blood group A- and H-like antigens in germfree rats. *Journal of Experimental Medicine*, 122, 1075–1086.

Hammarström, S., Perlmann, P., Gustafsson, B. E. & Lagercrantz, R. (1969) Autoantibodies to colon in germfree rats monocontaminated with Clostridium difficile. *Journal of Experimental Medicine*, 129, 747–756.

Hammer, B., Ashurst, P. & Naish, J. (1968) Diseases associated with ulcerative colitis and Crohn's disease. *Gut*, 9, 17–21.

Haneberg, B. & Aarskog, D. (1975) Human faecal immunoglobulins in healthy infants and children, and in some with diseases affecting the intestinal tract or the immune system. *Clinical and Experimental Immunology*, 22, 210–222.

Haneberg, B. & Endresen, C. (1976) Fragments of immunoglobulins in human faeces. *Acta Pathologica et Microbiologica Scandinavica*, Section C 84, 31–36.

Hannuksela, M., Alkio, H., Selroos, O. (1971) Kveim reaction in Crohn's disease. *Lancet*, ii, 974.

Happel, K. R. & Hershfield, N. B. (1974) An association between ulcerative colitis and Salmonella infection. *Clinical Research*, 22, 589A.

Hardy Smith, A. & Macphee, I. W. (1971) A clinico-immunological study of ulcerative colitis and ulcerative proctitis. *Gut*, 12, 20–26.

Harrison, W. J. (1965) Autoantibodies against intestinal and gastric mucous cells in ulcerative colitis. *Lancet*, i, 1346–1350.

Haslock, I. (1973) Arthritis and Crohn's disease. A family study. *Annals of Rheumatic Diseases*, 32, 479–486.

Hausamen, T. U., Halcrow, D. A. & Taylor, K. B. (1969) Biological effects of gastrointestinal antibodies. III. The effects of heterologous and autoantibodies on deoxyribonucleic acid synthesis in the stomach and colon of guinea pigs and rabbits. *Gastroenterology*, 56, 1071–1077.

Healy, G. R. & Kraft, S. C. (1972) The indirect hemagglutination test for amebiasis in patients with inflammatory bowel disease. *American Journal of Digestive Diseases*, **17**, 97–103.

Heatley, R. V., Bolton, P. M., Owen, E., Jones Williams, W. & Hughes, L. E. (1975a) A search for a transmissible agent in Crohn's disease. *Gut*, **16**, 528–532.

Heatley, R. V., Calcraft, B. J., Rhodes, J., Owen, E. & Evans, B. (1974) Treatment of chronic proctitis with disodium cromoglycate. *Gut*, **15**, 829.

Heatley, R. V., Rhodes, J., Calcraft, B. J., Whitehead, R. H., Fifield, R. & Newcombe, R. G. (1975b) Immunoglobulin E in rectal mucosa of patients with proctitis. *Lancet*, **ii**, 1010–1012.

Heaton, K. W., McCarthy, C. F., Horton, R. E., Cornes, J. S. & Read, A. E. (1967) Miliary Crohn's disease. *Gut*, **8**, 4–7.

Helms, R. A., Miller, S. E., Grendell, J. H. & Bull, D. M. (1974) Anti-inflammatory drugs: differential effects on lymphoblastic transformation and antibody-dependent cellular cytotoxicity. *Clinical Research*, **22**, 702A.

Henry, C., Bernard, D. & Depieds, R. (1968) Étude biochimique et immunochimique des antigènes solubles de la muqueuse du gros intestin humain. I. Extraction et fractionnement. *Annales de l'Institut Pasteur*, **114**, 395–416.

Hess, E. V., Fink, C. W., Taranta, A. & Ziff, M. (1964) Heart muscle antibodies in rheumatic fever and other diseases. *Journal of Clinical Investigation*, **43**, 886–893.

Hiatt, R. B. & Katz, L. (1962) Mast cells in inflammatory conditions of the gastrointestinal tract. *American Journal of Gastroenterology*, **37**, 541–545.

Hinz, C. F., Jr, Perlmann, P. & Hammarström, S. (1967) Reactivity *in vitro* of lymphocytes from patients with ulcerative colitis. *Journal of Laboratory and Clinical Medicine*, **70**, 752–759.

Hobbs, J. R. & Hepner, G. W. (1968) Immunoglobulins and alimentary disease. *Lancet*, **ii**, 47.

Hodgson, H. J. F., Potter, B. J. & Jewell, D. P. (1975) Complement in inflammatory bowel disease. *Gut*, **15**, 833–834.

Høj, L. & Sørensen, S. F. (1976) Lymphocyte subpopulations in chronic inflammatory bowel disease. *Scandinavian Journal of Gastroenterology*, **11**, Suppl. 38, 91.

Holm, G. & Palmblad, J. (1976) Acute energy deprivation in man: effect on cell-mediated immunological reactions. *Clinical and Experimental Immunology*, **25**, 207–211.

Holmgren, J., Hammarström, S., Holm, S. E., Ahlmén, J., Attman, P. O. & Jodal, U. (1972) An antigenic relationship between human kidney, colon and the common antigen of Enterobacteriaceae. *International Archives of Allergy and Applied Immunology*, **43**, 89–97.

Hunt, P. S. (1972) The action of autologous lymphocytes against colon cells from patients with acute ulcerative colitis: *in vitro* studies. *British Journal of Surgery*, **59**, 911.

Hunt, P. S. & Trotter, S. (1973) Lymphoblastic response to autologous colon epithelial cells in ulcerative colitis *in vitro*. *Gut*, **14**, 875–879.

Hunt, P. S. & Trotter, S. (1975) The *in-vitro* action of lymphocytes on autologous colon epithelial cells in ulcerative colitis. *Australian and New Zealand Journal of Surgery*, **45**, 214–219.

Hurley, T. H. & Lane, W. R. (1971) The Kveim controversy. *Lancet*, **ii**, 1373.

Hurley, T. H., Sullivan, J. R. & Hurley, J. V. (1975) Reaction to Kveim test material in sarcoidosis and other diseases. *Lancet*, **i**, 494–496.

Isaacson, P. (1976) Tissue demonstration of

carcinoembryonic antigen (CEA) in ulcerative colitis. *Gut*, **17**, 561–567.

Ishizaka, K. (1970) Human reaginic antibodies. *Annual Review of Medicine*, **21**, 187–200.

Ishizaka, K. & Ishizaka, T. (1968) Reversed type allergic skin reactions by anti-γE-globulin antibodies in humans and monkeys. *Journal of Immunology*, **100**, 554–562.

Israel, H. L. & Goldstein, R. A. (1971) Relation of Kveim-antigen reaction to lymphadenopathy. Study of sarcoidosis and other diseases. *New England Journal of Medicine*, **284**, 345–349.

Jacoby, R. K. & Jayson, M. I. V. (1974) HL-A 27 in Crohn's disease. *Annals of the Rheumatic Diseases*, **33**, 422–424.

James, D. G. (1975) Kveim revisited, reassessed. *New England Journal of Medicine*, **292**, 859–860.

Janowitz, H. D. & Sachar, D. B. (1976) New observations in Crohn's disease. *Annual Review of Medicine*, **27**, 269–285.

Jarnum, S. & Jensen, K. B. (1975) Fecal radioiodide excretion following intravenous injection of ^{131}I-albumin and ^{125}I-immunoglobulin G in chronic inflammatory bowel disease. An aid to topographic diagnosis. *Gastroenterology*, **68**, 1433–1444.

Jensen, K. B., Goltermann, N., Jarnum, S., Weeke, B. & Westergaard, H. (1970) IgM turnover in Crohn's disease. *Gut*, **11**, 223–228.

Jewell, D. P. & MacLennan, I. C. M. (1973) Circulating immune complexes in inflammatory bowel disease. *Clinical and Experimental Immunology*, **14**, 219–226.

Jewell, D. P. & Truelove, S. C. (1972a) Circulating antibodies to cow's milk proteins in ulcerative colitis. *Gut*, **13**, 796–801.

Jewell, D. P. & Truelove, S. C. (1972b) Reaginic hypersensitivity in ulcerative colitis. *Gut*, **13**, 903–906.

Jewell, D. P. & Truelove, S. C. (1972c) Azathioprine in ulcerative colitis: an interim report on a controlled therapeutic trial. *British Medical Journal*, **i**, 709–712.

Jewell, D. P. & Truelove, S. C. (1974) Azathioprine in ulcerative colitis: final report of controlled therapeutic trial. *British Medical Journal*, **iv**, 627–630.

Jewell, D. P., MacLennan, I. C. M. & Truelove, S. C. (1972) Circulating immune complexes in ulcerative colitis and Crohn's disease. *Gut*, **13**, 839–840.

Jones, E. G., Beeken, W. L., Roessner, K. D. & Brown, W. R. (1976) Serum and intestinal fluid immunoglobulins and jejunal IgA secretion in Crohn's disease. *Gut*, **14**, 12–19.

Jones Williams, W. (1965) A study of Crohn's syndrome using tissue extracts and the Kveim and Mantoux tests. *Gut*, **6**, 503–505.

Jones Williams, W. (1971) The Kveim controversy. *Lancet*, **ii**, 926–927.

Joynson, D. H. M., Jacobs, A., Murray Walker, D. & Dolby, A. E. (1972) Defect of cell-mediated immunity in patients with iron-deficiency anaemia. *Lancet*, **ii**, 1058–1059.

Kagnoff, M. F. (1974) Induction and paralysis: a conceptual framework from which to examine the intestinal immune system. *Gastroenterology*, **66**, 1240–1256.

Karlish, A. J., Cox, E. V., Hampson, F. & Hemsted, E. H. (1972) The Kveim test in Crohn's disease, ulcerative colitis, and coeliac disease. *Lancet*, **i**, 438–439.

Katsaros, D. & Truelove, S. C. (1969) Regional enteritis and glucose-6-phosphate dehydrogenase deficiency. *New England Journal of Medicine*, **281**, 295–296.

Katz, S. I., Mann, D. L., Nelson, D. L., Abelson, L. D. &

Strober, W. (1976) Non-H-complex-linked B-lymphocyte antigens in gluten -sensitive enteropathy and dermatitis herpetiformis. *Clinical Research*, **24**, 447A.

Kelin, M., Binder, H. J., Mitchell, M., Aaronson, R. & Spiro, H. (1974) Treatment of Crohn's disease with azathioprine: a controlled evaluation. *Gastroenterology*, **66**, 916–922.

Kellermeyer, R. W. & Graham, R. C., Jr (1968) Kinins – possible physiologic and pathologic roles in man. *New England Journal of Medicine*, **279**, 754–759, 802–807, 859–866.

Keren, D. F., Milligan, F. D., Strandberg, J. D. & Yardley, J. H. (1975) Intercurrent cytomegalovirus colitis in a patient with ulcerative colitis. *Johns Hopkins Medical Journal*, **136**, 178–182.

Kirk, B. W. & Freedman, S. O. (1967) Hypogammaglobulinemia, thymoma and ulcerative colitis. *Canadian Medical Association Journal*, **96**, 1272–1277.

Kirsner, J. B. (1965) The immunologic response of the colon. *Journal of the American Medical Association*, **191**, 809–814.

Kirsner, J. B. (1970) Ulcerative colitis 1970 – recent developments. *Scandinavian Journal of Gastroenterology*, Suppl. 6, 63–91.

Kirsner, J. B. (1971) Ulcerative colitis. Mysterious, multiplex and menacing. *Journal of Chronic Diseases*, **23**, 681–684.

Kirsner, J. B. (1973) Genetic aspects of inflammatory bowel disease. *Clinics in Gastroenterology*, **2**, 557–575.

Kirsner, J. B. & Palmer, W. L. (1954) Ulcerative colitis: considerations of its etiology and treatment. *Journal of the American Medical Association*, **155**, 341–346.

Koffler, D., Minkowitz, S., Rothman, W. & Garlock, J. (1962) Immunocytochemical studies in ulcerative colitis and regional ileitis. *American Journal of Pathology*, **41**, 733–745.

Kohler, P. F. (1973) Clinical immune complex disease. Manifestations in systemic lupus erythematosus and hepatitis B virus infection. *Medicine*, **52**, 419–429.

Korelitz, B. I. & Sommers, S. C. (1974) Differential diagnosis of ulcerative and granulomatous colitis by sigmoidoscopy, rectal biopsy and cell counts of rectal mucosa. *American Journal of Gastroenterology*, **61**, 460–469.

Korsmeyer, S., Strickland, R. G., Wilson, I. D. & Williams, R. C., Jr (1974) Serum lymphocytotoxic and lymphocytophilic antibody activity in inflammatory bowel disease. *Gastroenterology*, **67**, 578–583.

Korsmeyer, S. J., Williams, R. C., Jr, Wilson, I. D. & Strickland, R. G. (1975) Lymphocytotoxic antibody in inflammatory bowel disease. A family study. *New England Journal of Medicine*, **293**, 1117–1120.

Korsmeyer, S. J., Williams, R. C., Jr, Wilson, I. D. & Strickland, R. G. (1976) Lymphocytotoxic and RNA antibodies in inflammatory bowel disease: a comparative study in patients and their families. *Annals of the New York Academy of Sciences*, **278**, 574–584.

Kovács, A. (1974) Titre of anti-*E. coli* antibodies in ulcerative colitis. *Digestion*, **10**, 205–209.

Kovács, A., Onody, K. & Petranyi, G. (1975) Untersuchungen über die Zytotoxizität der Lymphozyten bei Colitis ulcerosa. *Zeitschrift für Gastroenterologie*, **13**, 573–576.

Kraft, S. C. (1967) Comments on Selected Summaries. *Gastroenterology*, **53**, 799–800.

Kraft, S. C. (1971a) Cellular immunity in Crohn's disease. *Gastroenterology*, **61**, 544–548.

Kraft, S. C. (1971b) Crohn's disease and sarcoidosis. *New England Journal of Medicine*, **285**, 1259–1260.

Kraft, S. C. (1974) Immunosuppressive drug therapy in inflammatory bowel disease. *Drug Therapy*, **4**, 55–59, 65–66.

Kraft, S. C. (1976) Pathogenesis of ulcerative colitis. In *Gastrointestinal Emergencies*, 34th Hahnemann Symposium, ed. Clearfield, H. R. & Dinoso, V. P., Jr, pp. 169–180. New York: Grune & Stratton.

Kraft, S. C. & Kirsner, J. B. (1960) Mast cells and the gastrointestinal tract: a review. *Gastroenterology*, **39**, 764–770.

Kraft, S. C. & Kirsner, J. B. (1966) Present status of immunological mechanisms in ulcerative colitis. *Gastroenterology*, **51**, 788–797.

Kraft, S. C. & Kirsner, J. B. (1968) Some considerations of immunologic mechanisms in non specific ulcerative colitis. *Israel Journal of Medical Sciences*, **4**, 122–129.

Kraft, S. C. & Kirsner, J. B. (1971a) Ulcerative colitis. In *Immunological Diseases*, 2nd edn, ed. Samter, M., Vol. II, Ch. 82, pp. 1346–1366. Boston: Little, Brown.

Kraft, S. C. & Kirsner, J. B. (1971b) Immunological apparatus of the gut and inflammatory bowel disease. *Gastroenterology*, **60**, 922–951.

Kraft, S. C. & Kirsner, J. B. (1975) The immunology of ulcerative colitis and Crohn's disease: clinical and humoral aspects. In *Inflammatory Bowel Disease*, ed. Kirsner, J. B. & Shorter, R. G., pp. 60–80. Philadelphia: Lea and Febiger.

Kraft, S. C. & Kirsner, J. B. (1976) Immunology in gastroenterology. In *Gastroenterology*, 3rd edn, ed. Bockus, H. L., Vol. IV, Ch. 176, pp. 601–628. Philadelphia: Saunders.

Kraft, S. C. & Wall, A. J. (1976) Ulcerative colitis and Crohn's colitis. In *The Science and Practice of Clinical Medicine*, ed.-in-chief, Sanford, J. P., Vol. 1, *Disorders of the Gastrointestinal Tract/Disorders of the Liver/Nutritional Disorders*, ed. Dietschy, J. M., pp. 144–151. New York: Grune & Stratton.

Kraft, S. C., Bregman, E. & Kirsner, J. B. (1962) Criteria for evaluating autoimmune phenomena in ulcerative colitis. *Gastroenterology*, **43**, 330–336.

Kraft, S. C., Ford, H. E., McCleery, J. L. & Kirsner, J. B. (1968) Serum immunoglobulin levels in ulcerative colitis and Crohn's disease. *Gastroenterology*, **54**, 1251.

Kraft, S. C., Rimpila, J. J., Fitch, F. W. & Kirsner, J. B. (1966) Immunohistochemical studies of the colon in ulcerative colitis. *Archives of Pathology*, **82**, 369–378.

Kunin, C. M. (1962) Antibody distribution against nonenteropathic *E. coli*. Relation to age, sex and breast feeding. *Archives of Internal Medicine*, **110**, 676–686.

Kunin, C. M. (1963) Separation, characterization, and biological significance of a common antigen in *Enterobacteriaceae*. *Journal of Experimental Medicine*, **118**, 565–586.

Lagercrantz, R., Perlmann, P. & Hammarström, S. (1971) Immunological studies in ulcerative colitis. V. Family studies. *Gastroenterology*, **60**, 381–389.

Lagercrantz, R., Hammarström, S., Perlmann, P. & Gustafsson, B. E. (1966) Immunological studies in ulcerative colitis. III. Incidence of antibodies to colon-antigen in ulcerative colitis and other gastro-intestinal diseases. *Clinical and Experimental Immunology*, **1**, 263–276.

Lagercrantz, R., Hammarström, S., Perlmann, P. & Gustafsson, B. E. (1968) Immunological studies in ulcerative colitis. IV. Origin of autoantibodies. *Journal of Experimental Medicine*, **128**, 1339–1352.

Laham, M. N., Panush, R. S. & Caldwell, J. R. (1976) Modulation of peripheral blood lymphocyte (PBL) responses by complement (C). *Clinical Research*, 24, 331A.

Law, D. W. (1964) Serum complement in ulcerative colitis. *Clinical Research*, 12, 31.

Lawton, A. R., Royal, S. A., Self, K. S. & Cooper, M. D. (1972) IgA determinants on B-lymphocytes in patients with deficiency of circulating IgA. *Journal of Laboratory and Clinical Medicine*, 80, 26–33.

Lehner, T., Wilton, J. M. A. & Ivanyi, L. (1976) Double-blind crossover trial of levamisole in recurrent aphthous ulceration. *Lancet*, ii, 926–929.

Lev, R. & Orlic, D. (1974) Histochemical and radioautographic studies of normal human fetal colon. *Histochemistry*, 39, 301–311.

Levine, R. S., Warner, N. E. & Johnson, C. F. (1964) Cytomegalic inclusion disease in the gastrointestinal tract of adults. *Annals of Surgery*, 159, 37–48.

Lewkonia, R. M. & McConnell, R. B. (1976) Familial inflammatory bowel disease – heredity or environment? *Gut*, 17, 235–243.

Lewkonia, R. M., Woodrow, J. C., McConnell, R. B. & Price Evans, D. A. (1974) HL-A antigens in inflammatory bowel disease. *Lancet*, i, 574–575.

Lindblad, J. H. & Farr, R. S. (1961) The incidence of positive intradermal reactions and the demonstration of skin-sensitizing antibody to extracts of ragweed and dust in humans without history of rhinitis or asthma. *Journal of Allergy*, 32, 392–401.

Lloyd, G., Green, F. H. Y., Fox, H., Mani, V. & Turnberg, L. A. (1975) Mast cells and immunoglobulin E in inflammatory bowel disease. *Gut*, 16, 861–866.

Lo Gerfo, P., Krupey, J. & Hansen, H. J. (1971) Demonstration of an antigen common to several varieties of neoplasia. Assay using zirconyl phosphate gel. *New England Journal of Medicine*, 285, 138–141.

LoGrippo, G. A., Anselm, K., Hayashi, H. & Priest, R. J. (1970) Immunologic competence in idiopathic ulcerative colitis (Humoral aspects of immunity). *Henry Ford Hospital Medical Journal*, 18, 249–256.

Lorber, M., Schwartz, L. I. & Wasserman, L. R. (1955) Association of antibody-coated red blood cells with ulcerative colitis: report of four cases. *American Journal of Medicine*, 19, 887–894.

Loygue, J., Sandor, G., Levy, M., Malafosse, M., Huguet, C., Huguier, M. & Levy, E. (1972) Étude comparative de diverses protéines sériques chez des malades atteints de recto-colite hémorragique et de maladie de Crohn. *Archives Françaises des Maladies de l'Appareil Digestif*, 61, 649–662.

Lurhuma, A. Z., Cambiaso, C. L., Masson, P. L. & Heremans, J. F. (1976) Detection of circulating antigen–antibody complexes by their inhibitory effect on the agglutination of IgG-coated particles by rheumatoid factor or C1q. *Clinical and Experimental Immunology*, 25, 212–226.

McCaffery, T. D., Jr, Kraft, S. C. & Rothberg, R. M. (1972) The influence of different techniques in characterizing human antibodies to cow's milk proteins. *Clinical and Experimental Immunology*, 11, 225–234.

MacDermott, R. P., Donaldson, R. M., Jr & Trier, J. S. (1974) Glycoprotein synthesis and secretion by mucosal biopsies of rabbit colon and human rectum. *Journal of Clinical Investigation*, 54, 545–554.

McDevitt, H. O. & Bodmer, W. F. (1974) HL-A, immune-response genes, and disease. *Lancet*, i, 1269–1275.

McGiven, A. R., Ghose, T. & Nairn, R. C. (1967) Autoantibodies in ulcerative colitis. *British Medical Journal*, ii, 19–23.

McHattie, J., Magil, A., Jeejeebbhoy, K. & Falk, R. E. (1971) Immunoresponsiveness of lymphocytes from patients with regional ileocolitis (Crohn's disease) by *in vitro* testing. *Clinical Research*, 19, 779.

Maclaurin, B. P., Cooke, W. T. & Ling, N. R. (1972) Impaired lymphocyte reactivity against tumour cells in patients with Crohn's disease. *Gut*, 13, 614–620.

MacLennan, I. C. M. (1972) Competition for receptors for immunoglobulin on cytotoxic lymphocytes. *Clinical and Experimental Immunology*, 10, 275–283.

MacPherson, B. R., Albertini, R. J. & Beeken, W. L. (1976) Immunological studies in patients with Crohn's disease. *Gut*, 17, 100–106.

Magalhaes, A. F. N., Peters, T. J. & Doe, W. F. (1974) Studies on the nature and significance of connective tissue antibodies in adult coeliac disease and Crohn's disease. *Gut*, 15, 284–288.

Mani, V., Lloyd, G., Green, F. H. Y., Fox, H. & Turnberg, L. A. (1976) Treatment of ulcerative colitis with oral disodium cromoglycate. A double-blind controlled trial *Lancet*, i, 439–441.

Manns, J. J. (1972) Military Crohn's disease. *British Medical Journal*, iv, 152.

Marcussen, H. (1974) Histological liver disorder and anti-colon antibodies in ulcerative colitis. *Acta Pathologica et Microbiologica Scandinavica*, Section A, 82, 714–718.

Marner, I.-L., Friborg, S. & Simonsen, E. (1975) Disease activity and serum proteins in ulcerative colitis. Immunochemical quantitation. *Scandinavian Journal of Gastroenterology*, 10, 537–544.

Martin, F. & Martin, M. S. (1970) Demonstration of antigens related to colonic cancer in the human digestive system. *International Journal of Cancer*, 6, 352–360.

Mavligit, G. M., Jubert, A. V., Gutterman, J. U., McBride, C. M. & Hersh, E. M. (1974) Immune reactivity of lymphoid tissues adjacent to carcinoma of the ascending colon. *Surgery, Gynecology and Obstetrics*, 139, 409–412.

Meuwissen, S. G. M., Schellekens, P. T. A., Huismans, L. & Tytgat, G. N. (1975) Impaired anamnestic cellular response in patients with Crohn's disease. *Gut*, 16, 854–860.

Meuwissen, S. G. M., Feltkamp-Vroom, T. M., Brutel de la Riviere, A., van der Borne, A. E. G. K. & Tytgat, G. N. (1976) Analysis of the lympho-plasmocytic infiltrate in Crohn's disease by means of thymocyte- and lymphocyte-specific antisera. *Gastroenterology*, 70, 919.

Michael, J. G. & Rosen, F. S. (1963) Association of 'natural' antibodies to gram-negative bacteria with the γ_1-macroglobulins. *Journal of Experimental Medicine*, 118, 619–626.

Mitchell, A. B. S., Gill, A. M., Orchard, R. T. & Parkins, R. A. (1975) Carcinoembryonic antigen in patients suffering from ulcerative proctocolitis. *American Journal of Digestive Diseases*, 20, 407–417.

Mitchell, D. N. & Rees, R. J. W. (1969) A transmissible agent from sarcoid tissue. *Lancet*, ii, 81–84.

Mitchell, D. N. & Rees, R. J. W. (1970) Agent transmissible from Crohn's disease tissue. *Lancet*, ii, 168–171.

Mitchell, D. N., Rees, R. J. W. & Goswami, K. K. A. (1976) Transmissible agents from human sarcoid and Crohn's disease tissues. *Lancet*, ii, 761–765.

Mitchell, D. N., Cannon, P., Dyer, N. H., Hinson, K. F. W. & Willoughby, J. M. T. (1970) Further observations on Kveim test in Crohn's disease. *Lancet*, **ii**, 496–498.

Mitchell, M. S. (1976) Role of 'suppressor' T lymphocytes in antibody-induced inhibition of cytophilic antibody receptors. *Annals of the New York Academy of Sciences*, **276**, 229–241.

Mitelman, F., Hartley-Asp, B. & Ursing, B. (1976) Chromosome aberrations and metronidazole. *Lancet*, **ii**, 802.

Molnar, I. G., Vandevoorde, J. P. & Gitnick, G. L. (1976) CEA levels in fluids bathing gastrointestinal tumors. *Gastroenterology*, **70**, 513–515.

Monteiro, E., Fossey, J., Shiner, M., Drasar, B. S. & Allison, A. C. (1971) Antibacterial antibodies in rectal and colonic mucosa in ulcerative colitis. Lancet, **i**, 249–251.

Moore, T. L., Kantrowitz, P. A. & Zamcheck, N. (1972) Carcinoembryonic antigen (CEA) in inflammatory bowel disease. *Journal of the American Medical Association*, **222**, 944–947.

Morganroth, J. & Watson, D. W. (1970) Sensitivity to atypical mycobacterial antigens in patients with Crohn's disease. *American Journal of Digestive Diseases*, **15**, 653–657.

Morris, P. J. (1974) Histocompatibility systems, immune response, and disease in man. In *Contemporary Topics in Immunobiology*, ed. Cooper, M. D. & Warner, N. L., Vol. 3, Ch. 6, pp. 141–169. New York: Plenum Press.

Morris, R. I., Metzger, A. L., Bluestone, R. & Terasaki, P. I. (1974) HL-A-W27 – A useful discriminator in the arthropathies of inflammatory bowel disease. *New England Journal of Medicine*, **290**, 1117–1119.

Mowat, N. A. G., Douglas, A. S., Brunt, P. W., McIntosh, J. A. R., King, P. C. & Boddy, K. (1973) Epsilon-aminocaproic acid therapy in ulcerative colitis. *American Journal of Digestive Diseases*, **18**, 959–965.

Mowbray, J. F., Hoffbrand, A. V., Holborow, E. J., Seah, P. P. & Fry, L. (1973) Circulating immune complexes in dermatitis herpetiformis. *Lancet*, **i**, 400–402.

Mul, N. A. J., de Boer, L. E. M., Taminiau, J. A. & Ballieux, R. E. (1975) Light chain type ratio of IgA-producing cells in human jejunal biopsies. *European Journal of Clinical Investigation*, **5**, 63–67.

Nagle, G. J. & Kurtz, S. M. (1967) Electron microscopy of the human rectal mucosa. A comparison of idiopathic ulcerative colitis with inflammation of known etiologies. *American Journal of Digestive Diseases*, **12**, 541–567.

Nahir, M., Gideoni, O., Eidelman, S. & Barzilai, A. (1976) HLA antigens in ulcerative colitis. *Lancet*, **ii**, 573.

Nairn, R. C. & de Boer, W. G. R. M. (1966) Species distribution of gastrointestinal antigens. *Nature (London)*, **210**, 960–962.

Nairn, R. C., Fothergill, J. E., McEntegart, M. G. & Porteous, I. G. (1962) Gastro-intestinal-specific antigen: an immunohistological and serological study. *British Medical Journal*, **i**, 1788–1790.

Najjar, V. A. (1974) The physiological role of γ-globulin. *Advances in Enzymology*, **41**, 129–178.

Nász, I., Kulcsár, G., Dán, P., Sallay, K., Vertes, L., Geck, P., Keskeny, S. & Horvath, J. (1973) Aetiological significance of viruses and role of lymphocytes in certain gastrointestinal diseases. *Acta Microbiology of the Academy of Sciences of Hungary*, **20**, 191–203.

Nelson, D. L., Falchuk, Z. M., Kasarda, D. & Strober, W. (1974) Gluten-sensitive enteropathy: correlation of organ culture behaviour with HL-A status. *Clinical Research*, **22**, 695A.

Ng, R. P. & Vicary, F. R. (1976) Cell-mediated immunity

and transfer factor in Crohn's disease. *British Medical Journal*, **iii**, 87–88.

Nilsson, B. S. (1971) *In vitro* lymphocyte reactivity to PPD and phytohaemagglutinin in relation to PPD skin reactivity and age. *Scandinavian Journal of Respiratory Diseases*, **52**, 39–47.

Orr, M. M., Tamarind, D. L., Cook, J., Fincham, W. J., Hawley, P. R., Quilliam, J. P. & Irving, M. H. (1975) Chronic lesions of rabbit bowel due to contact with antiseptic skin preparation. *Gut*, **16**, 401.

Otto, H. F. (1973) The interepithelial lymphocytes of the intestinum. Morphological observations and immunologic aspects of intestinal enteropathy. *Current Topics in Pathology (Berlin)*, **57**, 81–121.

Padilla, A. J. & Sparberg, M. (1972) Regional enteritis and sarcoidosis in one patient. A case report. *Gastroenterology*, **63**, 153–160.

Pardo Gilbert, A. & Zamacoma Ravelo, G. (1968) Serum proteins and endotoxins in chronic ulcerative colitis. *Diseases of the Colon and Rectum*, **11**, 124–126.

Parent, K. & Mitchell, P. D. (1976) Bacterial variants: etiologic agent in Crohn's disease? *Gastroenterology*, **71**, 365–368.

Parent, K., Barrett, J. & Wilson, I. D. (1971) Investigation of the pathogenic mechanisms in regional enteritis with *in-vitro* lymphocyte cultures. *Gastroenterology*, **61**, 431–439.

Pascual, R. S., Gee, J. B. L. & Finch, S. C. (1973) Usefulness of serum lysozyme measurement in diagnosis and evaluation of sarcoidosis. *New England Journal of Medicine*, **289**, 1074–1076.

Pepys, M. B., Wansbrough-Jones, M. H., Dash, A. C. & Mirjah, D. D. (1975) Complement dependence of IgA antibody production. *Gut*, **16**, 827.

Perlmann, P. & Broberger, O. (1963) *In-vitro* studies of ulcerative colitis. II. Cytotoxic action of white blood cells from patients on human fetal colon cells. *Journal of Experimental Medicine*, **117**, 717–735.

Perlmann, P. & Broberger, O. (1969) Lower gastrointestinal system. In *Textbook of Immunopathology*, ed. Miescher, P. A. & Muller-Eberhard, H. J., Vol. II, Ch. 44, pp. 551–561. New York: Grune & Stratton.

Perlmann, P., Hammarström, S., Lagercrantz, R. & Campbell, D. (1967) Autoantibodies to colon in rats and human ulcerative colitis: cross reactivity with *Escherichia coli* 0:14 antigen. *Proceedings of the Society for Experimental Biology and Medicine*, **125**, 975–980.

Perlmann, P., Hammarström, S., Lagercrantz, R. & Gustafsson, B. E. (1965) Antigen from colon of germfree rats and antibodies in human ulcerative colitis. *Annals of the New York Academy of Sciences*, **124**, 377–394.

Perrett, A. D., Higgins, G., Johnston, H. H., Massarella, G. R., Truelove, S. C. & Wright, R. (1971) The liver in Crohn's disease. *Quarterly Journal of Medicine*, **40**, 187–209.

Persson, S. (1974) Studies on Crohn's disease. III. Concentrations of immunoglobulins G, A, and M in the mucosa of the terminal ileum. *Acta Chirurgica Scandinavica*, **140**, 64–67.

Persson, S. & Danielsson, D. (1973) Studies on Crohn's disease. II. Immunoglobulin-containing cells in the terminal ileum. *Acta Chirurgica Scandinavica*, **139**, 735–738.

Phear, D. N. (1958) The relation between regional ileitis and sarcoidosis. *Lancet*, **ii**, 1250–1251.

Poen, H., Ballieux, R. E., Mul, N. A. J., Stoop, J. W., ten Thije, O. J. & Zegers, B. J. M. (1969) Increased serum

IgA in intestinal disease. In *Protides of the Biological Fluids*, ed. Peeters, H. Vol. 16, pp. 485–489. Oxford: Pergamon Press.

Polčák, J. & Skálová, M. (1968) Immunologic manifestations of healthy consanguineous relatives of patients suffering from ulcerative colitis. *American Journal of Proctology*, 19, 197–203.

Polčák, J., Vokurka, V. & Skalova, M. (1967) Immunologische Phänomene in Familien mit Colitis ulcerosa. *Gastroenterologia*, 107, 164–167.

Powell, R. D., Warner, N. E., Levine, R. S. & Kirsner, J. B. (1961) Cytomegalic inclusion disease and ulcerative colitis. Report of a case in a young adult. *American Journal of Medicine*, 30, 334–340.

Priest, R. J., Rebuck, J. W. & Havey, G. T. (1960) A new qualitative defect of leukocyte function in ulcerative colitis. *Gastroenterology*, 38, 715–720.

Quie, P. G., White, J. G., Holmes, B. & Good, R. A. (1967) *In-vitro* bactericidal capacity of human polymorphonuclear leukocytes: diminished activity in chronic granulomatous disease of childhood. *Journal of Clinical Investigation*, 46, 668–679.

Rachail, M., Pellet, D., Bruttmann, G., Coulomb, M. & Faure, H. (1973) Le traitement de la maladie de Crohn par le BCG selon la méthode de Geffroy. A propos de 8 observations. *Semaine des Hôpitaux (Paris)*, 49, 3067–3071.

Ramachandar, K., Sachar, D. B., Janowitz, H. D., Forman, S. P., Douglas, S. D. & Taub, R. N. (1974) B Lymphocytes in inflammatory bowel disease. *Lancet*, ii, 45–46.

Ranlöv, P., Nielsen, M. H. & Wanstrup, J. (1972) Ultrastructure of the ileum in Crohn's disease. Immune lesions and mastocytosis. *Scandinavian Journal of Gastroenterology*, 7, 471–476.

Rao, S. N. (1973) Mast cells as a component of the granuloma in Crohn's disease. *Journal of Pathology*, 109, 79–82.

Rebuck, J. W., Hodson, J. M., Priest, R. J. & Barth, C. L. (1963) Basophilic granulocytes in inflammatory tissues of man. *Annals of the New York Academy of Sciences*, 103, 409–426.

Remacle-Bonnet, M. & Depieds, R. (1974) Study of the antigenic constituents of human colon connective tissue. *Pathologie et Biologie*, 22, 113–117.

Renz, M., Ward, M., Eastwood, M. A. & Harkness, R. A. (1976) Neutrophil function and myeloperoxidase activity in inflammatory bowel disease. *Lancet*, ii, 584.

Rhodes, J., Bainton, D., Beck, P. & Campbell, H. (1971) Controlled trial of azathioprine in Crohn's disease. *Lancet*, ii, 1273–1276.

Richens, E. R., Gough, K. R. & Williams, M. J. (1973) Leucocyte migration studies with spleen preparations in Crohn's disease. *Gut*, 14, 376–379.

Richens, E. R., Williams, M. J., Gough, K. R. & Ancill, R. J. (1974a) Leucocyte migration studies in Crohn's disease using Crohn's colon homogenate and mitochondrial and microsomal fractions. *Gut*, 15, 19–23.

Richens, E. R., Williams, M. J., Gough, K. R. & Ancill, R. J. (1974b) Mixed-lymphocyte reaction as a measure of immunological competence of lymphocytes from patients with Crohn's disease. *Gut*, 15, 24–28.

Rimpila, J. J., O'Neal, S. T., Diab, I. M., Roth, L. J. & Kraft, S. C. (1976) Immunohistochemical studies of inflammatory bowel disease using a freeze-dried tissue technique. *Gastroenterology*, 70, 929.

Rippey, J. H. & Sommers, S. C. (1967) Hypertrophied plasma cells in regional enteritis. *American Journal of Digestive Diseases*, 12, 465–467.

Röpke, C. (1972) Lymphocyte transformation and delayed hypersensitivity in Crohn's disease. *Scandinavian Journal of Gastroenterology*, 7, 671–677.

Rosenberg, J. L., Kraft, S. C. & Kirsner, J. B. (1976) Inflammatory bowel disease in all three members of one family. *Gastroenterology*, 70, 759–760.

Rosenberg, J. L., Levin, B., Wall, A. J. & Kirsner, J. B. (1975a) A controlled trial of azathioprine in Crohn's disease. *American Journal of Digestive Diseases*, 20, 721–726.

Rosenberg, J. L., Wall, A. J., Levin, B., Binder, H. J. & Kirsner, J. B. (1975b) A controlled trial of azathioprine in the management of chronic ulcerative colitis. *Gastroenterology*, 69, 96–99.

Rosenthal, A. S., Lipsky, P. E. & Shevach, E. M. (1975) Macrophage-lymphocyte interaction and antigen recognition. *Federation Proceedings*, 34, 1743–1748.

Rothberg, R. M. & ten Bensel, R. W. (1967) Thymic alymphoplasia with immunoglobulin synthesis. *American Journal of Diseases of Children*, 113, 639–648.

Rothberg, R. M., Kraft, S. C., Farr, R. S., Kriebel, G. W., Jr, & Goldberg, S. S. (1971) Local immunologic responses to ingested protein. In *The Secretory Immunologic System*, ed. Dayton, D. H., Jr, Small, P. A., Jr, Chanock, R. M., Kaufman, H. E. & Tomasi, T. B., Jr, pp. 293–307. Washington: U.S. Government Printing Office.

Rudzik, O. & Bienenstock, J. (1974) Isolation and characteristics of gut mucosal lymphocytes. *Laboratory Investigation*, 30, 260–266.

Rule, A. H., Goleski-Reilly, C., Sachar, D. B., Vandevoorde, J. & Janowitz, H. D. (1973) Circulating carcinoembryonic antigen (CEA): relationship to clinical status of patients with inflammatory bowel disease. *Gut*, 14, 880–884.

Russell, A. S., Schlaut, J., Percy, J. S. & Dossetor, J. B. (1974) HL-A (transplantation) antigens in ankylosing spondylitis and Crohn's disease. *Journal of Rheumatology*, 1, 203–209.

Russell, A. S., Percy, J. S., Schlaut, J., Sartor, V. E., Goodhart, J. M., Sherbaniuk, R. W. & Kidd, E. G. (1975) Transplantation antigens in Crohn's disease: linkage of associated ankylosing spondylitis with HL-AW27. *American Journal of Digestive Diseases*, 20, 359–361.

Saba, T. M. (1970) Physiology and physiopathology of the reticuloendothelial system. *Archives of Internal Medicine*, 126, 1031–1052.

Sachar, D. B., Taub, R. N., Brown, S. M., Present, D. H., Korelitz, B. I. & Janowitz, H. D. (1973) Impaired lymphocyte responsiveness in inflammatory bowel disease. *Gastroenterology*, 64, 203–209.

Sachar, D. B., Taub, R. N., Ramachandar, K., Meyers, S., Forman, S. P., Douglas, S. D. & Janowitz, H. D. (1976) T and B lymphocytes and cutaneous anergy in inflammatory bowel disease. *Annals of the New York Academy of Sciences*, 278, 565–572.

Salter, R. H. & Read, A. E. (1970) Epsilon-aminocaproic acid therapy in ulcerative colitis. *Gut*, 11, 585–587.

Samson, R. R., McClelland, D. B. L. & Shearman, D. J. C. (1973) Studies on the quantitation of immunoglobulin in human intestinal secretions. *Gut*, 14, 616–626.

Sanders, R. C. (1964) An attempt to devise a skin test for regional enteritis. *Gut*, 5, 194–195.

Sandtor, G., Levy, E., Malafosse, M., Huguet, C., Huguier, M. & Loygue, J. (1975) Some serum protein studies in

Crohn's disease and ulcerative colitis. *Research Communications in Chemical Pathology and Pharmacology*, **11**, 129–145.

Scadding, J. G. (1971) The Kveim controversy. *Lancet*, **ii**, 1372–1373.

Schachter, H. & Kirsner, J. B. (1975) Definitions of inflammatory bowel disease of unknown aetiology. *Gastroenterology*, **68**, 591–600.

Schachter, H., Goldstein, M. J., Rappaport, H., Fennessy, J. J. & Kirsner, J. B. (1970) Ulcerative and 'granulomatous' colitis – validity of differential diagnostic criteria. A study of 100 patients treated by total colectomy. *Annals of Internal Medicine*, **72**, 841–851.

Schein, P. S. & Winokur, S. H. (1975) Immunosuppressive and cytotoxic chemotherapy: long-term complications. *Annals of Internal Medicine*, **82**, 84–95.

Schlegel, R. J. (1975) Chronic granulomatous disease 1974. *Journal of the American Medical Association*, **231**, 615–617.

Schlosstein, L., Terasaki, P. I., Bluestone, R. & Pearson, C. M. (1973) High association of an HL-A antigen, W27, with ankylosing spondylitis. *New England Journal of Medicine*, **288**, 704–706.

Scott, B. B., Swinburne, M. L., Rajah, S. M. & Losowsky, M. S. (1974) HL-A8 and the immune response to gluten *Lancet*, **ii**, 374–377.

Segal, A. W. & Loewi, G. (1976) Neutrophil dysfunction in Crohn's disease. *Lancet*, **ii**, 219–221.

Sewell, P., Cooke, W. T., Cox, E. V. & Meynell, M. J. (1963) Milk intolerance in gastrointestinal disorders. *Lancet*, **ii**, 1132–1135.

Sheehan, R. G., Necheles, T. F., Lindeman, R. J., Meyer, H. J. & Patterson, J. F. (1967) Regional enteritis and granulomatous colitis associated with erythrocyte glucose-6-phosphate dehydrogenase deficiency. *New England Journal of Medicine*, **277**, 1124–1126.

Shorter, R. G., Huizenga, K. A. & Spencer, R. J. (1972a) A working hypothesis for the etiology and pathogenesis of nonspecific inflammatory bowel disease. *American Journal of Digestive Diseases*, **17**, 1024–1032.

Shorter, R. G., Cardoza, M., Spencer, R. J. & Huizenga, K. A. (1969) Further studies of *in vitro* cytotoxicity of lymphocytes from patients with ulcerative and granulomatous colitis for allogeneic colonic epithelial cells, including the effects of colectomy. *Gastroenterology*, **56**, 304–309.

Shorter, R. G., Huizenga, K. A., ReMine, S. G. & Spencer, R. J. (1970) Effects of preliminary incubation of lymphocytes with serum on their cytotoxicity for colonic epithelial cells. *Gastroenterology*, **58**, 843–850.

Shorter, R. G., Huizenga, K. A., Spencer, R. J. & Guy, S. K. (1972b) Inflammatory bowel disease. The role of lymphotoxin in the cytotoxicity of lymphocytes for colonic epithelial cells. *American Journal of Digestive Diseases*, **17**, 689–696.

Shorter, R. G., Huizenga, K. A., Spencer, R. J. & Weedon, D. (1973) Lymphotoxin in nonspecific inflammatory bowel disease lymphocytes. *American Journal of Digestive Diseases*, **18**, 79–83.

Shorter, R. G., Spencer, R. J., Huizenga, K. A. & Hallenbeck, G. A. (1968) Inhibition of *in-vitro* cytotoxicity of lymphocytes from patients with ulcerative colitis and granulomatous colitis for allogeneic colonic epithelial cells using horse anti-human thymus serum. *Gastroenterology*, **54**, 227–231.

Shorter, R. G., Cardoza, M., Huizenga, K. A., ReMine, S. G. & Spencer, R. J. (1969) Further studies of *in-vitro*

cytotoxicity of lymphocytes for colonic epithelial cells. *Gastroenterology*, **57**, 30–35.

Shorter, R. G., Cardoza, M. R., ReMine, S. G., Spencer, R. J. & Huizenga, K. A. (1970) Modification of *in-vitro* cytotoxicity of lymphocytes from patients with chronic ulcerative colitis or granulomatous colitis for allogenic colonic epithelial cells. *Gastroenterology*, **58**, 692–698.

Shorter, R. G., Huizenga, K. A., Spencer, R. J., Aas, J. & Guy, S. K. (1971) Inflammatory bowel disease. Cytophilic antibody and the cytotoxicity of lymphocytes for colonic cells *in vitro*. *American Journal of Digestive Diseases*, **16**, 673–680.

Shorter, R. G., Tomasi, T. B., Huizenga, K. A., Spencer, R. J. & Stobo, J. D. (1976) The immunology of chronic ulcerative colitis and Crohn's disease. *Annals of the New York Academy of Sciences*, **278**, 586–591.

Siltzbach, L. E. (1976) Qualities and behavior of satisfactory Kveim suspensions. *Annals of the New York Academy of Sciences*, **278**, 665–668.

Siltzbach, L. E., Vieira, L. O. B. D., Topilsky, M. & Janowitz, H. D. (1971) Is there Kviem responsiveness in Crohn's disease? *Lancet*, **ii**, 634–636.

Silverman, N. A., Potvin, C., Alexander, J. C., Jr & Chretien, P. B. (1975) *In-vitro* lymphocyte reactivity and T-cell levels in chronic cigarette smokers. *Clinical and Experimental Immunology*, **22**, 285–292.

Simonowitz, D., Block, G. E., Riddell, R. H., Kraft, S. C. & Kirsner, J. B. (1977) The production of an unusual tissue reaction in rabbit bowel injected with Crohn's disease homogenates. *Surgery*, **82**, 211–218.

Singer, H. C., Anderson, J. G. D., Frischer, H. & Kirsner, J. B. (1971) Familial aspects of inflammatory bowel disease. *Gastroenterology*, **61**, 423–430.

Singleton, J. W. (1976) The National Cooperative Crohn's Disease Study (NCCDS): Preliminary results of Part I. *Gastroenterology*, **70**, 938.

Sion, A. & Friedell, M. T. (1974) Autolymphocytotoxins in ulcerative colitis and carcinoma of the colon. A lesion of tolerance. *International Surgery*, **59**, 141–146.

Skinner, J. M. & Whitehead, R. (1974a) A morphological assessment of immunoreactivity in colonic Crohn's disease and ulcerative colitis by a study of the lymph nodes. *Journal of Clinical Pathology*, **27**, 202–206.

Skinner, J. M. & Whitehead, R. (1974b) The plasma cells in inflammatory disease of the colon: a quantitative study. *Journal of Clinical Pathology*, **27**, 643–646.

Sloan, W. P., Bargen, J. A., & Gage, R. P. (1950) Life histories of patients with chronic ulcerative colitis: a review of 2000 cases. *Gastroenterology*, **16**, 25–38.

Søborg, M. & Bendixen, G. (1967) Human lymphocyte migration as a parameter of hypersensitivity. *Acta Medica Scandinavica*, **181**, 247–256.

Soltis, R. D. & Wilson, I. D. (1975) Serum immunoglobulin M concentrations following bowel resection in chronic inflammatory bowel disease. *Gastroenterology*, **69**, 885–892.

Soltis, R. D. & Wilson, I. D. (1976) The effect of heat inactivation of serum on the detection of immune complexes. *Clinical Research*, **24**, 576A.

Söltoft, J. (1969) Immunoglobulin-containing cells in normal jejunal mucosa and in ulcerative colitis and regional enteritis. *Scandinavian Journal of Gastroenterology*, **4**, 353–360.

Söltoft, J., Binder, V. & Gudmand-Höyer, E. (1973) Intestinal immunoglobulins in ulcerative colitis. *Scandinavian Journal of Gastroenterology*, **8**, 293–300.

Söltoft, J., Petersen, L. & Kruse, P. (1972)

Immunoglobulin deficiency and regional enteritis. *Scandinavian Journal of Gastroenterology*, 7, 233–236.

Sommers, S. C. (1966) Mast cells and Paneth cells in ulcerative colitis. *Gastroenterology*, 51, 841–850.

Spector, W. G. & Heesom, N. (1969) The production of granulomata by antigen–antibody complexes. *Journal of Pathology*, 98, 31–39.

Spiegelberg, H. L. (1974) Biological activities of immunoglobulins of different classes and subclasses. *Advances in Immunology*, 19, 259–294.

Springer, G. F. & Horton, R. E. (1969) Blood group isoantibody stimulation in man by feeding blood group-active bacteria. *Journal of Clinical Investigation*, 48, 1280–1291.

Stefani, S. & Fink, S. (1967) Effect of *E. coli* antigens, tuberculin, and phytohaemagglutinin upon ulcerative colitis lymphocytes. *Gut*, 8, 249–252.

Steinfeld, J. L., Davidson, J. D., Gordon, R. S., Jr, & Greene, F. E. (1960) The mechanism of hypoproteinemia in patients with regional enteritis and ulcerative colitis. *American Journal of Medicine*, 29, 405–415.

Ste-Marie, M. T., Lee, E. M. & Brown, W. R. (1974) Radioimmunologic measurements of naturally occurring antibodies. III. Antibodies reactive with *Escherichia coli* or *Bacteroides fragilis* in breast fluids and sera of mothers and newborn infants. *Pediatric Research*, 8, 815–819.

Sterns, E. E. & Sheppard, M. S. (1974a) The clearance of interstitial albumin from the colon. *Clinical Research*, 22, 737A.

Sterns, E. E. & Sheppard, M. S. (1974b) The different capacity for albumin transport by intestinal lymphatics. *Clinical Research*, 22, 738A.

Stobo, J. D., Tomasi, T. B., Huizenga, K. A., Spencer, R. J. & Shorter, R. G. (1976) *In-vitro* studies of inflammatory bowel disease. Surface receptors of the mononuclear cell required to lyse allogeneic colonic epithelial cells. *Gastroenterology*, 70, 171–176.

Stoebner, R. & Patterson, M. (1965) Lymphocytic skin testing in ulcerative colitis and regional enteritis: a preliminary report. *Clinical Research*, 13, 32.

Straus, E., Vernace, S., Janowitz, H. & Paronetto, F. (1975) Migration of peripheral leukocytes in the presence of carcinoembryonic antigen. Studies in patients with chronic inflammatory diseases of the intestine and carcinoma of the colon and pancreas. *Proceedings of the Society for Experimental Biology and Medicine*, 148, 494–497.

Straus, E., Rule, A., Grotsky, H., Janowitz, H. D. & Glade, P. (1972) *In-vitro* migration of leucocytes in the presence of meconium antigen in patients with inflammatory bowel disease and cancer of the colon. *Gastroenterology*, 62, 817.

Strickland, R. G. & Williams, R. C., Jr (1975) T cells in Crohn's disease. *Gastroenterology*, 69, 275–276.

Strickland, R. G., Husby, G., Black, W. C. & Williams, R. C., Jr (1975) Peripheral blood and intestinal lymphocyte subpopulations in Crohn's disease. *Gut*, 16, 847–853.

Strickland, R. G., Friedler, E. M., Henderson, C. A., Wilson, I. D. & Williams, R. C., Jr (1975) Serum lymphocytotoxins in inflammatory bowel disease. Studies of frequency and specificity for lymphocyte subpopulations. *Clinical and Experimental Immunology*, 21, 384–393.

Strickland, R. G., Korsmeyer, S., Soltis, R. D., Wilson, I. D. & Williams, R. C., Jr (1974) Peripheral blood T and B cells in chronic inflammatory bowel disease. *Gastroenterology*, 67, 569–577.

Strober, W., Wochner, R. D., Carbone, P. P. & Waldmann, T. A. (1967) Intestinal lymphangiectasia: a protein-losing enteropathy with hypogammaglobulinemia, lymphocytopenia and impaired homograft rejection. *Journal of Clinical Investigation*, 46, 1643–1656.

Strober, W., Falchuk, Z. M., Rogentine, G. N., Nelson, D. L. & Klaeveman, H. L. (1975) The pathogenesis of gluten-sensitive enteropathy. *Annals of Internal Medicine*, 83, 242–256.

Svejgaard, A. & Ryder, L. P. (1976) Interaction of HLA molecules with non-immunological ligands as an explanation of HLA and disease associations. *Lancet*, ii, 547–549.

Tada, T. & Ishizaka, K. (1970) Distribution of γE-forming cells in lymphoid tissues of the human and monkey. *Journal of Immunology*, 104, 377–387.

Taguchi, K., Gordon, J. & MacLean, L. D. (1974) Suppressed cell-mediated immunity due to a serum factor in bacterial sepsis. *Surgical Forum*, 25, 35–36.

Tamura, H. (1973) Acute ulcerative colitis associated with cytomegalic inclusion virus. *Archives of Pathology*, 96, 164–167.

Taub, R. N., Sachar, D., Janowitz, H. & Siltzbach, L. E. (1976) Induction of granulomas in mice by inoculation of tissue homogenates from patients with inflammatory bowel disease and sarcoidosis. *Annals of the New York Academy of Sciences*, 278, 560–563.

Taub, R. N., Sachar, D., Siltzbach, L. E. & Janowitz, H. D. (1975) Transmission of ileitis and sarcoid granulomas to mice. *Transactions of the Association of American Physicians*, 87, 219–224.

Taylor, K. B. & Truelove, S. C. (1961) Circulating antibodies to milk proteins in ulcerative colitis. *British Medical Journal*, ii, 924–929.

Taylor, K. B. & Truelove, S. C. (1962) Immunological reactions in gastrointestinal disease: a review, *Gut*, 3, 277–288.

Taylor, K. B., Truelove, S. C. & Wright, R. (1964) Serologic reactions to gluten and cow's milk proteins in gastrointestinal disease. *Gastroenterology*, 46, 99–108.

Teisberg, P. & Gjone, E. (1975) Humoral immune system activity in inflammatory bowel disease. *Scandinavian Journal of Gastroenterology*, 10, 545–549.

Thayer, W. R., Jr (1970) Crohn's disease (regional enteritis). A look at the last four years. *Scandinavian Journal of Gastroenterology*, Suppl. 6, 165–185.

Thayer, W. R., Jr & Spiro, H. M. (1963a) Persistence of serum complement in sera of patients with ulcerative colitis. *Journal of Laboratory and Clinical Medicine*, 62, 24–30.

Thayer, W. R., Jr & Spiro, H. M. (1963b) Protein abnormalities in ulcerative colitis patients and their families. *Gastroenterology*, 44, 444–447.

Thayer, W. R., Jr, Charland, C. & Field, C. E. (1976) The subpopulations of circulating white blood cells in inflammatory bowel disease. *Gastroenterology*, 71, 379–384.

Thayer, W. R., Jr, Brown, M., Sangree, M. H., Katz, J. & Hersh, T. (1969) *Escherichia coli* 0:14 and colon hemagglutinating antibodies in inflammatory bowel disease. *Gastroenterology*, 57, 311–318.

Thomas, L. (1961) Role of endotoxins in immune and vascular reactions. *Gastroenterology*, 40, 364–366.

Thomas, L. (1964) Circulating autoantibodies and human disease. *New England Journal of Medicine*, 270, 1157–1159.

Thomas, L. (1971) The Kveim test. *New England Journal of Medicine*, 284, 388–389.

Thompson, R. A., Asquith, P. & Cooke, W. T. (1969) Secretory IgA in the serum. *Lancet*, **ii**, 517–519.

Thorsby, E. & Lie, S. O. (1971) Relationship between the HL-A system and susceptibility to disease. *Transplantation Proceedings*, **3**, 1305–1307.

Tomasi, T. B., Jr (1972) Secretory immunoglobulins. *New England Journal of Medicine*, **287**, 500–506.

Tomasi, T. B., Jr & Bienenstock, J. (1968) Secretory immunoglobulins. *Advances in Immunology*, **9**, 1–96.

Tomasi, T. B. & Grey, H. M. (1972) Structure and function of immunoglobulin A. *Progress in Allergy*, **16**, 81–213.

Tomasi, T. B., Jr, Bull, D., Tourville, D., Montes, M. & Yurchak, A. (1971) Distribution and synthesis of human secretory components. In *The Secretory Immunologic System*, ed. Dayton, D. H., Jr, Small, P. A., Jr, Chanock, R. M., Kaufman H. E. & Tomasi, T. B., Jr, pp. 41–54. Washington: U.S. Government Printing Office.

Townsend, C. M., Jr, Sakai, H., Fish, J. C. & Ritzmann, S. E. (1973) T-cell functions in patients with inflammatory bowel disease. *Clinical Research*, **21**, 97.

Turk, J. L. (1969) Cell-mediated immunological processes in leprosy. *Bulletin of the World Health Organization*, **41**, 779–792.

Ursing, B. & Kamme, C. (1975) Metonidazole for Crohn's disease. *Lancet*, **i**, 775–777.

Verrier Jones, J., Housley, J., Ashurst, P. M. & Hawkins, C. F. (1969) Development of delayed hypersensitivity to dinitrochlorobenzene in patients with Crohn's disease. *Gut*, **10**, 52–56.

Verrier Jones, J., Cumming, R. H., Asplin, C. M., Laszlo, G. & White, R. J. (1976) Evidence for circulating immune complexes in erythema nodosum and early sarcoidosis. *Annals of the New York Academy of Sciences*, **278**, 212–217.

Victor, R. G., Kirsner, J. B. & Palmer, W. L. (1950) Failure to induce ulcerative colitis experimentally with filtrates of feces and rectal mucosa: a preliminary report. *Gastroenterology*, **14**, 398–400.

Vince, A., Dyer, N. H., O'Grady, F. W. & Dawson, A. M. (1972) Bacteriological studies in Crohn's disease. *Journal of Medical Microbiology*, **5**, 219–229.

Waldmann, T. A., Durm, M., Broder, S., Blackman, M., Blaese, R. M. & Strober, W. (1974) Role of suppressor T cells in pathogenesis of common variable hypogammaglobulinaemia. *Lancet*, **ii**, 609–613.

Walker, J. G. & Greaves, M. F. (1969) Delayed hypersensitivity and lymphocyte transformation in Crohn's disease and proctocolitis. *Gut*, **10**, 414.

Walker, W. A. & Isselbacher, K. J. (1974) Uptake and transport of macromolecules by the intestine. Possible role in clinical disorders. *Gastroenterology*, **67**, 531–550.

Wall, A. J. & Kraft, S. C. (1976) Regional enteritis. In *The Science and Practice of Clinical Medicine*, ed.-in-chief Sanford, J. P., Vol. 1, *Disorders of the Gastrointestinal Tract/Disorders of the Liver/Nutritional Disorders*, ed. Dietschy, J. M., pp. 138–144. New York: Grune & Stratton.

Ward, M. & Eastwood, M. A. (1975) Serum C_3 and C_4 complement components in ulcerative colitis and Crohn's disease. *Digestion*, **13**, 100–103.

Ward, M. & Eastwood, M. A. (1976) The nitroblue tetrazolium test in Crohn's disease and ulcerative colitis. *Digestion*, **14**, 179–183.

Warren, K. S. (1976) A functional classification of granulomatous inflammation. *Annals of the New York Academy of Sciences*, **278**, 7–18.

Warren, K. S., Domingo, E. O. & Cowan, R. B. T. (1967) Granuloma formation around schistosome eggs as a manifestation of delayed hypersensitivity. *American Journal of Pathology*, **51**, 735–756.

Watson, D. & Martucci, R. (1974) Cell-mediated immunity to *E. coli* 0119:B14 antigen in patients with chronic inflammatory bowel disease (CIBD) and normal individuals. *Clinical Research*, **22**, 120A.

Watson, D. & Martucci, R. (1975) Sensitivity to mycobacterial antigens in patients with chronic inflammatory bowel disease. *Clinical Research*, **23**, 100A.

Watson, D. W. (1969) Immune responses and the gut. *Gastroenterology*, **56**, 944–965.

Watson, D. W. & Pinedo, G. (1971) Lymphocyte stimulation by colonic and fecal antigens in patients with ulcerative colitis and Crohn's disease. *Clinical Research*, **19**, 177.

Watson, D. W., Quigley, A. & Bolt, R. J. (1966) Effect of lymphocytes from patients with ulcerative colitis on human adult colon epithelial cells. *Gastroenterology*, **51**, 985–993.

Watson, D. W., Styler, H. J. & Bolt, R. J. (1965) The autologous leukocyte skin test in patients with ulcerative colitis. *Gastroenterology*, **49**, 649–655.

Webster, L. T., Jr, Butterworth, A. E., Mahmoud, A. A. F., Mngola, E. N. & Warren, K. S. (1975) Suppression of delayed hypersensitivity in schistosome-infected patients by niridazole. *New England Journal of Medicine*, **292**, 1144–1147.

Weeke, B. & Jarnum, S. (1971) Serum concentration of 19 serum proteins in Crohn's disease and ulcerative colitis. *Gut*, **12**, 297–302.

Weetman, A. P., Haggith, J. & Douglas, A. P. (1974) Enteric loss of lymphocytes in coeliac disease and in Crohn's disease. *Gut*, **15**, 823.

Weiden, P. L., Blaese, R. M., Strober, W., Block, J. B. & Waldmann, T. A. (1972) Impaired lymphocyte transformation in intestinal lymphangiectasia: evidence for at least two functionally distinct lymphocyte populations in man. *Journal of Clinical Investigation*, **51**, 1319–1325.

Wenckert, A., Kristensen, M., Eklund, A. E., Barany, F., Jarnum, S., Worning, H., Folkenborg, O., Holtz, A., Bonnevie, O. & Riis, P. (1976) The long-term prophylactic effect of salazosulphapyridine (Salazopyrin^R) in primarily resected patients with Crohn's disease. A controlled double-blind trial. *Scandinavian Journal of Gastroenterology*, **11**, Suppl. 38, 93.

Whorwell, P. J., Baldwin, R. C. & Wright, R. (1976) Ferritin in Crohn's disease tissue: detection by electron microscopy. *Gut*, **17**, 696–699.

Williams, M. J., Richens, E. R., Gough, K. R. & Ancill, R. J. (1975) Leukocyte migration test in Crohn's disease, ulcerative colitis, and ankylosing spondylitis using Crohn's colon homogenate, mitochondrial, and microsomal fractions. *American Journal of Digestive Diseases*, **20**, 425–429.

Williams, R. C., Jr & Law, D. H., IV (1958) Serum complement in connective tissue disorders. *Journal of Laboratory and Clinical Medicine*, **52**, 273–281.

Willoughby, J. M. T. & Mitchell, D. N. (1971) *In-vitro* inhibition of leucocyte migration in Crohn's disease by a sarcoid spleen suspension. *British Medical Journal*, **iii**, 155–157.

Willoughby, J. M. T., Mitchell, D. N. & Wilson, J. D. (1971) Sarcoidosis and Crohn's disease in siblings. *American Review of Respiratory Disease*, **104**, 249–254.

Willoughby, J. M. T., Kumar, P. J., Beckett, J. & Dawson,

A. M. (1971) Controlled trial of azathioprine in Crohn's disease. *Lancet*, **ii**, 944–947.

Wilson, I. D. (1972) Human serum antibodies specific for secretory IgA. *Immunology*, **22**, 1001–1011.

Winstone, N. E., Henderson, A. J. & Brooke, B. N. (1960) Blood groups and secretor status in ulcerative colitis. *Lancet*, **ii**, 64–65.

Wolf-Jürgensen, P., Anthonisen, P. & Riis, P. (1965) Cutaneous bacterial inflammatory reaction in patients with ulcerative colitis. *Gut*, **6**, 221–224.

Wright, R. (1970) Ulcerative colitis. *Gastroenterology*, **58**, 875–897.

Wright, R. & Truelove, S. C. (1966) Autoimmune reactions in ulcerative colitis. *Gut*, **7**, 32–40.

Xavier, R. G., Prolla, J. C., Bemvenuti, G. A. & Kirsner, J. B. (1974) Tissue cytogenetic studies in chronic ulcerative colitis and carcinoma of the colon. *Cancer*, **34**, 684–695.

Yogman, M. W., Touloukian, R. J. & Gallagher, R. (1974) Intestinal granulomatosis in chronic granulomatous disease and in Crohn's disease. *New England Journal of Medicine*, **290**, 228.

Zeromski, J., Perlmann, P., Lagercrantz, R. & Gustafsson, B. E. (1970a) Immunological studies in ulcerative colitis. VI. Light microscopic studies with peroxidase conjugated antibodies. *Clinical and Experimental Immunology*, **7**, 463–467.

Zeromski, J., Perlmann, P., Lagercrantz, R., Hammarström, S. & Gustafsson, B. E. (1970b) Immunological studies in ulcerative colitis. VII. Anti-colon antibodies of different immunoglobulin classes. *Clinical and Experimental Immunology*, **7**, 469–475.

Zweibaum, A. & Bouhou, E. (1970) Iso- et hétéro-systemes naturels de groupe digestif chez l'homme. *Annales de l'Institut Pasteur*, **118**, 547–561.

Zweibaum, A., Oudea, P., Halpern, B. & Veyre, C. (1966) Presence in colic glandular cells of various mammalian species of an antigen cross-reacting with human blood group A substance. *Nature (London)*, **209**, 159–161.

8. Animal models for coeliac disease and inflammatory bowel disease

M. R. Haeney, R. Ferguson and P. Asquith

INTRODUCTION

Immunological mechanisms are thought to play a role, of varying significance, in the aetiopathogenesis of coeliac disease (Ch. 6) and inflammatory bowel disease, i.e. ulcerative colitis and Crohn's disease (Ch. 7). The search for animal models encompassing this spectrum of disease is difficult since one cannot precisely and objectively define each condition. In general, pathology will result from a dynamic interaction between an individual (endogenous factors) and his environment (exogenous factors) which produces structural and biochemical changes in tissues, and which, if severe or extensive enough, will result in altered physiology and symptoms and signs of clinical disease (Mottet, 1972). Intestinal illness may result from abnormal patient responsiveness, exposure to a harmful agent, or a combination of these factors. A small dose of exogenous agent(s) in an individual with impaired intestinal responses or a large dose in a relatively resistant individual are two extremes of many possible combinations. This can be further complicated when one agent precipitates the destructive process and another promotes its progression even though the initiator no longer exists. These dynamic interactions have a direct bearing on the problems of developing valid experimental animal models.

Researchers attempting to produce experimental models have used three basic approaches: (1) studies of naturally occurring animal diseases resembling human disease, (2) administration of exogenous agents to animals and (3) alteration of animal–host reactivity.

ANIMAL MODELS FOR COELIAC DISEASE

NATURALLY OCCURRING DISEASES

Morphological changes in the jejunal mucosa resembling those found in coeliac disease have been found in a variety of animal diseases (Table 8.1).

1. Pigs

White scours occurs in suckling piglets from 2 to 4 weeks old (Mouwen, 1974) with resulting fat malabsorption and steatorrhoea (Mouwen, 1972; Mouwen, Schotman, Wensing and Kijkuit, 1972). The small-intestinal mucosa is affected, the most severe changes being seen in the duodenum and distal jejunum, the latter contrasting with human coeliac disease, where the maximal damage is in the proximal jejunum (Rubin and Dobbins, 1965). Dissecting microscopic appearances of the mucosa of piglets with white scours vary from isolated areas with fewer large villi than normal, to severer changes consisting of convolutions or even a flat mucosa with a mosaic pattern. Corresponding histological changes are noted, with shortening and broaden-

Table 8.1 Naturally occurring diseases resembling coeliac disease

Animal	Description	Cause	Reference
Pig	White scours – affects duodenum and distal jejunum, varying degrees of villous atrophy	Unknown, although *E. coli* are found in increased numbers	Mouwen *et al.*, 1972
Pig	Transmissible gastroenteritis – villous atrophy with lymphocyte infiltration of the lamina propria	Virus	Thake, 1968 Olson *et al.*, 1973 Haeltermann, 1972
Turkey	Bluecomb – transmissible gastroenteritis. Shortening of jejunal microvilli	Coronavirus	Adams *et al.*, 1972
Dog	Villous abnormality, including inflammatory cell infiltration of the lamina propria	Unknown	Vernon, 1962 Kaneko *et al.*, 1965
Mice	Villous atrophy, ileum more affected than jejunum	Sensitized thymus-derived lymphocytes	Reilly and Kirsner, 1965

ing of the villi, increased cell mitoses, and crypt hyperplasia. Mucosal depth, however, remains unaltered. The epithelium is also damaged, with flattening of the cells and narrowing of the brush border. There is increased cellular infiltration of the lamina propria, consisting predominantly of plasma cells, lymphocytes, histiocytes and eosinophils, and the numbers of intraepithelial lymphocytes appear increased. Electron-microscopic studies (Mouwen, 1972) show abnormal microvilli while histochemistry reveals decreased activities of alkaline phosphatase, leucine aminopeptidase, acid phosphatase, succinate dehydrogenase and NADH-oxydoreductase (Mouwen, 1972).

The aetiology of white scours is not proven; although *Escherichia coli* are found in increased numbers in the luminal contents (Mouwen, 1974), the significance of this is in doubt. Clearly, further investigations are merited as the intestinal changes in many respects are comparable with those of coeliac disease.

Pigs suffering from transmissible gastroenteritis (TGE) develop villous atrophy (Thake, 1968) and a decreased number of microvilli, histological changes comparable to those seen in human coeliac disease. Also, like coeliac disease, the villous epithelium becomes cuboidal, jejunal villi shorten and crypts deepen (Kerzner, Kelly, Gall, Butler and Hamilton, 1977), but in contrast to the coeliac mucosa where plasma cell infiltration of the lamina propria occurs (Ferguson, Asquith and Cooke, 1974), lymphocyte infiltration of the lamina propria is a feature in the pigs. TGE is caused by a virus which Olson, Watler and Roberts (1973) have given orally to gnotobiotic pigs. Eighteen hours later they noted a uniform and consistent atrophy of villi in both the jejunum and ileum. Scanning electron-microscopy 48 hours after ingestion of the virus showed the villi to be virtually absent. Shortening of jejunal villi correlates with deterioration in glucose-mediated jejunal sodium flux (Kerzner *et al.*, 1977). An interesting finding is that, in contrast to coeliac disease, duodenal involvement is rare (Olson *et al.*, 1973). It has been concluded that the 'villous atrophy' is dependent upon the quantity of infecting virus given, the age of the pig, and the virulence of the infecting virus (Haelterman, 1972). Support for this conclusion has been provided by Stone, Stark and Phillips (1974). Their work also reflects the importance of a normally functioning immunological apparatus in the protection of the small-intestinal mucosa against antigens. (One assumes that the latter argument is also relevant to the human situation, and, in this context, to coeliac disease and the defence against intraluminal gluten.) Newborn pigs are agammaglobulinaemic (Stone *et al.*, 1974), any im-immunoglobulins being derived initially from maternal colostrum. It appears that if newborn pigs receive a reasonably high level of maternal antibodies from colostrum these will be absorbed from the intestine into the serum, offering a high degree of protection against the TGE virus.

In pigs, a malabsorption syndrome can also occur after abrupt weaning, the steatorrhoea being seemingly independent of intraluminal *E. coli* (Kenworthy and Allen, 1966). It is also apparent that when germ-free pigs are placed in a normal environment, morphological changes occur in the small intestine. The changes described include a broadening and shortening of the villi, replacement of columnar epithelium with cuboidal, the epithelial 'brush border' is lost, and the cellularity of the lamina propria increases. Furthermore, when certain strains of *E. coli* are introduced into the proximal small bowel of germ-free or gnotobiotic piglets, there is an increase in the plasma cell population of the lamina propria and the number of intraepithelial lymphocytes (Kenworthy, 1970; Kenworthy, 1971). He concluded that the villous and epithelial cell changes could follow on the increased inflammatory reaction in the lamina propria.

2. Turkeys

Turkey poults can suffer a transmissible enteritis (Bluecomb disease) which is now considered to be caused by a corona virus (King, 1975). The jejunal morphology is altered, with shortened microvilli, and an associated malabsorption syndrome occurs. Adams, Ball, Annis and Hofstad (1972) gave a strain of the transmissible enteritis virus to turkey poults orally, and to turkey embryos via the amniotic sac. In a predominantly electron-microscopic study they noted, in both poults and embryos, shortened epithelial microvilli in the upper small intestine. The poults showed, however, no gross changes in either the epithelial cell layer or lamina propria, but in the embryos the epithelial cells became shorter. Although interesting, the changes described have few features in common with coeliac disease.

3. Other species

A malabsorption syndrome resembling coeliac disease has been described in dogs (Vernon, 1962; Kaneko, Moulton, Brodey and Perryman, 1965), and in cats (Miller, 1963). Coeliac-like villous damage has also been reported in mice with runt intestinal disease (Reilly and Kirsner, 1965), but this latter is discussed below.

The animal models so far described show that transmissible agents can damage the intestinal mucosa. It is not clear whether this is a primary response to the agent or whether it is consequent to secondary bacterial infection or to damage by other intraluminal agents, such as food products. If the latter be true, then a more relevant 'natural' animal model for coeliac disease would exist.

A wide range of chemicals, drugs, dietary proteins and other agents has been administered to animals in the search for a contrived model of coeliac disease, with varying degrees of success.

1. Infused chemicals (Table 8.2)

Williams (1963), in an extensive study, injected a variety of agents into the small intestine of young adult Wistar rats, including 0.2 N-HCl, varying concentrations of formic acid, formaldehyde and ethyl alcohol, ferric chloride, half-saturated picric acid, trypsin,

continuously infused the proximal jejunum of rats with either 0.3M or 0.35M lactic acid at a rate of 48 ml/24 hours for 12 days. With the lesser concentration of acid, villous elongation and crypt lengthening developed, but at the higher concentration at the infusion site the villi became shorter, whilst the crypts elongated further. Reicken et al. (1972) concluded alteration in jejunal morphology took place in two stages: an initial stage of mucosal hypertrophy representing a transitional situation to compensate for epithelial cell loss, and a subsequent stage of decompensation in which the villi were reduced in size, in spite of an increase in crypt

Table 8.2 Jejunal mucosal disease induced by infused chemicals

Animal	Method	Result	Reference
Rat	Hydrochloric acid, formic acid and formaldehyde	Jejunal ulceration and necrosis	Williams, 1963
	Ferric chloride, picric acid	Cuboidal epithelial cells, shortened microvilli	
Rat	Lactic acid	Decreased villous height, increased crypt length	Hamilton, 1967 Riecken et al., 1972
Dog	Hydrochloric acid	'Flat' mucosa, plasma cell infiltration of the lamina propria	Townley et al., 1964

glycerol, 10 per cent Tween 80, Teepol, *Staphylococcus* enterotoxin and purified *E. coli* endotoxin. Each substance was injected into a 2-cm length of jejunum at laparotomy, the segment was clamped for 2 minutes after which the clamps were removed and normal saline flushed through the segment. The animals were killed 24 to 48 hours later, and jejunal tissue obtained for histological and electron-microscopic studies. Hydrochloric acid, formic acid and formaldehyde application resulted in jejunal ulceration or necrosis. Teepol, Tween 80, trypsin and the two bacterial toxins appeared to have no effect. Both ferric chloride and half-saturated picric acid caused morphological changes, the normal jejunal columnar epithelium being altered to cuboidal and, in addition, shortened microvilli were noted on electron-microscopic study. HCL was also used by Townley, Cass and Anderson (1964). Following intermittent instillation into an isolated jejunal segment of a dog, a 'flat' mucosa developed, with irregularity and flattening of the surface epithelium and plasma cell infiltration of the lamina propria.

Early experiments with lactic acid, using a prolonged (10-day) continuous-infusion system into the rat jejunum, were carried out by Hamilton (1967). After this period, mucosal zonation without ulceration occurred, consisting of a decrease in villous height and an increase in crypt length. Associated with this was an increased faecal fat excretion. Other workers (Riecken, Bloch, Menge, Idelberger, Kramer, Miller and Lorenz-Meyer, 1972) have extended these observations. They

length and mitotic counts. Hyper-regeneration was not fully proven, however, because only mitotic counts were estimated. In contrast to these morphological differences between the effect of 0.3M and 0.35M lactic acid, on the basis of glucose absorption, function was depressed in both groups of rats. Subsequently, Robinson (1972) questioned the usefulness of this particular experimental model because very severe experimental conditions were required to elicit a typical response.

2. Drugs

Several therapeutic agents used in humans have intestinal side-effects which have subsequently been evaluated in animals (Table 8.3).

Antimitotic agents

A single oral dose of aminopterin in rats produces degenerative changes in the jejunal villi (Millington, Finean, Forbes and Frazer, 1962), although these are not comparable to coeliac disease. Similarly, intramuscular aminopterin and 5-fluorouracil and oral colchicine all produce degenerative changes in rat jejunal mucosa. There is initial broadening and then disappearance of villi (Williams, 1963). In the mongoose, colchicine causes villous oedema and round-cell infiltration at low doses, the main effect being on the differentiating cells of the villi without damage to crypt cells (Stemmermann and Hayashi, 1971). At higher doses, colchicine causes arrest in metaphase of cells undergoing mitosis in the crypts and severe villous atrophy

Table 8.3 Jejunal mucosal disease induced by drugs

Animal	Method	Result	Reference
Rats	Aminopterin, colchicine, fluoro-uracil	Broadening of villi	Millington et al., 1962
Rats	Methotrexate	Broadening of villi	Robinson et al., 1966
Rats	Vinblastine and mustine	Villous atrophy	Tibbutt and Holt, 1974
Rats	Cyclophosphamide	Smaller villi, fewer mitotic figures per crypt	Ecknauer and Lohrs, 1976
Rats	Triparanol	Flattened villi with inflammatory cell infiltration, but ileum more affected than jejunum	McPherson and Shorter, 1965
Rats	Triparanol	Glucose malabsorption, responding to a gluten-free diet	Bloch et al., 1972
Rats	Triparanol	No gross morphological changes, but increased mitotic activity	Riecken and Menge, 1974
Mice	Triparanol	Reduced villous height and increased plasma cell infiltration	Ferguson et al., 1978
Mice	Adriamycin	Smaller villi, fewer mitotic figures per crypt	Burholt et al., 1977
Guinea-pigs	Vincristine	Villous atrophy	Hobson et al., 1974
Mongoose	Colchicine	Villous atrophy	Stemmermann and Hayashi, 1971
Monkeys	Neomycin	Functional impairment with normal morphology	Gilat et al., 1967 Dobbins et al., 1968

may follow (Stemmermann and Hayashi, 1971). Single systemic injections of vincristine sulphate in guinea-pigs (Hobson, Jervis, Kingry and Wallace, 1974) or vinblastine and mustine in rats (Tibbutt and Holt, 1974) cause severe villous atrophy, flattening of epithelial cells and reduced alkaline phosphatase activity in the epithelium. Less marked changes have been seen following single doses of cyclophosphamide in rats (Ecknaur and Löhrs, 1976) or adriamycin in mice (Burholt, Hagemann, Schenken and Lesher, 1977). In these latter studies, treatment resulted in a transient decrease in proliferative activity in the jejunum, with fewer mitotic figures per crypt and smaller villi. This was followed by a compensatory proliferative phase within 48 to 72 hours of administration of the drug. It seems likely that the mechanism of the tissue damage of these various substances is by inducing mitotic arrest, yet their effect on function may be delayed, or not as obvious as the morphological effects. Thus, oral methotrexate administration in rats (Robinson, Antonioli and Vannotti, 1966) does not reduce intestinal transport capacity in vivo or in vitro until 48 hours after treatment. They also noted that the extremely abnormal-appearing mucosa was still able to function relatively normally, and that during recovery there was often a delay in functional normalization despite apparent morphological recovery.

Neomycin
In man, oral neomycin produces a malabsorption syndrome associated with clubbing of intestinal villi,

increased lymphocyte and plasma cell infiltration of the lamina propria and brush border fragmentation (Jacobson, Prior and Faloon, 1960; Dobbins, Herrerro and Mansbach, 1968; Keusch, Troncale and Plaut, 1970). In contrast, neomycin does not appear to produce severe morphological alterations in animals (Gilat, Morin and Binder, 1967; Dobbins, Herrerro and Mansbach, 1968).

Triparanol
Normal animals. An acute malabsorption syndrome with reversible jejunal mucosal atrophy was reported as a side-effect of the drug Triparanol during its clinical use for treating hypercholesterolaemia (McPherson and Summerskill, 1963; McPherson and Shorter, 1965). Stimulated by these observations, McPherson and Shorter, (1965) administered this drug orally to adult Sprague-Dawley rats. After a week, definite morphological changes were noted in the small intestine, but, in contrast to coeliac disease, the changes in the ileum were more obvious than the jejunum. A moderate to severe inflammatory reaction was noted in the lamina propria, and in areas of the ileum severe flattening of villi occurred. The mucosa recovered on withdrawal of the drug. The changes seen in the jejunum in no way approached the severity of the lesions seen in coeliac disease. McPherson and Shorter (1965) also performed mitotic counting in areas of abnormal jejunum and ileum. In addition, estimates were made of the ratio of mature to immature crypt cells. They noted a change

in the ratio of adult to immature cells in the absence of any change of mitotic activity, consistent with a maturation defect. Concerning intestinal function, Bloch, Menge, Martini and Riecken (1972) showed glucose malabsorption occurred in Triparanol-fed rats, but of much greater interest was their additional finding of a return to normal of glucose malabsorption in the Triparanol-damaged rat jejunum when the animals were placed on a gluten-free diet!

The mechanism by which Triparanol damages the intestinal mucosa of the rat is not known, but further investigations have been undertaken by Riecken and Menge (1974). Triparanol administered in a dose of 50 mg/kg/day for 10 days did not reduce villous height, but crypt length and villous width were increased. These changes were accompanied by increased mitotic activity,

gross T-cell deficiency and heterozygous litter-mates of the same genetic background were compared with respect to jejunal mucosal cell populations; no significant differences were found. These two groups of mice were then exposed to routines of oral Triparanol and/or oral gluten, and in some cases intraperitoneal gluten, in order to compare the separate and cumulative effects of the two reagents in immunologically normal and T-cell-deficient animals. Oral administration of gluten resulted in significant increases in plasma cells and a decrease in lymphocytes in the lamina propria, and reduction in villous height, in both groups of mice. These changes were less marked after administration of Triparanol alone. In combined treatment (intraperitoneal gluten and oral Triparanol) a relatively massive increase in lamina propria plasma cells and significant increases also

Table 8.4 The cellular population of the proximal jejunal mucosa in each experimental group of heterozygote mice. (Nude mice and their 'normal' heterozygote litter mates were derived by heterozygote intercross of animals bred into a BALB/C genetic background)

Lamina propria cells/sq mm	Heterozygote normal-diet mice, n=7		Gluten-fed heterozygote mice. Oral gluten 500 mg/kg/day, n=5		Triparanol-fed heterozygote mice. Oral Triparanol 50 mg/kg day, n=5		I/P gluten (1 × 500 mg/kg) and gluten- and Triparanol-fed heterozygote mice, n=8	
	Mean	SD	Mean	SD	Mean	SD	Mean	SD
Plasma cells	737	883	2884	420	1336	923	640	406
Lymphocytes	5857	1545	4052	568	3488	524	3405	1376
Eosinophils	14	30	0	0	88	96	10	19
Reticulum cells	309	179	108	52	408	148	251	103
Miscellaneous cells	5714	1777	4328	229	7744	885	6098	2186
Total cells	12786	2312	11372	913	13072	1340	10346	2876
Epithelium cells/mm length								
Lymphocytes	20	15	26	13	36	18	12	6

I/P = intraperitoneal.

suggesting a structurally compensated stage of an altered mucosal zonation of the hyper-regenerative type. Riecken and Menge (1974) did not find any distinct changes in the gross cellular morphology of the rat jejunum; however, cytochemical and electron-microscopic studies indicated that Triparanol administration damages lysosomes. The fact that glucose malabsorption was affected by gluten intake might suggest that, in the human situation, gluten may be a secondary factor in the production of the mucosal abnormality found in coeliac disease. There is some evidence that gluten administered *per se* to rats does not induce any changes in the jejunal mucosa (see below).

Immunodeficient animals. To further explore the possible damaging effect of Triparanol and the mechanism of any damage, a further study has recently been completed (Ferguson, Catty, Asquith and Cooke, 1978). The jejunal mucosa of genetically athymic (nude) mice with

in intraepithelial lymphocytes and in villous widths were observed only in the nude mice (Table 8.4–8.7).

The overall results could indicate that plasma cells in the lamina propria of the mouse jejunal mucosa were triggered into differentiation and antibody synthesis by a T-cell-independent process, and in the absence of T-cell activity (namely in the nude mice) gluten may be a more powerful stimulator of this differentiation. By analogy, it was concluded that suppressor T-cell function may be impaired in the jejunal mucosa of patients with coeliac disease.

3. Gluten feeding (Table 8.8)

In addition to the evaluation of gluten in the Triparanol model, it has also been studied in isolation. An initial observation (Ribeiro, Sobrinho-Simoes and Mesquita, 1957) suggested that the addition of gluten to the diet of rats increased faecal fat output. However,

Table 8.5 Mucosal measurements of the proximal jejunum of heterozygote mice in each experimental group

Mucosal measurement (microns)	Heterozygote normal-diet mice n=7		Gluten-fed heterozygote mice. Oral gluten 500 mg/kg/day, n=5		Triparanol-fed heterozygote mice Oral Triparanol 50 mg/kg day, n=5		I/P gluten (1 × 500 mg/kg) and gluten- and Triparanol-fed heterozygote mice, n=8	
	Mean	SD	Mean	SD	Mean	SD	Mean	SD
Villous height	347	63	284	10	280	33	281	43
Villous width	78	5	77	25	99	10	89	17
Epithelial cell height	23	5	24	2	28	4	24	2
Crypt depth	68	20	48	4	79	22	79	13

Table 8.6 The cellular population of the proximal jejunal mucosa in each experimental group of nude mice

Lamina propria cells/sq. mm	Nude mice, normal diet, n=6		Gluten-fed nude mice. Oral gluten 500 mg/kg/day, n=5		Triparanol-fed nude mice. Oral Triparanol 50 mg/kg/day n=5		I/P gluten (1 × 500 mg/kg) and gluten- and Triparanol-fed nude mice, n=7	
	Mean	SD	Mean	SD	Mean	SD	Mean	SD
Plasma cells	147	234	1774	756	736	710	2548	793
Lymphocytes	5707	903	3304	926	4216	1428	2594	1023
Eosinophils	13	33	16	36	0	0	11	20
Reticulum cells	273	99	200	147	336	299	249	193
Miscellaneous cells	5853	657	4672	1165	5924	1835	5631	1191
Total cells	12 017	951	9976	1626	11 300	2738	11 057	2352
Epithelium cells/mm length Lymphocytes	17	4	15	2	12	9	34	16

Table 8.7 Mucosal measurements of the proximal jejunum of nude mice in each experimental group

Mucosal Measurement (microns)	Nude mice, normal diet, n=6		Gluten-fed nude mice. Oral gluten 500 mg/kg/day, n=5		Triparanol-fed nude mice. Oral Triparanol 50 mg/kg/day n=5		I/P gluten (1 × 500 mg/kg) and gluten- and Triparanol-fed nude mice, n=7	
	Mean	SD	Mean	SD	Mean	SD	Mean	SD
Villous height	343	53	278	19	264	53	302	90
Villous width	68	9	85	17	71	16	86	11
Epithelial cell height	24	4	23	4	22	4	22	3
Crypt depth	76	23	88	15	70	12	59	11

Table 8.8 Experimental effects of gluten feeding

Animal	Result	Reference
Rats	Increased faecal fat excretion	Ribeiro *et al.*, 1957
Rats	No effect on faecal fat excretion or morphology	Williams and Laster, 1963 Althausen and Grodsky, 1961 Bloch *et al.*, 1972
Mice	Reduced villous height, increased plasma cell infiltration	Ferguson *et al.*, 1978

attempts made to produce steatorrhea in adult male albino rats by feeding them diets containing 2 and 4 per cent gliadin or 4 per cent gluten were unsuccessful (Williams and Laster, 1963). Althausen and Grodsky (1961) have reported studies in which the daily feeding of 400 mg of wheat gluten or an equivalent amount of gluten to rats 5 days a week for 18 to 22 months failed to cause malabsorption of fats, carbohydrates or amino acids. This insensitivity of the rat to gluten has been confirmed by other workers (Bloch, Menge, Martini and Riecken, 1972).

Gluten fed in a dose of 500 mg/kg body weight to normal and athymic nude mice led in both groups to a reduction in villous height, and a decreased population of lamina propria lymphocytes (Ferguson, Catty, Asquith and Cooke, 1978). In the nude mice, crypt hyperplasia occurred. If one assumes that these changes resulted from an immunological reaction to gluten, functioning T-cells do not appear to be necessary for this to occur.

4. Infestations

Altered jejunal morphology is found in helminth parasite infestations such as infestation of the rat with the nematode *Nippostrongylus brasiliensis* (Symons and Fairbairn, 1962; 1963; Symons, 1965). The histological appearances in severely infested animals in some ways resemble those seen in coeliac disease, with shortened or absent villi, crypt lengthening, and an increase in mitotic figures. Symons (1965) studied cell kinetics in infested animals using tritiated thymidine, and demonstrated increased cell production in the crypts, and an increase in cell migration on the villi. Cell loss, measured by DNA loss and excretion of radiolabelled iron, shows a considerable increase on the ninth day of infestation. Loehry and Creamer (1969) have also examined the small-intestinal mucosa by the technique of autolysis 9 days after infestation with *Nippostrongylus brasiliensis*. It seems that increased cell loss may be associated with shortening of the villi, and the increased cell production with hypertrophy of intervillous ridges. On dissecting microscopy, convolutions and a 'flat' mucosa were seen. The presence of partial villous atrophy in normal rats infested with this nematode has been confirmed by others (Ferguson, 1974; Ferguson and Jarrett, 1975). However, when the infested rats had been previously depleted of thymus-derived lymphocytes by thymectomy and irradiation, the expected villous atrophy was absent in 70 per cent of experimental animals (Ferguson and Jarrett, 1975). This implies that villous damage was directly related to functioning T-cells, either by direct T-cell cytotoxicity, thymus-dependent antibody production, or by other mechanisms. As passive immunization of the thymus-deprived animals with hyperimmune anti-*Nippostrongylus* serum did not restore the capacity

of the infestation to damage the small-bowel mucosa (Ferguson and Jarrett, 1975), it suggests that T-cell factors, rather than antibodies, are involved in the pathogenesis of the villous atrophy in this model. These findings, however, cannot be directly related to coeliac disease.

ALTERATION OF HOST REACTIVITY

1. Lymphatic obstruction

Williams (1963) studied the jejunal mucosa of the rat following obstruction of the lymphatic drainage with silk sutures and noted that 24 hours after such a procedure the villi became swollen and oedematous. Later, occasional inflammatory reactions were noted, while 30 weeks following this procedure the only histological abnormality demonstrated was an excess of lymphocytes, plasma cells and eosinophils in the stroma, the changes generally being of mild degree. It is difficult to assess the importance of these changes or their relevance to coeliac disease.

2. Explantation and autolysis

Zetterlund (1962) demonstrated flattening of the mucosa in segments of small intestine transplanted onto the abdominal wall of rats. Similar changes have been described (Stephens, Finckh and Milton, 1964) in the duodenal mucosa of dogs after exteriorization of 10–12 cm of duodenum with an intact blood supply onto the abdominal wall. Six fully grown mongrel dogs of both sexes were used. Twenty-four hours after explantation the overall histological appearances of the mucosa differed little from normal. However, Stephens and his co-workers (1964) noted that the lamina propria contained many plasma cells and occasional lymphocytes and polymorphs (they do not, however, provide data with respect to the normal canine duodenum). One week after explantation, villous shortening occurred, and in some areas the normally columnar epithelium appeared cuboidal. By 6 weeks, villi were sparse in number, and much reduced in length, the mucosa being almost entirely made up of elongated intestinal glands and their supporting stroma. The lamina propria close to the surface contained fibroblastic spindle cells and polymorphs, but elsewhere were thought normal. Recovery of the mucosa took place after covering the isolated duodenum with skin, suggesting that trauma, rather than vascular impairment, was the cause of the mucosal changes.

Confirmation of the findings was provided by Townley, Cass and Anderson (1964) who exteriorized a jejunal loop in a dog. The jejunal mucosa assumed a 'flat' appearance and there was irregularity and flattening of the surface epithelium along with plasma cell infiltration of the lamina propria. The time that it took for these changes to appear is not, however, apparent. Similar explant experiments have been performed on rats (Loehry and Grace, 1974). Small pieces of rat jejunum, with the blood supply preserved, were explanted onto the anterior abdominal wall. After 6 weeks, areas of the mucosa appeared totally 'flat' when examined with the dissecting microscope. Histologically, the lesion was also patchy, in that some parts were devoid of villi and others had shortened and broadened villi. The crypts became long and hyperplastic. A dynamic study (Loehry and Grace, 1974) using intraperitoneally-injected tritium-labelled thymidine demonstrated a considerably increased turnover in the flat mucosa, with some disorganization of cell production and migration. Mitotic activity was also found to be raised. These changes probably represent a compensatory reaction for increased cell loss, and the histological and dissecting microscopic changes found by Loehry and Grace (1974) are similar to the villous abnormalities and long hyperplastic crypts seen in coeliac disease.

Finally, using a different technique – 'autolysis' – Loehry and Creamer (1969) found a flattened mucosa which appeared to consist entirely of hypertrophied intervillous ridges. They thought it comparable to coeliac disease.

3. Immunological mechanisms

The possibility that an immunological hypersensitivity reaction to dietary gluten is the primary cause of coeliac disease has been the stimulus for considerable clinical investigation.

In the majority of models discussed so far, although in some respects they resemble coeliac disease, the 'primary' effector mechanism was non-immunological, for example lactic acid infusion. Immunological mechanisms may have contributed to the tissue damage, but in this context, they are therefore 'secondary'. Little progress has been made in finding a 'primary' immunological model of coeliac disease. Where mucosal abnormality has been experimentally produced, dietary antigen has played no role in the pathogenesis of the lesion and hence the relationship of these models to coeliac disease remains indirect.

Cytotoxic antibody production

Rabin and Rogers (1976) immunized rabbits with intestinal extracts prepared from rabbits, guinea-pigs and germ-free rats. The resultant serum antibody response to intestinal antigen was determined by gel-precipitation and direct tissue-immunofluorescence. Forty-eight hours prior to sacrifice, local haemorrhage was induced in the duodenum using a non-traumatic vascular clamp. Of 20 rabbits immunized with rabbit intestinal extracts (8 with duodenum, 8 with ileum, 4 with colon) 6 had abnormal duodenal histology,

characterized by stunted villi and infiltration of plasma cells and lymphocytes in the lamina propria. These changes are similar to those of coeliac disease in man. However, the abnormal histology seen in the rabbits did not correlate with the presence of circulatory anti-intestinal antibody in immunized animals, nor was there any difference in the histology of traumatized areas of the duodenum of normal and actively-immunized rabbits.

Cell-mediated immune reactions (Table 8.9)

Allograft rejection. When small intestinal grafts are transplanted into genetically dissimilar recipients of the same species, the transplanted tissue retains normal appearance and function for some days, but is then rejected. Holmes, Klein, Winawer and Fortner (1971) reported small-intestinal allograft rejection when transplanted into Thiry-Vella loops in dogs. Subsequently, this work was confirmed and extended. One group has studied the rejection of foetal mouse small intestine transplanted under the renal capsule of normal, adult, syngeneic or allogeneic mice (Ferguson and Parrott, 1972a, b, 1973; MacDonald and Ferguson, 1976). Transplanted foetal intestine should be sterile with no intraluminal bacteria, hence any resulting pathological changes can be attributed to rejection. In allogeneic recipients, the grafts developed normally for a few days after implantation, having well-defined crypts, normal villi and regular columnar epithelium. Early rejection is characterized by lymphocyte infiltration of the lamina propria and lymphocyte accumulation in lymphatics. When rejection is established, the lymphocyte infiltration extends into the epithelium and submucosa, in addition to involving the lamina propria. Late rejection shows complete mucosal destruction, the grafts consisting of smooth muscle infiltrated with lymphocytes and some plasma cells (MacDonald and Ferguson, 1976). Rejection of grafts by thymus-deprived, allogeneic hosts is significantly delayed, indicating that the rejection of small intestine in this model is thymus-dependent (Ferguson and Parrott, 1973). Mucosal destruction precedes the appearance of anti-graft antibodies in the host serum (Elves and Ferguson, 1975), confirming the cellular nature of the rejection process. Although in established rejection the lesions described resemble the jejunal histology in untreated coeliac disease, the enterocytes appear normal until a late stage and plasma cell infiltration of the lamina propria is not a particularly noticeable feature, in contrast to the findings in coeliac disease (Holmes, Asquith, Stokes and Cooke, 1974; Ferguson, Asquith and Cooke, 1974).

Graft-versus-host disease. Graft-versus-host (or runt) disease occurs when immunocompetent lymphocytes are injected into an allogeneic host which is either immunodeficient or specifically tolerized to donor cells.

Table 8.9 Immunologically mediated experimental villous atrophy

Hypersensitivity reaction	Animal	Method	Result	Reference
Cell-mediated	Dog	Allograft rejection	Mucosal atrophy	Holmes et al., 1971
Cell-mediated	Mouse	Allograft rejection	Lymphocytic infiltration, but relatively normal enterocytes until late stage.	Ferguson and Parrott, 1972 MacDonald and Ferguson, 1976
Cell-mediated	Mouse	Graft-versus-host disease	Villous atrophy, crypt hyperplasia, but sparse cellular infiltrate	Reilly and Kirsner, 1965
Cell-mediated	Guinea-pig	Contact sensitivity (DNCB)	Villous destruction, xylose malabsorption	Bicks et al., 1967

Wasting and diarrhoea occur, accompanied by malabsorption (Hedberg, Reiser and Reilly, 1968), protein-losing enteropathy (Cornelius, 1970), and bile-salt depletion (Palmer and Reilly, 1971). In a classical experiment, Reilly and Kirsner (1965) reported small-intestinal changes in F_1 hybrid mice which had been injected with parental-strain spleen cells within 18 hours of birth. The mice were sacrificed when gross runting was present, usually between 10 and 14 days after injection. Although pathological changes were more pronounced in the ileum than in the jejunum, gross villous atrophy of the jejunum was present in places, together with crypt hyperplasia. In addition, a sparse cellular infiltration of the lamina propria occurred.

Contact sensitivity. Contact skin sensitivity to 2,4-dinitro-1-chlorobenzene (DNCB) is a function of sensitized T-lymphocytes. Skin sensitization of guinea-pigs with DNCB, followed by feeding of DNCB in an inert adhesive paste (Orabase), resulted in marked changes in the small intestine, characterized by villous destruction, local infection and a fibrino-purulent exudate. The morphological changes were accompanied by a malabsorption of *d*-xylose (Bicks, Azar and Rosenberg, 1967a).

ANIMAL MODELS FOR INFLAMMATORY BOWEL DISEASE

NATURALLY OCCURRING DISEASES (Table 8.10)

1. Dogs

A clinicopathological spectrum of spontaneous canine colitides, consisting of ileitis, colitis and proctitis, has been described by Van Kruiningen (1972). Four of the 8 cases described demonstrated a range of manifestations of 'regional enteritis' similar to that in man, namely, terminal ileitis, procto-colitis and segmental granulomatous proctitis. A rectal stricture was reported. A range of pathology was seen in other tissues apart from bowel, including perianal fistulae and hepatic granulomata. Van Kruningen thought that one dog had

changes comparable to those seen in ulcerative colitis in man. This latter point is difficult to comment on, as the reported crypt abscesses, mucosal hypertrophy and capillary congestion are not in themselves always diagnostic of ulcerative colitis (Mottet, 1972). The regional enteritis-like lesions closely resembled two previously reported cases of inflammatory bowel disease in cocker spaniel dogs (Strande, Sommers and Petrak, 1954).

Of particular interest is the chronic relapsing histiocytic type of canine colitis that occurs predominantly in boxer dogs (Kennedy and Cello, 1966). This colitis has a female : male ratio of 2 : 1 and usually begins in puppies. The affected dogs have a history of diarrhoea prior to the onset of bloody, mucus-covered stools. The disease is characterized by remissions and exacerbations, many of the relapses being triggered by pregnancy and changes in food or environment. The initial lesions occur in the rectum and, with progression, the disease spreads proximally. The involved mucosa is thickened, and there is ulceration and re-epithelialization. The unique microscopical feature of the chronic lesion is an infiltration of the lamina propria and submucosa by periodic acid-Schiff (PAS)-positive macrophages (Kennedy and Cello, 1966). No crypt abscesses or pseudopolyps are seen. Mild to moderate disease has been effectively controlled with Salazopyrine, though in the more severe forms systemic antibiotics and steroids are needed, but with variable results (Kennedy and Cello, 1966).

The condition shares features of both Crohn's disease of the colon and ulcerative colitis, but is probably not an experimental model for either. Histologically, the similarity appears closer to Whipple's disease in man and even closer to Johne's disease in cattle.

Mottet (1972) has suggested that canine colitis is not a specific disease but that dogs suffer from a spectrum of inflammatory bowel diseases. When considering possible pathogenetic mechanisms in man, it is noteworthy that the dog was the first species to suffer a range of spontaneous colonic disease similar to humans. Furthermore, it is the pedigree dogs, resulting

Table 8.10 Naturally occurring inflammatory bowel disease in animals. (Modified from MacPherson and Pfeiffer, 1976)

Animal	Description	Cause	Reference
Dog	Terminal ileitis, hepatic granulomata, perianal fistulae	Unknown	Strande et al., 1954 van Kruiningen, 1972
Dog	Chronic, relapsing, histiocytic canine colitis resembling human ulcerative colitis	Unknown	Kennedy and Cello, 1966
Horse	Colitis, acute toxaemic features	? Endotoxin	Rooney et al., 1963
Horse	Ileitis, granulomatous infiltration and features similar to human regional enteritis	Unknown, but Mycobacterium avium isolated in one case	Cimprich, 1974
Cattle	Ileitis and colitis resembling regional enteritis. Granulomatous lesions present	Mycobacterium johnei	Johne and Frothingham, 1895 Bang, 1906 Patterson and Allen, 1972
Pig	Terminal ileitis, occasionally colon involved	Unknown	Emsbo, 1951
Hamster	Ileitis, hyperplastic mucosa and lymphocytic infiltration	Transmissible agent from diseased tissue. Slow lactose-fermenting E. coli cultured	Boothe and Cheville, 1967 Amend et al., 1976
Rat	Caecitis, predominantly perivascular with occasional strictures	Unknown	Stewart and Jones, 1941
Mouse	Colitis with rectal prolapse. High mortality	Citrobacter freundii	Brennan et al., 1965 Ediger et al., 1974
Gibbon	Acute colitis	Associated with stress	Stout and Snyder, 1969
Gorilla	Acute colitis	Associated with stress	Scott and Keymer, 1975

from generations of inbreeding, that possess the disease susceptibilities (Van Kruiningen, 1972).

2. Horses

Equine colitis is a sporadic, acute, fatal disease of unknown aetiology, characterized by severe diarrhoea and toxaemia (Rooney, Bryans and Doll, 1963). Experimental studies suggest that the manifestations of the disease are due to endotoxaemia, since intravenous injections of *Escherichia coli* endotoxin produce a similar disease. The pathology is most severe in the caecum and colon where the mucosa is intensely hyperaemic, with oedema and haemorrhage in the submucosa. Microscopically, there is a marked arterial vasoconstriction, variable epithelial necrosis and a moderate acute inflammatory cell infiltrate.

A spontaneous granulomatous enteritis bearing a resemblance to Crohn's disease also occurs in horses. Cimprich (1974) reported 10 cases presenting with chronic weight loss, hypoalbuminaemia and either no or intermittent diarrhoea. Macroscopically, the ileum was most severely affected with serosal granular plaques, omental adhesions, a thickened, corrugated mucosal surface and marked mesenteric lymphadenopathy. Histologically, there was a diffuse, granulomatous-cell infiltrate with prominent giant cells in the lamina propria and submucosa. All horses had marked villous atrophy. Detailed microbiological investigations were negative except for one horse in whom *Mycobacterium avium*

was isolated from the faeces. The features of the disease are similar to Crohn's disease in man, Johne's disease of cattle and histiocytic colitis in boxer dogs.

3. Cattle

In 1895, Johne and Frothingham observed an unusual form of intestinal tuberculosis in cattle and Bang (1906) described this condition as chronic pseudotuberculosis. It is now termed paratuberculosis, or Johne's disease of cattle. Oral infection with *Mycobacterium johnei* is the cause. The disease may affect any ruminant species and presents as cachexia, chronic diarrhoea and bowel changes comparable with regional enteritis in man. Indeed, Johne's disease lends substance to the idea that Crohn's disease may be caused by a mycobacterium; the large and small bowel may be affected, and a 'cobblestone' apearance due to submucosal thickening may be observed (Patterson and Allen, 1972). Aggregation of epithelioid cells into granulomatous lesions are also seen. While no specific organism has ever been implicated in the aetiology of Crohn's disease, it is important to note that even in cattle experimentally infected with *M. johnei* it is often difficult to demonstrate bacilli in the intestinal tissues.

4. Pigs

Terminal ileitis, resembling regional enteritis, has been described in Scandinavian pigs (Emsbo, 1951). The disease incidence is approximately 1 per cent of all animals slaughtered. Thickening of the terminal ileum occurs, with the length of ileum involved varying from 25 to 160 cm. Emsbo noted, in several animals, perforation of the ileum and a diffuse peritonitis. An interesting observation, confirmed by others (Field, Buntain and Jennings, 1953), was that litter-mates of affected animals were sometimes diseased. Nevertheless, attempts by Emsbo to demonstrate an infectious agent in the lesions, or to transmit the condition experimentally, either by inoculation or by contact, were unsuccessful. With respect to any comparison with human Crohn's disease, giant cell systems in the diseased intestine have been reported by Emsbo (1951), but not by other workers (Field et al., 1953). However, the latter group did note increased cellularity of the lamina propria and the presence of epithelioid cells. An additional feature appears to be prominent muscular hypertrophy of the ileum. This is not so in human Crohn's, yet the 'enteritis' described in pigs may involve the colon (Emsbo, 1951) as does Crohn's disease.

5. Rodents

Hamsters

Acute and chronic ileitis have been reported in the Golden Syrian hamster (Boothe and Cheville, 1967). The lesion is restricted to the ileum, which is enlarged, thickened and rigid, but it has a friable wall. Histologically, there is hyperplasia of the ileal mucosa with lymphocyte infiltration. The enteritis can be reproduced in healthy hamsters by oral inoculation of homogenized ileum and distal jejunum from diseased animals and leads to death in less than 5 weeks (Amend, Loeffler, Ward and van Hoosier, 1976). Cultures grow a slow lactose-fermenting E. coli.

Rats

Stewart and Jones (1941) reported a naturally occurring disease in the caecum of rats. The inflammatory process was mainly perivascular with a periarteritis and endarteritis obliterans. After healing there was scarring at the ulcer sites, occasionally with stricture formation.

Runt disease in rats also has colonic manifestations (Singer, Spiro and Thayer, 1966). This will be discussed in a subsequent section of this chapter.

Mice

A large spontaneous outbreak of colitis in a conventional mouse colony has been described (Ediger, Kovatch and Rabstein, 1974). It was characterized by both a high mortality and a high incidence of rectal prolapse. Interestingly, one previous report had described experimentally induced colitis and diarrhoea in mice using the bacteria Citrobacter freundii (Brennan, Fritz and Flynn, 1965). This same organism was isolated by Ediger et al.

(1974) from the colon of mice affected with spontaneous colitis.

6. Apes

Stout and Snyder (1969) reported a fatal, ulcerative colitis-like lesion in 4 Siamang gibbons. Clinically, the symptoms resembled acute Shigella dysentery, but none of the animals' cage-mates developed diarrhoea. In all cases, the onset of the colitis coincided with 'socio-environmental upheaval'. More recently, acute ulcerative colitis leading to death has been described in 2 young gorillas and an orang-utan (Scott and Keymer, 1975). The absence of any defined infective agent and the association in 2 apes of preceding stressful experiences suggest that the syndrome may be examples of ulcerative colitis comparable to the human disease. However, 2 of the animals had been given antibiotics for intercurrent illness prior to death. The antibiotic was not named, hence it is interesting to speculate that one known to induce colitis in humans was used (Price and Davies, 1977). Therefore an alternative possibility of antibiotic-induced colitis arises. These higher apes are rare, precluding from an organizational point of view their use as a naturally occurring model of inflammatory bowel disease.

EXOGENOUS AGENTS PRODUCING MODELS RESEMBLING INFLAMMATORY BOWEL DISEASE

1. Sulphated polyanions

Following the ingestion of carrageenan, ulcerative colitis-like lesions develop in the caecum and colon of rabbits, guinea-pigs, rats and, to a lesser degree, mice (Marcus and Watt, 1969). Rhesus monkeys have also been shown to be susceptible (Benitz, Goldberg and Coulston, 1973).

Carrageenan is an extract of various red seaweeds, commonly Chondrus crispus and Euchema spinosum, and is used as a food additive. Native carrageenan is a sulphated polysaccharide with a molecular weight between 100 000 and 800 000. Mild acid hydrolysis results in degraded carrageenan (MW 30 000), but the original sulphate content and polyanionic properties are retained. If one compares toxicity in guinea-pigs and rabbits, the degraded product was more ulcerogenic than native undegraded carrageenan. Animals fed 0.1 per cent, 1.0 per cent or 5 per cent degraded carrageenan in the drinking water developed colonic ulceration. Of those given a mean daily dose of 0.07 g for 12 weeks, 60 per cent developed ulcers, while of those given a mean daily dose of 1.4 g for 30 days, 100 per cent developed ulcers. Clinical manifestations were loss of weight, diarrhoea and bleeding (Watt and Marcus, 1970; Marcus and Watt, 1971; Anver and Cohen, 1976). The ulcers first appeared in the caecum, then the colon and rectum. Histology showed caecal mucosal haemorrhages, acute or subacute inflammatory cell infiltrates, oedema, crypt abscesses and degeneration of surface epithelium (Watt and Marcus, 1973; Anver and Cohen, 1976). A prominent feature was the marked epithelial hyperplastic changes, including pseudopolyps associated with ulcerations. When carrageenan was given parenterally, there was no effect, hence it was postulated that degraded oral carrageenan induces mucosal damage by a local action rather than by acting systemically (Watt and Marcus, 1973).

Mucosal granulomas can also occur. Guinea-pigs fed degraded carrageenan develop them in the caecum and colon, followed by mucosal ulceration of the affected area (Sharratt, Grasso, Carpanini and Gangolli, 1970). No lesions are present in the small intestine (Anver and Cohen, 1976). The inflammatory infiltrate surrounding the ulcer consists mostly of macrophages, accompanied by lymphocytes, plasma cells and polymorphonuclear cells. Treatment of the animals with 0.1 per cent neomycin in addition to the carrageenan limits the infiltrate to macrophages. Furthermore, with respect to mechanisms of tissue damage, Abraham, Fabian, Goldberg and Coulston (1974) have shown that the ability of macrophage lysosomes in the lamina propria to endocytose and store the substance is closely related to caecal ulceration. If macrophage lysosomes do not endocytose the carrageenan, ulcers do not occur (Abraham et al., 1974). Presumably, following uptake, carrageenan stimulates lysosomal enzyme release with resultant local tissue damage and ulceration. It is interesting that ulceration is absent in guinea-pigs fed carrageenan in milk (Abraham et al., 1974). This can be explained by the fact that carrageenan is known to bind to milk (Anderson, 1967) and hence is unavailable for macrophage endocytosis (Abraham et al., 1974).

With respect to sulphated compounds in general, other high molecular weight sulphated polyanions such as sulphated amylopectin and sodium lignosulphonate produce damage in guinea-pigs. Even 0.1 per cent sulphated amylopectin, a synthetic polysaccharide derived from potato starch, causes colonic ulcers (Watt and Marcus, 1972). Sodium lignosulphonate, a molecule of sulphonated phenylpropane units of molecular weight 20 000, also produces an 80–100 per cent incidence of lesions, depending on the concentration used and the duration of exposure (Watt and Marcus, 1973).

To extrapolate from any animal model to human disease is dangerous since different species may react differently to exogenous agents such as carrageenan, and any one of a variety of agents may have a primary role in the genesis of human colitis. However, in man there is no evidence that carrageenan is involved; thus Bonfils (1970) stated that in 200 patients receiving carrageenan daily for up to 2 years in the treatment of peptic ulceration, there was no evidence of ulcerative colitis. The major criticism levelled by Sharratt et al. (1971) against the carrageenan model relates to the different anatomical site of the lesions compared with human ulcerative colitis. Nevertheless, Mottet (1972) felt the macroscopical and histological similarities to human inflammatory bowel disease were impressive. For example, there is mucosal ulceration, loss of haustration, mucosal granularity, pseudo-polyp and stricture formation. This last feature is, of course, more a characteristic of Crohn's disease, but benign strictures also occur in ulcerative colitis. Also the microscopic picture is analogous to human colitis: inflammatory changes in the mucosa, crypt abscess formation, cystic dilatation of mucosal glands and hyperplastic changes of the glandular epithelium.

These sulphated compounds do therefore produce intestinal lesions resembling inflammatory bowel disease; however, the damage does seem to depend on continuous feeding. But perhaps this is the situation in humans where an unknown dietary agent, for example Cornflakes (James, 1977) or refined carbohydrates (Martini and Brandes, 1976), acting either alone or in association with an infectious agent, viral or bacterial (see below), is unwittingly responsible for IBD.

2. Other dietary agents

Long, Kolmer and Swalm (1935) fed inert materials such as kaolin to rats and, at autopsy, noted pathological abnormalities in the intestinal mucosa of animals fed large amounts. However, lesions were not produced regularly. Rats fed diets including karaya gum, bran or psyllium were susceptible to the development of caecal lesions (Hoelzel, Da Costa and Carlson, 1941). Placing sand and talc in isolated ileal loops, and including these substances as part of the diet of dogs (Chess, Olander, Puestow, Benner and Chess, 1950), did give rise to granulomatous lesions of the small intestine, although the overall morphological changes were not comparable with those of Crohn's disease.

3. Infectious agents and their products

Many of the clinico-pathological features of inflammatory bowel disease in man could be explained on an infectious basis. Efforts to identify the suspected causative organism have taken two major paths: (1) immunization of experimental animals with a variety of bacteria or bacterial products in the hope of understanding basic mechanisms of bacterial invasion and the associated host inflammatory response; in most experiments it is not possible to consider these two effects separately: (2) transmission experiments, where homogenates of diseased human tissue have been injected into experimental animals in the hope of reproducing the disease. Recent information regarding the transmission of inflammatory bowel disease to animals, together with serological data and virological findings, have provided a basis for renewed interest in the role of infectious agents in the aetiology of inflammatory bowel disease (Beeken, Mitchell and Cave, 1976).

Bacterial immunization (Table 8.11)

Broberger and Perlmann (1959) found autoantibodies to human colon in the sera of patients with ulcerative colitis and suggested that their occurrence was a result of stimulation by bowel bacteria. It was then shown that these sera also reacted with a polysaccharide antigen extracted from a sterile rat colon and that the reaction could be inhibited by antigen from certain strains of *E. coli* (Perlmann, Hammarström, Lagercrantz and Gustafsson, 1965). They suggested that stimulation, perhaps by the Kunin antigen, might be responsible for the formation of anticolon antibodies in ulcerative colitis.

Zweibaum, Morard and Halpern (1968) immunized rats with certain strains of *E. coli* and produced an experimental colitis similar to human ulcerative colitis in terms of symptoms, course, site of lesions and histological features. This experimental disease could also be prevented by oral administration of the appropriate *E. coli* strain.

Colonic autoantibodies were induced in over 50 per cent of rabbits immunized with *E. coli* derived from patients with ulcerative colitis (Cooke, Filipe and Dawson, 1968). Although enzyme histochemistry suggested early mucosal damage there were no obvious morphological changes.

Germ-free rats monocontaminated with anaerobic *Clostridium* species also produced autoantibodies to colon antigen (Hammarström, Perlmann, Gustafsson and Lagercrantz, 1969). These antibodies were not found in the sera of germ-free rats, germ-free rats mono-

Table 8.11 Inflammatory bowel disease induced by bacteria. (Modified from MacPherson and Pfeiffer, 1976)

Animal	Method	Result	Reference
Rabbits	Injection of live and dead *E. coli* into footpads	Chronic ulcerative disease of caecum	Halpern *et al.*, 1967
Rabbits	Immunization with *E. coli* derived from patients with ulcerative colitis	Histochemical changes suggesting early mucosal damage, but no morphological changes	Cooke *et al.*, 1968
Rabbits	Intra-ileal injection of L-form of *Streptococcus faecalis*	Focal granulomatous lesions in terminal ileum	Orr *et al.*, 1974
Rats	Immunization with *E. coli* strains	Features similar to human ulcerative colitis	Zweibaum *et al.*, 1968
Pigs	Monocontaminated with *E. coli*	Mild enteritis and colitis	Staley *et al.*, 1970
Mice	Contaminated with *Citrobacter freundii*	Colitis with diarrhoea	Brennan *et al.*, 1965 Brynjolfsson and Haley, 1967
Rhesus monkeys	Peroral *Shigella flexneri*	Acute fulminant colitis	Takeuchi *et al.*, 1968

Asherson and Holborow (1966) injected rabbits with dead bacteria in Freund's complete adjuvant. After one month, autoantibodies were present in the serum which reacted with a mucus-like antigen detected in the colon and sometimes in the ileum and stomach.

Injection of some strains of *E. coli* into the footpads of rats produced a colonic inflammatory disease characterized by diarrhoea, bleeding and colonic ulceration (Halpern, Zweibaum, Oriol-Palou and Morard, 1967). The disease was produced by both living and dead bacteria, and the symptoms and lesions were chronic. No cross-reaction was observed between the *E. coli* producing the disease and any colonic tissue antigen. The authors felt that the experimental colitis was the result of an immunological breakdown of colonic bacterial balance. They supported this hypothesis by showing that the disease could be prevented by daily oral administration of live *E. coli* to these animals (Halpern *et al.*, 1967).

contaminated with other bacteria, conventional rats of germ-free origin, or conventional Sprague–Dawley rats. The anticolon antibodies of *Clostridium*-infected rats reacted with the same faecal extract as the antibodies of ulcerative colitis patients, but there was no cross-reactivity between clostridial antigen and colon antigen. The authors considered that the mechanism of autoantibody production in this model could be: immunogenic alteration of gastrointestinal mucins by bacterial degradation, adjuvant effects of bacterial products, or a combination of these two mechanisms.

Colitis in young pigs has been reported, neonatal pigs monocontaminated with *E. coli* producing a mild enteritis and colitis (Staley, Corley and Jones, 1970). Cellular changes were minimal until oedema of the lamina propria developed approximately 6 days after monocontamination. The response sequence involved macrophage accumulation in the lamina propria, swollen terminal capillary endothelium, extravascular fibrin and platelet deposition, oedema of the lamina propria and submucosa, lymphangiectasis and perilymphangitis. In neonatal pigs, the attachment and penetration of *E. coli* onto ileal and colonic epithelium was similar in both areas and occurred with equal frequency. Experimental colitis in mice was also induced by a bacterium, *Citrobacter freundii* (Brennan, Fritz and Flynn, 1965; Brynjolfsson and Haley, 1967). Takeuchi, Formal and Sprinz (1968) described an acute colitis in rhesus monkeys following per-oral injection of *Shigella flexneri*. The colitis was acute, fulminant and limited to the mucosa, with epithelial cell invasion, micro-ulcer formation and crypt abscesses. A chronic state of colitis could not be established.

Recently, it has been shown that L-forms of bacteria can induce granulomatous changes in the intestine (Orr, Tamarind, Cook, Fincham, Hawley, Quilliam and Irving, 1974). These workers injected suspensions of the stable L-form of *Streptococcus faecalis* (strain B9) into the wall of rabbit terminal ileum. As a control, 'parent' organisms or sterile medium were injected into other groups of rabbits. Focal granulomatous lesions, consisting of epithelioid and giant cells, were found in the ileal submucosa of rabbits injected with L-forms but not in the remaining groups of animals. Variant bacteria have also been implicated in the aetiology of inflammatory bowel disease by finding bacterial variants of *Pseudomonas maltophilia* and *Pseudomonas*-like bacteria in tissue removed during surgery from 3 patients with Crohn's disease and another patient with features of both Crohn's disease and ulcerative colitis (Parent and Mitchell, 1976). Bacterial variants were not cultured from colonic specimens of 1 patient with chronic ulcerative colitis or from 2 patients with colonic carcinoma. The authors hypothesize that the infectious agent in inflammatory bowel disease is a bacteriophage-induced L-form or similar variant. Such forms may invade the bowel, so providing immunogenic stimulation, and subsequently antigen–antibody complexes may be deposited at sites of bowel inflammation (Parent and Mitchell, 1976).

Transmissible agents, ? viral, in Crohn's disease
One of the most exciting developments in the field of animal models relevant to Crohn's disease is the recent work on 'transmissible agents'.

In 1970, Mitchell and Rees described results of controlled experiments in which homogenates of Crohn's tissue obtained from intestine or lymph nodes were injected into footpads of normal and immunologically deficient mice. Some footpads developed histological changes typical of the focal granulomata of Crohn's disease. Following on from this, rabbits were inoculated intra-ileally with Crohn's tissue homogenates (Cave, Mitchell, Kane and Brooke, 1973; Cave and Mitchell,

1974). In the recipient rabbits focal epithelioid and giant cell granulomata were observed in the submucosa, other areas of the bowel, and in mesenteric lymph nodes, the work strongly suggesting that there was a transmissible agent in Crohn's disease. Subsequent studies (Mitchell, Rees and Goswami, 1976) have shown that starting with mouse tissue inoculae the 'transmissible' agent can produce disseminated granulomata, which survive homogenization and ultrafiltration, but not initial autoclaving.

When considering the significance of these findings, it is noteworthy, however, that Taub, Sachar, Janowitz and Silzbach (1976) not only produced granulomas using Crohn's tissue but also using tissue from patients with ulcerative colitis and unrelated gastrointestinal conditions. One other major problem is that other workers (Bolton, Owen, Heatley, Jones-Williams and Hughes, 1973; Heatley, Bolton, Owen, Jones-Williams and Hughes, 1975) have not been able to induce granuloma formation at the innoculation site of Crohn's tissue homogenates. These workers concluded that their negative results might indicate that a 'transmissible agent' was not universally present in Crohn's disease. Nevertheless, it is important to recall that they used different animals, namely, rats, guinea-pigs and mice, and that the techniques and reagents were also different.

In most of the above 'positive' experiments it has been assumed that the 'transmissible' agent was a virus, yet on some of the data provided other infectious agents cannot be excluded, for example *Mycobacteria*. Certainly the consideration that Crohn's is due to a virus was given considerable impetus by the finding of virus particles in human Crohn's tissue (Aronson, Phillips, Beeken and Forsyth, 1975; Cave, Mitchell and Brooke, 1975; Gitnick, Arthur and Shibata, 1976; Gitnick and Rosen, 1976). That particles have not been found in other laboratories (Cook and Turnbull, 1975; Whorwell, Baldwin and Wright, 1976) could easily be explained if one assumes that the disease is not homogeneous or the virus is only present intermittently. A final cautionary note is the finding of many viruses in the normal human alimentary tract (Flewett and Bloxall, 1976), a point which should always be borne in mind in interpreting such data.

ALTERATION OF HOST REACTIVITY

1. Lymphatic obstruction
Many of the changes which follow lymphatic obstruction in animals resemble Crohn's disease. Reichert and Mathes (1936) cannulated the intestinal lymphatics in dogs and injected sclerosing agents. Changes of lymph-oedema with thickening of the intestinal muscular and submucosal layer followed, changes that were enhanced by intravenous injection of *Escherichia coli*. The mucosa

did not, however, become ulcerated, nor were granulomata detected.

Lymphatic obstruction in pigs was produced by injecting formalin into the mesenteric lymph nodes (Kalima, Saloniemi and Rahko, 1976). After one week, the terminal ileum became hyperaemic and oedematous. Microscopically, oedema of all intestinal layers with lymphangiectasia and abundant inflammatory cells in the lamina propria were observed. In the subserosa and mesentery, granuloma-like collections of round cells were present, consisting of lymphocytes, macrophages and multinucleate giant cells. Between 1 and 3 weeks later, many of the pigs had developed internal fistulae. Microscopically, there were numerous epithelial erosions, deep ulcers and crypt abscesses. In the most severely affected regions, there was villous atrophy. Three weeks to 3 months after lymphatic destruction, all the pigs had numerous adhesions while some had fistulae, ulceration and lymphoid hyperplasia. Again numerous granulomas were present in the submucosa and subserosa.

2. Vascular impairment

In contrast to lymphatic obstruction and its relevance to understanding Crohn's disease, vascular impairment has been suggested by many workers seeking an aetiological explanation for ulcerative colitis.

Mechanical obstruction of colonic blood flow in dogs resulted in varying degrees of mucosal ulceration (Marston, Marcuson, Chapman and Arthur, 1969). Earliest changes included radiological 'thumbprinting', due to mucosal oedema and haemorrhage, which reverted to normal within a few weeks. Increased numbers of polymorphonuclear leucocytes were noted and were directly related to the extent of devascularization and mucosal necrosis. In contrast, Matthews and Parks (1972) gradually reduced the calibre of the middle colic and inferior mesenteric arteries in dogs by the application of Ameroid casein plastic around the artery. This induced a slowly progressive, complete occlusion, but ischaemic colitis rarely occurred.

Using a different approach, Kirsner (1961) reported that injection of cholinergic compounds in dogs produces a bloody diarrhoea resembling early ulcerative colitis in man. The symptoms rapidly subsided after stopping these agents. The histological appearance of the colon showed hyperaemia, vascular dilatation and haemorrhage. The colitis observed after prolonged administration of histamine or the histamine releaser, compound 40/80, in dogs (Kirsner, 1961) is of interest in the light of recent evidence that stabilization of mast cell degranulation by sodium cromoglycate improves proctitis in man (Heatley, Calcraft, Rhodes, Owen and Evans, 1974).

3. Immunological mechanisms

Experimental models attempting to reproduce each of the 4 major hypersensitivity reactions (Coombs and Gell, 1976) have been devised for the investigation of inflammatory bowel disease (Table 8.12).

Immediate hypersensitivity reactions

Gray and Walzer (1938) passively sensitized the skin and rectal mucosa of subjects to peanut protein by the local injection of human serum containing reaginic antibody to peanuts. Twenty-four to 48 hours later, the peanut protein was either ingested orally or applied directly to the rectum. Immediate hypersensitivity reactions developed at the sensitized cutaneous and mucous membrane sites within 5 to 25 minutes. In the rectum, reactions consisted of blanching and oedema lasting approximately 5 minutes, followed by hyperaemia intensifying over 15 to 20 minutes. No eosinophilia was found at biopsied reaction sites. Subjective symptoms included pruritus, rectal burning and the urge to defaecate. Subsequently, Gray, Harten and Walzer (1940) passively sensitized exposed ileum and colon in 2 humans with ileocolostomies. Oral and local allergenic challenge resulted in macroscopic effects identical to those previously seen in the rectum by Gray and Walzer (1938). In similar experiments in rhesus monkeys, local passive anaphylaxis in the small and large intestines was accomplished by intramucosal injection of reaginic antibody to cotton seed, cow's milk or horse serum (Walzer, Gray, Straus and Livingston, 1938). Intravenous challenge with specific allergen caused blanching, oedema, hyperperistalsis and spasm at sensitized sites, while histologically there was submucosal oedema and infiltration with eosinophils and lymphocytes (Walzer et al., 1938; Grayzel and Walzer, 1939).

Cytotoxic antibody production

The finding of autoantibodies to human colon in the sera of patients with ulcerative colitis (Broberger and Perlmann, 1959) prompted many workers to investigate the effects of anticolon autoantibody production in animals by immunization with colonic tissue.

Richardson and Leskowitz (1961) failed to produce gastrointestinal lesions in rabbits, guinea-pigs, rats or mice following the injection of normal homologous whole stomach, small intestine, or colon with Freund's adjuvant given either intradermally or by footpad injection over periods of 2 to 10 weeks. Le Veen, Falk and Schatman (1961) prepared an antigen from sterile, homogenized dog colon mucosa, raised an antiserum in rabbits and ducks and then injected the antiserum into several dogs. A bloody diarrhoea developed within 1 to 2 days associated with ulcerating lesions similar to those seen in acute ulcerative colitis. The disease was subject to remissions and relapses, but chronic disease could not

Table 8.12 Immunologically mediated inflammatory bowel disease

Hypersensitivity reaction	Animal	Method	Result	Reference
Type I – immediate hypersensitivity	Monkey	Local passive anaphylaxis	Submucosal oedema with eosinophilic and lymphocytic infiltration	Walzer et al., 1938 Grayzel and Walzer, 1939
Type II – cytotoxic antibody	Rabbits, mice, rats and guinea-pigs	Immunization with homologous colon	No effect	Richardson and Leskowitz, 1961
	Dogs	Injection of anti-dog colon serum raised in rabbits and ducks	Acute relapsing ulcerative colitis. Chronic disease not produced	LeVeen et al., 1961 Shean et al., 1964 Bicks and Walker, 1962
	Rats	Autoantibodies induced by immunization with dog colonic mucus	Colitis resembling human disease	Oriol Palou et al., 1967
	Rabbits	Injection of guinea-pig colon in complete Freund's adjuvant	Mild capillary dilatation in colon	Hausamen et al., 1969
	Rabbit	Immunization with rabbit, guinea-pig or germ-free rat small and large intestine	Lack of correlation between histological changes and presence of anti-intestinal antibody	Rabin and Rogers, 1976
Type III – immune complex deposition	Rabbit	Intramucosal injection of egg albumin into sensitized recipient	Oedema, polymorph infiltration, vasculitis and focal necrosis	Goldgraber and Kirsner, 1959 Kirsner, 1961
	Rabbit	Auer reaction – antigenic challenge of sensitized animal after non-specific irritation of colon	Colitis	Kirsner et al., 1959 Ford and Kirsner, 1964 Hodgson et al., 1976
Type IV – delayed	Guinea-pig	Contact sensitivity to DNCB	Mucosal ulceration with necrosis and mononuclear cell infiltration	Bicks and Rosenberg, 1964 Bicks et al., 1965; 1967
	Mouse	Allograft rejection	Features dissimilar to human colitis	Holden and Ferguson, 1976
	Rats	Graft-versus-host disease	Features dissimilar to human colitis	Singer, Spiro and Thayer, 1966

be induced. Similar studies by other workers (Shean, Barker and Fonkalsrud, 1964) incorporated Freund's adjuvant to develop adequate titres of rabbit anti-dog colon antibodies. These experiments showed that pre-cipitating antibodies against dog colon cross-reacted with all gastrointestinal tissues. Attempts to induce chronic colitis by long-term injection of autologous colon were unsuccessful. The use of Freund's adjuvant increased the difficulty of interpretation of the experi-mental findings (Kraft, Bregman and Kirsner, 1962).

Bicks and Walker (1962) attempted to show that an immune reaction could be localized to the colon without prior sensitization. They succeeded in producing colitis in dogs by intravenous injections of rabbit anticolon serum. An acute immunological reaction developed primarily limited to the colon but with evidence of

systemic involvement. Mucosal infiltration, submucosal oedema and perivascular cuffing were the dominant histological features.

Oriol Palou, Halpern, Zweibaum, Morard, Veyre and Abadie (1967) produced experimental colitis with auto-antibodies in rats immunized with dog colonic mucus. The lesions were confined to the colon, symptoms were similar to human disease and elevated titres of specific antibody to colon glandular cells were found. Symptoms and macroscopic and histological findings resembled proctocolitis.

An antiserum prepared by injections into rabbits of aqueous extracts of adult and foetal guinea-pig colon in Freund's complete adjuvant induced only a mild capil-lary dilatation on subsequent injection into the guinea-pig. Also no histological changes in the mucosa were seen in rabbits with circulating autoantibodies against constituents of colonic mucosa (Hausamen, Halcrow and Taylor, 1969).

Recently, Rabin and Rogers (1976) have immunized rabbits with rabbit, guinea-pig or germ-free rat duodenum, ileum or colon. The resultant antibody response to intestinal antigen was determined by gel-precipitation and direct tissue immunofluorescence. Two days prior to sacrifice of each immunized animal, a part of the duodenum, ileum and colon was traumatized to bring any circulating antibody into contact with the tissue. As a control, normal rabbits were also traumatized. Sections were taken from the area of trauma, and at points 1 cm and 10 cm distant from it. Six out of 20 rabbits immunized with rabbit intestinal extracts had abnormal histology of the ileum, characterized by a mixed cell infiltrate in the lamina propria and an oedematous submucosa with a perivascular inflammatory cell infiltrate. However, of the 6 rabbits with abnormal histology, only 3 had circulating anti-intestinal antibody detectable. Similarly, in rabbits immunized with guinea-pig or germ-free rat tissue, the presence of antibody did not correlate with histological changes. The histology of traumatized areas of the intestine of normal and actively immunized rabbits did not differ and tissue 1 cm distant from the area of trauma in actively immunized animals did not differ histologically from tissue 10 cm distant from the area of trauma. Thus allowing serum antibody to come into contact with the intestine did not accentuate tissue damage. This study reproduced some features of human inflammatory bowel disease, namely circulating anti-intestinal antibody in the absence of pathological changes in the intestine (Lagercrantz, Hammarström, Perlmann and Gustafsson, 1966).

Thus, while showing that animal colon can participate in direct antigen-antibody reactions, no model has produced a diffuse, chronic, self-perpetuating or progressive inflammatory disease of the intestinal mucosa. It is recognized that the presence of circulating anticolon antibodies in humans does not necessarily imply an immunological aetiology for IBD but may represent the effects of tissue damage.

Immune complex deposition

Arthus-type reactions are due to antigen–antibody complexes formed in moderate antigen excess. They can be produced in the gastrointestinal tract by intramucosal injection, or local application of antigen in an animal already producing specific antibody. Thus intramucosal injection of egg albumin into a sensitized rabbit produced an intensely haemorrhagic, necrotizing reaction in the colon (Goldgraber and Kirsner, 1959; Kirsner, 1961). Mucosal oedema, vascular congestion and a polymorph infiltrate present 6 hours after injection were replaced by oedema, vasculitis and focal necrosis after 3

days, and local granuloma formation after 1 week. Tissue damage can also be produced by direct local application of antigen to the intestinal mucosa of an animal passively sensitized with specific antibody. This eliminates the chance that local cell-mediated reactions could contribute to the changes induced. Bellamy and Nielsen (1974) showed that guinea-pigs sensitized passively to BSA and then locally challenged with that antigen produced a marked emigration of large numbers of neutrophils into the intestinal lumen.

The Auer reaction. Experiments suggest that once the colon is inflamed, the deposition of locally produced or systemically derived immune complexes may produce severe ulcerative disease. In 1920, Auer injected a large dose of specific antigen into a sensitized animal and produced severe inflammation at the site of a previously induced non-specific irritation. This 'Auer reaction' was reproduced by others by sensitizing rabbits to egg albumin, and then giving intravenous or intraperitoneal specific antigen after irritating the distal colon with dilute formalin (Kirsner, Elchlepp, Goldgraber, Ablaza and Ford, 1959). A form of colitis was produced, characterized by superficial ulceration and haemorrhage, with infiltration of polymorphonuclear cells, plasma cells and lymphocytes. Ford and Kirsner (1964) also showed that intrarectal administration of specific antigen in sensitized rabbits induced a colitis in the distal colon previously exposed to mild formalin solution. More recently, Hodgson, Skinner, Potter and Jewell (1976) prepared HSA-anti-HSA immune complexes *in vitro*. After first exposing rabbit rectum to a 1 per cent formalin solution, the rabbits were then given soluble immune complexes intravenously and serial rectal biopsies were taken. Control animals, given formalin, were injected with saline, antigen or antibody alone. These animals showed minimal lesions which healed within 24 hours. In contrast, rabbits given immune complexes developed a severe inflammatory response within 3 hours, and which was maximal at 1 week. Histologically, the changes were those of severe, acute ulcerative colitis.

Delayed hypersensitivity reactions

Contact sensitivity. Bicks and Rosenberg (1964), in guinea-pig colon, demonstrated a contact type of chronic delayed hypersensitivity reaction. They skin-sensitized animals to DNCB and then challenged the guinea-pig locally with DNCB in an inert adhesive paste. Daily rectal challenge produced mucosal ulceration with necrosis, oedema, vascular congestion and infiltration with lymphocytes, plasma cells and macrophages (Bicks and Rosenberg, 1964; Bicks, Brown, Hickey and Rosenberg, 1965; Bicks, Azar, Rosenberg, Dunham and Luther, 1967b). The severity of the reaction was dependent on the frequency of application of the contact allergen and could be modified, but not predictably or completely, by azathioprine. The reaction, which was specific, could be transferred to non sensitized recipient animals by lymphocytes but not by serum (Bicks *et al.*, 1967b). A similar, but less intense, lesion could be produced by prolonged primary contact of DNCB with colonic mucosa without prior skin sensitization. The *in-vitro* specific inhibition of macrophage-migration inhibition confirmed the presence of cellular immune reactivity.

Allograft rejection. Rejection of small-intestinal allografts has been discussed as a model for jejunal mucosal atrophy; allografts of mouse colon are also rejected, although more slowly than small-intestinal grafts (Holden and Ferguson, 1976). There is, however, no crypt hyperplasia during rejection of colonic tissue and over all the changes found do not resemble those of inflammatory large-bowel disease in man.

Graft-versus-host disease. Singer, Spiro and Thayer (1966) produced graft-versus-host (runt) disease in 67 per cent of CDF neonatal rats 15 to 23 days after the injection of $20–25 \times 10^6$ spleen cells from hooded rats. Of the runted animals, 25 per cent had diarrhoea. Their colons showed epithelial cell atrophy with an inflammatory cell infiltrate in the lamina propria and submucosa consisting of lymphocytes, plasma cells and eosinophils. These colonic lesions did not resemble the lesions seen in human ulcerative colitis.

4. Other factors

Finally colonic abnormalities have also been created in a number of different animals by diverse methods. Mucosal oedema and haemorrhage have been described in monkeys subjected to deficiencies of vitamin A, folic acid and pyridoxine (Kirsner, 1961). Local necrosis has also been noted in dogs receiving intrarectal instillation of collagenase or intra-arterial lysozyme (Kirsner, 1961). Intracerebral electrodes with self-administered stimulation, under conditions promoting indecision and frustration, have produced a bloody diarrhoea in dogs (Kirsner, 1961). A lesion similar to ulcerative colitis has been produced by irradiation of rats and rabbits (Friedman and Warren, 1942; Sommers and Warren, 1958). Crypt abscesses were found in 9 per cent of irradiated rats and were very similar to the lesions of the human disease. Tween 80 appears to cause colonic inflammation when administered as an enema to rats (Lutzger and Factor, 1976).

CONCLUSION

Immunological mechanisms are thought to play a part in, or even be causative in, coeliac disease and inflammatory bowel disease. Naturally occurring animal diseases or contrived animal models which resemble the above conditions may define such mechanisms more clearly in 4 major ways. Firstly, naturally occurring diseases in animals can be fully analysed with respect to their essential components and in particular any significant immunological ones studied, hence the parallel situation in man can be better understood. Secondly, studies of maturing, germ-free gnotobiotic animals help in the understanding of the normal development and functional organization of the immunological apparatus of the intestine. This information may then be related to the intestine of man. Thirdly, the successful search for exogenous agents which reproduce a lesion in a 'convenient' experimental animal, structurally and functionally similar to the human pathological process, can provide tissues for detailed dissection and analysis. And fourthly, animal models can be useful in separating, in the diseased state, the features of the primary response from the effect of secondary epiphenomena.

Many of the animal models described and summarized in this chapter employ immune-independent precipitating agents, for example hydrochloric acid. Yet, it is often difficult to decide how many of the end-pathological features are due to the agent or the secondary involvement of other immune-independent or -dependent mechanisms. It seems inconceivable that in a tissue like the intestine, where all components of the individual's immunological apparatus are so well represented, that at some stage immune mechanisms are not activated and that resultant effector mechanisms do not contribute to the pathological features of the disease.

Finally, 2 major problems keep recurring in any studies of intestinal diseases, either in humans or via animal models: (1) there is the increasing conviction that in diseases such as coeliac disease, Crohn's disease and ulcerative colitis, it is unlikely that we are dealing with 3 tightly definable homogeneous diseases and (2) there is often the impression from animal models that whatever the 'trigger-mechanism', the intestine has only a limited number of major ways in which it can react. Minor features can and do, however, vary enormously. Nevertheless, accepting that we soon will have more precise definitions of human intestinal diseases (including any sub-types) and given the massive increase in knowledge of immune mechanisms in the intestine, further studies of animal models, both natural and contrived, will make a major contribution to the understanding of these common and disabling human diseases.

REFERENCES

Abraham, R., Fabian, R. J., Goldberg, L. & Coulston, F. (1974) Role of lysosomes in carrageenan-induced caecal ulceration. *Gastroenterology*, **67**, 1169–1181.

Adams, N. R., Ball, R. A., Annis, C. L. & Hofstad, M. S. (1972) Ultrastructural changes in the intestines of turkey poults and embryos affected with transmissible enteritis. *Journal of Comparative Pathology*, **82**, 187–192.

Althausen, T. L. & Grodsky, G. M. (1961) Effect of wheat proteins on intestinal absorption in rats. *Gastroenterology*, **40**, 665

Amend, N. K., Loeffler, D. G., Ward, B. C. & Van Hoosier, G. L., Jr (1976) Transmission of enteritis in the Syrian hamster. *Laboratory Animal Science*, **26**, 566–572.

Anderson, W. (1967) Carrageenan. Structure and biological activity. *Canadian Journal of Pharmacological Science*, **2**, 81–90.

Anver, M. R. & Cohen, B. J. (1976) Animal model: ulcerative colitis induced in guinea pigs with degraded carrageenan. *American Journal of Pathology*, **84**, 431–435.

Aronson, M. D., Phillips, C. A., Beeken, W. L. & Forsyth, B. R. (1975) Isolation and characterization of a viral agent from intestinal tissue of patients with Crohn's disease and other chronic intestinal disorders. *Progress in Medical Virology*, **21**, 165–176.

Asherson, G. L. & Holborow, E. J. (1966) Autoantibody production in rabbits. VIII. Autoantibodies to gut produced by the injection of bacteria. *Immunology*, **10**, 161–167.

Auer, J. (1920) Local autoinoculation of the sensitized organism with foreign protein as a cause of abnormal reactions. *Journal of Experimental Medicine*, **32**, 427–444.

Bang, B. (1906) Chronic mycobacterial enteritis in ruminants as a model of Crohn's disease. *Proceedings of the Royal Society of Medicine*, **65**, 998–1001.

Beeken, W. L., Mitchell, D. N. & Cave, D. R. (1976) Evidence for a transmissible agent in Crohn's disease. *Clinics in Gastroenterology*, **5**, 2, 289–302.

Bellamy, J. E. C. & Nielsen, N. O. (1974) Immune-mediated emigration of neutrophils into the lumen of the small intestine. *Infection and Immunity*, **9**, 615–619.

Benitz, K. F., Goldberg, L. & Coulston, F. (1973) Intestinal effects of carrageenans in the rhesus monkey (Macaca mulatta). *Food and Cosmetics Toxicology*, **11**, 565–575.

Bicks, R. O. & Rosenberg, E. W. (1964) A chronic delayed hypersensitivity reaction in the guinea pig colon. *Gastroenterology*, **46**, 543–549.

Bicks, R. O. & Walker, R. H. (1962) Immunologic 'colitis' in dogs. *American Journal of Digestive Disease*, **7**, 574–584.

Bicks, R. O., Azar, M. M. & Rosenberg, E. W. (1967) Delayed hypersensitivity reactions in the intestinal tract. II. Small intestinal lesions associated with xylose malabsorption. *Gastroenterology*, **53**, 437–443.

Bicks, R. O., Brown, G., Hickey, H. D., Jr & Rosenberg, E. W. (1965) Further observations on a delayed hypersensitivity reaction in the guinea pig colon. *Gastroenterology*, **48**, 425–429.

Bicks, R. O., Azar, M. M., Rosenberg, E. W., Dunham, W. G. & Luther, J. (1967) Delayed hypersensitivity reactions in the intestinal tract. I. Studies of 2,4-dinitrochlorobenzene-caused guinea pig and swine colon lesions. *Gastroenterology*, **53**, 422–436.

Bloch, R., Menge, H., Martini, G. A. & Riecken, E. O. (1972) Effect of gluten on glucose absorption from the small intestine in experimentally induced malabsorption in rats. *Digestion*, **7**, 139–146.

Bolton, P. M., Owen, E., Heatley, R. V., Jones-Williams, W. & Hughes, L. E. (1973) Negative findings in laboratory animals for a transmissible agent in Crohn's disease. *Lancet*, **ii**, 1122–1124.

Bonfils, S. (1970) Carrageenan and the human gut. *Lancet*, **ii**, 414.

Boothe, A. D. & Cheville, N. F. (1967) The pathology of proliferative ileitis of the golden Syrian hamster. *Pathologia Veterinaria (Basel)*, **4**, 31–44.

Brennan, P. C., Fritz, T. E. & Flynn, R. J. (1965) *Citrobacter freundii* associated with diarrhoea in laboratory mice. *Laboratory Animal Care*, **15**, 266–275.

Broberger, O. & Perlmann, P. (1959) Autoantibodies in human ulcerative colitis. *Journal of Experimental Medicine*, **110**, 657–674.

Brynjolfsson, G. & Haley, H. B. (1967) Experimental enteritis cystica in rats. *American Journal of Clinical Pathology*, **47**, 69–73.

Burholt, D. R., Hagemann, R. F., Schenken, L. L. & Lesher, S. (1977) Influence of adriamycin and adriamycin-radiation combination on jejunal proliferation in the mouse. *Cancer Research*, **31**, 22–27.

Cave, D. R. & Mitchell, D. N. (1974) An experimental animal model of Crohn's disease. *Gut*, **15**, 345.

Cave, D. R., Mitchell, D. N. & Brooke, B. N. (1975) Experimental animal studies of the etiology and pathogenesis of Crohn's disease. *Gastroenterology*, **69**, 618–624.

Cave, D. R., Mitchell, D. N., Kane, S. P. & Brooke, B. N. (1973) Further animal evidence of a transmissible agent in Crohn's disease. *Lancet*, **ii**, 1120–1122.

Chess, S., Olander, G., Puestow, C. B., Benner, W. & Chess, D. (1950) Regional enteritis. Clinical and experimental observations. *Surgery, Gynaecology and Obstetrics*, **91**, 343–350.

Cimprich, R. E. (1974) Granulomatous enteritis in horses. *Veterinary Pathology*, **11**, 535–547.

Cook, M. G. & Turnbull, G. J. (1975) A hypothesis for the pathogenesis of Crohn's disease based on an ultrastructural study. *Virchows Archiv A: Pathological Anatomy and Histology*, **365**, 327–336.

Cooke, E. M., Filipe, M. I. & Dawson, I. M. P. (1968) The production of colonic autoantibodies in rabbits by immunisation with *Escherichia coli*. *Journal of Pathology and Bacteriology*, **96**, 125–130.

Coombs, R. R. A. & Gell, P. G. H. (1976) Classifications of allergic reactions responsible for clinical hypersensitivity and disease. In *Clinical Aspects of Immunology*, 3rd edn, ed. Gell, P. G. H., Coombs, R. R. A. & Lachmann, P. J., pp. 761–782. Oxford: Blackwell Scientific Publications.

Cornelius, E. A. (1970) Protein-losing enteropathy in the graft-versus-host reaction. *Transplantation*, **9**, 247–252.

Dobbins, W. O., III, Herrero, B. A. & Mansbach, C. M. (1968) Morphologic alterations associated with neomycin induced malabsorption. *American Journal of the Medical Sciences*, **255**, 63–77.

Ecknauer, R. & Löhrs, U. (1976) The effect of a single-dose of Cyclophosphamide on the jejunum of specified pathogen-free and germ-free rats. *Digestion*, **14**, 269–280.

Ediger, R. D., Kovatch, R. M. & Rabstein, M. M. (1974) Colitis in mice with a high incidence of rectal prolapse. *Laboratory Animal Science*, **24**, 488–494.

Elves, M. W. & Ferguson, A. (1975) The humoral immune response to allografts of foetal small intestine in mice. *British Journal of Experimental Pathology*, **56**, 454–458.

Emsbo, P. (1951) Terminal or regional ileitis in swine. *Nordisk Veterinaer Medicin*, **3**, 1–28.

Ferguson, A. (1974) Lymphocytes in coeliac disease. In *Coeliac Disease. Proceedings of the Second International Coeliac Symposium*, ed. Hekkens, W. Th. J. M. & Peña, A. S., pp. 265–276. Leiden: Stenfert Kroese.

Ferguson, A. & Jarrett, E. E. E. (1975) Hypersensitivity reactions in the small intestine. I. Thymus dependence of experimental partial villous atrophy. *Gut*, **16**, 114–117.

Ferguson, A. & Parrott, D. M. V. (1972) Growth and development of 'antigen-free' grafts of foetal mouse intestine. *Journal of Pathology*, **106**, 95–101.

Ferguson, A. & Parrott, D. M. V. (1972b) The effect of antigen deprivation on thymus-dependent and thymus-independent lymphocytes in the small intestine of the mouse. *Clinical and Experimental Immunology*, **12**, 477–488.

Ferguson, A. & Parrott, D. M. V. (1973) Histopathology and time course of rejection of allografts of mouse small intestine. *Transplantation*, **15**, 546–554.

Ferguson, R., Asquith, P. & Cooke, W. T. (1974) The jejunal cellular infiltrate in coeliac disease complicated by lymphoma. *Gut*, **15**, 458–461.

Ferguson, R., Catty, D., Asquith, P. & Cooke, W. T. (1978) B-cell differentiation in the jejunal mucosa of athymic (nude) and normal mice. Plasma cell induction by gluten and triparanol treatment. In preparation.

Field, H. I., Buntain, D. & Jennings, A. R. (1953) Terminal or regional ileitis in pigs. *Journal of Comparative Pathology*, **63**, 153–158.

Flewett, T. H. & Boxall, E. (1976) The hunt for viruses in infections of the alimentary systems. *Clinics in Gastroenterology*, **5**, 2, 359–385.

Ford, H. & Kirsner, J. B. (1964) 'Auer colitis' in rabbits induced by intrarectal antigen. *Proceedings of the Society for Experimental Biology and Medicine*, **116**, 745–748.

Friedman, N. B. & Warren, S. (1942) Evolution of experimental radiation ulcers of the intestine. *Archives of Pathology*, **33**, 326–333.

Gilat, T., Morin, J. E. & Binder, H. J. (1967) The effect of neomycin in the small intestinal mucosa of the monkey. *Laval Médical*, **38**, 352–355.

Gitnick, G. L. & Rosen, V. J. (1976) Electron microscopic studies of viral agents in Crohn's disease. *Lancet*, **ii**, 217–219.

Gitnick, G. L., Arthur, M. H. & Shibata, I. (1976) Cultivation of viral agents from Crohn's disease. A new sensitive system. *Lancet*, **ii**, 215–217.

Goldgraber, M. B. & Kirsner, J. B. (1959) The Arthus phenomenon in the colon of rabbits. A serial histological study. *Archives of Pathology*, **67**, 556–571.

Gray, I. & Walzer, M. (1938) Studies in mucous membrane hypersensitiveness. III. The allergic reaction of the passively sensitized rectal mucous membrane. *American Journal of Digestive Disease and Nutrition*, **4**, 707–712.

Gray, I., Harten, M. & Walzer, M. (1940) Studies in mucous membrane hypersensitiveness. IV. The allergic reaction in the passively sensitized mucous membranes of the ileum and colon in humans. *Annals of Internal Medicine*, **13**, 2050–2056.

Grayzel, D. & Walzer, M. (1939) The pathology of the allergic reactions in the passively sensitised tissues of the Macacus Rhesus monkey. *Journal of Allergy*, **10**, 478.

Haelterman, E. O. (1972) On the pathogenesis of transmissible gastroenteritis of swine. *Journal of the American Veterinary Medical Association*, **160**, 534–540.

Halpern, B., Zweibaum, A., Oriol-Palou, R. & Morard, J. C.

(1967) Experimental immune ulcerative colitis. In *Mechanisms of Inflammation induced by Immune Reactions*, Immunopathology, Fifth International Symposium. ed. Miescher, P. A. & Grabder, P., pp. 161–178. New York: Grune & Stratton.

Hamilton, J. R. (1967) Prolonged infusion of the small intestine of the rat – effect of dilute lactic acid on fat absorption and mucosal morphology. *Pediatric Research*, **1**, 341–353.

Hammarström, S., Perlmann, P., Gustafsson, B. E. & Lagercrantz, R. (1969) Autoantibodies to colon in germ free rats monocontaminated with *Clostridium difficile*. *Journal of Experimental Medicine*, **129**, 747–756.

Hausamen, T. U., Halcrow, D. A. & Taylor, K. B. (1969) Biological effects of gastrointestinal antibodies. I. The production of antibodies to components of adult and foetal guinea pig gastric and colonic mucosa. *Gastroenterology*, **56**, 1053–1061.

Heatley, R. V., Bolton, P. M., Owen, E., Jones Williams, W. & Hughes, L. E. (1975) A search for a transmissible agent in Crohn's disease. *Gut*, **16**, 528–532.

Heatley, R. V., Calcraft, B. J., Rhodes, J., Owen, E. & Evans, B. (1974) Treatment of chronic proctitis with disodium cromoglycate. *Gut*, **15**, 829.

Hedberg, C. A., Reiser, S. & Reilly, R. W. (1968) Intestinal phase of the runting syndrome in mice. II. Observations on nutrient absorption. *Transplantation*, **6**, 104–110.

Hobson, R. W., Jervis, H. R., Kingry, R. L. & Wallace, J. R. (1974) Small bowel changes associated with Vincristine sulfate treatment. An experimental study in the guinea pig. *Cancer*, **34**, 1888–1896.

Hodgson, H. J. F., Skinner, J. M., Potter, B. J. & Jewell, D. P. (1976) Immune complexes in ulcerative colitis – an experimental model. *Gut*, **17**, 399.

Hoelzel, F., DaCosta, E. & Carlson, A. J. (1941) Production of intestinal lesions by feeding Karaya gum and other material to rats. *American Journal of Digestive Disease*, **8**, 266–270.

Holden, R. J. & Ferguson, A. (1976) Histopathology of cell mediated immune reaction in mouse colon–allograft rejection. *Gut*, **17**, 661–670.

Holmes, G. K. T., Asquith, P., Stokes, P. L. & Cooke, W. T. (1974) Cellular infiltrate of jejunal biopsies in adult coeliac disease in relation to gluten withdrawal. *Gut*, **15**, 278–283.

Holmes, J. T., Klein, M. S., Winawer, S. J. & Fortner, J. G. (1971) Morphological studies of rejection in canine jejunal allografts. *Gastroenterology*, **61**, 693–706.

Jacobson, E. D., Prior, J. T. & Faloon, W. W. (1960) Malabsorption syndrome induced by neomycin: morphologic alterations in the jejunal mucosa. *Journal of Laboratory and Clinical Medicine*, **56**, 245–250.

James, A. H. (1977) Breakfast and Crohn's disease. *British Medical Journal*, **i**, 943–945.

Johne, H. A. & Frothingham, I. (1895) Chronic mycobacterial enteritis in ruminants as a model of Crohn's disease. *Proceedings of the Royal Society of Medicine*, **65**, 998–1001.

Kalima, T. V., Saloniemi, H. & Rahko, T. (1976) Experimental regional enteritis in pigs. *Scandinavian Journal of Gastroenterology*, **11**, 353–362.

Kaneko, J. J., Moulton, J. E., Brodey, R. S. & Perryman, V. D. (1965) Malabsorption syndrome resembling non-tropical sprue in dogs. *Journal of the American Veterinary Medical Association*, **146**, 463–473.

Kennedy, P. C. & Cello, R. M. (1966) Colitis of Boxer dogs. *Gastroenterology*, **51**, 926–931.

Kenworthy, R. (1970) Effect of *Escherichia coli* on germ-free and gnotobiotic pigs. I. Light and electron microscopy of the small intestine. *Journal of Comparative Pathology*, **80**, 53–63.

Kenworthy, R. (1971) Observations on the reaction of the intestinal mucosa to bacterial challenge. *Journal of Clinical Pathology*, **24**, Supplement (Royal College of Pathologists), 5, 138–145.

Kenworthy, R. & Allen, W. D. (1966) Influence of diet and bacteria on small intestinal morphology, with special reference to early weaning and *Escherichia coli*. Studies with germ free and gnotobiotic pigs. *Journal of Comparative Pathology*, **76**, 291–296.

Kerzner, B., Kelly, M. H., Gall, D. G., Butler, D. G. & Hamilton, J. R. (1977) Transmissible gastroenteritis: sodium transport and the intestinal epithelium during the course of viral enteritis. *Gastroenterology*, **72**, 457–461.

Keusch, G. T., Troncale, F. J. & Plaut, A. G. (1970) Neomycin-induced malabsorption in a tropical population. *Gastroenterology*, **58**, 197–202.

King, D. J. (1975) Comments on the etiology and immunity of transmissible (coronaviral) enteritis of turkeys (Bluecomb). *American Journal of Veterinary Research*, **36**, 555–565.

Kirsner, J. B. (1961) Experimental 'colitis' with particular reference to hypersensitivity reactions in the colon. *Gastroenterology*, **40**, 307–312.

Kirsner, J. B., Elchlepp, J. E., Goldgraber, M. B., Ablaza, J. & Ford, H. (1959) Production of an experimental ulcerative 'colitis' in rabbits. *Archives of Pathology*, **68**, 392–408.

Kraft, S. C., Bregman, E. & Kirsner, J. B. (1962) Criteria for evaluating autoimmune phenomena in ulcerative colitis. *Gastroenterology*, **43**, 330–336.

Lagercrantz, R., Hammarström, S., Perlmann, P. & Gustafsson, B. E. (1966) Immunologic studies in ulcerative colitis. III. Incidence of antibodies to colon-antigen in ulcerative colitis and other gastrointestinal diseases. *Clinical and Experimental Immunology*, **1**, 263–276.

LeVeen, H. H., Falk, G. & Schatman, B. (1961) Experimental ulcerative colitis produced by anticolon sera. *Annals of Surgery*, **154**, 275–280.

Loehry, C. A. & Creamer, B. (1969) Three-dimensional structure of the rat small intestinal mucosa related to mucosal dynamics. *Gut*, **10**, 112–120.

Long, C. F., Kolmer, J. A. & Swalm, W. A. (1935) Observations on intestines of rats fed inert materials. *Journal of Laboratory and Clinical Medicine*, **20**, 475–481.

Lutzger, L. G. & Factor, S. M. (1976) Effects of some water-soluble contrast media on the colonic mucosa. *Radiology*, **118**, 545–548.

MacDonald, T. T. & Ferguson, A. (1976) Hypersensitivity reactions in the small intestine. II. Effects of allograft rejection on mucosal architecture and lymphoid cell infiltrate. *Gut*, **17**, 81–91.

MacPherson, B. & Pfeiffer, C. J. (1976) Experimental colitis. *Digestion*, **14**, 424–452.

McPherson, J. R. & Shorter, P. G. (1965) Intestinal lesions associated with Triparanol. A clinical and experimental study. *American Journal of Digestive Diseases*, **10**, 1024–1033.

McPherson, J. R. & Summerskill, W. H. J. (1963) An acute malabsorption syndrome with reversible mucosal atrophy. *Gastroenterology*, **44**, 900–904.

Martini, G. A. & Brandes, J. W. (1976) Increased consumption of refined carbohydrates in patients with Crohn's disease. *Klinische Wochenschrift*, **54**, 367–371.

Marcus, R. & Watt, J. (1969) Seaweeds and ulcerative colitis in laboratory animals. *Lancet*, **ii**, 489–490.

Marcus, R. & Watt, J. (1971) Experimental ulceration of the colon induced by non-algal sulphated products. *Gut*, **12**, 868.

Marston, A., Marcuson, R. W., Chapman, M. & Arthur, J. F. (1969) Experimental study of devascularization of the colon. *Gut*, **10**, 121–130.

Matthews, J. G. W. & Parks, T. G. (1972) Production of ischaemic colitis experimentally in the dog by vasoconstriction and hypotensive techniques. *Gut*, **13**, 323.

Miller, R. M. (1963) Coeliac disease in a kitten. *Small Animal Clinics*, **3**, 483–484.

Millington, P. F., Finean, J. B., Forbes, O. C. & Frazer, A. C. (1962) Studies of the effects of aminopterin on the small intestine of rats. I. The morphological changes following a single dose of aminopterin. *Experimental Cell Research*, **28**, 162–178.

Mitchell, D. N. & Rees, R. J. W. (1970) Agent transmissible from Crohn's disease tissue. *Lancet*, **ii**, 168–171.

Mitchell, D. N., Rees, R. J. W. & Goswami, K. K. (1976) Transmissible agents from human sarcoid and Crohn's disease tissues. *Lancet*, **ii**, 761–765.

Mottet, N. K. (1972) On animal models for inflammatory bowel disease. *Gastroenterology*, **62**, 1269–1271.

Mouwen, J. M. V. M. 'White scours in piglets at three weeks of age.' Unpublished MD Thesis, Utrecht, 1972.

Mouwen, J. M. V. M. (1974) Villous atrophy in piglets. In *Coeliac Disease. Proceedings of the Second International Coeliac Symposium*, ed. Hekkens, W. Th. J. M. & Peña, A. S. pp. 277–284. Leiden: Stenfert Kroese.

Mouwen, J. M. V. M., Schotman, A. J. H., Wensing, T. & Kijkuit, C. J. (1972) Some biochemical aspects of white scours in piglets. *Tijdschrift voor Diergeneeskunde*, **97**, 65–91.

Olson, D. P., Waxler, G. L. & Roberts, A. W. (1973) Small intestinal lesion of transmissible gastroenteritis in gnotobiotic pigs: a scanning electron microscopic study. *American Journal of Veterinary Research*, **34**, 1239–1245.

Oriol Palou, R., Halpern, B., Zweibaum, A., Morard, C. J., Veyre, C. & Abadie, A. (1967) Experimental production of haemorrhagic ulcerative colitis with autoantibodies. *Medical Hygiene*, **23**, 62–64.

Orr, M. M., Tamarind, D. L., Cook, J., Fincham, W. J., Hawley, P. R., Quilliam, J. P. & Irving, M. H. (1974) Preliminary studies on the response of rabbit bowel to intramural injections of L-form bacteria. *British Journal of Surgery*, **61**, 921.

Palmer, R. H. & Reilly, R. W. (1971) Bile salt depletion in the runting syndrome. *Transplantation*, **12**, 479–483.

Parent, K. & Mitchell, P. D. (1976) Bacterial variants: etiologic agent in Crohn's disease? *Gastroenterology*, **71**, 365–368.

Patterson, D. S. P. & Allen, W. M. (1972) Chronic mycobacterial enteritis in ruminants as a model of Crohn's disease. *Proceedings of the Royal Society of Medicine*, **65**, 998–1001.

Perlmann, P., Hammarström, S., Lagercrantz, R. & Gustafsson, B. E. (1965) Antigen from colon of germfree rats and antibodies in human ulcerative colitis. *Annals of the New York Academy of Sciences*, **124**, 377–394.

Price, A. B. & Davies, D. R. (1977) Pseudomembranous colitis. *Journal of Clinical Pathology*, **30**, 1–12.

Rabin, B. S. & Rogers, S. J. (1976) Nonpathogenicity of anti-intestinal antibody in the rabbit. *American Journal of Pathology*, **83**, 269–277.

Reichert, F. L. & Mathes, M. E. (1936) Experimental

lymphedema of the intestinal tract and its relation to regional cicatrizing enteritis. *Annals of Surgery*, **104**, 601–616.

Reilly, R. W. & Kirsner, J. B. (1965) Runt intestinal disease. *Laboratory Investigation*, **14**, 102–107.

Ribeiro, E., Sobrinho-Simões, M. & Mesquita, A. M. (1957) Effect of dietary gluten on the faecal fat in the rat. *Metabolism*, **6**, 378–380.

Richardson, G. S. & Leskowitz, S. (1961) An attempt at production of autoimmunity to tissue of the gastrointestinal tract. *Proceedings of the Society for Experimental Biology and Medicine*, **106**, 357–359.

Riecken, E. O. & Menge, H. (1974) Atrophic changes in rats. In *Coeliac Disease. Proceedings of the Second International Coeliac Symposium*, ed. Hekkens, W. Th. J. M. & Peña, A. S., pp. 292–308. Leiden: Stenfert Kroese.

Riecken, E. O., Bloch, R., Menge, H. Idelberger, K., Kramer, F., Miller, B. & Lorenz-Meyer, H. (1972) Morphologische und funktionelle Befunde nach Milchsäuredauer-infusion in das Jejunum der Ratte. *Zeitschrift fur Zeltforschung und Mikroskopische Anatomie (Berlin)*, **132**, 107–129.

Robinson, J. W. L. (1972) Intestinal malabsorption in the experimental animal. *Gut*, **13**, 938–945.

Robinson, J. W. L., Antonioli, J.-A. & Vannotti, A. (1966) The effect of oral methotrexate on the rat intestine. *Biochemical Pharmacology*, **15**, 1479–1489.

Rooney, J. R., Bryans, J. T. & Doll, E. R. (1963) Colitis 'X' of horses. *Journal of the American Veterinary Medical Association*, **142**, 510–511.

Rubin, C. E. & Dobbins, W. O., III (1965) Peroral biopsy of the small intestine: a review of its diagnostic usefulness. *Gastroenterology*, **49**, 676–697.

Scott, G. B. D. & Keymer, J. F. (1975) Ulcerative colitis in apes: a comparison with the human disease. *Journal of Pathology*, **115**, 241–244.

Sharratt, M., Grasso, P., Carpanini, F. & Gangolli, S. D. (1970) Carrageenan ulceration as a model for human ulcerative colitis. *Lancet*, **ii**, 932.

Sharratt, M., Grasso, P., Carpanini, F. & Gangolli, S. D. (1971) Carrageenan ulceration as a model for human ulcerative colitis. *Lancet*, **i**, 192–193.

Shean, F. C., Barker, W. F. & Fonkalsrud, E. W. (1964) Studies on active and passive antibody induced colitis in the dog. *American Journal of Surgery*, **107**, 337–339.

Singer, J. B., Spiro, H. M. & Thayer, W. R. (1966) Colonic manifestations of runt disease. *Yale Journal of Biology and Medicine*, **39**, 106–112.

Sommers, S. C. & Warren, S. (1955) Ulcerative colitis lesions in irradiated rats. *American Journal of Digestive Diseases*, **22**, 109–111.

Staley, T. E., Corley, L. D. & Jones, E. W. (1970) Early pathogenesis of colitis in neonatal pigs monocontaminated with *Escherichia coli*. Fine structural changes in the colonic epithelium. *American Journal of Digestive Diseases*, **15**, 923–935.

Stemmermann, G. N. & Hayashi, T. (1971) Colchicine intoxication: a reappraisal of its pathology based on a study of three fatal cases. *Human Pathology*, **2**, 321–332.

Stephens, F. O., Finckh, E. S. & Milton, G. W. (1964) Changes in exteriorised duodenal mucosa. Loss of villi, with recovery after skin coverage of explant. *Gastroenterology*, **47**, 626–630.

Stewart, H. L. & Jones, B. F. (1941) Pathologic anatomy of chronic ulcerative cecitis: a spontaneous disease of the rat. *Archives of Pathology*, **31**, 37–54.

Stone, S. S., Stark, S. L. & Phillips, M. (1974) Transmissible gastroenteritis virus in neonatal pigs; intestinal transfer of colostral immunoglobulins containing specific antibodies. *American Journal of Veterinary Research*, **35**, 339–345.

Stout, C. & Snyder, R. L. (1969) Ulcerative colitis-like lesion in Siamang gibbons. *Gastroenterology*, **57**, 256–261.

Strande, A., Sommers, S. C. & Petrak, M. (1954) Regional enterocolitis in cocker spaniel dogs. *Archives of Pathology*, **57**, 357–362.

Symons, L. E. A. (1965) Kinetics of the epithelial cells, and morphology of villi and crypts in the jejunum of the rat infected by the nematode *Nippostrongylus brasiliensis*. *Gastroenterology*, **49**, 158–168.

Symons, L. E. A. & Fairbairn, D. (1962) Pathology, absorption, transport, and activity of digestive enzymes in rat jejunum parasitized by the nematode *Nippostrongylus brasiliensis*. *Federation Proceedings*, **21**, 913–918.

Symons, L. E. A. & Fairbairn, D. (1963) Biochemical pathology of the rat jejunum parasitized by the nematode *Nippostrongylus brasiliensis*. *Experimental Parasitology*, **13**, 284–304.

Takeuchi, A., Formal, S. B. & Sprinz, H. (1968) Experimental acute colitis in the Rhesus monkey following peroral infection with *Shigella flexneri*. An electron microscope study. *American Journal of Pathology*, **52**, 503–529.

Taub, R. N., Sachar, D., Janowitz, H. & Siltzbach, L. E. (1976) Induction of granulomas in mice by inoculation of tissue homogenates from patients with inflammatory bowel disease and sarcoidosis. *Annals of the New York Academy of Sciences*, **278**, 560–563.

Thake, D. C. (1968) Jejunal epithelium in transmissible gastroenteritis of swine. An electron microscopic and histochemical study. *American Journal of Pathology*, **53**, 149–168.

Tibbutt, D. A. & Holt, J. M. (1974) Observations on the effect of vinblastine and mustine on the small intestine. *British Journal of Haematology*, **28**, 150.

Townley, R. R. W., Cass, M. H. & Anderson, C. M. (1964) Small intestinal mucosal patterns of coeliac disease and idiopathic steatorrhoea seen in other situations. *Gut*, **5**, 51–55.

Van Kruiningen, H. J. (1972) Canine colitis comparable to regional enteritis and mucosal colitis of man. *Gastroenterology*, **62**, 1128–1142.

Vernon, D. F. (1962) Idiopathic sprue in a dog. *Journal of the American Veterinary Medical Association*, **140**, 1062–1067.

Walzer, M., Gray, I., Straus, H. W. & Livingston, S. (1938) Studies in experimental hypersensitiveness in the Rhesus monkey. IV. The allergic reactions in passively locally sensitized abdominal organs (preliminary report). *Journal of Immunology*, **34**, 91–95.

Watt, J. & Marcus, R. (1970) Ulcerative colitis in rabbits fed degraded carrageenan. *Journal of Pharmacy and Pharmacology*, **22**, 130–131.

Watt, J. & Marcus, R. (1971) Carrageenan-induced ulceration of the large intestine in the guinea pig. *Gut*, **12**, 164–171.

Watt, J. & Marcus, R. (1972) Ulceration of the colon in rabbits fed sulphated amylopectin. *Journal of Pharmacy and Pharmacology*, **24**, 68–69.

Watt, J. & Marcus, R. (1973) Progress report. Experimental ulcerative disease of the colon in animals. *Gut*, **14**, 506–510.

Whorwell, P. J., Baldwin, R. O. & Wright, R. (1976) Ferritin in Crohn's disease tissue: detection by electron microscopy. *Gut*, **17**, 696–699.

Williams, A. W. (1963) Experimental production of altered jejunal mucosa. *Journal of Pathology and Bacteriology*, **85,** 467–472.

Williams, J. N., Jr & Laster, L. (1963) Investigation of the use of the albino rat for studying gliadin-induced steatorrhoea. *Metabolism*, **12,** 467–471.

Zetterlund, C. G. (1962) Buried strip of intestinal wall. Process of healing studied in the rat. *Acta Chirurgia Scandinavica*, **124,** 467–473.

Zweibaum, A., Morrard, J.-Cl. & Halpern, B. (1968) Réalisation d'une colite ulcéro-hémorrhagique expérimentale par immunisation bactérienne. *Pathologie-Biologie (Paris)*, **16,** 813–823.

9. Primary immune deficiency

I. N. Ross and P. Asquith

INTRODUCTION

The normal gastrointestinal tract contains numerous immunocompetent cells derived from the B-cell and T-cell series. It is assumed that many of these are involved in the defence of the intestinal mucosa against intraluminal antigens, for example ingested foods and also microorganisms. Alteration in the delicate balance between the immune apparatus and the 'internal' environment of the intestine could lead to gastrointestinal disease. In theory one factor which may be of major consequence in this respect is the absence (congenital or acquired) of one or more components of the immune system. This chapter considers primary immune deficiency and the intestine.

It has become increasingly difficult logically to classify immune defects, even into the broad subdivisions based on B-cell and T-cell abnormalities. Also diseases which not long ago were thought relatively homogeneous, for example selective IgA deficiency, have now been shown to be complex. In addition, the question as to whether an abnormality of immune hyporesponsiveness is congenital or acquired is much more difficult to answer. In this review the widely accepted WHO classification of primary immune defects (Table 9.1) has been used with patients subdivided into those with (1) antibody (B-cell) defects, (2) cellular (T-cell) defects, (3) combined B- and T-cell defects, and (4) phagocyte abnormalities.

ANTIBODY (B-CELL) DEFECTS

X-LINKED INFANTILE CONGENITAL HYPOGAMMAGLOBULINAEMIA

Main immunological features

1. IgG less than 0·2 g/l, reduced or absent IgA, IgD, IgE and IgM.
2. Absence of plasma cells and B-lymphocytes in bone marrow and peripheral blood.
3. Recurrent pyogenic infection usually by 6 months of age.

The syndrome was first described by Bruton in 1952 and is characterized by very low serum levels of all 5 immunoglobulin classes and an absence of secretory immunoglobulins. Only infrequently are normal levels of IgD or IgE found. Inheritance is by a sex-linked recessive gene, the genetic defect being carried by the female whose sons will have a 1:2 chance of being affected, and the daughters a 1:2 chance of being carriers. Occasionally, female infants have hypogammaglobulinaemia and some of these may represent a homozygous form of the condition (Bernheim, Creyssel, Gilly and Fournier, 1959; Diamont, Kallós and Rubensohn, 1961). The finding of an HLA haplotype difference between 2 siblings with this condition suggests that the immune deficit is not linked to the major histocompatibility complex (Buckley, MacQueen and Ward, 1976).

Investigation usually shows a complete absence of plasma cells and B-lymphocytes from the bone marrow, peripheral blood and lymphoid tissues. It is believed that the mammalian equivalent of the avian Bursa of Fabricius fails to develop, resulting in a lack of the correct microenvironment for the differentiation of primitive stem cells into B-lymphocytes (Abdou, Cassella, Abdou and Abrahamsohn, 1973). T-cell function is usually normal as assessed by delayed type cutaneous hypersensitivity reactions and lymphocyte transformation to PHA and allogeneic cells.

Patients usually present about 5 to 6 months of age with recurrent bacterial infections causing bronchitis, otitis media and meningitis; it is during this period that placentally transferred maternal IgG antibody has been catabolized and therefore is no longer protective. Infants with transient 'physiological' hypogammaglobulinaemia may also present with infections and gastrointestinal symptoms (Ochs and Ament, 1976) at this age; however, the presence of circulating B-lymphocytes and plasma cells in jejunal and rectal biopsies differentiates it from X-linked hypogammaglobulinaemia.

Gastrointestinal symptoms (Table 9.2)

Many early descriptions of X-linked hypogammaglobulinaemia recorded individuals with various gastrointestinal symptoms. Bruton (1952) described vomiting and gastrointestinal upset in his patient and steatorrhoea occurring in two brothers was reported by Allen and Hadden (1964). A peroral jejunal biopsy from one showed thickening of the mucosa with oedema of the lamina propria and there was also shortening of the villi and an excess cellular infiltrate. Gluten withdrawal

Table 9.1 Classification of primary deficiency syndromes. (Based on a report of a World Health Organization Committee: Fudenberg, Good, Goodman, Hitzig, Kunkel, Roitt, Rosen, Rowe, Seligmann and Soothill, 1971)

Type of immunodeficiency	Main gastrointestinal features
Antibody (B-cell) defects	
X-linked (congenital) hypogammaglobulinaemia	Malabsorption and diarrhoea
Transient hypogammaglobulinaemia of infancy	Malabsorption and diarrhoea
Common variable (late-onset) acquired hypogammaglobulinaemia	Pernicious anaemia, hypogammaglobulinaemic sprue, *Giardia lamblia* infestation, bacterial overgrowth of the small intestine, nodular lymphoid hyperplasia, colitis, proctitis, malignancy
Deficiency of κ or λ type immunoglobulins	Achlorhydria, malabsorption and diarrhoea
X-linked immunodeficiency with hyper-IgM	Diarrhoea, *Candida* infection, malignant infiltration of the gastrointestinal tract
Selective IgA deficiency	Pernicious anaemia, coeliac disease, Crohn's disease
Secretory component deficiency	Diarrhoea, *Candida* infection
Selective IgM deficiency	Ulcerative colitis, Crohn's disease, Whipple's disease
Selective IgE deficiency	
Selective IgD deficiency	Coeliac disease
Cellular (T-cell) defects	
Congenital thymic aplasia (Di George syndrome)	Malabsorption and diarrhoea
Chronic mucocutaneous candidiasis	Mouth ulcers, oesophageal disease, diarrhoea
Combined B- and T-cell defects	
Severe combined immunodeficiency disease (autosomal recessive, X-linked, sporadic)	Malabsorption and diarrhoea
Immunodeficiency with enzyme deficiency	
Immunodeficiency with short-limbed dwarfism	
Immunodeficiency with thymoma	
Immunodeficiency with ataxia telangiectasia	Vitamin B_{12} malabsorption, gastric carcinoma
Cellular immunodeficiency with abnormal immunoglobulin synthesis (Nezelof's syndrome)	Malabsorption, candidiasis
Immunodeficiency with eczema and thrombocytopaenia (Wiskott–Aldrich syndrome)	Recurrent bloody diarrhoea and malabsorption
Graft-versus-host disease	Diarrhoea
Phagocyte dysfunction	
Chronic granulomatous disease	Gastrointestinal obstruction, malabsorption and diarrhoea

was tried in both patients without substantial improvement and there was no deterioration on reintroduction of gluten. Bernheim, Creyssel, Gilly and Fournier (1959) noted steatorrhoea in a twin brother and sister with X-linked hypogammaglobulinaemia, whilst Diamant, Kallós and Rubensohn (1961) reported diarrhoea in an affected boy. Of 6 patients with hypogammaglobulinaemia and continuous or chronic intermittent diarrhoea (Dubois, Roy, Fulginiti, Merrill and Murray, 1970) only 1 had steatorrhoea. Three of the 6 had lactase or disaccharidase deficiency. In contrast, Ament, Ochs and Davis (1973) found diarrhoea in only 1 of 8 patients with X-linked hypogammaglobulinaemia. The symptomatic patient had giardiasis with steatorrhoea, lactase

intolerance and vitamin B_{12} malabsorption, reversed by treatment with metronidazole (Ochs, Ament and Davis, 1972). However, even in the asymptomatic patients there was evidence of subclinical gastrointestinal abnormality. Thus 5 had bacterial overgrowth of the small intestine and in 6 a rectal biopsy showed the histological appearance of colitis with numerous crypt abscesses and infiltration of the lamina propria with polymorphonuclear leucocytes (Ament, Ochs and Davis, 1973).

There is an increased risk of developing a malignancy in X-linked hypogammaglobulinaemia (approximately 6 per cent), usually lymphoreticular tumours or leukaemia (Kirkpatrick, 1976a). Finally Thomas, Ochs and

Table 9.2 Gastrointestinal and other diseases occurring in X-linked (congenital) hypogammaglobulinaemia

Disease	Reference
1. Malabsorption syndrome	1–5
2. Isolated lactase and disaccharidase deficiency	5, 6
3. Bacterial overgrowth of small intestine	6
4. *Giardia lamblia* infestation	6, 7
5. Appearance of colitis on rectal biopsy	7
6. Crohn's disease	8
7. Chronic hepatitis and HB$_s$Ag infection	9
8. Increased incidence of malignancy	10

References to Table 9.2

1. Bruton (1952).
2. Allen and Hadden (1964).
3. Bernheim, Creyssel, Gilly and Fournier (1959).
4. Diamant, Kallós and Rubensohn (1961).
5. Dubois, Roy, Fulginiti, Merrill and Murray (1970).
6. Ochs, Ament and Davis (1972).
7. Ament, Ochs and Davis (1973).
8. Eggert, Wilson and Good (1969).
9. Thomas, Ochs and Wedgwood (1974).
10. Kirkpatrick (1976a).

Wedgwood (1974) described a male patient who was found to be a chronic carrier of HB$_s$Ag following an episode of hepatitis.

Treatment

Replacement therapy with commercial human gamma-globulin injections or fresh frozen plasma infusions reduces the number of infections and may also help the diarrhoea. Antibiotics are usually reserved for clinical attacks of infection.

COMMON VARIABLE (LATE ONSET) ACQUIRED HYPOGAMMAGLOBULINAEMIA

Main immunological features

1. IgG less than 2–5 g/l (normal in adults 6–16 g/l); IgA may be undetectable or present in variable amounts.
2. Increased incidence of autoimmune disease and T-cell defects.
3. Recurrent pyogenic infections.

This condition, like X-linked hypogammaglobulin-aemia, usually presents with recurrent infections; however, in contrast, symptoms can develop at any age and up to 60 per cent complain of gastrointestinal problems, usually chronic or frequently occurring diarrhoea (Rosen and Janeway, 1966; Gitlin, Gross and Janeway, 1959; Ament, Ochs and Davis, 1973; Hermans, Diaz-Buxo and Stobo, 1976). Over half of these patients have evidence of malabsorption with a raised faecal fat, often related to *Giardia lamblia* infestation (Ament, Ochs and Davis, 1973; Hermans, Diaz-Buxo and Stobo, 1976).

Common variable hypogammaglobulinaemia is usu-ally sporadic, but in some families an autosomal reces-sive mode of inheritance is apparent and an increased incidence of autoimmune disease is found in relatives of affected individuals. The finding of an HLA haplotype difference in a pair of siblings with this condition sug-gests that the immune deficit is not linked to the major histocompatibility complex (Buckley, MacQueen and Ward, 1976). The lifetime prevalence of hypogam-maglobulinaemia with IgG levels below 2 g/l has been estimated as 15 per million in men and 4 per million in women (Medical Research Working Party on Hypogam-maglobulinaemia, 1971).

Immunological investigation shows normal or reduced numbers of circulating peripheral blood B-lymphocytes (Cooper, Lawton and Bockman, 1971; Abdou, Cassela, Abdou and Abrahamsohn, 1973; Webster and Asher-son, 1974; Preud'Homme, Griscelli and Seligmann, 1973). Unlike some cases of selective IgA deficiency, these peripheral B-lymphocytes do not usually produce immunoglobulin on *in-vitro* stimulation (Wu, Lawton and Cooper, 1973; Broom, de la Concha, Webster, Loewi and Asherson, 1975). Although lymph node biopsies can show lymphoid hyperplasia, there is usually a marked absence of cells in the B-cell dependent areas (Cooper, Lawton and Bockman, 1971) and the majority of patients have reduced plasma cells and immuno-globulin-containing cells in their small intestine (Ger-son, Janowitz and Paronetto, 1972) and in other organs such as the gall-bladder (Twomey, Jordan, Jarrold, Trubowitz, Ritz and Conn, 1969). However, in some patients immunoglobulin-containing cells may be seen in significant numbers in the small intestinal tract, some resembling normal plasma cells (Broom, de la Concha, Webster, Loewi and Asherson, 1975), and trace amounts of immunoglobulins may be detected in jejunal juice (Webster *et al.*, 1977). In rectal biopsies, although plasma cells are usually absent, cells with intracytoplasmic immunoglobulin, particularly IgA, may be found (Webster, 1975).

Waldman *et al.* (1974), Sampson, Rodey, Finik, Junkerman and Metzig (1977) and Whitemeyer, Bank-hurst and Williams (1976) have suggested that excessive suppressor T-cell activity is responsible for the B-cell defect in that there is suppression of *in-vitro* immuno-globulin production from poke-weed mitogen (PWM) stimulated normal B-cells when T-cells from affected individuals are added to the culture. Further support is given to these findings by the report from Keightly, Cooper and Lawton (1976) that, even in normal in-dividuals, *in-vitro* B-cell stimulation by PWM is de-pendent upon T-cell suppressor/helper activity. Other tests of T-cell function are usually normal in common variable hypogammaglobulinaemia, but one-third to one-half of patients may show cutaneous anergy, de-creased or normal T-cell rosettes and a depressed response of peripheral blood lymphocyte transformation

Table 9.3 Gastrointestinal and hepatic conditions occurring in common variable acquired hypogammaglobulinaemia

Disease	Reference
1. Pernicious anaemia	1–20
2. Gastric carcinoma	21, 22
3. Pancreatic insufficiency	1, 20–23
4. Cholelithiasis	20, 24
5. Hypogammaglobulinaemic sprue	8, 21, 23, 25–40
6. *Giardia lamblia* infection	6, 18, 14, 17, 29, 30, 37, 39, 41–51.
7. Bacterial overgrowth of small intestine	14, 23, 34, 37, 39, 42, 45, 46, 50–52.
8. Nodular lymphoid hyperplasia	6, 14, 17, 20, 23, 36, 39, 43–45, 48, 49, 51, 53–59.
9. Disaccharidase deficiency	50, 58, 60
10. Protein-losing enteropathy	28, 39, 61, 62
11. Non-granulomatous ulcerative jejuno-ileitis	63
12. Crohn's disease	64, 65
13. Ulcerative colitis	46, 66–68
14. Colitis and proctitis	23, 26, 39, 40, 69, 70
15. Staphylococcal enterocolitis	20
16. Chronic salmonella and shigella infections	13, 34, 42, 63, 70–72
17. Liver disease	73, 74
18. Amyloidosis	70, 75

References to Table 9.3

1. Lewis and Brown (1957).
2. Crowder, Thompson and Kupfer (1959).
3. Gibbs and Pryor (1961).
4. Larsson, Hagelquist and Cöster (1961).
5. Lee, Jenkins, Hughes and Kazantzis (1964).
6. Hermans, Huizenga, Hoffman, Brown and Markowitz (1966).
7. Clark, Tornyos, Herbert and Twomey (1967).
8. Hoskins, Winawer, Broitman, Gottlieb and Zamcheck (1967).
9. Goodman, Smith and Northey (1967).
10. Conn, Binder and Burns (1968).
11. Twomey, Jordan, Jarrold, Trubowitz, Ritz and Conn (1969).
12. Douglas, Goldberg, Fudenberg and Goldberg (1970).
13. Twomey, Jordan, Laughter, Meuwissen and Good (1970).
14. Ajdukiewicz, Youngs and Bouchier (1972).
15. Gelfand, Berkel, Godwin, Rocklin, David and Rosen (1972).
16. Hughes, Brooks and Conn (1972).
17. Cowling, Strickland, Ungar, Whittingham and Rose (1974).
18. Twomey (1975).
19. Ehtessabian, Cassidy, Thomas, Matthews and Tubergen (1976).
20. Hermans, Diaz-Buxo and Stobo (1976).

21. Cooke, Weiner and Shinton (1957).
22. Hudson and Aldor (1970).
23. Hughes, Cerda, Holtzapple and Brooks (1971).
24. Diaz-Buxo, Hermans and Elveback (1975)
25. Sanford, Favour and Tribeman (1954).
26. Zelman and Lewin (1958).
27. Kabler (1960).
28. Vesin, Troupel, Acar, Renault, Desbuquois and Cattan (1960).
29. Cohen, Paley and Janowitz (1961).
30. Huizenga, Wollaeger, Green and McKenzie (1961).
31. Green and Sperber (1962).
32. Swift (1962).
33. Pelkonen, Siurala and Vuopio (1963).
34. Collins and Ellis (1965).
35. Johnson, Van Arsdel, Tobe and Ching (1967).
36. Cooper, Lawton and Bockman (1971).
37. Ament and Rubin (1972).
38. Gerson, Janowitz and Paronetto (1972).
39. Ament, Ochs and Davis (1973).
40. Webster (1975).
41. Zamcheck, Hoskins, Winawer, Broitman and Gottlieb (1963).
42. McCarthy, Austad and Read (1965).
43. Grise (1968).
44. Bird, Jacobs, Silbiger and Wolff (1969).
45. Anderson, Pellegrino and Schaefer (1970).
46. Hersh, Floch, Binder, Conn, Prizont and Spiro (1970).
47. Cooper, Lawton and Bockman (1971).
48. Johnson, Goldberg, Pops and Weiner (1971).
49. Michaels, Go, Humbert, Dubois, Stewart and Ellis (1971).
50. Brown, Butterfield, Savage and Tada (1972).
51. Parkin, McClelland, O'Moore, Percy-Robb, Grant and Shearman (1972).
52. Brown, Savage, Dubois, Alp, Mallory and Kern (1972).
53. Firkin and Blackburn (1958).
54. Frik, Heinkel and Zeitler (1963).
55. Hodgson, Hoffman and Huizenga (1967).
56. Kirkpatrick, Waxman, Smith and Schimke (1968).
57. Penny (1969).
58. Dubois, Roy, Fulginiti, Merrill and Murray (1970).
59. De Smet, Tubergen and Martel (1976).
60. Caplinger and Boellner (1968).
61. Waldmann and Laster (1964).
62. Bjernulf, Johansson and Parrow (1971).
63. Corlin and Pops (1972).
64. Söltoft, Petersen and Kruse (1972).
65. Jones, Beeken, Roessner and Brown (1976).
66. Squire (1962).
67. Kirk and Freedman (1967).
68. Kopp, Trier, Stiehm and Foroozan (1968).
69. Rosecan, Trobaugh and Danforth (1955).
70. Conn and Quintiliani (1966).
71. Douglas, Goldberg and Fudenberg (1970).
72. Stites, Levin, Lauer, Costom and Fudenberg (1973).
73. Thomas, Ochs and Wedgwood (1974).
74. Webster (1976).
75. Mawas, Sors and Bernier (1969).

to mitogens such as PHA (Kopp, Trier, Stiehm and Foroozan, 1968; Douglas, Goldberg and Fudenberg, 1970; Gajl-Peczalska, Park, Biggar and Good, 1973; Webster and Asherson, 1974; Webster and Brostoff, 1976). Some of these T-cell defects may be due to nutritional deficiency resulting from malabsorption and if so they could be reversible (Jose, Welch and Doherty, 1970; Edelman, Suskind, Olson and Sirisinha, 1973; Levin, Lipsky, Kirkpatrick, 1975). A protein-losing enteropathy, often found in immunodeficiency, could also contribute to the cellular abnormality (Vesin, Troupel, Acar, Renault, Desbuquois and Cattan, 1960; Waldmann and Laster, 1964; Ament, Ochs and Davis, 1973). More recently, an enzyme defect has been described with lowered lymphocyte levels of purine 5′-nucleotidase (Johnson, North, Asherson, Allsop, Watts and Webster, 1977).

Gastrointestinal disease

A variety of gastrointestinal and hepatic conditions have been described in common variable immune deficiency (Table 9.3).

Stomach

Pernicious anaemia-like syndrome. Achlorhydria is present in about half of the patients (Twomey, Jordan, Jarrold, Trubowitz, Ritz and Conn, 1969; Hermans, Diaz-Buxo and Stobo, 1976; Webster, 1976) and gastric atrophy with a pernicious anaemia (PA)-like syndrome may develop (Van Leeuwen and Van Dommelen, 1956; Lewis and Brown, 1957; Crowder, Thompson and Kupfer, 1959; Gibbs and Pryor, 1961; Larsson, Hagelquist and Cöster, 1961; Lee, Jenkins, Hughes and Kazantzis, 1964; Waldmann and Laster, 1964; Hermans, Huizenga, Hoffman, Brown and Markowitz, 1966; Clark, Tornyos, Herbert and Twomey, 1967; Hoskins, Winawer, Broitman, Gottlieb and Zamcheck, 1967; Goodman, Smith and Northey, 1967; Conn, Binder and Burns, 1968; Twomey, Jordan, Jarrold, Trubowitz, Ritz and Conn, 1969; Douglas, Goldberg, Fudenberg and Goldberg, 1970; Twomey, Jordan, Laughter, Meuwissen and Good, 1970; Ajdukiewicz, Youngs and Bouchier, 1972; Gelfand, Berkel, Godwin, Rocklin, David and Rosen, 1972; Hughes, Brooks and Conn, 1972; Cowling, Strickland, Ungar, Whittingham and Rose, 1974; Twomey, 1975; Ehtessabian, Cassidy, Thomas, Matthews and Tubergen, 1976). Nevertheless, recorded cases of vitamin B_{12} malabsorption may be secondary to giardia infection (Ament, Ochs and Davis, 1973). The syndrome differs from classical PA in several respects (Table 9.4).

The PA occurring in immunodeficiency is rare in children but more commonly occurs in older patients. Biopsy of the stomach shows loss of parietal and chief cells, intestinalization of the mucosa, a mononuclear cell infiltrate, but an absence of plasma cells (Twomey, Jordan, Laughter, Meuwissen and Good, 1970). The lack of a plasma cell infiltrate and also the absence of autoantibodies suggests that in Addisonian PA autoantibodies are secondary phenomena and that the actual mucosal damage is caused by a cell-mediated immune mechanism. Indeed, some patients with either Addisonian PA or the PA syndrome associated with immune deficiency have circulating lymphocytes that produce a migration-inhibition factor and undergo lymphocyte transformation in the presence of human or hog intrinsic factor and human mitochondria from liver and stomach (Fixa, Thiele, Komárková and Nožička, 1972; Gelfand, Berkel, Godwin, Rocklin, David and Rosen, 1972; James, Asherson, Chanarin, Coghill, Hamilton, Himsworth and Webster, 1974). Serum gastrin levels are raised in Addisonian PA compared to immunodeficient PA (Hughes, Brooks and Conn, 1972), presumably due to preservation of antral tissue in the former and complete gastric atrophy in the latter.

Malignancy. Malignancy occurs much more frequently in patients with common variable hypogammaglobulinaemia than in the normal population (Forssman and Herner, 1964; Twomey, Jordan, Jarrold, Trubowitz, Ritz and Conn, 1969; Hersh, Floch, Binder, Conn, Prizont and Spiro, 1970; Gatti and Good, 1971; Huizenga and Hermans, 1972; Creagan and Fraumeni, 1973; Kersy, Spector and Good, 1973; Hermans, Diaz-Buxo and Stobo, 1976). Hermans, Diaz-Buxo and Stobo (1976) reported 8 malignant tumours in a series of 50 patients, and of these 8 (cases), 4 had tumours of the stomach and in 2 of these patients there was no evidence of atrophic gastritis. Carcinoma of the colon, lym-

Table 9.4 Comparison of classical pernicious anaemia and pernicious anaemia associated with common variable hypogammaglobulinaemia

	Classical pernicious anaemia	*Pernicious anaemia associated with common variable hypogammaglobulinaemia*
Age of onset	40–60 years	20–40 years
Gastric histology	Plasma cell infiltrate; atrophy may spare antrum	Mononuclear cell infiltrate only, no plasma cells
Intrinsic factor	Absent	Absent
Male/female relationship	1:2	1:1
Serum gastrin	Raised	Normal
Parietal and intrinsic factor antibodies	Present	Absent

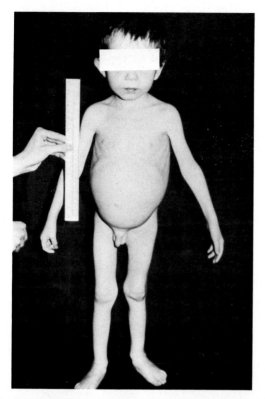

Fig. 9.1 Patient aged 5 years with recurrent chest infections, malabsorption and common variable acquired hypogammaglobulinaemia showing short stature, wasting and malnutrition (photograph courtesy of Dr M. J. Tarlow).

phoma of the colon and rectum, and polyposis of the colon were also found in the same series. In most of these patients the tumour occurred several years after the onset of their immune deficiency.

Small intestine

Over half the patients with common variable immunodeficiency show evidence of malabsorption, frequently secondary to giardial infestation. Treatment of the giardiasis usually reverses the symptoms of malabsorption. However, there remains a group of patients who have persistent malabsorption (Fig. 9.1), a condition termed hypogammaglobulinaemic sprue (Sanford, Favour and Tribeman, 1954; Cooke, Weiner and Shinton, 1957; Zelman and Lewin, 1958; Kabler, 1960; Vesin, Troupel, Acar, Renault, Desbuquois and Cattan, 1960; Cohen, Paley and Janowitz, 1961; Huizenga, Wollaeger, Green and McKenzie, 1961; Swift, 1962; Green and Sperber, 1962; Pelkonen, Siurala and Vuopio, 1963; Collins and Ellis, 1965; Hoskins, Winawer, Broitman, Gottlieb and Zamcheck, 1967; Johnson, Van Arsdel, Tobe and Ching, 1967; Cooper, Lawton and Bockman, 1971; Hughes, Cerda, Holtzapple and Brooks, 1971; Ament and Rubin, 1972; Gerson, Janowitz and Paronetto, 1972; Ament, Ochs and Davis, 1973; Webster, 1975). The jejunal biopsy on dissecting microscopy (Fig. 9.2) and routine histology resembles coeliac disease (CD), often with total villous atrophy (Fig. 9.3a and b), but unlike CD there is an absence of plasma cells. Much debate exists whether these patients respond to a gluten-

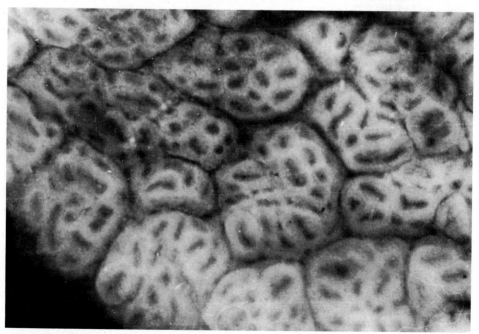

Fig. 9.2 Dissecting microscopic appearance of jejunal biopsy from patient with common variable (late onset) acquired hypogammaglobulinaemia, showing mosaic appearance.

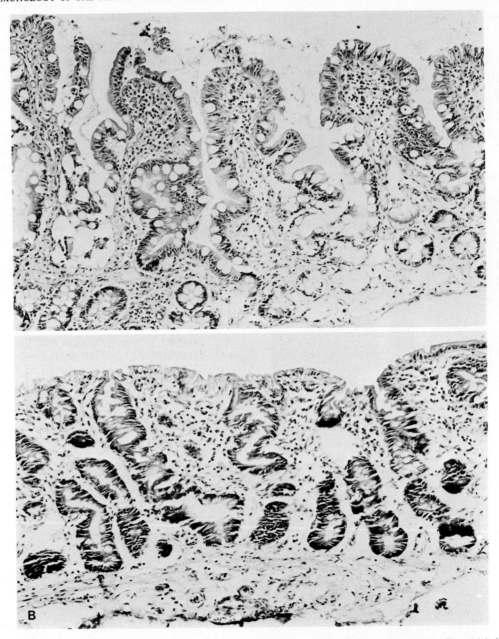

Figs 9.3a and 9.3b Jejunal biopsy from patient illustrated in Figure 9.1 initially showing 'normal' villi (Fig. 9.3a), but a repeat 6 months later showed a 'flat' mucosa (Fig. 9.3b). His malabsorption failed to respond to gammaglobulin injections, antibiotics and a gluten-free diet.

free diet (GFD) (Kabler, 1960; Hoskins, Winawer, Broitman, Gottlieb and Zamcheck, 1967; Johnson, Van Arsdel, Tobe and Ching, 1967; Hughes, Cerda, Holtzapple and Brooks, 1971; Ament and Rubin, 1972; Ament, Ochs and Davis 1973; Eidelman, 1976). Cases purporting to show an improvement on a GFD have often concurrently been treated with gammaglobulin injections and antibiotics and follow-up jejunal biopsies after gluten withdrawal have not been performed (Vesin,

Troupel, Acar, Renault, Desbuquois and Cattan, 1960; Huizenga, Wollaeger, Green and McKenzie, 1961; Green and Sperber, 1962; Swift, 1962; Mann, Brown and Kern, 1970; Cooper, Lawton and Bockman, 1971). Indeed some patients have restarted a normal diet and even had a gluten challenge without deterioration in gastrointestinal function (Hughes, Cerda, Holtzapple and Brooks, 1971). Nevertheless, Webster (1976) described a patient who showed improvement in malabsorption and jejunal morphology on a GFD. Gluten rechallenge was not carried out. A patient with a severe mucosal lesion which returned to normal over a period of 6 years without elimination of gluten was reported by Hughes, Cerda, Holtzapple and Brooks (1971). This coincided with a long period free of significant infection. Dobbins and Sahba (1972) suggest that a chronic viral enteritis might be a causative factor in the malabsorption of hypogammaglobulinaemic sprue, but this remains to be substantiated. Alternatively, the occasional improvement on GFD could be due to a state of transient gluten intolerance (Visakorpi and Immonen, 1967; Walker-Smith, 1970; *Lancet* editorial, 1976b).

Steroids have also been used with success in hypogammaglobulinaemic sprue (Hughes, Cerda, Holtzapple and Brooks, 1971; Diaz-Buxo, Hermans and Huizenga, 1975) although often other therapy, such an antibiotics, was administered. Gammaglobulin replacement is also beneficial in improving diarrhoea (Conn and Quintiliani, 1966; Binder and Reynolds, 1967).

Illustrative case history. A male Caucasian was first seen at the age of 16 years with *Haemophilus influenza* meningitis. Six years later, after complaints of diarrhoea, he was diagnosed as suffering from coeliac disease and treated with a GFD. When 26 he developed a pneumococcal meningitis and hypogammaglobulinaemia was detected. In his family history his maternal grandmother and a sister suffered from ulcerative colitis.

Examination showed a severe peripheral sensory neuropathy and evidence of folic acid, vitamin B_{12} and thiamine deficiency. Further investigation revealed abnormal xylose absorption, a faecal fat of 37.5 mmol/24 h (normally less than 17.5 mmol/24 h) and a jejunal biopsy showed partial villous atrophy with infiltration of the lamina propria with polymorphonuclear leucocytes, eosinophils and lymphocytes. The jejunal aspirate grew *Escherichia coli*, *Proteus mirabilis* and *Streptococcus pyogenes*, but there was no giardia infestation. A small amount of IgG was present in the fluid. An increased loss of $^{51}CrCl_3$-labelled albumin in his faeces indicated a protein-losing enteropathy. He improved considerably on vitamin replacement, a course of co-trimoxazole, a gluten-free diet and gammaglobulin replacement. However, a jejunal biopsy performed 4 months later showed no morphological improvement.

By most definitions (Ch. 6), this patient does not have CD. He also illustrates how difficult it is to decide what response can be attributable solely to gluten withdrawal in such cases. On currently available data the descriptive term hypogammaglobulinaemic sprue would seem to be still useful.

With respect to the mechanism of mucosal damage Webster *et al.* (1977) reported trace amounts of immunoglobulins in the jejunal juice of hypogammaglobulinaemic patients and suggested that they may be capable of producing a local humoral response to dietary antigens such as gluten, sufficient to cause a disease resembling CD. Finally, non-granulomatous jejunoileitis responsive to antibiotics and gammaglobulin therapy has also been reported in hypogammaglobulinaemia (Corlin and Pops, 1972). This seems to be a separate entity with probably a different pathogenesis to that occurring in the sprue patients.

Protein-losing enteropathy

There are several reports of a protein-losing enteropathy in common variable hypogammaglobulinaemia (Vesin, Troupel, Acar, Renault, Desbuquois and Cattan, 1960; Waldmann and Laster, 1964; Bjernulf, Johansson and Parrow, 1971; Ament, Ochs and Davis, 1973). Again, administration of a GFD has apparently improved tests of *in-vivo* protein loss in such cases (Waldmann and Laster, 1964).

Nodular lymphoid hyperplasia

Nodular lymphoid hyperplasia (NLH) was first reported in a patient at autopsy by Firkin and Blackburn in 1958 but did not receive much prominence until its inclusion as one aspect of a syndrome by Hermans, Huizenga, Hoffman, Brown and Markowitz (1966). Since then NLH has been described in between 19 and 60 per cent of patients with common variable hypogammaglobulinaemia (Frik, Heinkel and Zeitler, 1963; Hermans, Huizenga, Hoffman, Brown and Markowitz, 1966; Hodgson, Hoffman and Huizenga, 1967; Grise, 1968; Kirkpatrick, Waxman, Smith and Schimke, 1968; Bird, Jacobs, Silbiger and Wolff, 1969; Penny, 1969; Anderson, Pellegrino and Schaefer, 1970; Davis, Eidelman and Loop, 1970; Dubois, Roy, Fulginiti, Merrill and Murray, 1970; Cooper, Lawton and Bockman, 1971; Hughes, Cerda, Holtzapple and Brooks, 1971; Johnson, Goldberg, Pops and Weiner, 1971; Michaels, Go, Humbert, Dubois, Stewart and Ellis, 1971; Ajdukiewicz, Youngs and Bouchier, 1972; Parkin, McClelland, O'Moore, Percy-Robb, Grant and Shearman, 1972; Ament, Ochs and Davis, 1973; Cowling, Strickland, Ungar, Whittingham and Rose, 1974; De Smet, Tubergen and Martel, 1976; Hermans, Diaz-Buxo and Stobo, 1976; Webster *et al.* 1977). A condition resembling NLH may occur in children possibly related to transient defective immunoglobulin production (Fieber and Schaefer, 1966; Capitanio and Kirkpatrick, 1970) and it has been reported in an adult patient without hypogammaglobulinaemia (Webster, 1976).

NLH usually occurs in adults but is occasionally found in children and adolescents (Firkin and Blackburn, 1958; Goldstein, Krivit and Hong, 1969; Dubois, Roy, Fulginiti, Merrill and Murray, 1970). Currently, there appears to be some controversy about the incidence of intestinal nodules in immune deficiency disease, but it is doubtful that they are an invariable accompaniment. One of the characteristic features of NLH is the 1–3 mm diameter nodules in the lamina propria of the small intestine, although, less commonly, they have also been found in the stomach, colon and rectum (Hodgson, Hoffman and Huizenga, 1967; Bird, Jacobs, Silbiger and Wolff, 1969; De Smet, Tubergen and Martel, 1976). These aggregates of lymphoid tissue appear as nodular or polypoid protrusions on endoscopy and as multiple-filling defects on barium studies. The lesions are large enough to produce distortion of the neighbouring villi, but the villi between the nodules are normal in shape. They may or may not be found on jejunal biopsy when present radiologically and vice versa (Webster et al., 1977). Histology shows germinal centres within these lymphoid follicles in contrast to the appearance of the small lymphoid collections seen in normal individuals. Plasma cells are characteristically absent or markedly reduced in the lamina propria (Hermans, Huizenga, Hoffman, Brown and Markowitz, 1966) both on immunofluorescent (Johnson, Goldberg, Pops and Weiner, 1971) and immunoperoxidase studies (Webster et al., 1977). The latter study also showed that IgM can be detected in the nodules and jejunal fluid but it is absent from other secretions such as saliva.

Giardia lamblia infestation occurs in 60–100 per cent of patients with NLH but only in about 30 per cent of patients with common variable hypogammaglobulinaemia without detectable NLH (Hughes, Cerda, Holtzapple and Brooks, 1971; Ajdukiewicz, Youngs and Bouchier, 1972; Ament, Ochs and Davis, 1973; Hermans, Diaz-Buxo and Stobo, 1976). Eradication of giardiasis does not result in regression of NLH. When comparing the incidence of giardiasis in different series, it is important to recall that the absence of this protozoan in the stool may be misleading. Examination of jejunal biopsies and mucosal scrapings is more reliable.

Gastrointestinal malignancy would appear to occur more often in patients with NLH than in those without. Hermans, Diaz-Buxo and Stobo (1976) described 13 patients with NLH and 5 of these developed malignancy in the intestine.

The basic mechanisms underlying NLH are unknown, but it is postulated that chronic intraluminal antigen stimulation of the intestinal mucosa results in proliferation of B-cells carrying a surface antigen recognition site. Because of the accompanying basic defect in hypogammaglobulinaemia, in spite of this stimulation and B-cell proliferation, secretion does not occur. IgG antibody (Uhr and Möller, 1968) and perhaps antigen elimination may be important in the feedback control of lymphocyte proliferation and the absence of this feedback results in a piling up of plasma-cell percursors in the lymphoid tissues, although intestinal mucosa from hypogammaglobulinaemic patients may secrete immunoglobulin *in vitro* (McClelland, Shearman and Van Furth, 1976). The role of T-cell mediated mechanisms in NLH are unknown but there does not appear to be a major functional defect (Webster et al., 1977).

Gastrointestinal infection

G. lamblia is commonly found in patients with common variable hypogammaglobulinaemia and is frequently implicated as the cause of diarrhoea, malabsorption and any jejunal mucosal lesions (Cohen, Paley and Janowitz, 1961; Huizenga, Wollaeger, Green and McKenzie, 1961; Zamcheck, Hoskins, Winawer, Broitman and Gottlieb, 1963; McCarthy, Austad and Read, 1965; Hermans, Huizenga, Hoffman, Brown and Markowitz, 1966; Hoskins, Winawer, Broitman, Gottlieb and Zamcheck, 1967; Grise, 1968; Bird, Jacobs, Silbiger and Wolff, 1969; Anderson, Pellegrino and Schaefer, 1970; Hersh, Floch, Binder, Conn, Prizont and Spiro, 1970; Hughes, Cerda, Holtzapple and Brooks, 1971; Johnson, Goldberg, Pops and Weiner, 1971; Michaels, Go, Humbert, Dubois, Stewart and Ellis, 1971; Ajdukiewicz, Youngs and Bouchier, 1972; Ament and Rubin, 1972; Brown, Butterfield, Savage and Tada, 1972; Parkin, McClelland, O'Moore, Percy-Robb, Grant and Shearman, 1972; Ament, Ochs and Davis, 1973; Cowling, Strickland, Ungar, Whittingham and Rose, 1974). The reason the protozoan is found so frequently in this form of immunodeficiency and yet only rarely or not at all in other primary immunodeficiency syndromes is unknown. It is possible that in these other syndromes the correct microenvironment is not present for the development of a giardial infection; genetic factors, such as blood groups, may also be relevant (Barnes and Kay, 1977).

This protozoan occurs in 33–64 per cent of immunodeficient patients with diarrhoea. *Trichomonas hominis* is also found, but probably does not cause symptoms (Hermans, Diaz-Buxo and Stobo, 1976) while coccidial infections could also be a cause of malabsorption in immunodeficiency (Meisel, Perera, Meligios and Rubin, 1976).

Bacterial overgrowth of the small intestine is also increased in common variable hypogammaglobulinaemia and variously consists of anaerobic organisms such as bacteroides, lactobacillus and clostridia, and aerobes such as streptococcus, staphylococcus, haemophilus, diptheroides, coliforms and yeasts (Collins and Ellis, 1965; McCarthy, Austad and Read, 1965; Anderson, Pellegrino and Schaefer, 1970; Hersh, Floch, Binder, Conn, Prizont and Spiro, 1970; Hughes, Cerda, Holtzapple and Brooks, 1971; Ajdukiewicz, Youngs and Bouchier, 1972; Ament and Rubin, 1972; Brown, Butterfield, Savage and Tada, 1972; Brown, Savage, Dubois, Alp, Mallory and Kern, 1972; Parkin, McClelland, O'Moore, Percy-Robb, Grant and Shearman, 1972;

Ament, Ochs and Davis, 1973). The bacterial counts rarely reach the numbers found in blind loop syndromes where counts are more than 1×10^5 organisms per ml. Unconjugated bile salts are not usually found in jejunal contents (Ament, Ochs and Davis, 1973) and glycine-1-^{14}C labelled glycocholate breath tests are normal (Webster, 1976). Whether the intraluminal organisms contribute to any of the gastrointestinal manifestations found in the patients is controversial, but organisms may be found in jejunal mucosa (Webster, 1976) – as in tropical sprue (Tomkins, Drasar and James, 1975) – and symptomatic improvements can be effected with antibiotic treatment, and occasionally cholestyramine (Gleich and Hofmann, 1971).

The isolated lactase deficiency and disaccharidase deficiency occurring in hypogammaglobulinaemia are probably often secondary to giardia infestation or small intestine bacterial overgrowth (Caplinger and Boellner, 1968; Dubois, Roy, Fulginiti, Merrill and Murray, 1970; Brown, Butterfield, Savage and Tada, 1972). Perhaps surprisingly, salmonella and shigella infections are unusual, being reported only in occasional patients with immune deficiency; nevertheless, the infections are often resistant to therapy (Freundlich, 1957; Waldmann and Laster, 1964; Collins and Ellis, 1965; McCarthy, Austad and Read, 1965; Conn and Quintiliani, 1966; Douglas, Goldberg and Fudenberg, 1970; Twomey, Jordan, Laughter, Meuwissen and Good, 1970; Stites, Levin, Lauer, Costom and Fudenberg, 1973).

Colon and rectum

Ament *et al.* (1973) have described 2 patients who developed watery diarrhoea unrelated to giardia infestation. Sigmoidoscopy showed an oedematous mucosa with contact bleeding, and histology of the rectal biopsy showed oedema, haemorrhage and a polymorphonuclear leucocyte cell infiltrate of the lamina propria, but no crypt abscesses. Prednisone produced clinical remission and reversal of the sigmoidoscopic appearances. A further patient with proctitis and crypt abscesses on biopsy was unresponsive to sulphasalazine and systemic steroids (Ochs and Ament, 1976). Symptoms of colitis have also been noted in other patients (Zelman and Lewin, 1958; Conn and Quintiliani, 1966). Conversely, Webster (1975) found early crypt abscesses in rectal biopsies from 7 of 17 patients, of whom only 2 complained of diarrhoea. Classical Crohn's disease and ulcerative colitis also occur (Squire, 1962; Kirk and Freedman, 1967; Kopp, Trier, Stiehm, Foroozan, 1968; Hersh, Floch, Binder, Conn, Prizont and Spiro, 1970; Söltoft, Petersen and Kruse, 1972; Jones, Beeken, Roessner and Brown, 1976).

Cholelithiasis and pancreatic disease

Cholelithiasis is increased in hypogammaglobulinaemia and pancreatitis may contribute to subsequent malabsorption (Cooke, Weiner and Shinton, 1957; Hudson and Aldor, 1970; Hughes, Cerda, Holtzapple and Brooks, 1971; Diaz-Buxo, Hermans and Elvebaur, 1975; Hermans, Diaz-Buxo and Stobo, 1976). The pancreatic disease may affect both endocrine as well as exocrine pancreatic function, causing insulin-dependent diabetes mellitus (Webster, 1976).

DEFICIENCY OF KAPPA OR LAMBDA TYPE IMMUNOGLOBULINS

About 65 per cent of the immunoglobulins in the serum of normal adults contain kappa (κ)-light chains, and the rest lambda (λ)-light chains. Although physiologic variations of the κ/λ ratio occur in infants and some alteration of the ratio may be found in primary immunodeficiency syndromes (Yount, Hong, Seligmann, Good and Kunkel, 1970; Skvaril, Barandun, Morell, Kuffer and Probst, 1975), a marked reduction or an absence of one particular light chain class is rare. However, several patients have now been reported with a marked alteration in the κ/λ-light chain ratio, usually with an associated immunodeficiency syndrome and gastrointestinal pathology (Bernier, Gunderman and Ruymann, 1972; Barandun, Morell, Skvaril and Oberdorfer, 1976; Zegers, Maertzdorf, van Loghem, Mul, Stoop, van der Laag, Vossen and Ballieux, 1976). These individuals have reduced plasma cells in their bone marrow and gastrointestinal mucosa with an altered κ/λ ratio corresponding to that observed in the immunoglobulins of the peripheral blood and secretions.

Barandun, Morell, Skvaril and Oberdorfer (1976) reported one patient with pernicious anaemia and chronic diarrhoea responding to antibiotics who had a κ-chain deficiency and another patient with achlorhydria and gastric atrophy who had a λ-chain deficiency. Both individuals had a panhypogammaglobulinaemia. Bernier, Gunderman and Ruymann (1972) described a female who had diarrhoea and an isolated lactase deficiency associated with a slightly decreased serum IgA and markedly reduced κ-chain type immunoglobulin. Finally, Zegers, Maertzdorf, van Loghem, Mul, Stoop, van der Laag, Vossen and Ballieux (1976) described a male who had cystic fibrosis, malabsorption and diabetes mellitus associated with IgA deficiency and undetectable κ-chain type immunoglobulin.

These cases may represent the extremes of the mild variations of the κ/λ ratio sometimes seen in primary immunodeficiency and further patients need to be studied before this can be claimed as a distinct immunodeficiency syndrome.

Main immunological features

1. Decreased levels of IgA and IgG with raised levels of IgM.
2. Increased susceptibility to infection and malignancy.

This condition is characterized by reduced serum IgA and IgG and usually grossly elevated IgM levels, the latter reaching 1.5–10 g/l. The IgM fraction is not a monoclonal protein and contains antibody activity. In some patients an elevated IgD may be found. Although predominantly affecting males, female cases occur which may represent a primary acquired form. The syndrome is also frequently associated with chronic rubella (South, Montgomery and Rawls, 1975).

Patients usually present at 1 to 2 years of age with recurrent pyogenic infections and associated thrombocytopaenia and neutropaenia; aplastic and haemolytic anaemias and renal disease may also develop. Chronic diarrhoea can be present and monilial infection of the gastrointestinal tract has been described (Rosen, Kevy, Merler, Janeway and Gitlin, 1961; Hong, Schubert, Perrin and West, 1962; Stiehm and Fundenberg, 1966; Rosen, 1974). One such patient developed oesophageal ulcers, from which *Candida parapsilosis* was isolated, and subsequently developed an oesophageal stenosis (Ament, 1975). Malignant infiltration of the gastrointestinal tract and viscera with IgM-producing cells may occur (Rosen, 1974). It is noteworthy that some patients with X-linked immunodeficiency can be asymptomatic (Hong, Schubert, Perrin and West, 1962; Ament, Ochs and Davis, 1973).

SELECTIVE IgA DEFICIENCY

Main immunological features

1. Serum IgA less than 0.05 g/l (normal in adults 0.75–5.20 g/l).
2. Cell-mediated immunity normal.
3. Associated with allergy, recurrent sinopulmonary infection, autoimmune disease and numerous gastrointestinal and hepatic disorders.

Selective IgA deficiency is the commonest primary immunodeficiency disorder in man, occurring in between 1:500 to 1:700 of individuals (Bachman, 1965; Bull and Tomasi, 1968; Hanson, 1968; Hobbs, 1968, Johansson, Högman and Killander, 1968). It can occur sporadically, but autosomal dominant, autosomal recessive, intermediate and polygenic modes of inheritance have also been reported (Koistinen, 1976). Although IgA deficiency can occur in monozygotic twins (Bjernulf, Johannson and Parrow, 1971) only one twin may be affected (Lewkonia, Gairdner and Doe, 1976). This finding together with the fact that IgA deficiency may

follow penicillamine or phenytoin therapy (Seager, Jamison, Wilson, Hayward and Soothill, 1975; Proesmans, Jaeken, Eekels, 1976; Hjalmarson, Hanson and Nilsson, 1977; Stanworth, Johns, Williamson, Shadforth, Felix-Davies and Thompson, 1977) suggests that environmental factors can also be important in its development. IgA deficiency has been associated with a number of chromosomal abnormalities, including deletion of the long or short arms of chromosome 18 (Stewart, Elliot and Robinson, 1970; Grundbacher, 1972; Faed, Whyte, Paterson, McCathie and Robertson, 1972; Leisti, Leisti, Perheentupa, Savilahti, and Aula, 1973).

A low or undetectable serum IgA is usually found in conjunction with the absence of secretory IgA (S IgA) from body secretions, such as saliva and jejunal fluid (Bull and Thomasi, 1968; Haneberg and Aarskog, 1975) and a reduction of IgA-containing plasma cells in the gastrointestinal tract. However, a small number of individuals may have normal S IgA production with normal numbers of IgA-fluorescing cells in their intestine (Bellanti, Artenstein and Buescher, 1966; Hazenberg, Hoedmaeker, Niewenhuis and Mandema, 1968; Ammann and Hong, 1971b; Brown, Savage, Dubois, Alp, Mallory and Kern, 1972; Jones, Beeken, Roessner and Brown, 1976). Alternatively, a selective deficiency of S IgA may be found in the presence of a normal serum IgA (Krakauer, Zinneman and Hong, 1975; Strober, Krakauer, Klaeveman, Reynolds and Nelson, 1976).

IgA-deficient subjects usually have normal numbers of circulating surface IgA-bearing lymphocytes in their blood, although in occasional patients these cells are reduced or absent (Lawton, Royal, Self and Cooper, 1972). *In-vitro* stimulation of peripheral blood lymphocytes from IgA-deficient individuals with PWM results in release of immunoglobulin A (Wu and Lawton, 1972) and IgA may be synthesized from small-intestinal mucosa in culture together with SC although the two do not appear to combine properly (McClelland, Shearman and Van Furth, 1976). These findings suggest that IgA deficiency may result from (1) a failure of B-lymphocytes to differentiate into IgA cells from their IgG or IgM precursors, (2) arrested development of IgA cells due to metabolic abnormalities, or (3) disturbance of factors extrinsic to the B-lymphocyte which are essential for normal induction of plasma cell maturation.

Although many IgA-deficient individuals are allegedly asymptomatic, some develop immunological abnormalities or significant disease in time (Ammann and Hong, 1971b; Koistinen and Sarna, 1976). In particular, IgA deficiency occurs in 40 per cent of individuals with ataxia telangiectasia and the serum abnormality may occur several years before the onset of sinopulmonary

Table 9.5 Gastrointestinal and hepatic disease occurring in IgA-deficient individuals

Disease	Reference
1. Gingival hyperplasia	1
2. Oesophageal carcinoma	2
3. Pernicious anaemia	3–5
4. Gastric carinoma	6, 7
5. Post-vagotomy diarrhoea	8
6. Cystic fibrosis of the pancreas	9
7. Coeliac disease with response to gluten withdrawal	10–23
8. Coeliac disease-like syndrome without response to gluten withdrawal	24–26
9. Primary intestinal lymphangiectasia	27
10. Intestinal nodular lymphoid hyperplasia	28–30
11. Tropical sprue	31
12. Cow's milk intolerance	32
13. Isolated lactase deficiency	33
14. Disaccharidase deficiency	33
15. Bacterial overgrowth of the small intestine	8, 30, 34, 35
16. *Giardia lamblia* infestation	29, 35, 36
17. Crohn's disease	12, 37–41
18. Ulcerative colitis	12, 16, 35
19. Colonic carcinoma	42, 43
20. Hepatitis B antigen positivity	44
21. Haemachromatosis	45
22. Active chronic hepatitis	45
23. Alcoholic cirrhosis	46
24. Wilson's disease in association with penicillamine therapy	47,48
25. Chronic mucocutaneous candidiasis	49–51
26. Secretory component deficiency with normal serum IgA, but secretory IgA deficiency	52, 53

References to Table 9.5

1. Aarli and Tönder (1975).
2. Ammann and Hong (1973a).
3. Spector (1974).
4. Ginsberg and Mullinax (1970).
5. Castleman and McNeely (1971).
6. Fraser and Rankin (1970).
7. Kirkpatrick (1976a).
8. McLoughlin, Bradley, Chapman, Temple, Hede and McFarland (1976).
9. Ammann and Hong (1971b).
10. Crabbé and Heremans (1966).
11. Bjernulf, Johansson and Parrow (1971).
12. Claman, Merrill, Peakman and Robinson (1970).
13. Mann, Brown and Kern (1970).
14. Savilahti, Pelkonen and Visakorpi (1971).
15. Carroll, Silverman, Isobe, Brown, Kelts and Brooke (1976).
16. Falchuk and Falchuk (1975).
17. Le Bodic, Le Bodic, Dedieu and Mussini-Montpellier (1975).
18. Ansaldi, Santini and Marengo (1974).
19. Crabbé and Heremans (1967).
20. Hong and Ammann (1972).
21. Hobbs and Hepner (1968).
22. Asquith, Thompson and Cooke (1969).
23. Brown, Ferguson, Carswell, Horne and MacSween (1973).
24. Anderson, Finlayson and Deschner (1974).
25. Dedieu, Le Bodic, Simon, Le Mevel, de Lisle and Miniconi (1975).
26. Ament (1975).
27. Eisner and Bralow (1968).
28. Hermans, Huizenga, Hoffman, Brown and Markowitz (1966).
29. Gryboski, Self, Clemett and Herskovic (1968).
30. Hersh, Floch, Binder, Conn, Prizont and Spiro (1970).
31. Samuel and Jarnum (1971).
32. Harrison, Kilby, Walker-Smith, France and Wood (1976).
33. Dubois, Roy, Fulginiti, Merrill and Murray (1970).
34. Cattan, Debray, Crabbé, Seligmann, Marche and Danon (1966).
35. Brown, Savage, Dubois, Alp, Mallory and Kern (1972).
36. Hoskins, Winawer, Broitman, Gottlieb and Zamcheck (1967).
37. Weeke and Jarnum (1971).
38. Bergman, Johansson and Krause (1973).
39. Jones, Beeken, Roessner and Brown (1976).
40. Ross and Asquith (1977).
41. Söltoft, Petersen and Kruse (1972).
42. Miller, Holland, Sugarbaker, Strober and Waldmann (1970).
43. Ertel (1973).
44. Benbassat, Keren and Zlotnic (1973).
45. Joske (1975).
46. Wilson, Onstad and Williams (1968).
47. Proesmans, Jaeken and Eekels (1976).
48. Hjalmarson, Hanson and Nilsson (1977).
49. Schlegel, Bernier, Bellanti, Maybee, Osbourne, Stewart, Pearlman, Ouelette and Biehusen (1970).
50. Claman, Hartley and Merrill (1966).
51. Fulginiti, Sieber, Claman and Merrill (1966).
52. Krakauer, Zinneman and Hong (1975).
53. Strober, Krakauer, Klaeveman, Reynolds and Nelson (1976).

or gastrointestinal symptoms. Transient IgA deficiency is present in many infants and in some is thought to predispose to atopy, possibly by allowing penetration of foreign antigens through mucosal membranes. It has been suggested that these antigens then involve the IgE system with resultant atopy (Taylor, Norman, Orgel, Stokes, Turner and Soothill, 1973; Soothill, 1974). Such a mechanism has also been implicated in cow's milk intolerance (Harrison, Kilby, Walker-Smith, France and Wood, 1976).

Gastrointestinal disease (Table 9.5)

In general IgA deficiency appears to be an association with, rather than a cause of, gastrointestinal disease. Even gastrointestinal infection is not a major factor in IgA-deficient subjects, perhaps due to a compensatory production of secretory IgM (Thompson, 1970; Coelho, Pereira, Virella and Thompson, 1974). Nevertheless, in certain diseases, for example CD, the incidence of IgA deficiency seems greater than in the so-called normal population (Asquith, Thompson and Cooke, 1969).

Stomach

Pernicious anaemia (PA) associated with selective IgA deficiency is similar in some respects to classical Addisonian PA in that gastric atrophy and elevation of serum gastrin levels occur (Ginsberg and Mullinax, 1970; Spector, 1974). Gastric carinoma has been reported in IgA deficiency, but may reflect the known increased incidence of gastric tumours in PA (Fraser and Rankin, 1970; Kirkpatrick, 1976a). However, in IgA-deficient patients, gastrointestinal tract tumours appear more frequently than in other sites, and oesophageal and colonic neoplasms have been described (Ammann and Hong, 1973a; Miller, Holland, Sugarbaker, Strober and Waldmann, 1970; Ertel, 1973).

serum IgM (Asquith, Thompson and Cooke, 1969) the serum IgA is very low or absent, with a reduction of IgA plasma cells in the small intestine and a concomitant increase of IgM-fluorescing cells (Hobbs and Hepner, 1968). These patients have positive immunofluorescent staining for reticulin antibodies in the basement membrane underlying the surface epithelial cells (Ammann and Hong, 1971a).

In a starting population of coeliacs approximately 1:40 have IgA deficiency (Hobbs and Hepner, 1968; Asquith, Thompson and Cooke, 1969; Savilahti, Pelkonen and Visakorpi, 1971; Ansaldi, Santini and Marengo, 1974; Brown, Ferguson, Carswell, Horne and MacSween, 1973) and most of these respond to gluten

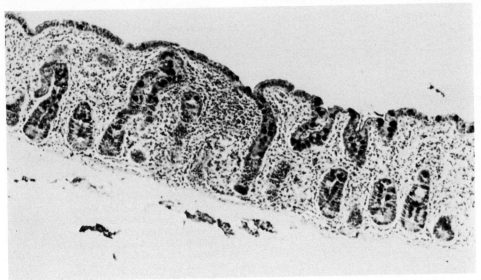

Fig. 9.4 Histological appearance of jejunal biopsy from patient with coeliac disease and selective IgA deficiency, showing subtotal villous atrophy. The epithelial cells are cuboidal and there are excess inflammatory cells in the lamina propria.

Small intestine

Malabsorption and diarrhoea are common in IgA deficiency (West, Hong and Holland, 1962). The condition resembles CD with a jejunal biopsy showing subtotal (Fig. 9.4) or total villous atrophy (Crabbé and Heremans, 1966; Crabbé and Heremans, 1967; Hobbs and Hepner, 1968; Asquith, Thompson and Cooke, 1969; Claman, Merrill, Peakman and Robinson, 1970; Mann, Brown and Kern, 1970; Bjernulf, Johansson and Parrow, 1971; Savilahti, Pelkonen and Visakorpi, 1971; Hong and Ammann, 1972; Brown, Ferguson, Carswell, Horne and MacSween, 1973; Anderson, Finlayson and Deschner, 1974; Ansaldi, Santini and Marengo, 1974; Ament, 1975; Dedieu, Le Bodic, Simon, Le Mevel, de Lisle, Miniconi, 1975; Falchuk and Falchuk, 1975; Le Bodic, Le Bodic, Dedieu, Mussini-Montpellier, 1975; Carrol, Silverman, Isobe, Brown, Kelts and Brooke, 1976). However, unlike CD where there is often an elevated serum IgA and reduced

withdrawal as in classical CD (Fig. 9.5). A few patients fail to respond to a GFD alone and require milk withdrawal (Asquith, 1970; Asquith, 1974), while others continue with a sometimes fatal malabsorption in spite of therapy with steroids or fresh frozen plasma infusions (Anderson, Finlayson, Deschner, 1974; Dedieu, Le Bodic, Simon, Le Mevel, de Lisle and Miniconi, 1975; Ament, 1975). Some of these individuals show progressive villous atrophy of the small intestine and it is possible that this group of non gluten-sensitive patients are sensitized to dietary antigens other than gluten (Dedieu, Le Bodic, Simon, Le Mevel, de Lisle and Miniconi, 1975). Certainly the intestine is more permeable to a variety of dietary antigens in selective IgA deficiency as reflected by increased serum antibody titres to dietary proteins (Buckley and Dees, 1969; Huntley, Robins, Lyerly and Buckley, 1971).

Illustrative case history. A 29-year-old Caucasian male was found to have no detectable serum IgA. As a child he had had three episodes of meningitis followed by epilepsy and he was started on phenytoin. In his family, 3 out of 7 brothers had a low or undetectable serum IgA and a cousin suffered from common variable hypogammaglobulinaemia. When aged 27 he began to lose weight and developed intermittent diarrhoea and constipation. Investigation shows a prolonged prothrombin time, reduced red-cell folate and abnormal xylose absorption. A peroral jejunal biopsy showed total villous atrophy, excess IgM-fluorescing plasma cells and only a few IgA cells present in the lamina propria. IgA-bearing lymphocytes were absent from the bone marrow and reduced in the peripheral blood. Gluten withdrawal resulted in an increase in weight and a correction of his

ported in several individuals with IgA deficiency (Hoskins, Winawer, Broitman, Gottlieb and Zamcheck, 1967; Gryboski, Self, Clement and Herskovic, 1968; Brown, Savage, Dubois, Alp, Mallory and Kern, 1972), one with intestinal nodular lymphoid hyperplasia. Zinneman and Kaplan (1972) found a selective reduction in secretory IgA levels in the jejunal aspirate in 10 patients with chronic giardia infections. On this basis it was implied that giardia infection may be secondary to defective mucosal IgA production, but their methods of estimation of IgA have been criticized (McClelland, Warwick and Shearman, 1973) and further studies of giardiasis by Jones and Brown (1974) found no evidence of immunoglobulin deficiency in either serum or secretions.

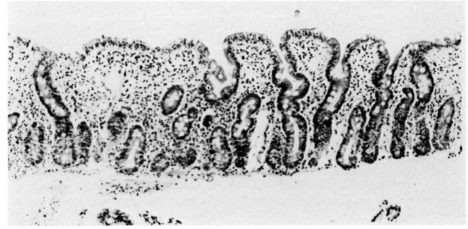

Fig. 9.5 Repeat jejunal biopsy from patient described in Figure 9.4 following a gluten-free diet. Villi are now present, the epithelial cells are columnar and there are fewer inflammatory cells in the lamina propria.

vitamin deficiencies and xylose malabsorption; his serum IgA remained undetectable. This individual therefore has five previously reported associations of IgA deficiency – recurrent infections involving the meninges, epilepsy, phenytoin medication (Grob and Herold, 1972; Seager, Jamison, Wilson, Hayward and Soothill, 1975), a family history of primary immunodeficiency (Van der Giessen, Reerink-Brongers and Algra-van Veen, 1967; Koistinen, 1976), and finally, of prime importance to his intestinal symptoms and malabsorption, he has coeliac disease.

Gastrointestinal infection

Chronic bacterial or parasitic infections of the small intestine, although commonly found in other primary deficiency syndromes, are rare in IgA deficiency (Cattan, Debray, Crabbé, Seligmann, Marche, Danon, 1966; Gryboski, Self, Clemett and Herskovic, 1968; Hersh, Floch, Binder, Conn, Prizont and Spiro, 1970; Brown, Savage, Dubois, Alp, Mallory and Kern, 1972; McLoughlin, Bradley, Chapman, Temple, Hede and McFarland, 1976). Giardiasis has, however, been re-

The notable absence of intestinal infection in IgA deficiency suggests that mechanisms other than local IgA secretion are important in intestinal immunity, possibly secretory IgM production and cell-mediated immune responses (Thompson, 1970; Boorman, Lina, Zurcher and Nieuwerkerk, 1973; Coelho, Pereira, Vierella and Thompson, 1974).

Disaccharidase and lactase deficiency

Lactase deficiency with or without associated deficiencies of maltase and sucrase have been occasionally documented in IgA deficiency (Dubois, Roy, Fulginiti, Merrill and Murray, 1970). In common variable hypogammaglobulinaemia, the enzyme changes are thought to be secondary to bacterial contamination of the bowel. However, this is rare in IgA deficiency and in this latter condition the mucosal defect may be no more than a chance finding.

Post-vagotomy diarrhoea

Severe diarrhoea following vagotomy was found to be associated with IgA deficiency in 6 out of 14 patients

(McLoughlin, Bradley, Chapman, Temple, Hede and McFarland, 1976). They all, in addition, had a deficiency of IgM and IgE. Jejunal biopsies were performed and were normal. However, all of the IgA- deficient patients had evidence of small-bowel bacterial colonization as assessed by culture of the jejunal aspirate and urinary indicans. A definitive cause of malabsorption, such as CD, was not established in these 6 patients.

Inflammatory bowel disease
Both Crohn's disease and ulcerative colitis have been reported in patients with IgA deficiency. In Crohn's disease this association is impressive. Of 471 Crohn's-disease patients reported in the literature, and 39 of our own patients, 7 patients were found to have IgA deficiency – an incidence of 1 : 73 (Ross and Asquith, 1977). The previous studies were those of Kraft, Ford, McCleery and Kirsner, 1968; Poen, Ballieux, Mul, Stoop, Ten Thije and Zegers, 1968; Deodhar, Michener and Farmer, 1969; Perret, Higgins, Johnston. Massarella, Truelove and Wright, 1971a; Weeke and Jarnum, 1971; Gellernt, Present and Janowitz, 1972; Bergman, Johansson and Krause, 1973; Bolton, James, Newcombe, Whitehead and Hughes, 1974; Persson, 1974; Soltis and Wilson, 1975; Jones, Beeken, Roessner and Brown, 1976; Pons Romero, Cabarcos, Uribarrena, Borda Celaya and Perez Miranda, 1976; Sailer, Ullmann and Berg, 1976. The incidence of IgA deficiency appears to be much less in ulcerative colitis. No cases were described among a series of 474 patients from the literature, nor found in 35 of our own patients (Kraft, Ford, McCleery and Kirsner, 1968; Deodhar, Michener and Farmer, 1969; Hardy-Smith and MacPhee, 1971; Perret, Higgins, Johnston, Massarella, Truelove and Wright, 1971b; Weeke and Jarnum, 1971; Gellernt, Present and Janowitz, 1972; Söltoft, Binder and Gudmand-Höyer, 1973; Bolton, James, Newcombe, Whitehead and Hughes, 1974; Soltis and Wilson, 1975; Sailer, Ullmann and Berg, 1976).

Three isolated case reports of IgA deficiency and ulcerative colitis were not included in the above analysis as all 3 patients had other diseases also known to be associated with IgA deficiency, namely, coeliac disease, hepatitis, and thyroiditis and biliary cirrhosis (Claman, Merrill, Peakman and Robinson, 1970; Brown, Savage, Dubois, Alp, Mallory and Kern, 1972; Falchuk and Falchuk, 1975). Furthermore, 2 other isolated cases of IgA deficiency have been described in Crohn's disease (Claman, Merrill, Peakman and Robinson, 1970; Söltoft, Petersen and Kruse, 1972), but the authors did not comment on how many of their other patients with inflammatory bowel disease had normal IgA levels.

In one patient with Crohn's disease from our series, a 29-year-old Caucasian female, there was a decrease in serum IgA over a period of 2 years from slightly low levels of 0.60 g/l to persistently undetectable levels – 13 years after the initial presentation of her disease. When her serum IgA was undetectable, there was an absence of S IgA, and IgA fluorescing plasma cells were not seen in the bone marrow or peripheral blood. These findings would add further support to the theory that environmental factors are important in some cases of IgA deficiency.

Treatment
Intravenous fresh frozen plasma is ineffective in the treatment of IgA deficiency, probably because infused IgA does not reach the secretory fluids, except perhaps saliva and then only if plasma is infused in large amounts (South, Cooper, Wollheim, Hong and Good, 1966; Goldberg, Barnett and Fudenberg, 1968). Some individuals with IgA deficiency have the potential of forming anti-IgA antibodies with resultant and sometimes fatal, anaphylactoid reactions on infusion of IgA-containing material (Vyas, Holmdahl, Perkins and Fudenberg, 1969; Invernizzi, Balestrieri, Consogno, Riboldi and Tincani, 1975). Anti-IgA antibodies of the IgG class have been described in ataxia telangiectasia by Strober, Wochner, Barlow, McFarlin and Waldmann (1968), resulting in increased catabolism of serum IgA. In IgA-deficient patients, fresh frozen plasma, pooled human gammaglobulin and unwashed red blood cells should not be given. Where transfusion is required the red cells should be packed and washed three times, alternatively blood from a compatible IgA-deficient individual should be used, or the patient's own blood prepared and frozen for future use. One therapy of promising value is the use of oral colostrum as described in the treatment of secretory IgA deficiency (Krakauer, Zinneman and Hong, 1975; Popović, Andjić and Paljm, 1976).

SECRETORY COMPONENT DEFICIENCY
There is a single case report of a Caucasian male patient with an absence of secretory component (SC) presenting with chronic intestinal candidiasis (Strober, Krakauer, Klaeveman, Reynolds and Nelson, 1976). Serum IgA levels were normal, but S IgA together with SC could not be detected in saliva or jejunal fluid. Also there was a failure of S IgA production on *in-vitro* culture of his jejunal mucosa. Krakauer, Zinneman and Hong (1975) described a further patient, a 52-year-old male, with only trace amounts of S IgA and SC in his jejunal fluid, an absence of these substances from his parotid saliva but with normal serum IgA levels. He had diarrhoea, abdominal cramps and a fungal infection of the small intestine on jejunal biopsy. Treatment with 20–30 ml of human colostrum produced symptomatic improvement.

These cases suggest that SC is necessary for the normal secretion of IgA into the intestinal lumen. With respect to extraintestinal sites, SC deficiency has also been described in the sudden infant-death syndrome, where it was found to be absent from the bronchial tissues in a proportion of individuals (Ogra, Ogra and Coppola, 1975).

Of additional importance is the description of a patient with recurrent pyogenic infections who had no intact serum IgA or S IgA (Moroz, Amir and De Vries, 1971). However, alpha heavy chain (HC) and SC were present in the saliva, free alpha HC in the serum and free alpha HC and light chains in the urine. These abnormalities were also present in two other asymptomatic family members. Presumably this abnormality represents failure of intracellular assembly of the molecular components of IgA and S IgA.

SELECTIVE IgE DEFICIENCY

IgE levels may be normal, low or absent in association with IgA deficiency (Michel, Guendon and Guerco, 1976), but isolated IgE deficiency has not been reported as an association with gastrointestinal disease (Brown, Lansford and Hornbrook, 1973).

SELECTIVE IgM DEFICIENCY

Severe selective IgM deficiency (arbitrarily defined as IgM levels of 10 per cent of the normal mean for age and sex) is rare; however, 1 patient with ulcerative colitis, with such a deficiency, has been documented (Ross and Thompson, 1976) and another with sclerosing intrahepatic cholangitis (Record, Eddleston, Shilkin and Williams, 1973). Moderate IgM deficiency is a frequent occurrence in coeliac disease, occurring in up to 60 per cent of patients on a normal diet. The values frequently improve on gluten withdrawal (Hobbs and Hepner, 1968; Asquith, Thompson and Cooke, 1969). Brown, Cooper and Hepner (1969) have shown that this may be due to reduced synthesis rather than increased gastrointestinal loss of IgM. IgM deficiency has also been reported in occasional patients with Crohn's disease, lymphoid nodular hyperplasia and Whipple's disease (Hobbs, 1975).

SELECTIVE IgD DEFICIENCY

An increased incidence of undetectable IgD has been found in coeliac disease, the significance of which is unknown (Asquith, Thompson and Cooke, 1969).

T-CELL DEFECTS

THE DI GEORGE SYNDROME (THYMIC HYPOPLASIA)

This syndrome results from failure of formation of the third and fourth pharyngeal pouches with a consequent hypoparathyroidism, cardiovascular abnormalities and absent T-cell function (Di George, 1968).

Clinical features are neonatal tetany, and if the patient survives recurrent infections, gastrointestinal problems may result from (1) associated congenital defects such as oesophageal atresia, (2) chronic monilial infection, (3) watery diarrhoea and malabsorption, and (4) failure to thrive. Thymic transplantation can be effective in reversing the T-cell abnormality and transfer factor has also been used (Cleveland, 1975).

CHRONIC MUCOCUTANEOUS CANDIDIASIS

Main presentations

1. Mucocutaneous candidiasis with or without a detectable defect of the cellular immune system.
2. Mucocutaneous candidiasis secondary to immunosuppression due to drugs or disease.

Chronic mucocutaneous candidiasis (CMC) is a condition with a heterogeneous aetiology in which there is chronic infection of mucous membranes, skin and nails with fungi of the *Candida* species, usually *Candida albicans*.

Patients are often difficult to classify, but usually they can be divided into four groups on clinical and genetic criteria (Table 9.6). These individuals may be further subdivided according to the presence or absence of immune defects, usually of the cellular immune system. Four patterns emerge on the basis of cutaneous delayed type hypersensitivity reactions to *Candida* and other antigens and *in-vitro* tests such as lymphocyte transformation and migration-inhibition factor (MIF) production (Table 9.7). CMC was first reported by Thorpe and Handley (1929) in an individual who also had hypoparathyroidism and since then many patients have been described with CMC and other forms of autoimmune endocrine disease, including hypothyroidism, diabetes mellitus, pernicious anaemia and Addison's disease (Ammann and Hong, 1973b).

Nature of the immunological defect in CMC

C. albicans can be cultured from the mouth, sputum and faeces of normal adults and children; however, the high incidence of delayed type hypersensitivity skin tests to *Candida* antigen within the normal population suggests that an active immune response is necessary to contain the fungus at a purely commensal level. Depression of immunity through immunosuppressive drugs (Kirkpatrick and Smith, 1974) or disease may allow *Candida* infection to occur either locally in skin and mucous membranes, or systemically. Many patients with CMC do not have any evidence of disease with acknowledged immunosuppressive features, but in at least 50 per cent or more of these individuals, abnormalities of the immune system, particularly cellular

Table 9.6 Clinicogenetic classification of patients with mucocutaneous candidiasis. (Derived from Higgs and Wells, 1972)

Group	Genetic group	Classification	Clinical features
1	Autosomal recessive	Familial chronic mucocutaneous candidiasis	Onset usually before 5 years
2	Unknown	Chronic mucocutaneous candidiasis with susceptibility to sinopulmonary infections	Early onset
3	Autosomal	Chronic mucocutaneous candidiasis with endocrinopathy	Early onset. Associated hypoparathyroidism, hypothyroidism, hypoadrenalism, diabetes mellitus and pernicious anaemia
4	Probably not genetically determined	Chronic mucocutaneous candidiasis	Onset in adult life; in one patient, associated malignant lymphoma and myopathy

immunity, can be demonstrated (Valdimarsson, Higgs, Wells, Yamamura, Hobbs and Holt, 1973; Higgs and Wells, 1972). The T-cell changes are distinct from the more severe T-cell defects found in other immuno-deficiency diseases such as in the Di George syndrome and in severe combined immunodeficiency. It is interesting that in some patients there is a dissociation between *in-vitro* and *in-vivo* tests of cellular immunity and this discordance might be explained by the fact that different populations of lymphocytes are responsible either for delayed type hypersensitivity skin reactions or lymphocyte transformation and MIF production (Bloom, Gaffney and Jimenez, 1972). Some patients have no evidence of immune deficiency while others appear to have cellular immune defects secondary to their *Candida* infection and which may be reversed by successful treatment with amphotericin B (Imperato, Buckley and Callaway, 1968; Kirkpatrick and Smith, 1974). Iron deficiency, commonly found in CMC, may be responsible for depressed lymphocyte function as the latter is reversed by iron therapy although the actual *Candida* infection does not necessarily improve (Higgs

and Wells, 1972; Fletcher, Mather, Lewis and Whiting, 1975; Nutritional Reviews, 1976).

Additional humoral abnormalities include selective IgA deficiency, and a decreased capacity to produce anti-*Candida* antibodies (Claman, Hartley and Merrill, 1966; Schlegel, Bernier, Bellanti, Maybee, Osbourne, Stewart, Pearlmann, Ouelette and Biehusen, 1970). In most patients, serum anti-*Candida* antibodies are present in high titre, but in some of these individuals the antibody appears to act as a serum blocking or inhibitory factor, as shown by its ability to suppress selectively the killing of *Candida in vitro* by normal sensitized lymphocytes (Valdimarsson, Higgs, Wells, Yamamura, Hobbs and Holt, 1973; Twomey, Waddell, Krantz, O'Reilly, L'Esperance and Good, 1975). *In vivo*, this serum factor could act by forming immune complexes with *Candida* antigen and thereby interfere with cellular responses to infection. Polymorphonuclear neutrophil leucocyte activity is usually normal, although myeloperoxidase deficiency and other enzyme changes have been reported in CMC (Lehrer and Cline, 1969; Bork and Denk, 1975; Van Scoy, Hill, Ritts and Quie, 1975).

Table 9.7 Immunological patterns in chronic mucocutaneous candidiasis. (Derived from Valdimarsson, Higgs, Wells, Yamamura, Hobbs and Holt, 1973; and Shuster and Eisen, 1976)

Immunological patterns	In-vivo tests (cutaneous delayed hypersensitivity reactions)			In-vitro tests		
	Candida	PPD	DNCB	PHA stimulation	MIF production	Candida-specific inhibitory serum factor
1	−	−	−	+	−	−
2	−	−	−	−	+	−
3	−	+	+	−	−	+
4	+	+	+	+	+	

Gastrointestinal manifestations (Table 9.8)

Candida infection has been associated with a number of gastrointestinal disorders. In some of these patients there may be a subtle cellular defect, as described above, or a secondary cause for their reduced immunity to *Candida*. In the mouth, *Candida* may be present as whitish plaques which may cause pain and discomfort during mastication (Ch. 4). *Candida* infection of the oesophagus is an unusual, but well-recognized clinical problem and may give rise to dysphagia, severe chest pain, haematemesis, oesophageal strictures and rupture (Ament, 1975; Lewicki and Moore, 1975; Ochs and Ament, 1976, Sehhat, Hazeghi, Bajoghli and Touri, 1976). Invasion of the tissues may result in monilial granuloma and it has been suggested that the intense inflammatory infiltrate found in tissues at the site of infection is due to direct activation of the alternative pathway (Ch. 2) by soluble products derived from *C. albicans* (Sohnle, Frank and Kirkpatrick, 1976).

Table 9.8 Gastrointestinal and other disorders associated with or caused by *Candida* infection

Disease	Reference
1. Oral ulcers	1
2. Oesophageal disease: dysphagia, chest pain, haematemesis, stricture and rupture	2–5
3. Gastric candidiasis	6, 7
4. Pernicious anaemia	8
5. Carbohydrate intolerance	9
6. Iron deficiency	1, 10
7. Diarrhoea	9, 11
8. Peritonitis	7
9. Anal fissures	9
10. Acute hepatic necrosis	2
11. Chronic active hepatitis and cirrhosis	2

References to Table 9.8
1. Fletcher, Mather, Lewis and Whiting (1975).
2. Ament (1975).
3. Lewicki and Moore (1975).
4. Ochs, and Ament (1976).
5. Sehhat, Hazeghi, Bajoghli and Touri (1976).
6. Nelson, Bruni and Goldstein (1975).
7. Staples, Boujak, Douglas and Leddy (1977).
8. Ammann and Hong (1973b).
9. Kumar, Chandrasekaran and Kumar (1976).
10. Higgs and Wells (1972).
11. Kane, Chretien and Garagusi (1976).

Illustrative case history
This case illustrates the range of immunological tests that may be performed in patients with *Candida* infection and the subtle T-cell defects that may be detected.

A 22-year-old Caucasian female (G. W.) had recurrent aphthous ulcers since her menarche at the age of 12. At the age of 20 years she developed dysphagia and a barium swallow showed multiple small ulcers extending

for 14 cm from the level of the carina, the distal 5 cm being narrowed. *Candida* species were grown from faeces, urine and a high vaginal swab, but not from a throat swab. She was treated with co-trimoxazole with improvement in her symptoms. However, she subsequently deteriorated, developing 1 cm diameter, punched-out ulcers on her tongue and buccal mucosa, which caused considerable pain on mastication or talking. She had a recurrence of dysphagia but no other gastrointestinal symptoms. There was a maternal family history of atopy, but no other immunological deficiency diseases, in particular 3 sisters were normal.

Oesophagoscopy showed a smooth, 'pin-hole' stricture at 31 cm (barium swallow shown in Fig. 9.6). Other investigations showed evidence of iron and folic acid deficiency, but there was no other evidence of intestinal malabsorption. Biopsy of an oral ulcer showed a dense inflammatory infiltrate consisting predominantly of lymphocytes, monocytes, neutrophils and eosinophils. Biopsy of the oesophagus showed excess inflammatory cells. A rectal biopsy was normal histologically but showed increased IgA-fluorescing cells in the lamina propria.

Treatment. After the recurrence of her *Candida* infection intravenous amphotericin B was administered

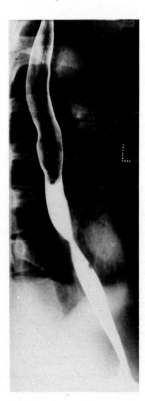

Fig. 9.6 Barium swallow in patient with dysphagia, *Candida* infection and a T-cell deficiency showing narrow stricture at 31 cm.

Table 9.9 Cellular immune function in a patient, G.W., suffering from oesophageal candidiasis

Test	G.W.	Normal subject	Comments
Peripheral blood			
T-cell quantitation	65%	68%	Normal values
B-cell quantitation	10%	14%	
Peripheral blood lymphocyte transformation (*ratio of test to control*) Mitogens:			
PHA 2.0 μg/ml	25	130	Impaired response to PHA and
PHA 0.2 μg/ml	7	39	pokeweed mitogens
Pokeweed	4	19	
Candida extract 1 mg/ml	1.7	1.3	Weak positive response to both
G.W.'s *Candida* organisms:			candida extract and the
1×10^6/ml	6	4	patient's own *Candida*
1×10^5/ml	1.3	4	organisms
PPD	3	16	Impaired PPD response
Leucocyte migration-inhibition test (*ratio of test to control*) G.W.'s *Candida* organisms:			
1×10^6/ml	0.90	0.84	Patient G.W. shows production
1×10^6/ml	1.00	1.00	of migration inhibition factor
Other *Candida* organisms:			to indifferent other *Candida*
1×10^6/ml	0.66	0.85	organisms, but not to her own
5×10^5/ml	0.68	0.88	*Candida* organisms.
Candida extract 1 mg/ml	0.69	0.85	
Candidacidal assay			
Percentage of *Candida* killed	26%	29%	Normal *in-vitro* candidacidal activity

with effect. She has been maintained on vitamin replacements, a gluten-free diet and Levamisole 150 mg daily. However, she has recently once again showed a deterioration.

Immunological investigations. *Humoral immunity.* There were normal levels of serum IgA, IgG, IgM and IgE, and a fluorescent antibody test for antibodies to *C. albicans* was positive at 1/25. In the saliva, IgA was within the normal range and there was a weak positive fluorescent antibody test for *Candida* antibodies of the IgA class only; secretory component was also present. Levels of serum C3 and C4 were grossly elevated; in addition, she showed no delayed skin reaction to PPD, *Candida* and Trichophyton.

Cellular immunity: summarized in Table 9.9.

Polymorphonuclear neutrophil leucocyte function. There was normal phagocytosis of *C. albicans*. The nitroblue tetrazolium test and tests of polymorphonuclear neutrophil leucocyte chemotaxis were normal.

Comment. This patient shows a basic lymphocyte defect with reduced *in-vitro* lymphocyte transformation to standard mitogens and *Candida* antigens, and also

cutaneous anergy, unimproved by treatment, suggesting a primary functional T-cell defect. She is, however, able to produce MIF to *Candida* antigen. The presence of normal *in-vitro* candidacial activity suggests the presence of a serum blocking factor *in vivo*.

Primary gastric candidiasis has been described with symptoms of nausea, vomiting, epigastric pain and in one case rupture of the stomach and subsequent peritonitis (Nelson, Bruni, Goldstein, 1975; Staples, Boujak, Douglas and Leddy, 1977).

C. albicans infection has also been implicated as a cause of abdominal cramps and watery diarrhoea without blood or mucus, and reversible by treatment with antifungal agents (Kane, Chretien and Garagusi, 1976; Kumar, Chandrasekaren and Kumar, 1976). Kumar *et al.* (1976) found evidence for *Candida*-induced diarrhoea in 2.5 per cent of children with diarrhoea and some of these patients also had associated carbohydrate intolerance and anal fissures. *Candida*-induced diarrhoea is often associated with malnutrition and is also described in patients who have had extensive antibiotic treatment, but in some individuals it may occur without any recognized predisposing causes (Kane *et al.* 1976).

Treatment of CMC

Apart from standard antifungal drugs such as nystatin and amphotericin B, various treatments to provide or boost an immune response to *Candida* have been tried. Transfer factor (TF) obtained from individuals showing strongly positive skin tests to *Candida* has been used successfully in association with amphotericin B, although in one patient there was a suppression of cellular immune function following the TF therapy (Kirkpatrick and Smith, 1974; Kirkpatrick and Gallin, 1975; Shulkind and Ayoub, 1975). Both foetal thymic transplantation and infusion of allogeneic lymphocytes from *Candida* skin-test positive individuals have also been tried (Kirkpatrick, 1976b). Levamisole has been shown *in vitro* to correct the failure of leucocyte migration-inhibition factor production found in some patients and could be useful in the clinical situation (Lieberman and Hsu, 1976).

COMBINED B- AND T-CELL DEFECTS

SEVERE COMBINED IMMUNODEFICIENCY DISEASE

Main immunological features

1. Profound deficit of both T- and B-cell immune systems.
2. Onset of severe recurrent infections during the first 6 months of life.

Severe combined immunodeficiency disease (SCID) consists of several disorders all characterized by a profound depression or an absence of T- and B-cell function (Hitzig, 1973). It is the second most common primary immunodeficiency syndrome and may be inherited either as an X-linked or autosomal recessive disorder (Swiss-type agammaglobulinaemia). The proportion of males to females affected is 3:1. The basic defect may be due either to an absence of stem cells, or to a failure of the thymus and bursa equivalent to develop. Approximately 50 per cent of patients with the autosomal recessive form of SCID have been found to have a deficiency of adenosine deaminase (ADA), an enzyme found in red blood cells, white cells and other tissues (Meuwissen, Pollara and Pickering, 1975; *Lancet* editorial, 1976a). Deficiency of this enzyme has been used as a marker for the carrier state of this form of SCID and as such may be useful in genetic counselling. One patient with SCID has been described with a possible membrane defect corrected *in vitro* by calcium ionophore (Kersey, Fish, Cox and August, 1977). In some but not all forms of SCID, the hypogammaglobulinaemia would appear to be secondary to the T-cell defect (Seeger, Robins,

Stevens, Klein, Waldmann, Zeltzer and Kessler, 1976; Geha, 1976).

Patients present usually within the first 6 months of life with recurrent bacterial, viral, fungal and protozoal infections which are often fatal. In particular, infections with *Candida* species, *Pneumocystis carinii* and *Cytomegalovirus* are common and it has been estimated that SCID accounts for 10 per cent of post-neonatal deaths (Rosen, 1972). Investigation shows thymus dysplasia, depletion of lymphocytes from lymphoid tissue and an absence of plasma cells in the gastrointestinal tract.

Gastrointestinal disease

Chronic diarrhoea with severe malabsorption and *Candida* infection are found in most patients (Gitlin and Craig, 1963; Hitzig, Barandun and Cottier, 1968; Rosen, 1971; Cederbaum, Niwayama, Stiehm, Neerhout, Ammann and Berman, 1974). Hitzig (1968), in a review of 70 patients, found severe diarrhoea in 86 per cent and *Candida* infection in 79 per cent. Lactose intolerance may be found initially (Dubois, Roy, Fulginiti, Merrill and Murray, 1970), but eventually severe malabsorption develops and parenteral alimentation may be required. Biopsy of the small intestine shows absent or abnormally shaped villi, crypt abscesses and, within the lamina propria, large vacuolated macrophages similar to those seen in Whipple's and chronic granulomatous disease (Horowitz, Lorenzsonn, Olsen, Albrecht and Hong, 1974). Plasma cells and lymphocytes are absent. Proctosigmoidoscopy may show a friable oedematous mucosa, while rectal biopsy shows the presence of crypt abscesses and the destruction of the surface epithelium; plasma cells are again absent.

The cause of the diarrhoea and malabsorption is not known; *Salmonella* or enteropathic *E. coli* organisms may be grown from stool cultures (Rosen, 1971), but even eradication of these infections and candidiasis may not improve the malabsorption syndrome.

Sclerosing cholangitis, cirrhosis due to large bile duct obstruction and hepatomegaly have been described in SCID and may represent the results of bacterial or viral infection of the biliary tract (Record, Eddleston, Shilkin and Williams, 1973; Thomas, Ochs and Wedgwood, 1974).

Treatment

Supportive

Appropriate antibiotics should be used for infections, and intravenous amphotericin B and topical antifungal agents may be required for *Candida* infection. Gammaglobulin replacements may be administered, but any blood products which are given and which contain viable lymphocytes should first be irradiated to avoid a graft-versus-host reaction (GVH).

Specific

These include foetal liver or thymus transplants and HLA matched or mixed lymphocyte culture (MLC) negative bone marrow grafts (Buckley, Whisnant, Schiff, Gilbertsen, Huang and Platt, 1976). These measures may lead to correction of the immune defect and a survival of up to 10 years has been reported using bone marrow grafts. However, the main danger is GVH reactions, which may be fatal, from incorrectly matched grafts. More recently, infusion of red blood cells containing normal amounts of ADA has been used to replace ADA in individuals with this enzyme-deficient form of SCID (Polmar, Stein, Schwartz, Wetzler, Chase and Hirschhorn, 1976).

ATAXIA TELANGIECTASIA

Ataxia telangiectasia may be inherited as an autosomal recessive condition and is characterized by an abnormality of mainly T-cell immunity, but 40 per cent of patients subsequently develop a selective serum IgA deficiency (Boder, 1975) although IgA may be present in secretions (Bellanti, Artenstein and Buesher, 1966). In some of these patients there is evidence of an IgG anti-IgA antibody which results in an increased catabolism of normal serum IgA (Strober, Wochner, Barlow, McFarlin and Waldmann, 1968).

Clinical onset usually occurs by 2 to 3 years, although appearance of the progressive ataxia and telangiectasia may be delayed for several years. As regards the immune-system defect, these patients are mainly subject to recurrent sinopulmonary infections and have a 10 per cent risk of developing a malignancy, usually a lymphoreticular tumour (Kirkpatrick, 1976a), but a gastric adenocarcinoma has also been described (Haerer, Jackson and Evers, 1969).

Gastrointestinal symptoms are not common, but Ament *et al.* (1973) have described mild vitamin B_{12} malabsorption in 3 of 6 patients. The malabsorption did not respond to intrinsic factor administration. Jejunal and rectal biopsies are usually normal morphologically, but IgA-fluorescing plasma cells are decreased. In IgA-deficient patients, IgA-bearing lymphocytes are present in the blood (Eidelman and Davis, 1968; Ament, Ochs and Davis, 1973). There is also evidence of hepatic dysfunction with elevated levels of alpha-fetoprotein detected in most patients (Waldmann and McIntire, 1972). This could represent a defect of liver mesenchymal tissue and it was suggested that the other manifestations of this condition are due to a generalized mesenchymal abnormality.

NEZELOF'S SYNDROME

Main immunological features

1. Absent or depressed T-cell immunity.
2. Increased susceptibility to infection.

3. Normal or near normal levels of immunoglobulins, with a variable antibody response to antigenic stimulus.

Nezelof's syndrome is a primary immunodeficiency disease characterized by markedly depressed T-cell function, but varying degrees of B-cell impairment (Nezelof, 1968). It may occur sporadically or have an autosomal recessive mode of inheritance. The cause of the condition is not known but could be due to a stem-cell defect or to thymic hypoplasia and consequent defective T-cell function. Patients usually present with recurrent infections as in SCID, but unlike the latter frequently have hepatosplenomegaly and lymphadenopathy (Lawlor, Ammann, Wright, La Franchi, Bilstrom and Stiehm, 1974). As in SCID generalized malabsorption, candidiasis and enterocolitis may be present.

Ament (1975) reported a case, that of a 6-year-old female with steatorrhoea, disaccharidase deficiency and vitamin B_{12} malabsorption. Small-intestinal biopsy showed total or partial villous atrophy with increased numbers of plasma cells together with polymorphonuclear leucocytes in the lamina propria. No pathogens or parasites were isolated from the intestine and the cause of her gastrointestinal disease was not ascertained.

Treatment

Apart from supportive therapy as described under SCID, bone marrow and thymus transplants have been tried as has the administration of transfer factor.

WISKOTT—ALDRICH SYNDROME — IMMUNODEFICIENCY WITH THROMBOCYTOPAENIA, ECZEMA AND RECURRENT INFECTION

Patients with this condition usually present in the first year of life with eczema, thrombocytopaenia and recurrent infections (Wiskott, 1937; Aldrich, Steinberg and Campbell, 1954; Huntley and Dees, 1957; Cooper, Chase, Lowman, Krivit and Good, 1968). The condition is inherited as an X-linked recessive one, but sporadic cases may also occur. T-cell function may initially be normal but deteriorates with age. A deficiency of IgM is often found and can be related to decreased synthesis. Synthesis of IgA and IgG are increased, also there appears to be an inability to respond to specific antigens as evidenced by a failure to form specific antibodies following immunization with polysaccharide antigens (Cooper, Chase, Lowman, Krivit and Good, 1968; Blaese, Strober and Waldman, 1975).

Bloody diarrhoea is a common symptom in early childhood; some patients show improvement with removal of animal protein from the diet (Wiskott, 1937; Aldrich, Steinberg and Campbell, 1954; Ament, Ochs and Davis, 1973). Ament, Ochs and Davis (1973) reported 1 patient with mild steatorrhoea and 3 patients with slightly abnormal vitamin B_{12} absorption.

Treatment

Apart from antibiotics for infections, fresh frozen plasma and transfer factor have also been utilized (Spitler, Levin, Stites, Fudenberg, Pirofsky, August, Stiehm, Hitzig and Gatti, 1972). Splenectomy, although improving the thrombocytopaenia, may be followed by a fatal infection.

PHAGOCYTE DYSFUNCTION

CHRONIC GRANULOMATOUS DISEASE

Chronic granulomatous disease is an inherited disorder characterized by recurrent infections of lymph nodes, skin, bone, liver and the gastrointestinal tract (Johnston and McMurray, 1967; Azimi, Bodenbender, Hintz and Kontras, 1968: Caldicott and Baehner, 1968; Johnston and Baehner, 1971; Baehner, 1975). The defect occurs mainly in males and may have an X-linked inheritance. The abnormality lies in polymorphonuclear leucocytes and monocytes, where phagocytosis can occur, but not killing of certain organisms. Patients usually present by 2 years of age and on examination are often found to have hepatosplenomegaly and lymphadenopathy. Diagnosis can be confirmed by bacteriocidal assay and using the quantitative nitroblue tetrazolium dye reduction assay. T- and B-cell function is normal with hypergammaglobulinaemia due to infection.

An unusual presenting feature may be upper gastrointestinal obstruction due to gastric antral narrowing caused by local granulomatous thickening of the stomach wall (Girdany, 1973). Ament and Ochs (1973) investigated 9 patients with chronic granulomatous disease and found that 4 complained of diarrhoea or vomiting. Steatorrhoea and vitamin B_{12} malabsorption were also present in some of their patients. In biopsies of the small bowel the villous architecture appeared normal; however, lipid-filled pigmented histiocytes were seen in the lamina propria – similar to those seen in Whipple's disease. The same appearance was seen in rectal biopsies, but in addition giant cells and granulomas were present in 5 patients. One of their patients had X-ray changes and histological abnormalities consistent with Crohn's disease involving the small intestine and colon. Other gastrointestinal findings are ulcerative stomatitis, fistulation and perianal abscesses in twenty per cent of patients (Johnston and McMurray, 1967; Johnston and Baehner, 1971). Other forms of neutrophil dysfunction may predispose to a carrier state for HB_sAg (Vierucci, de Martino, London and Blumberg, 1977).

Treatment

Infections should be treated with broad-spectrum antibiotics; continuous prophylactic infusions of white blood cells have also been used.

HLA HAPLOTYPES AND IMMUNODEFICIENCY DISEASE

The association of HLA and B-cell allo-antigen phenotypes with certain disease states suggests that either an increased susceptibility or an increased resistance to a particular disease is conferred by the genes of the major histocompatibility complex. Examination of the HLA phenotypes of patients with immunodeficiency diseases has shown conflicting results; this may in part be due to the different geographical populations studied and also due to the relatively small numbers of patients available.

Hors, Griscelli, Schmid and Dausset (1974) reported a significant increase of HLA-A1 in patients with a variety of primary immunodeficiency disorders, but without the classical HLA-A1, B8 linkage disequilibrium found in Caucasian populations. This absence of an HLA-A1, B8 linkage disequilibrium was confirmed by Hagle, Evers, Leven and Kruger (1976), who also found a decrease in HLA-B8. However, Buckley, MacQueen and Ward (1976) found a normal incidence of HLA-A1 in a similar group of patients, but an increased incidence of HLA-A2 and a decreased incidence of HLA-A3. They also reported the finding of a haplotype difference between a pair of siblings with X-linked hypogammaglobulinaemia and between a pair with common variable hypogammaglobulinaemia, suggesting that these immune deficits are not linked to the major histocompatibility complex.

In IgA deficiency an increased incidence of HLA-B8 together with HLA-A1 has been described (Bajtai, Hernadi and Ambrus, 1976). This is of interest in view of the association of HLA-A1 and B8, with autoimmune disease and with coeliac disease, in both of which IgA deficiency may be present (Wells, Michaeli and Fudenberg, 1975). It would be relevant to know whether or not patients with IgA deficiency and the HLA-A1, B8 haplotype have an increased tendency to disease compared to those IgA-deficient individuals without this haplotype, as this might allow identification of 'at risk' IgA-deficient individuals. Finally, Berkel and Ersoy (1976) reported an increase in HLA-BW17 and a decreased frequency of HLA-A1 and B8 in patients with hereditary ataxia telangiectasia.

In summary, this occurrence of an altered frequency of various HLA-A locus antigens in immunodeficiency disease compared to normal control populations suggests that a genetic locus closely associated or linked with the HLA-A locus could be involved in the control of immune differentiation.

CONCLUSIONS

Documentation of gastrointestinal disease in patients with immune deficiency is now extensive. In spite of this, the mechanism by which the defect produces disease is still not clear. Also, there is often a poor correlation between the extent of the deficiency and the results of laboratory findings with respect to gastrointestinal function. The variable appearance of jejunal biopsies in patients with apparently similar B-cell or T-cell abnormalities is one example. Sampling errors may account for this as the mucosal lesions may be patchy; multiple intestinal biopsies could overcome this difficulty. It is also possible that immune defects which appear similar on initial screening may, on further more detailed investigation, show important differences. Thus,

there may be several subgroups of patients, one being more susceptible to intestinal disease. The finding of an apparently normal intestine in patients with a major defect in mucosal IgA production is interesting and paradoxical in view of the importance of this immunoglobulin in mucosal defences. Presumably, other immunoglobulins, for example IgM, can compensate for the primary defect.

Finally, although the occurrence of pernicious anaemia, coeliac disease, inflammatory bowel disease, intestinal neoplasms and other intestinal diseases in patients with immune deficiency may be chance associations, the immune abnormality may be aetiologically important and studies of such patients could help in understanding the basic mechanisms underlying such diseases.

REFERENCES

Aarli, J. A. & Tönder, O. (1975) Effect of antiepileptic drugs on serum and salivary IgA. *Scandinavian Journal of Immunology*, **4**, 391–396.

Abdou, N. I., Cassela, S. R., Abdou, N. L. & Abrahamsohn, I. A. (1973) Comparative study of bone marrow and blood B cells in infantile and acquired agammaglobulinaemia. *Journal of Clinical Investigation*, **52**, 2218–2224.

Ajdukiewicz, A. B., Youngs, G. R. & Bouchier, I. A. D. (1972) Nodular lymphoid hyperplasia with hypogammaglobulinaemia. *Gut*, **13**, 589–595.

Aldrich, R. A., Steinberg, A. G. & Campbell, D. C. (1954) Pedigree demonstrating a sex-linked recessive condition characterised by draining ears, exczematoid dermatitis and bloody diarrhoea. *Pediatrics*, **13**, 133–139.

Allen, G. E. & Hadden, D. R. (1964) Congenital hypogammaglobulinaemia with steatorrhoea in two adult brothers. *British Medical Journal*, **ii**, 486–490.

Ament, M. E. (1975) Immunodeficiency syndromes and gastrointestinal disease. *Pediatric Clinics of North America*, **22**, 807–825.

Ament, M. E. & Ochs, H. D. (1973) Gastrointestinal manifestations of chronic granulomatous disease. *New England Journal of Medicine*, **288**, 382–387.

Ament, M. E. & Rubin, C. E. (1972) Relation of giardiasis to abnormal intestinal structure and function in gastrointestinal immunodeficiency syndromes. *Gastroenterology*, **62**, 216–226.

Ament, M. E., Ochs, H. D. & Davis, S. D. (1973) Structure and function of the gastrointestinal tract in primary immunodeficiency syndromes: a study of 39 patients. *Medicine*, **52**, 227–248.

Ammann, A. J. & Hong, R. (1971a) Unique antibody to basement membrane in patients with selective IgA deficiency and coeliac disease. *Lancet*, **i**, 1264–1266.

Ammann, A. J. & Hong, R. (1971b) Selective IgA deficiency. Presentation of 30 cases and a review of the literature. *Medicine*, **50**, 223–236.

Ammann, A. J. & Hong, R. (1973a) Selective IgA deficiency. *Immunologic Disorders in Infants and Children*, ed. Stiehm, E. R. and Fulginiti, V. A., Ch. 13, pp. 199–214. Philadelphia: Saunders.

Ammann, A. J. & Hong, R. (1973b) Cellular immunodeficiency disorders. *Immunologic Disorders in*

Infants and Children, ed. Stiehm, E. R. & Fulginiti, V. A., Ch. 15, pp. 236–272. Philadelphia: Saunders.

Anderson, K. E., Finlayson, N. D. C. & Deschner, E. E. (1974) Intractable malabsorption with a flat jejunal mucosa and selective IgA deficiency. *Gastroenterology*, **67**, 709–716.

Anderson, F. L., Pellegrino, E. D. & Schaefer, J. W. (1970) Dysgammaglobulinaemia associated with malabsorption and tetany. *American Journal of Digestive Diseases*, **15**, 279–286.

Ansaldi, N., Santini, B. & Marengo, M. L. (1974) Deficit selettivo di IgA e mallatia celiaca. *Minerva Pediatrica*, **26**, 651–655.

Asquith, P. (1970) 'Adult coeliac disease. A clinical morphological and immunological study.' M.D. Thesis, Birmingham University.

Asquith, P. (1974) Immunology. In *Clinics in Gastroenterology*, ed. Cooke, W. T. & Asquith, P., Vol. 3, No. 1, pp. 213–234. London: Saunders.

Asquith, P., Thompson, R. A. & Cooke, W. T. (1969) Serum-immunoglobulins in adult coeliac disease. *Lancet*, **ii**, 129–131.

Azimi, P. H., Bodenbender, J. G., Hintz, R. L., Kontras, S. B. (1968) Chronic granulomatous disease in three female siblings. *Journal of the American Medical Association*, **206**, 2865–2870.

Bachmann, R. (1965) Studies on the serum gamma A-globulin level. III. The frequency of A-gamma-A-globulinemia. *Scandinavian Journal of Clinical Laboratory Investigation*, **17**, 316–320.

Baehner, R. L. (1975) The growth and development of our understanding of chronic granulomatous disease. In: *The Phagocytic Cell in Host Resistance*, ed. Bellanti, J. A. & Dayton, D. M., pp. 173–200. New York: Raven Press.

Bajtai, G., Hernadi, E., Ambrus, M. (1976) HLA-A1 and B8 antigens in selective IgA deficiency. In *HLA and Disease. Abstracts*, Vol. 58, p. 193. Paris: Inserm.

Barandun, S., Morell, A., Skvaril, F. & Oberdorfer, A. (1976) Deficiency of κ- or λ-type immunoglobulins. *Blood*, **47**, 79–89.

Barnes, G. L. & Kay, R. (1977) Blood-groups in giardiasis. *Lancet*, **i**, 808.

Bellanti, J. A., Artenstein, M. S. & Buescner, E. L. (1966) Ataxia telangiectasia. Immunologic and virologic studies of serum and respiratory secretions. *Pediatrics*, **37**, 1924–1966.

Benbassat, J., Keren, L. & Zlotnic, A. (1973) Hepatitis in selective IgA deficiency. *British Medical Journal*, **iv**, 762–763.

Bergman, L., Johansson, S. G. O. & Krause, U. (1973) The immunoglobulin concentrations in serum and bowel secretion in patients with Crohn's disease. *Scandinavian Journal of Gastroenterology*, **8**, 401–406.

Berkel, A. I. & Ersoy, F. (1976) HLA antigens in ataxia-telangiectasia. In *HLA and Disease. Abstracts*, Vol. 58, p. 194. Paris: Inserm.

Bernheim, M., Creyssel, R., Gilly, R. & Fournier, P. (1959) Agammaglobulinémie congénitale avec stéatorrhée chez deux jumeux hétérozygotes de sexe différent. *Pédiatric*, **14**, 881–886.

Bernier, G. M., Gunderman, J. R., Ruymann, F. B. (1972) Kappa-chain deficiency. *Blood*, **40**, 795–805.

Binder, H. J. & Reynolds, R. D. (1967) Control of diarrhoea in secondary hypogammaglobulinaemia by fresh plasma infusions. *New England Journal of Medicine*, **277**, 802–803.

Bird, D. C., Jacobs, J. B., Silbiger, J. & Wolff, S. M. (1969) Hypogammaglobulinemia with nodular hyperplasia of the intestine. Report of a case with rectosigmoid involvement. *Radiology*, **92**, 1535–1536.

Bjernulf, A., Johansson, S. G. O. & Parrow, A. (1971) Immunoglobulin studies in gastrointestinal dysfunction with special reference to IgA deficiency. *Acta Medica Scandinavica*, **190**, 71–77.

Blaese, R. M., Strober, W. & Waldmann, T. A. (1975) Immunodeficiency in the Wiskott–Aldrich syndrome. *Birth Defects: Original Article Series*, **11**, 250–254.

Bloom, B. R., Gaffney, J. & Jimenez, L. (1972) Dissociation of MIF production and cell proliferation. *Journal of Immunology*, **109**, 1395–1398.

Boder, E. (1975) Ataxia-telangiectasia: some historic, clinical and pathologic observations. *Birth Defects*, **11**, 255–270.

Bolton, P. M., James, S. L., Newcombe, R. G., Whitehead, R. H. & Hughes, L. E. (1974) The immune competence of patients with inflammatory bowel disease. *Gut*, **15**, 213–219.

Boorman, G. A., Lina, P. H. C., Zurcher, C. & Nieuwerkerk, H. T. M. (1973) Hexamita and Giardia as a cause of mortality in congenital thymus-less (nude) mice. *Clinical and Experimental Immunology*, **15**, 623–627.

Bork, K. & Denk, R. (1975) Granulocytenfunktionsdefekte bei granulomatoser muco-cutaner candidiasis. *Archives for Dermatological Research*, **254**, 233–238.

Broom, B. C., de la Concha, E. G., Webster, A. D. B., Loewi, G. & Asherson, G. L. (1975) Dichotomy between immunoglobulin synthesis by cells in gut and blood of patients with hypogammaglobulinaemia. *Lancet*, **ii**, 253–256.

Brown, D. L., Cooper, A. G., Hepner, G. W. (1969) IgM metabolism in coeliac disease. *Lancet*, **i**, 858–861.

Brown, I. L., Ferguson, A., Carswell, F., Horne, C. H. W. & MacSween, R. N. M. (1973) Autoantibodies in children with coeliac disease. *Clinical and Experimental Immunology*, **13**, 373–382.

Brown, W. R., Lansford, C. L. & Hornbrook, M. (1973) Serum immunoglobulin E (IgE) concentrations in patients with gastrointestinal disorders. *American Journal of Digestive Diseases*, **18**, 641–645.

Brown, W. R., Butterfield, D., Savage, D. & Tada, T. (1972) Clinical, microbiological and immunological studies in patients with immunoglobulin deficiencies and gastrointestinal disorders. *Gut*, **13**, 441–449.

Brown, W. R., Savage, D. C., Dubois, R. S., Alp, M. H., Mallory, A. & Kern, F. (1972) Intestinal microflora of immunoglobulin-deficient and normal human subjects. *Gastroenterology*, **62**, 1143–1152.

Bruton, O. C. (1952) Agammaglobulinemia. *Pediatrics*, **9**, 722–728.

Buckley, R. H. & Dees, S. C. (1969) Correlation of milk precipitins with IgA deficiency. *New England Journal of Medicine*, **281**, 465–469.

Buckley, R. H., MacQueen, J. M. & Ward, F. E. (1976) HLA antigens in primary immunodeficiency diseases. *HLA and Disease. Abstracts*, Vol. 58, p. 195. Paris: Inserm.

Buckley, R. H., Whisnant, J. K., Schiff, R. I., Gilbertsen, R. B., Huang, A. T. & Platt, M. S. (1976) Correction of severe combined immunodeficiency by fetal liver cells. *New England Journal of Medicine*, **294**, 1076–1081.

Bull, D. M. & Tomasi, T. B. (1968) Deficiency of immunoglobulin A in intestinal disease. *Gastroenterology*, **54**, 313–320.

Caldicott, W. J. H. & Baehner, R. L. (1968) Chronic granulomatous disease of childhood. *American Journal of Roentgenology and Radium Therapy*, **103**, 133–139.

Capitanio, M. A. & Kirkpatrick, J. A. (1970) Lymphoid hyperplasia of the colon in children. *Radiology*, **94**, 323–327.

Caplinger, K. J. & Boellner, S. W. (1968) Primary acquired lactase deficiency with acquired hypogammaglobulinaemia. *American Journal of Diseases of Children*, **115**, 377–387.

Caroll, J. E., Silverman, A., Isobe, Y., Brown, W. R., Kelts, K. A. & Brooke, M. H. (1976) Inflammatory myopathy, IgA deficiency and intestinal malabsorption. *Journal of Pediatrics*, **89**, 216–219.

Castleman, B. & McNeely, B. U. (1971) Case records of the Massachusetts General Hospital, Case 1 – 1971. *New England Journal of Medicine*, **284**, 39–47.

Cattan, D., Debray, C., Crabbé, P., Seligmann, M., Marche, C. & Danon, F. (1966) Duodéno-jéjunite infectieuse chronique avec atrophie villositaire subtotale et stéatorrhée réversible par antibiothérapie prolongée. Carence isolée en γA-immunoglobuline sérique et salivaire. Étude histologique et immunohistochimique des muqueuses digestives. *Bulletins et Mémoires de la Société Medical des Hôpitaux de Paris*, **117**, 177–196.

Cederbaum, S. D., Niwayama, G., Stiehm, E. R., Neerhout, R. C., Ammann, A. J. & Berman, W. (1974) Combined immunodeficiency presenting as the Letterer–Siwe syndrome. *Journal of Pediatrics*, **85**, 466–471.

Claman, H. N., Hartley, T. F. & Merrill, D. (1966) Hypogammaglobulinemia, primary and secondary: immunoglobulin levels (γG, γA, γM) in one hundred and twenty-five patients. *Journal of Allergy*, **38**, 215–225.

Claman, H. N., Merrill, D. A., Peakman, D. & Robinson, A. (1970) Isolated severe gamma A deficiency: immunoglobulin levels, clinical disorders and chromosome studies. *Journal of Laboratory and Clinical Medicine*, **75**, 307–315.

Clark, R., Tornyos, K., Herbert, V. & Twomey, J. J. (1967) Studies on two patients with concomitant pernicious anaemia and immunoglobulin deficiency. *Annals of Internal Medicine*, **67**, 403–410.

Cleveland, W. W. (1975) Immunologic reconstitution in the Di George syndrome by fetal thymic transplant. *Birth Defects: Original Article Series*, **11**, 352–356.

Coelho, I. M., Pereira, M. T., Virella, G. & Thompson,

R. A. (1974) Salivary immunoglobulins in a patient with IgA deficiency. *Clinical and Experimental Immunology*, **18**, 685–699.

Cohen, N., Paley, D. & Janowitz, H. D. (1961) Acquired hypogammaglobulinemia and sprue: report of a case and review of the literature. *Journal of the Mount Sinai Hospital, New York*, **28**, 421–427.

Collins, J. R. & Ellis, D. S. (1965) Agammaglobulinemia, malabsorption and rheumatoid-like arthritis. *American Journal of Medicine*, **39**, 476–482.

Conn, H. O. & Quintiliani, R. (1966) Severe diarrhoea controlled by gamma globulin in a patient with agammaglobulinemia, amyloidosis and thymoma. *Annals of Internal Medicine*, **65**, 528–541.

Conn, H. O., Binder, H. & Burns, B. (1968) Pernicious anaemia and immunologic deficiency. *Annals of Internal Medicine*, **68**, 603–612.

Cooke, W. T., Weiner, W. & Shinton, N. K. (1957) Agammaglobulinaemia – report of two adult cases. *British Medical Journal*, **i**, 1151–1157.

Cooper, M. D., Lawton, A. R. & Bockman, D. E. (1971) Agammaglobulinaemia with B lymphocytes. Specific defect of plasma-cell differentiation. *Lancet*, **ii**, 791–795.

Cooper, M. D., Chase, H. P., Lowman, J. T., Krivit, W. & Good, R. A. (1968) Wiskott–Aldrich Syndrome. An immunologic deficiency disease involving the afferent limb of immunity. *American Journal of Medicine*, **44**, 499–513.

Corlin, R. F. & Pops, M. A. (1972) Nongranulomatous ulcerative jejunoileitis with hypogammaglobulinaemia. *Gastroenterology*, **62**, 473–478.

Cowling, D. C., Strickland, R. G., Ungar, B., Whittingham, S. & Rose, W. M. (1974) Pernicious-anaemia-like syndrome with immunoglobulin deficiency. *Medical Journal of Australia*, **1**, 15–17.

Crabbé, P. A. & Heremans, J. F. (1966) Lack of gamma A-immunoglobulin in serum of patients with steatorrhoea. *Gut*, **7**, 119–127.

Crabbé, P. A. & Heremans, J. F. (1967) Selective IgA deficiency with steatorrhoea. A new syndrome. *American Journal of Medicine*, **42**, 319–326.

Creagan, E. T. & Fraumeni, J. F. (1973) Familial gastric cancer and immunologic abnormalities. *Cancer*, **32**, 1325–1331.

Crowder, R. V., Thompson, W. T. & Kupfer, H. G. (1959) Acquired agammaglobulinemia with multiple allergies and pernicious anaemia. *Archives of Internal Medicine*, **103**, 445–452.

Davis, S. D., Eidelman, S. & Loop, J. W. (1970) Nodular lymphoid hyperplasia of the small intestine and sarcoidosis. *Archives of Internal Medicine*, **126**, 668–672.

Dedieu, P., Le Bodic, M. F., Simon, J., Le Mevel, B., de Lisle, L. R. & Miniconi, P. (1975) Entéropathie et déficit primaire en immunoglobuline A présentation d'un cas avec atrophie villositaire progressive. *Archives Françaises des Maladies de l'Appareil Digestif*, **64**, 347–357.

Deodhar, S. D., Michener, W. M. & Farmer, R. G. (1969) A study of the immunological aspects of chronic ulcerative colitis and transmural colitis. *American Journal of Clinical Pathology*, **51**, 591–597.

De Smet, A. A., Tubergen, D. G. & Martel, W. (1976) Nodular lymphoid hyperplasia of the colon associated with dysgammaglobulinaemia. *American Journal of Roentgenology*, **127**, 515–517.

Diamant, M., Kallós, P. & Rubensohn, G. (1961) Familial agammaglobulinemia. *International Archives of Allergy and Applied Immunology*, **19**, 193–201.

Diaz-Buxo, J. A., Hermans, P. E. & Elveback, L. R. (1975) Prevalence of cholelithiasis in idiopathic late-onset immunoglobulin deficiency. *Annals of Internal Medicine*, **82**, 213–214.

Diaz-Buxo, J. A., Hermans, P. E. & Huizenga, K. A. (1975) Gastrointestinal dysfunction in immunoglobulin deficiency. Effect of corticosteroids and tetracycline. *Journal of the American Medical Association*, **233**, 1189–1191.

Di George, A. M. (1968) Congenital absence of the thymus and its immunologic consequences: concurrence with congenital hypoparathyroidism. In *Immunologic Deficiency Diseases of Man*, ed. Good, R. A. & Bergsma, D. *Birth Defects: Original Article Series*, **4**, 116–121.

Dobbins, W. O. & Sahba, M. M. (1972) A possible explanation for the gastrointestinal mucosal lesion in immunoglobulin deficiency state. *American Journal of Digestive Diseases*, **17**, 23–25.

Douglas, S. D., Goldberg, L. S. & Fudenberg, H. H. (1970) Clinical, serologic and leukocyte function studies on patients with idiopathic 'acquired' agammaglobulinemia and their families. *American Journal of Medicine*, **48**, 48–53.

Douglas, S. D., Goldberg, L. S., Fudenberg, H. H. & Goldberg, S. B. (1970) Agammaglobulinaemia and co-existent pernicious anaemia. *Clinical and Experimental Immunology*, **6**, 181–187.

Dubois, R. S., Roy, C. C., Fulginiti, V. A., Merrill, D. A. & Murray, R. L. (1970) Disaccharidase deficiency in children with immunologic deficits. *Journal of Pediatrics*, **76**, 377–385.

Edelman, R., Suskind, R., Olson, R. E. & Sirisinha, S. (1973) Mechanisms of defective delayed hypersensitivity in children with protein-calorie malnutrition. *Lancet*, **i**, 506–509.

Eggert, R. C., Wilson, I. D. & Good, R. A. (1969) Agammaglobulinemia and regional enteritis. *Annals of Internal Medicine*, **71**, 581–585.

Ehtessabian, R., Cassidy, J. T., Thomas, M. R., Matthews, K. P. & Tubergen, D. G. (1976) Common variable immunodeficiency with pernicious anaemia, asthma, and reactions to gamma globulin; treatment with plasma. *Journal of Allergy and Clinical Immunology*, **58**, 337–350.

Eidelman, S. (1976) Intestinal lesions in immune deficiency. *Human Pathology*, **7**, 427–434.

Eidelman, S. & Davis, S. D. (1968) Immunoglobulin content of intestinal mucosal plasma-cells in ataxia telangiectasia. *Lancet*, **i**, 884–886.

Eisner, J. W. & Bralow, S. P. (1968) Intestinal lymphangiectasia with immunoglobulin A deficiency. *American Journal of Digestive Diseases*, **13**, 1055–1064.

Ertel, I. J. (1973) Yearbook of Pediatrics, ed. Gellis, S. S., pp. 107–108. Chicago: Year Book Medical Publishers.

Faed, M. J. W., Whyte, R., Paterson, C. R., McCathie, M. & Robertson, J. (1972) Deletion of the long arms of chromosome 18 (46,XX,18q−) associated with absence of IgA and hypothyroidism in an adult. *Journal of Medical Genetics*, **9**, 102–105.

Falchuk, K. R. & Falchuk, Z. M. (1975) Selective immunoglobulin A deficiency, ulcerative colitis and gluten-sensitive enteropathy – a unique association. *Gastroenterology*, **69**, 503–506.

Fieber, S. S. & Schaefer, H. J. (1966) Lymphoid hyperplasia of the terminal ileum – a clinical entity? *Gastroenterology*, **50**, 83–98.

Firkin, B. G. & Blackburn, C. R. B. (1958) Congenital and acquired agammaglobulinaemia. A report of four cases. *Quarterly Journal of Medicine*, **27**, 187–205.

Fixa, B., Thiele, H. G., Komárková, O. & Nožička, Z. (1972) Gastric autoantibodies and cell-mediated immunity in pernicious anaemia – a comparative study. *Scandinavian Journal of Gastroenterology,* **8,** 237–240.

Fletcher, J., Mather, J., Lewis, M. J. & Whiting, G. (1975) Mouth lesions in iron-deficient anaemia: relationship to *Candida albicans* in saliva and to impairment of lymphocyte transformation. *Journal of Infectious Diseases,* **131,** 44–50.

Forssman, O. & Herner, B. (1964) Acquired agammaglobulinaemia and malabsorption. *Acta Medica Scandinavica,* **176,** 779–786.

Fraser, K. J. & Rankin, J. G. (1970) Selective deficiency of IgA immunoglobulins associated with carcinoma of the stomach. *Australian Annals of Medicine,* **19,** 165–167.

Freundlich, E. (1957) Agammaglobulinemia. Report of a case. *Journal of Pediatrics,* **50,** 475–479.

Frik, W., Heinkel, K. & Zeitler, G. (1963) Vermehrung und Hyperplasie von Lymphfollikeln als Ursache granulärer Füllungsdefekte am Röntgenbild des gesamten Dunndarms. *Fortschritte Aufdem Gibiete der Röntgenstrahlen und der Nuklearmedizin,* **99,** 65–71.

Fudenberg, H. H., Good, R. A., Goodman, H. C., Hitzig, W., Kunkel, H. G., Roitt, I. M., Rosen, F. S., Rowe, D. S., Seligmann, M. & Soothill, J. R. (1971) Primary immunodeficiencies. Report of a World Health Organization Committee. *Pediatrics,* **47,** 927–946.

Fulginiti, V. A., Sieber, O. F., Claman, H. N., Merrill, D. (1966) Serum immunoglobulin measurement during the first year of life and in immunoglobulin deficiency states. *Journal of Pediatrics,* **68,** 723–730.

Gajl-Peczalska, K. J., Park, B. H., Biggar, W. D. & Good, R. A. (1973) B and T lymphocytes in primary immunodeficiency disease in man. *Journal of Clinical Investigation,* **52,** 919–928.

Gatti, R. A. & Good, R. A. (1971) Occurrence of malignancy in immunodeficiency diseases. *Cancer,* **28,** 89–98.

Geha, R. S. (1976) Is the B-cell abnormality secondary to T-cell abnormality in severe combined immuno-deficiency? *Clinical Immunology and Immunopathology,* **6,** 102–106.

Gelfand, E. W., Berkel, A. I., Godwin, H. A., Rocklin, R. E., David, J. R. & Rosen, F. S. (1972) Pernicious anaemia, hypogammaglobulinaemia and altered lymphocyte reactivity. A family study. *Clinical and Experimental Immunology,* **11,** 187–199.

Gellernt, I. M., Present, D. H. & Janowitz, H. D. (1972) Alterations in serum immunoglobulins after resection for ulcerative and granulomatous disease of the intestine. *Gut,* **13,** 21–23.

Gerson, C. D., Janowitz, H. D. & Paronetto, F. (1972) Hypogammaglobulinemia and malabsorption: immunofluorescent localization of immunoglobulins in the jejunal mucosa. *Mount Sinai Journal of Medicine, New York,* **39,** 158–164.

Gibbs, D. D. & Pryor, J. S. (1961) Hypogammaglobulinaemia ('acquired' adult form) and pernicious anaemia. *Proceedings of the Royal Society of Medicine,* **54,** 590–592.

Ginsberg, A. & Mullinax, F. (1970) Pernicious anemia and monoclonal gammopathy in a patient with IgA deficiency. *American Journal of Medicine,* **48,** 787–791.

Girdany, B. R. (1973) Chemical gastritis. In *Pediatric X-ray Diagnosis,* 6th edn. ed. Caffey, J., pp. 620–621. Chicago: Year Book Medical Publishers.

Gitlin, D. & Craig, J. M. (1963) The thymus and other lymphoid tissues in congenital agammaglobulinaemia. 1. Thymic alymphoplasia and lymphocytic hypoplasia and their relation to infection. *Pediatrics,* **32,** 517–530.

Gitlin, D., Gross, P. A. M. & Janeway, C. A. (1959) The gammaglobulins and their clinical significance. II. Hypogammaglobulinemia. *New England Journal of Medicine,* **260,** 72–76.

Gleich, G. J. & Hofmann, A. F. (1971) Use of cholestyramine to control diarrhoea associated with acquired hypogammaglobulinemia. *American Journal of Medicine,* **51,** 281–286.

Goldberg, L. S., Barnett, E. V. & Fudenberg, H. H. (1968) Selective absence of IgA: a family study. *Journal of Laboratory and Clinical Medicine,* **72,** 204–212.

Goldstein, G. W., Krivit, W. J. & Hong, R. (1969) Hypoimmunoglobulin G, hyperimmunoglobulin M, intestinal nodular hyperplasia and thrombocytopenia: an unusual association. *Archives of Diseases in Childhood,* **44,** 621–624.

Goodman, D. H., Smith, R. S. & Northey, W. T. (1967) Hypogammaglobulinemia, allergy and absence of intrinsic factor. *Journal of Allergy,* **40,** 131–134.

Green, I. & Sperber, R. J. (1962) Hypogammaglobulinemia, arthritis, sprue and megaloblastic anemia. *New York State Journal of Medicine,* **62,** 1679–1686.

Grise, J. W. (1968) Dysgammaglobulinemia with nodular lymphoid hyperplasia of the small intestine. *Radiology,* **90,** 579–580.

Grob, P. J. & Herold, G. E. (1972) Immunological abnormalities and hydantoins. *British Medical Journal,* **ii,** 561–563.

Grundbacher, F. J. (1972) Genetic aspects of selective immunoglobulin A deficiency. *Journal of Medical Genetics,* **9,** 344–347.

Gryboski, J. D., Self, T. W., Clemett, A. & Herskovic, T. (1968) Selective immunoglobulin A deficiency and intestinal nodular lymphoid hyperplasia. Correction of diarrhoea with antibiotics and plasma. *Pediatrics,* **42,** 833–837.

Haerer, A. F., Jackson, J. R. & Evers, C. G. (1969) Ataxia telangiectasia with gastric adenocarcinoma. Journal of the *American Medical Association,* **210,** 1884–1887.

Hagle, R., Evers, K. G., Leven, B. & Kruger, J. (1976) HLA frequencies in primary immunodeficiency diseases. *HLA and Disease. Abstracts,* Vol. 58, p. 200. Paris: Inserm.

Haneberg, B. & Aarskog, D. (1975) Human faecal immunoglobulins in healthy infants and children and in some with diseases affecting the intestinal tract or immune system. *Clinical and Experimental Immunology,* **22,** 210–222.

Hanson, L. A. (1968) Aspects of the absence of the IgA system. Ed. Begsma, D. & Good, R. A. *Birth Defects: Original Article Series,* **4,** 292–297.

Hardy Smith, A. & McPhee, I. W. (1971) A clinico-immunological study of ulcerative colitis and ulcerative proctitis. *Gut,* **12,** 20–26.

Harrison, M., Kilby, A., Walker-Smith, J. A., France, N. E. & Wood, C. B. S. (1976) Cows' milk protein intolerance; a possible association with gastroenteritis, lactose intolerance and IgA deficiency. *British Medical Journal,* **i,** 1501–1504.

Hazenberg, B. P., Hoedmaeker, P. J., Nieuwenhuis, P. & Mandema, E. (1968) Source of IgA in jejunal secretions. In *Protides of the Biological Fluids, 16th Colloquium,* ed. Peeters, H., pp. 491–497. Oxford: Pergamon Press.

Hermáns, P. E., Diaz-Buxo, J. A. & Stobo, J. D. (1976)

Idiopathic late-onset immunoglobulin deficiency. *American Journal of Medicine*, **61**, 221–237.

Hermans, P. E., Huizenga, K. A., Hoffman, H. N., Brown, A. L. & Markowitz, H. (1966) Dysgammaglobulinemia associated with nodular lymphoid hyperplasia of the small intestine. *American Journal of Medicine*, **40**, 78–89.

Hersh, T., Floch, M. H., Binder, H. J., Conn, H. O., Prizont, R. & Spiro, H. M. (1970) Disturbance of the jejunal and colonic bacterial flora in immunoglobulin deficiences. *American Journal of Clinical Nutrition*, **23**, 1595–1601.

Higgs, J. M. & Wells, R. S. (1972) Chronic muco-cutaneous candidiasis: associated abnormalities of iron metabolism. *British Journal of Dermatology*, **86**, Suppl. 8, 88–102.

Hitzig, W. H. (1968) The Swiss type of agammaglobulinemia. In *Immunologic Deficiency Diseases in Man*, ed. Good, R. A. & Gergsma, D. *Birth Defects: Original Article Series*, **4**, 82–87.

Hitzig, W. H. (1973) Congenital thymic and lymphocytic deficiency disorders. In *Immunologic Disorders in Infants and Children*, ed. Stiehm, E. R. & Fulgininiti, V., Ch. 14, pp. 215–235. Philadelphia: Saunders.

Hitzig, W. H., Barandun, S. & Cottier, H. (1968) Die schweizerische Form der Agammaglobulinämie. *Ergebnisse der Inneren Medizin und Kinderheilkunde*, **27**, 79–154.

Hjalmarson, O., Hanson, L. A. & Nilsson, L. Å. (1977) IgA deficiency during D.-penicillamine treatment. *British Medical Journal*, **i**, 549.

Hobbs, J. R. (1968) Immune imbalance in dysgammaglobulinaemia, type IV. *Lancet*, **i**, 110–114.

Hobbs, J. R. (1975) IgM deficiency. *Birth Defects: Original Article Series*, **11**, 112–116.

Hobbs, J. R. & Hepner, G. W. (1968) Deficiency of γM-globulin in coeliac disease. *Lancet*, **i**, 217–220.

Hodgson, J. R., Hoffman, H. N. & Huizenga, K. A. (1967) Roentgenologic features of lymphoid hyperplasia of the small intestine associated with dysgammaglobulinemia. *Radiology*, **88**, 883–888.

Hong, R. & Ammann, A. J. (1972) Selective absence of IgA, autoimmune phenomena and autoimmune disease. *American Journal of Pathology*, **69**, 491–495.

Hong, R., Schubert, W. K., Perrin, E. V. & West, C. D. (1962) Antibody deficiency syndrome associated with B-2 macroglobulinaemia. *Journal of Pediatrics*, **61**, 831–842.

Horowitz, S., Lorenzsonn, V. W., Olsen, W. A., Albrecht, R. & Hong, R. (1974) Small intestinal disease in T-cell deficiency. *Journal of Pediatrics*, **85**, 457–462.

Hors, J., Griscelli, C., Schmid, M., Dausset, J. (1974) HL-A antigens and immune deficiency states. *British Medical Journal*, **iv**, 45.

Hoskins, L. C., Winawer, S. J., Broitman, S. A., Gottlieb, L. S. & Zamcheck, N. (1967) Clinical giardiasis and intestinal malabsorption. *Gastroenterology*, **53**, 265–279.

Hudson, E. & Aldor, T. (1970) Pancreatic insufficiency and neutropenia with associated immunoglobulin deficit. *Archives of Internal Medicine*, **125**, 314–316.

Hughes, W. S., Brooks, F. P. & Conn, H. A. (1972) Serum gastrin levels in primary hypogammaglobulinemia and pernicious anemia. *American Journal of Medicine*, **77**, 746–750.

Hughes, W. S., Cerda, J. J., Holtzapple, P. & Brooks, F. P. (1971) Primary hypogammaglobulinemia and malabsorption. *Annals of Internal Medicine*, **74**, 903–910.

Huizenga, K. A. & Hermans, P. E. (1972) Association of gastric carcinoma with idiopathic late-onset immunoglobulin deficiency. *Annals of Internal Medicine*, **76**, 605–609.

Huizenga, K. A., Wollaeger, E. E., Green, P. A. & McKenzie, B. F. (1961) Serum globulin deficiencies in non-tropical sprue, with report of two cases of acquired agammaglobulinaemia. *American Journal of Medicine*, **31**, 572–580.

Huntley, C. C. & Dees, S. C. (1957) Eczema associated with thrombocytopenic purpura and purulent otitis media. Report of five fatal cases. *Pediatrics*, **19**, 351–361.

Huntley, C. C., Robins, J. B., Lyerly, A. D. & Buckley, R. H. (1971) Characterization of precipitating antibodies to ruminant serum and milk proteins in humans with selective IgA deficiency. *New England Journal of Medicine*, **284**, 7–10.

Imperato, P. J., Buckley, C. E., III & Callaway, J. L. (1968) Candida granuloma. *Archives of Dermatology*, **97**, 139–146.

Invernizzi, F., Balestrieri, G., Consogno, G., Riboldi, P. S. & Tincani, A. (1975) Anti-IgA antibodies in two brothers with selective IgA deficiency. *Acta Haematologica*, **54**, 312–320.

James, D., Asherson, G., Chanarin, I., Coghill, N., Hamilton, S., Himsworth, R. L. & Webster, D. (1974) Cell mediated immunity to intrinsic factor in autoimmune disorders. *British Medical Journal*, **iv**, 494–496.

Johansson, S. G. O., Högman, C. F. & Killander, J. (1968) Quantitative immunoglobulin determination. *Acta Pathologica et Microbiologica Scandinavica*, **74**, 519–530.

Johnson, B. L., Goldberg, L. S., Pops, M. A. & Weiner, M. (1971) Clinical and immunological studies in a case of nodular lymphoid hyperplasia of the small bowel. *Gastroenterology*, **61**, 369–374.

Johnson, R. L., Van Arsdel, P. P., Tobe, A. D. & Ching, Y. (1967) Adult hypogammaglobulinemia with malabsorption and iron deficiency anemia. *American Journal of Medicine*, **43**, 935–943.

Johnson, S. M., North, M. E., Asherson, G. L., Allsop, J., Watts, R. W. E. & Webster, A. D. B. (1977) Lymphocyte purine 5′-nucleotidase deficiency in primary hypogammaglobulinaemia. *Lancet*, **i**, 168–170.

Johnston, R. B. & Baehner, R. L. (1971) Chronic granulomatous disease: correlation between pathogenesis and clinical findings. *Pediatrics*, **48**, 730–739.

Johnston, R. B. & McMurray, J. S. (1967) Chronic familial granulomatosis: report of five cases and review of the literature. *American Journal of Diseases of Childhood*, **114**, 370–378.

Jones, E. G. & Brown, W. R. (1974) Serum and intestinal fluid immunoglobulins in patients with Giardiasis. *American Journal of Digestive Diseases*, **19**, 791–796.

Jones, E. G., Beeken, W. L., Roessner, K. D. & Brown, W. R. (1976) Serum and intestinal fluid immunoglobulins and jejunal IgA secretions in Crohn's disease. *Digestion*, **14**, 12–19.

Jose, D. G., Welch, J. S. & Doherty, R. L. (1970) Humoral and cellular immune responses to Streptococci, influenza and other antigens in Australian Aboriginal school children. *Australian Pediatric Journal*, **6**, 192–202.

Joske, R. A. (1975) Haemochromatosis, active chronic hepatitis and familial IgA deficiency. *Digestion*, **12**, 32–38.

Kabler, J. D. (1960) Rare malabsorption syndromes. *Annals of Internal Medicine*, **52**, 1221–1235.

Kane, J. G., Chretien, J. H. & Garagusi, V. F. (1976) Diarrhoea caused by Candida. *Lancet*, **i**, 335–336.

Keightly, R. G., Cooper, M. D. & Lawton, A. R. (1976) The T cell dependence of B cell differentiation induced by pokeweed mitogen. *Journal of Immunology*, **117**, 1538–1544.

Kersey, J. H., Spector, B. D. & Good, R. A. (1973) Primary immunodeficiency disease and cancer, the immune deficiency cancer-registry. *International Journal of Cancer*, **12**, 333–347.

Kersey, J. H., Fish, L. A., Cox, S. T., August, C. S. (1977) Severe combined immunodeficiency with response to calcium ionophore: a possible membrane defect. *Clinical Immunology and Immunopathology*, **7**, 62–68.

Kirk, B. W. & Freedman, S. O. (1967) Hypogammaglobulinemia, thymoma and ulcerative colitis. *Canadian Medical Association Journal*, **96**, 1272–1277.

Kirkpatrick, C. H. (1976a) Cancer and immunodeficiency diseases. *Birth Defects: Original Article Series*, **12**, 61–78.

Kirkpatrick, C. H. (1976b) Reconstitution of defective cellular immunity with foetal thymus and dialysable transfer factor. Long term studies in a patient with chronic mucocutaneous Candidiasis. *Clinical and Experimental Immunology*, **23**, 414–428.

Kirkpatrick, C. H. & Gallin, J. I. (1975) Suppression of cellular immune responses following transfer factor: report of a case. *Cellular Immunology*, **15**, 470–474.

Kirkpatrick, C. H. & Smith, T. K. (1974) Chronic mucocutaneous Candidiasis: immunologic and antibiotic therapy. *Annals of Internal Medicine*, **80**, 310–320.

Kirkpatrick, C. H., Waxman, D., Smith, O. D. & Schimke, R. N. (1968) Hypogammaglobinemia with nodular lymphoid hyperplasia of the small bowel. *Archives of Internal Medicine*, **121**, 273–277.

Koistinen, J. (1976) Familial clustering of selective IgA deficiency. *Vox Sanguinis*, **30**, 181–190.

Koistinen, J. & Sarna, S. (1976) Immunological abnormalities in the sera of IgA deficient blood donors. *Vox Sanguinis*, **29**, 203–213.

Kopp, W. L., Trier, J. S., Stiehm, E. R. & Foroozan, P. (1968) 'Acquired' agammaglobulinaemia with defective delayed hypersensitivity. *Annals of Internal Medicine*, **69**, 309–317.

Kraft, S. C., Ford, H. E., McCleery, J. L., Kirsner, J. B. (1968) Serum immunoglobulin levels in ulcerative colitis and Crohn's disease. *Gastroenterology*, **54**, 1251.

Krakauer, R., Zinneman, H. H. & Hong, R. (1975) Deficiency of secretory IgA and intestinal malabsorption. *American Journal of Gastroenterology*, **64**, 319–323.

Kumar, V., Chandrasekaran, R. & Kumar, L. (1976) Candida diarrhoea. *Lancet*, **i**, 752.

Lancet editorial (1976a) A.D.A. Deficiency. *Lancet*, **i**, 895–896.

Lancet editorial (1976b) Temporary gluten intolerance. *Lancet*, **ii**, 555.

Larsson, S. O., Hagelquist, E. & Cöster, C. (1961) Hypogammaglobulinaemia and pernicious anaemia. *Acta Haematologica*, **26**, 50–64.

Lawlor, G. J., Ammann, A. J., Wright, W. C., La Franchi, S. H., Bilstrom, D. & Stiehm, E. R. (1974) The syndrome of cellular immunodeficiency with immunoglobulins. *Journal of Paediatrics*, **84**, 183–192.

Lawton, A. R., Royal, S. A., Self, K. S. & Cooper, M. D. (1972) IgA determinants on B-lymphocytes in patients with deficiency of circulating IgA. *Journal of Laboratory and Clinical Medicine*, **80**, 26–33.

Le Bodic, M. F., Le Bodic, L., Dedieu, P. & Mussini-Montpellier, J. (1975) Entéropathies et déficit en IgA. A propos de deux observations. *Archives d'Anatomie Pathologique*, **23**, 159–166.

Lee, F. I., Jenkins, G. C., Hughes, D. T. D. & Kazantzis, G. (1964) Pernicious anaemia, myxoedema and hypogammaglobulinaemia – a family study. *British Medical Journal*, **i**, 598–602.

Lehrer, R. I. & Cline, M. J. (1969) Leucocyte myeloperoxidase deficiency and disseminated Candidiasis: the role of myeloperoxidase in resistance to Candida infection. *Journal of Clinical Investigation*, **48**, 1478–1488.

Leisti, J., Leisti, S., Perheentupa, J., Savilahti, G. & Aula, P. (1973) Absence of IgA and growth hormone deficiency associated with short arm deletion of chromosome 18. *Archives of Diseases in Childhood*, **48**, 320–322.

Levin, D. M., Lipsky, P. E. & Kirkpatrick, C. H. (1975) Selective hypogammaglobulinaemia with persistence of IgE, malabsorption and a nutritionally dependent reversible defect in cell-mediated immunity. *American Journal of Medicine*, **58**, 129–134.

Lewicki, A. M. & Moore, J. P. (1975) Esophageal moniliasis. *American Journal of Roentgenology and Radium Therapy*, **125**, 218–225.

Lewis, E. C. & Brown, H. E. (1957) Agammaglobulinemia associated with pernicious anaemia and diabetes mellitus. *Archives of Internal Medicine*, **100**, 296–299.

Lewkonia, R. M., Gairdner, D. & Doe, W. F. (1976) IgA deficiency in one of identical twins. *British Medical Journal*, **i**, 311–313.

Lieberman, R. & Hsu, M. (1976) Levamisole-mediated restoration of cellular immunity in peripheral blood lymphocytes of patients with immunodeficiency diseases. *Clinical Immunology and Immunopathology*, **5**, 142–146.

Mann, J. G., Brown, W. R. & Kern, F. (1970) The subtle and variable clinical expressions of gluten-induced enteropathy (adult celiac disease, nontropical sprue). *American Journal of Medicine*, **48**, 357–366.

Mawas, C., Sors, C. & Bernier, J.J. (1969) Amyloidosis associated with primary agammaglobulinemia, severe diarrhoea and familial hypogammaglobulinemia. *American Journal of Medicine*, **46**, 624–634.

McCarthy, C. F., Austad, W. I. & Read, A. E. (1965) Hypogammaglobulinemia and steatorrhoea. *American Journal of Digestive Diseases*, **10**, 945–957.

McClelland, D. B. L., Shearman, D. J. C. & Van Furth, R. (1976) Synthesis of immunoglobulin and secretory component by gastrointestinal mucosa in patients with hypogammaglobulinaemia or IgA deficiency. *Clinical and Experimental Immunology*, **25**, 103–111.

McClelland, D. B. L., Warrwick, R. R. G. & Shearman, D. J. C. (1973) IgA concentration. *American Journal of Digestive Diseases*, **18**, 347–348.

McLoughlin, G. A., Bradley, J., Chapman, D. M., Temple, J. G., Hede, J. E. & McFarland, J. (1976) IgA deficiency and severe post vagotomy diarrhoea. *Lancet*, **i**, 168–170.

Medical Research Working Party on Hypogammaglobulinaemia (1971) Hypogammaglobulinaemia in the United Kingdom. *Medical Research Council Special Report Series*, **310**, 125.

Meisel, J. L., Perera, D. R., Meligios, C. & Rubin, C. E. (1976) Overwhelming watery diarrhoea associated with a cryptosporidium in an immunosuppressed patient. *Gastroenterology*, **70**, 1156–1160.

Meuwissen, H. J., Pollara, B. & Pickering, R. J. (1975) Combined immunodeficiency disease associated with adenosine deaminase deficiency. *Journal of Pediatrics*, **86**, 169–181.

Michaels, D. L., Go, S., Humbert, J. R., Dubois, R. S., Stewart, J. M. & Ellis, E. F. (1971) Intestinal nodular lymphoid hyperplasia, hypogammaglobulinemia and hematologic abnormalities in a child with ring 18 chromosome. *Journal of Pediatrics*, **79**, 80–88.

Michel, F. B., Guendon, R. & Guerco, A. J. (1976) IgE sériques des sujets ayant un déficit en IgA avec ou sans atopie. *La Nouvelle Presse Médicale*, 5, 1811–1814.

Miller, W. V., Holland, P. V., Sugarbaker, E., Strober, W. & Waldmann, T. A. (1970) Anaphylactic reactions to IgA: a difficult transfusion problem. *American Journal of Clinical Pathology*, 54, 618–621.

Moroz, C., Amir, J. & De Vries, A. (1971) A hereditary immunoglobulin A abnormality: absence of light-heavy-chain assembly. *Journal of Clinical Investigation*, 50, 2726–2733.

Nelson, R. S., Bruni, H. C. & Goldstein, H. M. (1975) Primary gastric Candidiasis in uncompromised subjects. *Gastrointestinal Endoscopy*, 22, 92–94.

Nezelof, C. (1968) Thymic dysplasia with normal immunoglobulins and immunologic deficiency: pure alymphocytosis. In *Immunologic Deficiency Disease in Man*, ed. Good, R. A. & Bergman, D. *Birth Defects: Original Article Series*, 4, 104–112.

Nutritional reviews (1976) Mucocutaneous fungal lesions and iron deficiency. *Nutritional Reviews*, 34, 203–204.

Ochs, H. D. & Ament, M. E. (1976) Gastrointestinal tract and immunodeficiency. In *Immunological Aspects of the Liver and Gastrointestinal Tract*. ed. Ferguson, A. & MacSween, R. N. M., Ch. 3, pp. 83–120. Lancaster: MTP Press.

Ochs, H. D., Ament, M. E. & Davis, S. D. (1972) Giardiasis with malabsorption in X-linked agammaglobulinaemia. *New England Journal of Medicine*, 287, 341–342.

Ogra, P. L., Ogra, S. S. & Coppola, P. R. (1975) Secretory component and sudden-infant-death syndrome. *Lancet*, ii, 387–390.

Parkin, D. M., McClelland, D. B. L., O'Moore, R. R., Percy-Robb, I. W., Grant, I. W. B. & Shearman, D. J. C. (1972) Intestinal bacterial flora and bile salt studies in hypogammaglobulinaemia. *Gut*, 13, 182–188.

Pelkonen, R., Siurala, M. & Vuopio, P. (1963) Inherited agammaglobulinemia with malabsorption and marked alterations in the gastrointestinal mucosa. *Acta Medica Scandinavica*, 173, 549–555.

Penny, R. (1969) Nodular lymphoid hyperplasia of the small intestine and hypogammaglobulinemia. *Gastroenterology*, 56, 982–985.

Perret, A. D., Higgins, G., Johnston, H. H., Massarella, G. R., Truelove, S. C. & Wright, R. (1971a) The liver in Crohn's disease. *Quarterly Journal of Medicine*, 40, 187–209.

Perret, A. D., Higgins, G., Johnston, H. H., Massarella, G. R., Truelove, S. C. & Wright, R. (1971b) The liver in ulcerative colitis. *Quarterly Journal of Medicine*, 40, 211–238.

Persson, S. (1974) Studies on Crohn's disease. III. Concentrations of immunoglobulins G, A and M in the mucosa of the terminal ileum. *Acta Chirurgica Scandinavica*, 140, 64–67.

Poen, H., Ballieux, R. E., Mul, N. A. J., Stoop, J. W., Ten Thije, O. J., Zegers, B. J. M. (1968) Increased serum IgA in intestinal disease. *Protides of the Biological Fluids*, 16, 485–489.

Polmar, S. H., Stein, R. C., Schwartz, A. L., Wetzler, E. M., Chase, P. A. & Hirschhorn, R. (1976) Enzyme replacement therapy for adenosine deaminase deficiency and severe combined immunodeficiency. *New England Journal of Medicine*, 295, 1337–1343.

Pons Romero, F., Cabarcos, A., Uribarrena, R., Borda Celaya, F. & Perez Miranda, M. (1976) Immunidad celular y humoral en la ileitis regional. Hallazgos en siete observaciones. *Revista Clinica Española*, 142, 541–545.

Popović, O., Andjić, J. & Paljm, A. (1976) Treatment of malabsorption in patients with variable immune deficiency/VID and selective IgA deficiency/S IgAD. *Proceedings 10th International Congress of Gastroenterology, Budapest 1976*, A 609.

Preud'Homme, J. L., Griscelli, C. & Seligmann, M. (1973) Immunoglobulins on the surface of lymphocytes in fifty patients with primary immunodeficiency diseases. *Clinical Immunology and Immunopathology*, 1, 241–256.

Proesmans, W., Jaeken, J. & Eekels, R. (1976) D-penicillamine induced IgA deficiency in Wilson's Disease. *Lancet*, ii, 804–805.

Record, C. O., Eddleston, A. L. W. F., Shilkin, K. B. & Williams, R. (1973) Intrahepatic sclerosing cholangitis associated with a familial immunodeficiency syndrome. *Lancet*, ii, 18–20.

Rosecan, M., Trobaugh, F. E. & Danforth, W. H. (1955) Agammaglobulinemia in the adult. *American Journal of Medicine*, 19, 303–313.

Rosen, F. S. (1971) The thymus gland and the immune deficiency syndromes. In *Immunological Disease*, ed. Samter, M., Vol. 1, pp. 497–519. Boston: Little, Brown.

Rosen, F. S. (1972) Immunity deficiency in children. *British Journal of Clinical Practice*, 26, 315–322.

Rosen, F. S. (1974) Primary immunodeficiency. *The Pediatric Clinics of North America*, 21, 533–549.

Rosen, F. S. & Janeway, C. A. (1966) The gammaglobulins. III. The antibody deficiency syndromes. *New England Journal of Medicine*, 275, 709–715.

Rosen, F. S., Kevy, S. V., Merler, E., Janeway, C. A. & Gitlin, D. (1961) Recurrent bacterial infections and dysgammaglobulinemia: deficiency of 7S gammaglobulins in the presence of elevated 19S gammaglobulins. *Pediatrics*, 28, 182–205.

Ross, I. N. & Asquith, P. (1977) Selective IgA deficiency in a patient with Crohn's disease. Unpublished observations.

Ross, I. N. & Thompson, R. A. (1976) Severe selective IgM deficiency. *Journal of Clinical Pathology*, 29, 773–777.

Sailer, D., Ullmann, B. & Berg, G. (1976) Serum-immunoglobulinspiegel bei colitis ulcerosa und morbus Crohn. *Deutsche Medizinische Wochenschrift*, 101, 1214–1217.

Sampson, D., Rodey, G. E., Finik, J., Junkerman, C. L. & Metzig, J. (1977) Splenic suppressor cells in hypogammaglobulinaemia. *British Medical Journal*, i, 614.

Samuel, A. M. & Jarnum, S. (1971) Malabsorption syndrome with IgA deficiency. *Journal of the Indian Medical Association*, 57, 290–292.

Sanford, J. P., Favour, C. B. & Tribeman, M. S. (1954) Absence of serum gamma globulins in an adult. *New England Journal of Medicine*, 250, 1027–1029.

Savilahti, E., Pelkonen, P. & Visakorpi, J. K. (1971) IgA deficiency in children. A clinical study with special reference to intestinal findings. *Archives of Diseases of Childhood*, 46, 665–670.

Schlegel, R. J., Bernier, G. M., Bellanti, J. A., Maybee, D. A., Osbourne, G. B., Stewart, J. L., Pearlman, D. S., Ouelette, J. & Biehusen, F. C. (1970) Severe candidiasis associated with thymic dysplasia, IgA deficiency and plasma antilymphocyte effects. *Pediatrics*, 45, 926–936.

Seager, J., Jamison, D. L., Wilson, J., Hayward, A. R. & Soothill, J. F. (1975) IgA deficiency, epilepsy and phenytoin treatment. *Lancet*, ii, 632–635.

Seeger, R. C., Robins, R. A., Stevens, R. H., Klein, R. B., Waldmann, D. J., Zeltzer, P. M. & Kessler, S. W. (1976) Severe combined immunodeficiency with B lymphocytes: in vitro correction of defective immunoglobulin production by addition of normal T lymphocytes. *Clinical and Experimental Immunology*, **26**, 1–10.

Sehhat, S., Hazeghi, K., Bajoghli, M. & Touri, S. (1976) Oesophageal moniliasis causing fistula formation and lung abscess. *Thorax*, **31**, 361–364.

Shulkind, M. C. & Ayoub, E. M. (1975) Transfer factor as an approach to the treatment of immune deficiency disease. *Birth Defects: Original Article Series*, **11**, 436–440.

Shuster, J. & Eisen, A. H. (1976) Immunologic deficiency diseases. In *Clinical Immunology*, 2nd edn., ed. Freedman, S. O. & Gold, P., Ch. 13. London: Harper & Row.

Skvaril, F., Barandun, S., Morell, A., Kuffer, F. & Probst, M. (1975) Imbalance of κ/λ immunoglobulin light chain ratios in normal individuals and in immunodeficient patients. Twenty-third Colloquium, Brugge. *Protides of the Biological Fluids*, ed. Peeters, H., pp. 415–420. New York: Pergamon Press.

Sohnle, P. G., Frank, M. M. & Kirkpatrick, C. H. (1976) Deposition of complement components in the cutaneous lesions of chronic mucocutaneous candidiasis. *Clinical Immunology and Immunopathology*, **5**, 340–350.

Soltis, R. D. & Wilson, I. D. (1975) Serum immunoglobulin M concentrations following bowel resection in chronic inflammatory bowel disease. *Gastroenterology*, **69**, 885–892.

Söltoft, J., Binder, V. & Gudmand-Höyer, E. (1973) Intestinal immunoglobulins in ulcerative colitis. *Scandinavian Journal of Gastroenterology*, **8**, 293–300.

Söltoft, J., Petersen, L. & Kruse, P. (1972) Immunoglobulin deficiency and regional enteritis. *Scandinavian Journal of Gastroenterology*, **7**, 233–236.

Soothill, J. F. (1974) Immunodeficiency and allergy. *Clinical Allergy*, **3**, 511–519.

South, M. A., Montgomery, J. R. & Rawls, W. E. (1975) Immune deficiency in congenital rubella and other viral infections. *Birth Defects: Original Article Series*, **11**, 234–238.

South, M. A., Cooper, M. D., Wollheim, F. A., Hong, R. & Good, R. A. (1966) The IgA system. I. Studies of the transport and immunochemistry of IgA in the saliva. *Journal of Experimental Medicine*, **123**, 615–627.

Squire, J. R. (1962) Hypogammaglobulinaemia. *Proceedings of the Royal Society of Medicine*, **55**, 393–395.

Spector, J. I. (1974) Juvenile achlorhydric pernicious anemia with IgA deficiency. *Journal of the American Medical Association*, **228**, 334–336.

Spitler, L. E., Levin, A. S., Stites, D. P., Fudenberg, H. H., Pirofsky, B., August, C. S., Stiehm, E. R., Hitzig, W. H. & Gatti, R. A. (1972) The Wiskott–Aldrich syndrome. Results of transfer factor therapy. *Journal of Clinical Investigation*, **51**, 3216–3224.

Stanworth, D. R., Johns, P., Williamson, N., Shadforth, M., Felix-Davies, D. & Thompson, R. A. (1977) Drug-induced IgA deficiency in rheumatoid arthritis. *Lancet*, **i**, 1001–1002.

Staples, P. J., Boujak, J., Douglas, R. G. & Leddy, J. P. (1977) Disseminated candidasis in a previously healthy girl: implication of a leucocyte candidacidal defect. *Clinical Immunology and Immunopathology*, **7**, 157–167.

Stewart, J. M., Go, S., Elliot, E. & Robinson, A. (1970) Absent IgA and deletions of chromosome 18. *Journal of Medical Genetics*, **7**, 11–19.

Stiehm, E. R. & Fudenberg, H. H. (1966) Clinical and immunologic features of dysgammaglobulinemia Type I. *American Journal of Medicine*, **40**, 805–815.

Stites, D. P., Levin, A. S., Lauer, B. A., Costom, B. H. & Fudenberg, H. H. (1973) Selective 'dysgamma-globulinemia' with elevated serum IgA levels and chronic salmonellosis. *American Journal of Medicine*, **54**, 260–264.

Strober, W., Krakauer, R., Klaeveman, H. L., Reynolds, H. Y. & Nelson, D. L. (1976) Secretory component deficiency: a disorder of the IgA immune system. *New England Journal of Medicine*, **294**, 351–356.

Strober, W., Wochner, R. D., Barlow, M. H., McFarlin, D. E. T. & Waldmann, T. A. (1968) Immunoglobulin metabolism in ataxia telangiectasia. *Journal of Clinical Investigation*, **47**, 1905–1915.

Swift, P. N. (1962) Hypogammaglobulinaemia, steatorrhoea and megaloblastic anaemia. Response to gluten-free diet and folic acid. *Postgraduate Medical Journal*, **38**, 633–639.

Taylor, B., Norman, A. P., Orgel, H. A., Stokes, C. R., Turner, M. W. & Soothill, J. F. (1973) Transient IgA deficiency and pathogenesis of infantile atopy. *Lancet*, **ii**, 111–113.

Thomas, I. T., Ochs, H. D. & Wedgwood, R. J. (1974) Liver disease and immunodeficiency syndromes. *Lancet*, **i**, 311.

Thompson, R. A. (1970) Secretory piece linked to IgM in individuals deficient in IgA. *Nature*, **226**, 946–948.

Thorpe, E. S. & Handley, H. E. (1929) Chronic tetany and chronic mycelial stomatitis in a child aged four and one-half years. *American Journal of Diseases of Children*, **38**, 328–338.

Tomkins, A. M., Drasar, B. S. & James, W. P. T. (1975) Bacterial colonisation of jejunal mucosa in acute tropical sprue. *Lancet*, **i**, 59–62.

Twomey, J. J. (1975) An immunological classification of pernicious anemia. *Birth Defects: Original Article Series*, **11**, 215–218.

Twomey, J. J., Jordan, P. H., Laughter, A. H., Meuwissen, H. J. & Good, R. A. (1970) The gastric disorder in immunoglobulin deficient patients. *Annals of Internal Medicine*, **72**, 499–504.

Twomey, J. J., Jordan, P. H., Jarrold, T., Trubowitz, S., Ritz, N. D. & Conn, H. O. (1969) The syndrome of immunoglobulin deficiency and pernicious anaemia. *American Journal of Medicine*, **47**, 340–350.

Twomey, J. J., Waddell, C. L., Krantz, S., O'Reilly, R., L'Esperance, P. & Good, R. A. (1975) Chronic mucocutaneous candidiasis with macrophage dysfunction, a plasma inhibitor and co-existent aplastic anaemia. *Journal of Laboratory and Clinical Medicine*, **85**, 968–977.

Uhr, J. W. & Möller, G. (1968) Regulatory effect of antibody on the immune response. *Advances in Immunology*, **8**, 81–127.

Valdimarsson, H., Higgs, J. M., Wells, R. S., Yamamura, M., Hobbs, J. R. & Holt, P. J. L. (1973) Immune abnormalities associated with chronic mucocutaneous Candidiasis. *Cellular Immunology*, **6**, 348–361.

Van der Giessen, M., Reerink-Brongers, E. E. & Algra-Van Veen, T. (1976) Quantitation of Ig classes and IgG subclasses in sera of patients with a variety of immunoglobulin deficiencies and their relatives. *Clinical Immunology and Immunopathology*, **5**, 388–398.

Van Leeuwen, L., Van Dommelen, C. K. V. (1956) Agammaglobulinemie. *Nederlands Tijdschrift Voor Geneeskunde*, **100**, 1303–1307.

Van Scoy, R. E., Hill, H. R., Ritts, R. E. & Quie, P. G. (1975) Familial neutrophil chemotaxis defect, recurrent bacterial infections, mucocutaneous Candidiasis and hyperimmunoglobulinemia E. *Annals of Internal Medicine*, **82**, 766–771.

Vierucci, A., De Martino, M., London, W. T. & Blumberg, B. J. (1977) Neutrophil function in children who are carriers of hepatitis-B surface antigen. *Lancet*, **i**, 157–161.

Vesin, P., Troupel, S., Acar, J., Renault, H., Desbuquois, G. & Cattan, R. (1960) Entéropathie avec perte de protéines et stéatorrhée. Étude par le PVP-I^{131} et la trioléine-I^{131}. Action du régime sans gluten. *Bulletin et Mémoires de la Société Médicale des Hôpitaux de Paris*, **76**, 261–271.

Visakorpi, J. A. & Immonen, P. (1967) Intolerance to cow's milk and wheat gluten in the primary malabsorption syndrome in infancy. *Acta Paediatrica Scandinavica*, **56**, 49–56.

Vyas, G. N., Holmdahl, L., Perkins, H. A. & Fudenberg, H. H. (1969) Serologic specificity of human anti-IgA and its significance in transfusion. *Blood*, **34**, 573–581.

Waldmann, T. A. & Laster, L. (1964) Abnormalities of albumin metabolism in patients with hypogammaglobulinemia. *Journal of Clinical Investigation*, **43**, 1025–1035.

Waldmann, T. A. & McIntire, K. R. (1972) Serum-alpha-fetoprotein levels in patients with ataxia-telangiectasia. *Lancet*, **ii**, 1112–1115.

Waldmann, T. A., Durm, M., Broder, S., Blackman, M., Blaese, R. M. & Strober, W. (1974) Role of suppressor T cells in pathogenesis of common variable hypogammaglobulinaemia. *Lancet*, **ii**, 609–613.

Walker-Smith, J. (1970) Transient gluten intolerance. *Archives of Disease in Childhood*, **45**, 523–526.

Webster, A. D. B. (1975) Immune deficiency disease. In *Topics in Gastroenterology*, ed. Truelove, S. C. & Goodman, M. J., No. 3, pp. 245–258. Oxford: Blackwell.

Webster, A. D. B. (1976) The gut and immunodeficiency disorders. In *Immunology of GI and Liver Disease*, ed. Wright, R., London: Saunders. Ch. 7, pp. 323–340.

Webster, A. D. B. & Asherson, G. L. (1974) Identification and function of T cells in the peripheral blood of patients with hypogammaglobulinaemia. *Clinical and Experimental Immunology*, **18**, 499–504.

Webster, A. D. B. & Brostoff, J. (1976) DNCB contact sensitivity in primary hypogammaglobulinaemia. *Lancet*, **i**, 1302.

Webster, A. D. B., Kenwright, S., Ballard, J., Shiner, M., Slavin, G., Levi, A. J., Leowi, G. & Asherson, G. L. (1977) Nodular lymphoid hyperplasia of the bowel in primary hypogammaglobulinaemia: study of *in vivo* and *in vitro* lymphocyte function. *Gut*, **18**, 364–372.

Weeke, B. & Jarnum, S. (1971) Serum concentrations of 19 serum proteins in Crohn's disease and ulcerative colitis. *Gut*, **12**, 297–302.

Wells, J. V., Michaeli, D. & Fundenberg, H. H. (1975) Auto-immunity in selective IgA deficiency. *Births Defects: Original Article Series*, **11**, 144–146.

West, C. D., Hong, R. & Holland, N. H. (1962) Immunoglobulin levels from the newborn period to adulthood and in immunoglobulin deficiency states. *Journal of Clinical Investigation*, **41**, 2054–2064.

Whitemeyer, S. B., Bankhurst, A. D., Williams, R. C. (1976) Studies on the suppression of normal B-cell maturation by peripheral blood cells from patients with acquired hypogammaglobulinaemia and from normal neonates. *Clinical and Experimental Immunology*, **6**, 312–317.

Wilson, I. D., Onstad, G. R., Williams, R. C. (1968) Selective immunoglobulin A deficiency in two patients with alcoholic cirrhosis. *Gastroenterology*, **54**, 253–259.

Wiskott, A. 1937) Familiärer angeborener Morbus Werlhoffii. *Monatsschrift Kinderhood*, **68**, 212.

Wu, L. Y. F. & Lawton, A. R. (1972) Evaluation of human B lymphocyte differentiation using pokeweed mitogen stimulation: *in vitro* studies in antibody deficiency syndromes. *Clinical Research*, **20**, 798.

Wu, L. Y. F., Lawton, A. R. & Cooper, M. D. (1973) Differentiation capacity of cultured B lymphocytes from immunodeficient patients. *Journal of Clinical Investigation*, **52**, 3180–3189.

Young, W. J., Hong, R., Seligmann, M., Good, R., Kunkel, H. G. (1970) Imbalances of gamma globulin subgroups and gene defects in patients with primary hypogammaglobulinemia. *Journal of Clinical Investigation*, **49**, 1957–1966.

Zamcheck, N., Hoskins, L. C., Winawer, S. J., Broitman, S. A. & Gottlieb, L. S. (1963) Histology and ultrastructure of the parasite and the intestinal mucosa in human giardiasis: effects of Atrabine therapy (abstract). *Gastroenterology*, **44**, 860.

Zegers, B. J. M., Maertzdorf, W. J., van Loghem, E., Mul, N. A. J., Stoop, J. W., van der Laag, J., Vossen, J. J. & Ballieux, R. E. (1976) Kappa-chain deficiency: an immunoglobulin disorder. *New England Journal of Medicine*, **294**, 1026–1030.

Zelman, S. & Lewin, H. (1958) Adult agammaglobulinemia associated with multiple congenital anomalies. *American Journal of Medicine*, **25**, 150–154.

Zinneman, H. H. & Kaplan, A. P. (1972) The association of giardiasis with reduced intestinal secretory immunoglobulin A. *American Journal of Digestive Diseases*, **17**, 793–797.

10. Milk allergy and the gastrointestinal tract in children

J. K. Visakorpi

DEFINITION

Milk allergy, or more precisely cow's milk allergy, has been recognized as a cause of many clinical symptoms in children since the beginning of this century (Schlossman, 1905). Yet, in spite of many carefully performed clinical studies on the epidemiology and symptomatology of milk allergy, we have to admit that even today the diagnostic criteria are difficult to define. This is mainly because the exact mechanisms involved have not been clarified and the final diagnosis has to be based mainly on the results of clinical provocation tests.

In this context the term 'allergy' is used in its original meaning (von Pirquet, 1906), implying that the response to cow's milk is changed with the individual showing evidence of hypersensitivity. Since the pathogenesis of the allergic reaction to milk is poorly understood, the term 'cow's milk-induced illness' has been proposed as more appropriate (Gerrard *et al.*, 1973). The term 'cow's milk intolerance' has also been used by many authors, who wish to stress that the basic mechanism in this syndrome is not yet understood. It is assumed that the reaction is to the protein in cow's milk or related to some milk additive (*vide infra*); although adverse reactions to milk also occur as a result of lactose intolerance, we are not primarily concerned with this phenomenon in this chapter.

As has been said already, the diagnosis of milk allergy is based on the results of a clinical challenge after a favourable response to elimination of cow's milk. Usually, the diagnosis is accepted only after the demonstration of symptoms in repeated challenges. This is not always possible and may even be unethical if the clinical reaction is severe enough.

INCIDENCE

Widely varying figures have been presented for the incidence of milk allergy in childhood. In Canada a prevalence figure of 7.5 per cent has been presented (Gerrard *et al.*, 1973), whereas in Israel, Freier and Kletter (1970), on the basis of a prospective study, suggest an incidence of about 0.5 per cent. This variation may be due to the different hereditary background and different feeding habits (for instance breast feeding) in different populations. The main reasons, however, are probably the variable definitions employed and the imprecise techniques which are available for the diagnosis of this syndrome, Moreover, most of the patients have mild symptoms and in such cases the diagnosis is difficult to establish. Severe gastrointestinal reactions clearly caused by milk are uncommon; in an extensive series seen at the Children's Hospital, University of Helsinki, the ratio between coeliac disease and the cow's milk-induced malabsorption syndrome is about 3:1. Ratios of 2:1 or 1:1 have been observed in several European centres for paediatric gastroenterology. These ratios imply incidence figures of 0.3–1.0 per thousand newborn for the milk-induced malabsorption syndrome, while the average incidence of coeliac disease in Europe seems to be 1:1000. On the other hand, in countries where severe infectious diarrhoeas are rare, milk allergy is presumably one of the chief causes of intractable diarrhoea in infants (Hyman, Reiter, Rodnan and Drash, 1971).

CLINICAL SYNDROMES

Milk allergy usually becomes apparent in early infancy, soon after the first exposure to cow's milk. According to Gerrard *et al.* (1973), the first signs developed within 3 days in 28 per cent of patients and in 7 days in 41 per cent. In a series of patients with milk-induced malabsorption syndrome the mean interval between the introduction of cow's milk into the diet and the appearance of symptoms was 1 month (Kuitunen, Visakorpi, Savilahti and Pelkonen, 1975). The shortest interval in this series was 1 day and the longest 4 months. A typical feature of milk allergy is that the symptoms and reactivity usually disappear spontaneously within 2 years. The other characteristics common to patients with milk allergy are the high frequency of allergic disorders in the parents and siblings of the patients and the tendency of the patients to develop allergies to other foods besides cow's milk (Gerrard *et al.*, 1973).

Several clinical syndromes have been observed in association with milk allergy (Table 10.1). Gerrard *et al.* (1973) studied 59 consecutive patients with milk allergy.

Table 10.1 Milk-induced clinical syndromes

1. Acute anaphylactic reaction (Collins-Williams, 1955)
2. Recurrent respiratory symptoms (Clein, 1954)
   (a) Rhinorrhoea
   (b) Bronchitis
   (c) Asthma
3. Syndrome of rhinitis, pneumonia, otitis media, wheezing and haemoptysis (Heiner, Sears and Knicker, 1962)
4. Recurrent otitis media (Tonkin, 1970)
5. Skin manifestations (Goldman et al., 1963)
   (a) Atopic eczema
   (b) Urticaria
   (c) Periorbital oedema (Freier, 1973)
   (d) Dermatitis herpetiformis (Pock-Steen and Niordson, 1970)
6. Gastrointestinal manifestations
   (a) Prolonged diarrhoea
   (b) Repeated vomiting
   (c) Abdominal colic
   (d) Prolonged diarrhoea with failure to thrive, malabsorption syndrome (Kuitunen, Visakorpi and Hallman, 1966)
   (e) Colitis (Bryboski, Burkle and Hillman, 1966; Sacca, 1971)
   (f) Eosinophilic gastroenteropathy (Waldman, Wochner, Laster and Gordon, 1967)
   (g) Iron-deficiency anaemia due to intestinal bleeding (Wilson, Heiner and Lahey, 1964)
   (h) Neonatal pneumatosis intestinalis (Aziz, 1973)
   (i) Thrombocytopenia with absent radius (Whitfield and Barr, 1976)
7. Central nervous system symptoms (Goldman et al., 1963).
   (a) Lethargy
   (b) Irritability and excessive crying
8. Syndrome of eye signs in patients with allergic malabsorption induced by certain bovine milk proteins (Liu, Giday and Moore, 1973)
9. Acrodermatitis enteropathica.
10. Sudden death (Parish, Barrett and Coombs, 1960).

Their series gives some idea of the relative incidence of the various symptoms:

Recurrent diarrhoea	in 24 patients
Repeated vomiting	in 13 patients
Persistent colic	in 12 patients
Eczema	in 27 patients
Recurrent rhinorrhoea	in 18 patients
Recurrent bronchitis	in 10 patients
Asthma	in 7 patients

In 25 instances the baby presented with only one symptom and in the remaining 34 instances with two or more.

GASTROINTESTINAL MANIFESTATIONS IN MILK ALLERGY

As can be seen from the data presented above, gastrointestinal symptoms are relatively common in connection with milk allergy. The gastrointestinal syndromes induced by milk are as indefinite as the other milk-related allergies, and in spite of the copious clinical literature it is difficult to discern a common pattern in these syndromes. One particular difficulty is that another constituent of milk, lactose, often causes symptoms similar to those of milk protein allergy, especially when the patient is exposed to both these noxious agents simultaneously. Indeed one of the important causes of lactose deficiency is cow's milk protein allergy (Liu, Tsao, Moore and Giday, 1968).

The basic symptoms of milk allergy are vomiting and diarrhoea. Depending on the severity and duration of the symptoms, on the age and general condition of the patient, and on the diet and type of treatment, various complications develop, of which failure to thrive is one of the most important. According to which tests are applied, for example intestinal biopsy, mucosal disaccharidase levels, anti-milk antibodies, absorptive function, etc., different kinds of clinical syndromes have been built up. As long ago as 1953, Kundstater and Schultz described milk allergy in the coeliac syndrome. The first attempt to apply peroral small-bowel biopsy in infants revealed mucosal atrophy in a patient with cow's milk allergy (Lamy et al., 1963). This syndrome was verified in 6 infants by Kuitunen, Visakorpi and Hallman (1965). Milk-induced malabsorption was verified simultaneously by Fällström, Winberg and Andersen (1965) and Davidson, Burnstine, Kugler and Bauer (1965). Since these pioneer investigations, other reports have described several syndromes which, apart from some minor differences, appear to be basically the same (Silver and Douglas, 1968; Liu et al., 1968; Freier et al., 1969; Auricchio, Rubino and Barbieri, 1969; Self et al., 1969; Matsumura, Kuroume and Amada, 1971; Loeb et al., 1971; Berg et al., 1970; Fontaine, Navarro and Polonovski, 1974; Jodl, Lojda and Hoffman, 1974; Navarro et al., 1975; Fontaine and Navarro, 1975; Deleze and Nussle, 1975). The main finding that links all these studies is that milk allergy is associated with a variable degree of intestinal inflammation and damage, which again results in a malabsorption syndrome with a variety of symptoms.

Clearly different findings were described by Gryboski, Burkle and Hillman (1966). Although their patients showed clinical resemblances to those described in the aforementioned studies, sigmoidoscopy revealed changes simulating ulcerative colitis. However, the structure of the small-intestinal mucosa was not studied in these patients, and sigmoidoscopy was not done routinely in many of the other investigations. Thus this colitis syndrome may have been the same as that described under the name malabsorption syndrome. In fact, Silver and Douglas (1968) were able to produce eosinophilic infiltration in the rectum by instillation of milk in patients with the milk-induced malabsorption syndrome.

Eosinophilic gastroenteropathy (Waldmann, Wochner, Laster and Gordon, 1967) seems to be quite a different entity. The milk-induced enteropathy series seen at the Children's Hospital, Helsinki, included one patient with this syndrome. Eosinophilic gastroenteropathy is apparently very rare, severe protein-losing enteropathy being its main manifestation. On the other hand, there are no signs of malabsorption. These findings are consistent with the histological picture of the intestine, which shows a mucosa with heavy eosinophilic infiltration but otherwise almost normal structure. Although blood eosinophilia has often been found in 'ordinary' milk allergy, eosinophilic infiltration of the intestinal mucosa is not a typical finding (Kuitunen, 1966). The report of Silverberg, Davidson, Buiumsohn and Lavy (1972) complicates the clear distinction between the 'regular' milk-induced malabsorption syndrome and eosinophilic gastroenteropathy. These workers published a series of 14 infants of different ages, with rather mild symptomatology, peripheral eosinophilia and eosinophilic infiltration in an otherwise normal intestinal mucosa.

Milk-induced gastrointestinal bleeding is a well-documented phenomenon (Wilson, Heiner and Lahey, 1964). It may exist in all patients with intestinal milk allergy, but is not manifested so clearly if the duration of the disease is short, as is usually the case in the malabsorption syndromes. In older infants, however, where the disease is less acute, iron-deficiency anaemia and hypoproteinaemia may be the only manifestations of milk allergy. In a recent report Wilson, Lahey and Heiner (1974) have shown occult blood loss induced by milk in 17 out of 34 infants with iron-deficiency anaemia.

Acrodermatitis enteropathica seems clearly to be a separate entity in which cow's milk plays some role. This disease will not be discussed here.

MILK-INDUCED MALABSORPTION SYNDROME

CLINICAL FINDINGS

This clinical description is based on a series of 54 infants seen during a 10-year period at the Children's Hospital, University of Helsinki (Kuitunen *et al.*, 1975). The symptomatology is rather uniform, with a basic syndrome of diarrhoea, vomiting and failure to thrive. In about 10 per cent of the cases, macroscopic blood was found in the stools, indicating the colitis syndrome described by Gryboski (1967). In 25 per cent, the initial dehydration was severe, often necessitating parenteral nutrition and in 4 cases leading to an ileus-simulating situation, a complication which was also noted by Freier and Kletter (1972). Two other interesting comments can be made on this group of patients. First, a special subgroup, comprising about 20 per cent of the whole series,

could be distinguished by the symptoms. The malabsorption syndrome was usually mild, and intestinal atrophy only partial. Additionally, however, these patients had atopic eczema, and usually recurrent respiratory symptoms as well. They also had peripheral eosinophilia. They responded to the treatment in the same way as the other patients. The second interesting finding was that the prevalence of Down's syndrome was clearly increased.

Table 10.2 shows the results of the most important routine laboratory examinations. In addition, various tests showed that about half the patients also had secondary lactose malabsorption, which was transient, however, and did not usually require total elimination of lactose (mother's milk was always used for the diet).

Table 10.2 Initial laboratory findings in patients with malabsorption syndrome and cow's milk allergy

Faecal fat excretion, more than 3 g/day	42/51
D-xylose excretion, less than 15 per cent	38/53
Positive urinary FIGLU test	40/50
Haemoglobin less than 10 g/100 ml	11/53
Eosinophils in blood, more than 4 per cent	17/52
Serum total protein less than 5.5 g/100 ml	14/45
Increased serum IgA (= more than +2SD)	37/50
Precipitins to cow's milk	32/49
Precipitins to gluten	6/49

Bacteriological examinations revealed nothing noteworthy. Quantitative determinations of the intestinal microflora (Juntunen, 1974) revealed duodenal colonization in some cases, with a faecal type of microflora, but there was no difference in this respect between patients with milk allergy and those with chronic, nonspecific diarrhoea without milk allergy.

The diagnosis rests solely on the results of clinical provocations. In these challenges milk allergy was manifested in about half the patients by typical acute reactions, which in some cases were anaphylactic in type. In the other patients, however, the response was different; they had anorexia, bulky stools and poor gain in weight for weeks, resembling the reactions to gluten in coeliac disease. This type of reaction was apparently related to the age of the patient and the stage of activity of the disease, for some of the patients showed at first an acute reaction and then a slower one. These studies also showed, like many earlier reports, that these patients tend to develop sensitivities to other food proteins, as well, if exposed to them during the sensitive period.

Follow-up studies showed that the intestinal disease is transient. Clinical sensitivity disappeared at the age of about one year, and this was independent of the time when the patient was admitted for treatment. It is clear that great variation exists in the severity of the disease. Some of the patients reacted to a small quantity of milk with severe symptoms; they tended to develop other sensitivities, and recovered late. Others showed only mild symptoms and recovered early during the first year.

With respect to gluten sensitivity in patients with milk allergy, Fällström et al. (1965) and Visakorpi and Immonen (1967) have described reactions to wheat gluten in some milk-sensitive patients. Recent studies (Kuitunen et al., 1975) have shown, however, that this reactivity to gluten has nothing to do with coeliac disease as usually defined. In these patients although the gluten may damage the small-intestinal mucosa, the majority of these individuals have so-called transient gluten-induced enteropathy. About 10 per cent of the

milk allergy patients, however, later developed true coeliac disease (Kuitunen et al., 1975). On admission, these patients were already older than most of the children suffering solely from milk allergy, and they had received gluten before the onset of the illness. Therefore it seems more likely that the coeliac disease was the primary entity in these patients and the milk allergy a secondary or simultaneous phenomenon which may, of course, have aggravated the symptoms of coeliac disease. Relevant to the point is the interesting observation of Pock-Steen and Niordson (1970) that a 30-year-old patient with dermatitis herpetiformis and gluten-induced intestinal damage was also sensitive to cow's

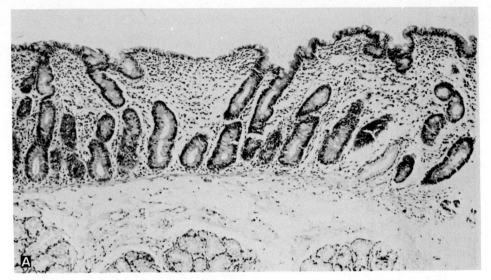

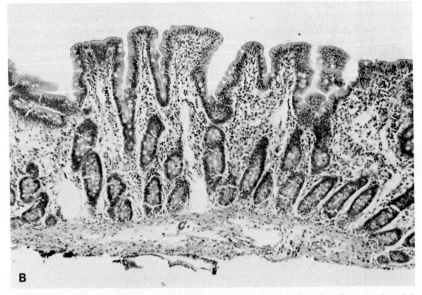

Fig. 10.1A and B Appearance of jejunal biopsy specimens in a child with cow's milk allergy and malabsorption syndrome before and during elimination of cow's milk. A. Before elimination, aged 3.5 months: subtotal villous atrophy. B. After elimination of cow's milk for 1 month: partial villous atrophy, round-cell infiltration and already normalized epithelium.

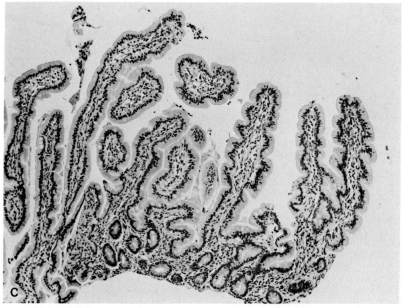

Fig. 10.1C Appearance of jejunal biopsy specimens in a child with cow's milk allergy and malabsorption syndrome before and during elimination of cow's milk. C. After elimination for 6 months: normal jejunal mucosa. (Kuitunen, Rapola, Savilahti and Visakorpi, 1973, reproduced by kind permission of the authors and also of the editor of *Scandinavica Acta Paediatrica* in which the figure first appeared.)

milk. The relations between milk allergy and coeliac disease have not, however, been fully elucidated.

MORPHOLOGICAL REACTIONS TO MILK

As mentioned earlier, various types of morphological changes have been described in association with milk allergy. Jejunal biopsies in the aforementioned 54 infants with the milk-induced malabsorption syndrome revealed the following changes:

Flat mucosa, subtotal villous atrophy in 27
Partial villous atrophy   in 17
Slight villous changes   in 3
Normal villous structure but
  intraepithelial round-cell
  infiltration   in 1

The findings in patients with subtotal villous atrophy are indistinguishable from those typical of coeliac disease regarding the shape of the villi, the epithelial cell damage and the round-cell infiltration (Fig. 10.1). Electron-micrographs show short microvilli, occasionally fused at the bases, abnormality in the shape and position of the nuclei, and thickening of the basement membranes (Fig. 10.2).

The direct effect of milk challenge on the small-intestinal mucosa has been investigated in 3 patients by Kuitunen, Rapola, Savilahti and Visakorpi (1973). Investigations of this kind are very difficult to perform, because the patients are so young, and usually sick, and investigations can be done only in connection with diagnostic provocations. One of these 3 patients was very sensitive and reacted acutely and strongly to a single dose of milk. A biopsy taken 20 hours after the challenge did not reveal much change in villous structure (partial villous atrophy), but there was clear round-cell infiltration into the surface epithelium and the lamina propria. Challenge also caused clear epithelial damage (Fig. 10.3). Electron-micrographs showed shortening of the microvilli, disorientation of the nuclei and some increase in the number of lysosomes. The other 2 patients reacted slowly. In one of these, increasing damage was seen after 4- and 38-day provocations, respectively; continuous accumulations of undulating and whirled collagen fibres at the thickened basal lamina were also seen. In the third patient the reactions, both clinical and morphological, were much less pronounced but nonetheless clear. Recently similar histological and ultrastructural changes have been reported in milk allergy both in infants reacting to cow's milk challenge with acute symptoms (Shiner, Ballard and Smith, 1975) and in infants not reacting acutely (Shiner, Ballard, Brook and Herman, 1975). The results of these studies show that a clinical reaction to milk is accompanied by morphological changes in the small-intestinal mucosa, indicating that the musocal lesion is induced by the milk itself.

Finally, morphological damage, produced by milk proteins (alpha-lactalbumin and beta-lactoglobulin), has also been demonstrated *in vitro* with the organ culture technique by Ritis and Jos (1974).

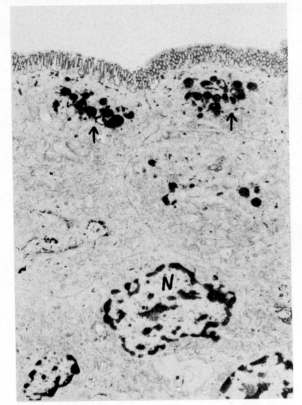

Fig. 10.2 Electron-micrograph of the surface epithelium of an infant with milk allergy and malabsorption syndrome after 38 days' provocation with cow's milk. The microvilli are short and fused at their bases. Large collections of lysosomes are seen in the apical part of the epithelial cells (arrows). × 4550. (Kuitunen, et al., 1973, reproduced by kind permission of the authors and also of the editor of *Scandinavica Acta Paediatrica* in which the figure first appeared.)

IMMUNOLOGY OF MILK ALLERGY

ANTIGENICITY OF MILK

The clinician is satisfied when he knows that cow's milk is the cause of his patient's disorder. However, a full understanding of the disease will only be possible when we know the exact nature of the allergen. Cow's milk contains more than 20 proteins, and in addition may contain contaminants such as antibiotics or preservatives which, alone or in combination with milk proteins, may act as allergens. Some basic knowledge of the nature of milk allergens has been gained through provocation tests performed with pure milk protein preparations. Goldman *et al.* (1963) performed oral provocations and skin tests in patients suffering from different kinds of milk allergy. Every patient gave an allergic reaction to one or more milk proteins. The frequencies of the reactions were as follows:

To beta-lactoglobulin   in 66 per cent
To casein   in 57 per cent
To alpha-lactalbumin   in 54 per cent and
To bovine serum albumin   in 51 per cent

Some of the patients with the milk-induced malabsorption syndrome in the series already cited (Kuitunen *et al.*, 1975) were challenged with pure milk proteins. Six out of 7 patients reacted to beta-lactoglobulin and 5 out of 6 to casein, whereas reactions to alpha-lactalbumin and to bovine serum proteins were rare. These patients were usually sensitive to more than one fraction. There are many case reports of sensitivity to beta-lactoglobulin, and Kletter *et al.* (1971) showed that this protein produces a positive reaction more often than the other milk proteins.

These findings indicate that some proteins are more

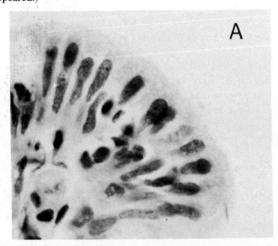

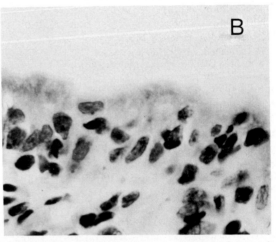

Fig. 10.3 Epithelial injury and changes in the round-cell infiltration of jejunal biopsy specimen of a child aged 7.3 months with cow's milk allergy and malabsorption syndrome: (A) Before provocation. (B) After 4 days' provocation with milk. (Visakorpi, 1974.) (Reprinted by kind permission of the author and also of H. E. Stenfert Kroese BV/Leiden. The figure first appeared in 'Definition of coeliac disease' in *Coeliac Disease*, ed. Hekkens, W. Th. J. M. and Peña, A. S., 1974, Leiden.)

allergenic than others, and that beta-lactoglobulin is one of the most potent of the milk protein antigens. Shapira, Tenebaum, Kletter and Russell (1971), however, suggested that alpha-lactalbumin might be the strongest antigen, because this fraction was responsible for precipitating antibodies in the patients they studied, who suffered from familial dysautonomia.

A new aspect of the problem of allergens is the observation that certain processes may increase the allergenicity of native milk proteins (Ch. 11). Bleumink (1970) has shown by intracutaneous tests that pasteurization, spray-drying and boiling of milk give rise to increased activity in susceptible persons. This increased activity is due to a non-enzymatic browning (Maillard) reaction which produces a lysine–carbohydrate linkage. Another mechanism which may play a role is the formation of new antigens in the digestive process. In fact, Spies (1973) has demonstrated new antigens generated by pepsin hydrolysis of milk proteins.

SERUM IMMUNOGLOBULINS

Changes in the serum immunoglobulin pattern in coeliac disease are well documented in many reports reviewed by Asquith (1974). Serum immunoglobulins have not been studied in all types of cow's milk allergy. In a series of 41 infants presenting with mainly gastro-intestinal symptoms due to milk allergy, Peleg, Mercazi and Freier (1974) demonstrated a rise of IgM in 25 per cent and a rise of IgA in 10 per cent of patients. In selected groups of patients with milk allergy Immonen (1968) made an extensive study of the serum immuno-globulins. She demonstrated that, as in coeliac disease in the same age group, there was a definite increase of IgA and normal levels of IgM in patients with milk-induced malabsorption syndrome and intestinal damage. In the series of 54 infants with this syndrome (Kuitunen et al., 1975) serum IgA was more than 2 SD above the normal mean level in 74 per cent of cases. Immonen (1968) also found rapid normalization of serum immunoglobulins during milk elimination and a clear increase of IgA and IgM after challenge, as can be seen from Figure 10.4. In these patients according to Savilahti (1973), serum IgE levels are low and no rise can be seen during challenge.

Although allergic diseases are commoner in patients with immunodeficiencies, as shown by Soothill and Steward (1973), there appeared to be no relationship between immunodeficiencies and milk-induced gastro-intestinal disorders.

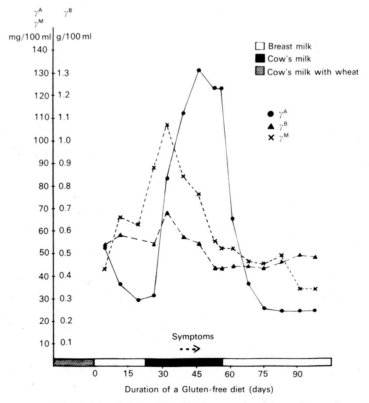

Fig. 10.4 Serum immunoglobulin levels in an infant with milk allergy and malabsorption syndrome during provocation with milk (Immonen, 1968). (Reproduced by kind permission of the author and also of the editor of *Annales Pediatrica Fenniae* in which the figure first appeared.)

INTESTINAL IMMUNOGLOBULINS

The distribution of immunoglobulin-containing round cells in the intestinal mucosa of infants suffering from the milk-induced malabsorption syndrome with damaged intestinal mucosa was studied extensively by Jos, Rey and Frézal (1972) and by Savilahti (1973), using peroral small-bowel biopsy and an immunofluorescence technique. In the former study the numbers of IgA-containing plasma cells were increased, although the numbers of other cells were normal. Savilahti (1973) studied the cell count during challenge, and observed a 2.4-fold rises in IgA and in IgM cells and a 1.8-fold rise in IgG cells, but found no consistent change in the number of IgE cells. The results were similar to those observed in children with active coeliac disease (Fig. 10.5).

of IgA and IgM during challenge. All these studies show that milk induces a strong local intestinal reaction, which is very similar to that seen in children suffering from coeliac disease. Primary errors of immunological responsiveness, however, have not been shown.

ANTIBODIES TO MILK

Serum antibodies to milk proteins were the first immunological abnormalities demonstrated in gastrointestinal milk allergy, and there have been numerous publications recording their presence in this situation. Heiner, Sears and Kniker (1962) noted the presence of strong precipitins to milk proteins in patients with recurrent pneumonia, gastrointestinal disorders and failure to thrive. The presence of precipitins seems to correlate fairly well with the intestinal damage, independently of

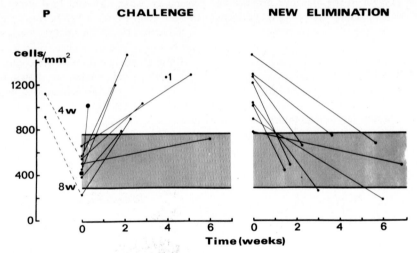

Fig. 10.5 IgA-containing jejunal mucosa cells in 8 patients with milk allergy and malabsorption syndrome during and after provocation (and in 2 patients before provocation). Shaded area, range of numbers of IgA-containing cells in 6 controls (Savilahti, 1973). (Reproduced by kind permission of the author and also of the editor of *Gut* in which the figure first appeared.)

In similar challenge investigations, Shiner *et al.* (1975a, 1975b), however, were able to show a clear increase in mucosal IgE-producing cells as well as degranulation of mast cells. The number of IgM-producing cells was also increased whereas the number of IgA-producing cells was unchanged. These differences in results may be due to the different timing of the post-challenge biopsies. It is also possible that the patients really reacted in different ways; the patients of Shiner *et al.* (1975a and b) exhibited typical reaginic reactions whereas the response of the patients of Savilahti (1973) was more chronic. Again, in similar patients, Kilby, Walker-Smith and Wood (1975) found an increase in IgA cells as well as an increase in IgM cells in their experiment.

Savilahti (1973) also studied the immunoglobulins in intestinal juice and faecal extract, and found increases

the cause of this damage. On the other hand, precipitins cannot usually be found in connection with anaphylactic milk allergy manifested by acute gastrointestinal symptoms, eczema, urticaria or asthma (Saperstein, Anderson, Goldman and Kniker, 1963). Sensitive tests, such as passive haemagglutination, very often detect circulating antibodies in normal infants. Kletter, Gery, Freier and Davies (1971) found haemagglutinating antibodies even in sera of newborns, but usually at levels lower than those of the mothers. If these infants were fed with cow's milk the titres then rose, the peak being reached at 3 months of age. Thereafter the titres gradually declined. These milk antibodies were shown by radioimmunodiffusion to be mainly IgG-class antibodies; IgA-class milk antibodies were present in lower titres, but rose gradually, reaching a peak at 7 months. IgM antibodies were rarely present.

With respect to milk antibodies in faeces, it has been suggested that the occurrence of precipitins and a high level of haemagglutinating antibodies indicates milk sensitivity or coeliac disease (Kletter, Freier, Davies and Gery, 1971). The coproantibodies to milk are mainly of class IgA.

Regarding the pathogenesis of milk allergy, investigations concerning IgE antibodies to milk are interesting. Heiner and Rose (1970) found raised levels of IgE in some individuals with food allergy, but Savilahti (1973), as already mentioned, could not verify this in patients with the milk-induced malabsorption syndrome. Kletter et al. (1971) found IgE antibodies to beta-lactoglobulin in 7 out of 26 infants with milk allergy. The experiments made by Parish (1971) may explain the discrepancies in these studies. He found that in milk-sensitive patients the antibodies were of two different types. About one-half to one-third of the patients reacting immediately with skin manifestations or asthma had reaginic antibodies, as shown by passive cutaneous anaphylaxis in monkeys. An even higher proportion of the patients had IgE antibodies that bound radioisotope-labelled beta-lactoglobulin and passively sensitized monkey basophils to anaphylactic degranulation. In another group of 9 children with milk-induced gastroenteritis occurring 12–36 hours after exposure, no anti-milk reagins could be found. In this group the allergy may be mediated by heat-stable IgG antibodies, because 3 sera conferred milk sensitivity on monkey skin for 2–4 hours. The 3 sera had high titres of IgG agglutinins, 1 to beta-lactoglobulin, 1 to alpha-lactalbumin and 1 to casein. All 3 fixed complement in the presence of milk.

COMPLEMENT CHANGES

As mentioned before, Parish (1971) observed complement consumption in 3 of his patients with milk-induced gastrointestinal disorders. This fits well with the findings of Matthews and Soothill (1970), who obtained evidence of complement activation in 5 patients with intestinal symptoms induced by milk, but not in 3 children with mainly cutaneous and respiratory manifestations. In 6 patients with the milk-induced malabsorption syndrome, however, Savilahti (1973) did not observe any changes in serum beta-1C/A levels during challenge whereas Shiner et al. (1975b) noted an increase of beta-1C/A in 2 patients, Shiner et al. (1975a and b) were also able to demonstrate C3 complement extracellularly at the basement membranes after challenge. These observations suggest that different mechanisms may operate in the pathogenesis of milk allergy.

CELLULAR REACTIVITY

Cell-mediated immune responses in milk-induced gastrointestinal disorders have not been investigated systematically. Borrone et al. (1970) investigated blast transformation of lymphocytes from peripheral blood of 2 children with milk allergy (chronic intestinal bleeding and urticaria). In both they found blast transformation. The test was negative in 11 control patients and in 4 patients with coeliac disease, but positive in 10 out of 21 patients suffering from chronic diarrhoea, which seemed to be related to cow's milk feeding.

A lymphocyte response has also been found by Brostoff (cited by Matthews and Soothill, 1970) in patients with milk allergy. On the other hand, Asquith, Housley and Cooke (1971) demonstrated marked in-vitro stimulation of lymphocytes from coeliac patients as well as from controls by two different preparations of beta-lactoglobulin, showing that cow's milk itself may contain mitogenic agents.

CONVENTIONAL ALLERGY TESTING

Efforts has been made to adapt conventional allergy tests for diagnostic purpose in food allergies. Immediate-onset food allergies are relatively simple to recognize from the clinical history, and the diagnosis can often be confirmed by allergy tests such as the skin test, allergen-induced leucocyte histamine release and skin window, as shown by Galant, Bullock and Frick (1973). Food sensitivity with delayed onset, which is the commonest form of milk-induced gastroenteropathy, causes many diagnostic problems. Unfortunately, the tests mentioned before are rarely helpful in the delayed type of food allergy.

COMMENTS AND CONCLUSIONS

During the past 10 years milk allergy has gained increasing recognition as an important cause of intestinal disorders. Severe forms of this syndrome are comparable in incidence to that of coeliac disease. Their incidence is increasing; this is partially due to improved diagnosis, but undoubtedly a true increase has also taken place. One of the causes is evidently the decline of breast feeding, but the formation of new antigens from natural milk proteins during food processing is a further possibility and may also have contributed to the increase.

One of the most typical features of gastrointestinal milk allergy is the age at onset, which clearly differs from the age of some other typical allergic phenomena. It is natural to speculate that this is connected with the physiologically weak defence mechanisms (i.e. increased permeability) of the intestinal mucosa during the first months of life. The development of milk antibodies found by Kletter et al. (1971) in normal infants could be explained by a physiological insufficiency of the intestinal mucosa of this kind. However, the modes of action of the defence mechanisms are obscure, although an immunological barrier has been suggested, for instance by Matthews and Soothill (1970). The IgA-producing system of the intestine is not fully developed in young infants (Savilahti, 1972). On theoretical grounds and also in practice it is important to know the types of allergic reaction which cause intestinal disorders. A full explanation of these reactions may facilitate the recognition of clinical syndromes, afford help in devising diagnostic tests, and even indicate methods of treatment. The many observations already cited suggest that reactions of at least two different kinds are involved. Type 1, i.e. anaphylactic or reaginic, reactions have been clearly shown clinically in some patients with milk allergy. Further evidence for Type 1 reactions is afforded by the presence of IgE-specific antibodies in these patients, as well as the good results obtained by treatment with disodium chromoglycate (Freier and Berger, 1973) and by the increase of IgE plasma cells (Shiner et al., 1975a and b; Kilby et al., 1975). It is also clear, however, that a Type 1 reaction occurring alone cannot explain the findings made in connection with challenge experiments. Even in patients with severe intestinal damage induced by milk the response seems mostly to be of a different type. The findings of Parish (1971) concerning delayed-onset gastroenteritis caused by complement-dependent, IgG antibody-mediated reactions may be relevant to these cases. The detection of complement activation by Matthews and Soothill (1970) and by Shiner et al. (1975a and b) favours this view, although Savilahti (1973) was unable to verify this observation. The findings concerning Type 4 responses are very preliminary so far.

Summarizing, it is evident that both clinically and experimentally several different types of reactions to milk occur in the gastrointestinal tract. We have as yet no clear understanding of the fundamental basis for such differences nor which reactions are primary and which represent secondary epiphenomena. Finally, it is important to note that the morphological reactions which milk proteins may induce in the intestinal mucosa are very similar to those seen in coeliac disease, from which we may infer that similar mechanisms are responsible for the damage in these two diseases.

REFERENCES

Asquith, P. (1974) Immunology. In *Coeliac Disease. Clinics in Gastroenterology*, 3rd edn, ed. Cooke, W. T. & Asquith, P., No. 1, pp. 213–234. London: Saunders.

Asquith, P., Houseley, J. & Cooke, W. T. (1971) Human lymphocyte stimulation by bovine β-lactoglobulin. *Gastroenterology*, **60**, 638.

Auricchio, S., Rubino, A., Barbieri, A., Ciccimarra, F., De Bellis, U. & Vetrella, M. (1969) L'intolleranza alle proteine del latte vaccino e la steatorrea indotta da beta-lattoglobulina. *Minerva Pediatrica*, **21**, 1809–1815.

Aziz, E. M. (1973) Neonatal pneumatosis intestinalis associated with milk intolerance. *American Journal of Diseases of Children*, **125**, 560–562.

Berg, N. O., Dahlqvist, A., Lindberg, T., Meeuwisse, G. W. & Akerman, M. (1970) Small intestinal mucosal structure, dissacharidases and dipeptidases in different types of malabsorption in childhood. A longitudinal study. In *Coeliac Disease*, ed. Booth, C. C. & Dowling, R. H. Edinburgh: Churchill Livingstone.

Bleumink, E. (1970) Food allergy; the chemical nature of the substances eliciting symptoms. *World Review of Nutrition and Dietetics*, **12**, 505–570.

Borrone, C., Dagna-Bricarelli, F., Massimo, L., Fossati-Guglielmoni, A. & Durand, P. (1970) Lymphocyte transformation in milk allergy. *Acta Paediatrica Scandinavica*, **59**, 449–450.

Clein, N. W. (1954) Cow's milk allergy in infants. *Pediatric Clinics of North America*, Pt 4, 949–962.

Collins-Williams, C. (1955) Acute allergic reaction to cow's milk. *Annals of Allergy*, **13**, 415–421.

Davidson, M., Burnstine, R. C., Kugler, M. M. & Bauer, C. H. (1965) Malabsorption defect induced by ingestion of beta-lactoglobulin. *Journal of Pediatrics*, **66**, 545–554.

Deleze, G. & Nussle, D. (1975) Cow's milk protein intolerance in childhood. *Helvetica paediatrica acta*, **30**, 135–139.

Fällström, S. P., Winberg, J. & Andersen, H. J. (1965) Cow's milk-induced malabsorption as a precursor of gluten intolerance. *Acta Paediatrica Scandinavica*, **54**, 101–115.

Fontaine, J. L. & Navarro, J. (1975) Small intestinal biopsy in cow's milk protein allergy in infancy. *Archives of Diseases in Childhood*, **50**, 357–362.

Fontaine, J. L., Navarro, J. & Polonovski, C. (1974) The intestinal biopsy in 20 cases of intolerance to cow's milk protein in infancy. *Acta Paediatrica Scandinavica*, **63**, 652–653.

Freier, S. (1973) Paediatric gastrointestinal allergy. *Clinical Allergy*, **3**, 597–618.

Freier, S. & Berger, H. (1973) Disodium cromoglycate in gastrointestinal protein intolerance. *Lancet*, **i**, 913–915.

Freier, S. & Kletter, B. (1970) Milk allergy in infants and young children. Current Knowledge. *Clinical Pediatrics (Phila.)*, **9**, 449–454.

Freier, S. & Kletter, B. (1972) Clinical and immunological aspects of milk protein intolerance. *Australian Paediatric Journal*, **8**, 140–146.

Freier, S., Kletter, B., Gery, I., Lebenthal, E. & Geifman, M. (1969) Intolerance to milk protein. *Journal of Pediatrics*, **75**, 623–631.

Galant, S. P., Bullock, J. & Frick, O. L. (1973) An immunological approach to the diagnosis of food sensitivity. *Clinical Allergy*, **3**, 363–372.

Gerrard, J. W., Mackenzie, J. W. A., Goluboff, N., Garson, J. Z. & Maningas, C. S. (1973) Cow's milk allergy: prevalence and manifestations in an unselected series of newborns. *Acta Paediatrica Scandinavica*, Suppl. 234, 1–21.

Goldman, A. S., Anderson, D. W., Jr, Sellers, W. A.,

Saperstein, S., Kniker, W. T. & Halpern, S. R. (1963) Milk allergy. I. Oral challenge with milk and isolated milk proteins in allergic children. *Pediatrics*, 32, 425–443.

Gryboski, J. D. (1967) Gastrointestinal milk allergy in infants. *Pediatrics*, 40, 354–362.

Gryboski, J. D., Burkle, F. & Hillman, R. (1966) Milk-induced colitis in an infant. *Pediatrics*, 38, 299–302.

Heiner, D. C. & Rose, B. (1970) Elevated levels of gamma E (IgE) in conditions other than classical allergy. *Journal of Allergy*, 45, 30–42.

Heiner, D. C., Sears, J. W. & Kniker, W. T. (1962) Multiple precipitins to cow's milk in chronic respiratory disease. *American Journal of Diseases of Children*, 103, 634–654.

Hyman, C. J., Reiter, J., Rodnan, J. & Drash, A. L. (1971) Parenteral and oral alimentation in the treatment of the non specific protracted diarrheal syndrome of infancy. *Journal of Pediatrics*, 78, 17–29.

Immonen, P. (1968) Levels of the serum immunoglobulins gamma A, gamma G and gamma M in the malabsorption syndrome in children. *Annales Paediatrie Fenniae*, 13, 115–153.

Jodl, J., Lojda, Z. & Hoffman, J. (1974) Intolerance to cow's milk proteins in children. *Acta Paediatrica Scandinavica*, 63, 653.

Jos, J., Rey, J. & Frézal, J. (1972) Étude immunohistochimique de la muqueuse intestinale chez l'enfant. I. Les syndromes de malabsorption. *Archives Françaises de Pédiatrie*, 29, 681–698.

Juntunen, K. (1974) Intestinal microflora of children with chronic diarrhoeal diseases and of children with IgA deficiency. Academic dissertation, University of Helsinki.

Kilby, A., Walker-Smith, J. A. & Wood, C. B. S. (1975) Small intestinal mucosa in cow's milk allergy. *Lancet*, i, 531.

Kletter, B., Freier, S., Davies, A. M. & Gery, I. (1971) The significance of coproantibodies to cow's milk proteins. *Acta Paediatrica Scandinavica*, 60, 173–180.

Kletter, B., Gery, I., Freier, S. & Davies, A. M. (1971) Immune responses of normal infants to cow's milk. I. Antibody type and kinetics of production. *International Archives of Allergy and Applied Immunology*, 40, 656–666.

Kletter, B., Gery, I., Freier, S., Noah, Z. & Davies, M. A. (1971) Immunoglobulin E antibodies to milk proteins. *Clinical Allergy*, 1, 249–255.

Kuitunen, P. (1966) Duodeno-jejunal histology in malabsorption syndrome in infants. *Annales Paediatriae Fenniae*, 12, 101–132.

Kuitunen, P., Visakorpi, J. K. & Hallman, N. (1965) Histopathology of duodenal mucosa in malabsorption syndrome induced by cow's milk. *Annales Paediatrici*, 205, 54–63.

Kuitunen, P., Rapola, J., Savilahti, E. & Visakorpi, J. K. (1973) Response of the jejunal mucosa to cow's milk in the malabsorption syndrome with cow's milk intolerance. A light- and electron-microscopic study. *Acta Paediatrica Scandinavica*, 62, 585–595.

Kuitunen, P., Visakorpi, J. K., Savilahti, E. & Pelkonen, P. (1975) Malabsorption syndrome with cow's milk intolerance: clinical findings and course in the light of 54 cases. *Archives of Disease in Childhood*, 50, 351–356.

Kunstadter, R. H. & Schultz, A. (1953) Gastrointestinal allergy and the celiac syndrome with particular reference to allergy to cow's milk. *Annals of Allergy*, 11, 426–434.

Lamy, M., Nezelof, C., Jos, J., Frézal, J. & Rey, J. (1963) La biopsie de la muqueuse intestinale chez l'enfants.

Premiers résultats d'une étude des syndrome de mal-absorption. *La Presse Médicale*, 71, 1267–1270.

Liu, H. Y., Giday, Z. & Moore, B. F. (1973) Certain bovine milk protein inducible eye signs in patients with allergic malabsorption. *Journal of Pediatric Ophthalmology*, 10, 7–11.

Liu, H.-Y., Tsao, M. U., Moore, B. & Giday, Z. (1968) Bovine milk protein-induced intestinal malabsorption of lactose and fat in infants. *Gastroenterology*, 54, 27–34.

Loeb, H., Vainsel, M., Cadranel, S., Dachy, A., Diederickx, M. & Wolter, R. (1971) Malabsorption and villous atrophy in 4 infants: relationship to cow's milk intolerance. *Acta Paediatrica Scandinavica*, 60, 372–373.

Matsumura, T., Kuroume, T. & Amada, K. (1971) Close relationship between lactose intolerance and allergy to milk protein. *Journal of Asthma Research*, 9, 13–29.

Matthews, T. S. & Soothill, J. F. (1970) Complement activation after milk feeding in children with cow's milk allergy. *Lancet*, ii, 893–895.

Navarro, J., Omanga, U., Mougenot, J.-F., Baudon, J.-J., Fontaine, J.-L., Polanovski, C. & Laplane, R. (1975) Gastrointestinal intolerance to cow milk proteins in infancy. I. Clinical study of 42 patients. *Archives Françaises de Pédiatrie*, 32, 773–779.

Parish, W. E. (1971) Detection of reaginic and short-term sensitizing anaphylactic or anaphylactoid antibodies to milk in sera of allergic and normal persons. *Clinical Allergy*, 1, 369–380.

Parish, W. E., Barrett, A. M., Coombs, R. R. A., Gunther, M. & Camps, F. E. (1960) Hypersensitivity to milk and sudden death in infancy. *Lancet*, ii, 1106–1110.

Peleg, R., Mercazi, M. & Freier, S. (1974) The natural history of milk allergy. In preparation.

Pock-Steen, O. C. H. & Niordson, A. M. (1970) Milk sensitivity in dermatitis herpetiformis. *British Journal of Dermatology*, 83, 614–619.

Ritis, G. de. & Jos, J. (1974) Organ culture of intestinal mucosa in coeliac disease and in cow's milk intolerance. Effects of protein fractions. *Acta Paediatrica Scandinavica*, 63, 162.

Sacca, J. D. (1971) Acute ischemic colitis due to milk allergy. *Annals of Allergy*, 29, 268–269.

Saperstein, S., Anderson, D. W., Jr, Goldman, A. S. & Kniker, W. T. (1963) Milk allergy. III. Immunological studies with sera from allergic and normal children. *Pediatrics*, 32, 580–587.

Savilahti, E. (1972) Immunoglobulin-containing cells in the intestinal mucosa and immunoglobulins in the intestinal juice in children. *Clinical and Experimental Immunology*, 11, 415–425.

Savilahti, E. (1973) Immunochemical study of the malabsorption syndrome with cow's milk intolerance. *Gut*, 14, 491–501.

Schlossmann, N. A. (1905) Uber die Giftwirkung des artfremden Eiweisses in der Milch auf den Organismus des Säuglings. *Archiv für Kinderheilkunde*, 41, 99–103.

Self, T. W., Herskovic, T., Czapek, E., Caplan, D., Schonberger, T. & Gryboski, J. D. (1969) Gastrointestinal protein allergy. Immunologic considerations. *Journal of the American Medical Association*, 207, 2393–2396.

Shapira, E., Tenebaum, R., Kletter, B. & Russell, A. (1971) Definition of cow's milk protein fraction evoking precipitating antibodies. *Journal of Laboratory and Clinical Medicine*, 77, 529–534.

Shiner, M., Ballard, J. & Smith, M. (1975a) The small-intestinal mucosa in cow's milk allergy. *Lancet*, i, 136–140.

Shiner, M., Ballard, J., Brook, C. G. D. & Herman, S. (1975b) Intestinal biopsy in the diagnosis of cow's milk protein intolerance without acute symptoms. *Lancet*, **ii**, 1060–1063.

Silver, H. & Douglas, D. M. (1968) Milk intolerance in infancy. *Archives of Disease in Childhood*, **43**, 17–22.

Silverberg, M., Davidson, M., Buiumsohn, A. & Lavy, U. (1972) Milk protein gastrointestinal hypersensitivity associated with eosinophilic gastroenteropathy in children. *Gastroenterology*, **62**, 812.

Soothill, J. F. & Steward, M. W. (1973) The relationship of allergic disease to immunodeficiency. *International Archives of Allergy and Applied Immunology*, **45**, 180–182.

Spies, J. R. (1973) Milk allergy. *Journal of Milk and Food Technology*, **36**, 225–231.

Tonkin, S. (1970) Maori infant health: 2. Study of morbidity and medico-social aspects. *New Zealand Medical Journal*, **72**, 229–238.

Visakorpi, J. K. (1974) Definition of coeliac disease in children. In *Coeliac Disease. Proceedings of the Second International Symposium*, ed. Hekkens, W. Th. J. M. & Pēna, A. S., pp. 10–16. Leiden: Stenfert Kroese.

Visakorpi, J. K. & Immonen, P. (1967) Intolerance to cow's milk and wheat gluten in the primary malabsorption syndrome in infancy. *Acta Paediatrica Scandinavica*, **56**, 49–56.

Von Pirquet, C. (1906) Allergie. *Munchener Medizinische Wochenschrift*, **53**, 1437–1438.

Waldmann, T. A., Wochner, R. D., Laster, L. & Gordon, R. S., Jr (1967) Allergic gastroenteropathy. A cause of excessive gastrointestinal protein loss. *New England Journal of Medicine*, **276**, 761–769.

Whitfield, M. F. & Barr, D. G. D. (1976) Cow's milk allergy in the syndrome of thrombocytopenia with absent radius. *Archives of Diseases in Childhood*, **51**, 337–343.

Wilson, J. F., Heiner, D. C. & Lahey, M. E. (1964) Milk-induced gastrointestinal bleeding in infants with hypochromic microcytic anemia. *Journal of the American Medical Association*, **189**, 568–572.

Wilson, J. F., Lahey, M. E. & Heiner, D. C. (1974) Studies on iron metabolism. 5. Further observations on cow's milk-induced gastrointestinal bleeding in infants with iron-deficiency anemia. *Journal of Pediatrics*, **84**, 335–344.

11. Food allergy and the gastrointestinal tract

E. Bleumink

INTRODUCTION

Food allergy is defined as an immunological reaction occurring after ingestion of substances in foodstuffs. Adverse reactions are also observed after epicutaneous contact with foods (for example, contact dermatitis caused by garlic or cinnamon) or after inhalation (of chlorogenic acid in coffee beans or wheat flour in bakers' asthma), but these fall outside the definition and are not considered here. There is a considerable overlap of allergic reactions provoked by foods in the gastro-intestinal tract on the one hand, and systemic reactions, skin symptoms and respiratory tract responses attributable to foods on the other. Gastrointestinal food allergy cannot therefore be easily isolated from reactions occurring in the circulation and in other organs.

Various mechanisms may underlie the adverse reactions which follow consumption of food: (1) toxic effects attributable to bacterial contamination and food additives, (2) intolerance phenomena (and/or idiosyncrasies) due to inborn errors (enzyme deficiencies). Examples are: lactose intolerance and hereditary haemolytic anaemia. The latter may occur in persons with glucose-6-phosphate-dehydrogenase deficiency after consumption of currants, gooseberries or the beans of *Ficia faba*, (3) allergic reactions mediated either by antibodies or committed T-lymphocytes, and (4) symptoms resembling allergic reactions but which are not elicited by immunological phenomena. To category (4) belong symptoms produced by substances which cause histamine release, or which activate the complement system, or which stimulate T-lymphocytes non-specifically.

In this chapter the two latter categories are mainly considered. Additional aspects of allergy to cow's milk are discussed in Chapter 10, while hypersensitivity reactions are classified in detail in Chapter 2. The most common allergic reactions to foods are caused by atopic phenomena (Type 1); Type IV phenomena to food constituents are probably rare, whilst controversy exists about the importance of Arthus reactions (Type III) in food allergy.

ATOPIC FOOD HYPERSENSITIVITY

Atopic hypersensitivities are observed to a great number of inhalants (pollen, house dust, human and animal danders, fungi) and to various common foods like milk, egg and fruits. Atopic people (about 10 per cent of the population) as a rule are hypersensitive to several substances. The patterns of allergies differ from patient to patient, but in adult life nearly all people who manifest atopic diseases are sensitive to human dander and house dust. During the first years of life particularly, clinical hypersensitivities to food are common. Often, however, the child 'outgrows' his food hypersensitivity (Lehmus and Roine, 1958; Morrison-Smith, 1973; Sherman, 1959). In adults allergic manifestations to foods are rare and positive skin reactions to food extracts, as a rule, are seen in combination with reactions to inhalant allergens (Bleumink, 1967; Young, 1965). Table 11.1 records positive skin reactions to egg, milk and human dander in several age groups of patients with atopic dermatitis. The percentage of positive skin reactions to egg and milk become lower with increasing age; on the other hand, the incidence of positive reactors to human dander (an inhalant allergen) increases.

INCIDENCE

Considerable controversy exists among allergists about the importance of foods as a cause of atopic diseases.

Table 11.1 Positive skin reactions in patients with atopic dermatitis (after Bleumink, 1970)

Age	Number of patients	Positive skin reactions to					
		Human dandruff		Egg		Cow's milk	
		Number	%	Number	%	Number	%
0–5 years	43	20	46	15	35	6	14
6–10 years	48	30	62	9	19	3	6
11–20 years	81	70	86	7	9	5	6
21–70 years	135	113	83	6	4.5	4	3

Estimates of the incidence of food allergy in asthma and atopic dermatitis range from 3 per cent to 40 per cent (compare review of Hedström, 1958, and Lehmus *et al.*, 1958). The main reason for this difference of opinion is the lack of a generally accepted and reliable test for atopic food allergy. Not uncommonly the diagnosis is based on the results of skin tests performed with poorly standardized and ill-defined food extracts which may contain an abundance of irritating substances and enzymes leading to non-specific (false) positive skin responses. Reliable data can only be obtained when well-standardized food extracts are used for skin testing and *in-vitro* assays.

From critical investigations (in which diet trials and food elimination and provocation methods were also used) it can be deduced that at least 10 per cent of children under the age of 6 with asthma, rhinitis and atopic dermatitis may show clinical symptoms of atopy after challenges with foods (especially milk, egg, fish, wheat and fruits), whereas in older atopic individuals, the incidence may be estimated at 1–3 per cent (Aas, 1966; Bachman and Dees, 1957; Collins-Williams, 1962; González de la Reguera, Iñigo and Oehling, 1971; Hedström, 1958; Hellerström and Raika, 1967; Gerrard *et al.*, 1967, 1973; Goldman *et al.*, 1963; Lehmus *et al.*, 1958; Osváth, Márton and Lehotzky, 1973; Wilken-Jensen, 1958, 1965; Young, 1965).

This means that in more than 0.2 per cent of the general population foods may provoke, or may lead to an aggravation of atopic symptoms.

FOODS INVOLVED IN ATOPY

Many handbooks and reviews on allergy contain long lists of foodstuffs to which people may become allergic. Although any food may be considered as potentially allergenic, only some are notorious, partly because of frequent encounter, partly because of a high content of allergenic material. Cow's milk, hen's eggs, and fish seem to be the most potent sensitizers followed by some fruits, tomatoes, oranges and bananas, and meat, nuts, chocolate and cereals; some reports mention atopic hypersensitivities to vegetables (peas, spinach) and potatoes, but apparently these are rare (Aas, 1966; Feinberg, Durham and Dragstedt, 1946; Gerrard *et al.*, 1973, González de la Reguera *et al.*, 1971; Hansen, 1957; Harris and Shure, 1957; Hedström, 1958; Lehmus, 1958; Wilken-Jensen, 1958; Young, 1965).

Of interest in this connection is the study of Gerrard *et al.* (1973) in which 787 babies were investigated for allergies to foods. The reactions observed are recorded in Table 11.2. Allergies to foods are often found in combination with other atopic hypersensitivities. For example, individuals allergic to bananas, as a rule, will be allergic to inhalants or other foods as well. The pattern of food hypersensitivities found in an individual person or in a group of patients is, of course, a reflection of the food habits of that group.

Fish allergy, particularly to cod, is very common in Norway, but not in many other countries (Aas, 1966). The incidence of hypersensitivities to soybean is high in individuals who use this as a substitute because of a milk allergy (May and Alberto, 1972a). Gerrard *et al.* (1973) observed, for example, that 20 per cent of his milk allergic infants had become allergic to soybean. In other groups of patients no soya allergy was observed. In a recent report, Horesh (1972) pointed to the importance of buckwheat sensitivity in children; the flour is employed, for example, in making griddle cakes and waffles. He tested 500 consecutive allergic patients living in Cleveland. Among them 37 showed positive skin tests, while 6 (1.2 per cent) were proven clinically sensitive to buckwheat. They have asthma, urticaria, angioedema and rhinitis after contact with the allergen. Buckwheat can provoke symptoms both as an ingestant and as an

Table 11.2 Reactions to foods noted in 787 babies suspected of having allergies to foods other than cow's milk (after Gerrard *et al.*, 1973)

	Eczema	*Diarrhoea*	*Vomiting*	*Urticaria*	*Bronchitis*
Orange	13	8	6	–	–
Egg	10	2	3	–	–
Rice	7	2	4	–	2
Tomato	10	2	–	1	–
Banana	4	2	3	–	–
Oats	3	3	2	–	1
Vitamin preparations	7	–	–	–	–
Chocolate	4	–	–	1	–
Pear	–	1	–	1	–
Wheat	1	–	–	–	–
Barley	2	2	–	–	–
Potato	1	–	–	–	–
Peanut	–	–	–	1	–
Totals	62	22	18	5	3

inhalant. Based on these and other reports, buckwheat therefore seems to be important in North America (and in Japan) as an eliciting factor of atopy, but in many other countries no buckwheat hypersensitivities have been observed.

Egg allergy

In addition to cow's milk (Ch. 10) two foods are worth special attention, namely egg and fish, of which egg hypersensitivity has been studied most intensively. Egg allergy predominantly occurs in infants and children. It is commonly associated with milk hypersensitivity (Oswath and Markus, 1968). From a literature review by Ratner and Untracht (1952) 38 per cent of the allergic children with atopic dermatitis and 13 per cent of the infants with asthma show positive skin reactions to egg. More recently Freedman (1961) performed skin tests in 50 children with dermatitis. He observed that 69 per cent of these children reacted after injection of an egg extract. Sedlis, Prose and Holt (1966) investigated 115 children with infantile eczema; 35 per cent responded with wheal and erythema reactions. Furthermore, Young (1965) observed that 20 of 51 atopic patients with positive skin reactions to food had positive skin reactions to egg white.

Several investigations have involved food trial tests with egg. Ratner et al. (1952), for example, did oral provocation tests in children with positive skin responses to egg. More than 25 per cent of them were found clinically hypersensitive to egg white. Stifler (1965) studied 40 children under the age of 2 with severe eczema. Twenty-three of a total of 27, who showed positive skin tests to foods, reacted after ingestion of an egg-white solution. The offending foods were eliminated, 3–8 weeks after which challenges were instituted; marked changes occurred in 10 of the 'egg-sensitive' children. They developed gastrointestinal upsets, urticaria and exacerbation of their eczema.

Sedlis et al. (1966) studied 115 children with infantile eczema. In 27 infants with a positive skin test to egg, oral challenge tests were performed after elimination of the food and a symptom-free period. Six of these patients showed no reaction, 16 reacted with urticaria and angioedema, 3 showed erythema and flare-ups of their eczema and two reacted with vomiting. Subsequently, Matsumura, Kuruome and Suzuki (1967) investigated 40 children with infantile eczema, papular urticaria, vomiting, diarrhoea and bronchial asthma. In 21 of these infants egg was shown as a causative agent by challenges, food diary and elimination diet methods. Further a total of 82 patients with atopic dermatitis were investigated by Gonzáles de la Reguera et al. (1971) for the presence of food hypersensitivity; 59 of them showed one or more positive skin reactions. Milk, egg and fish were found the most frequently occurring eliciting factors (Table 11.3). Finally, with respect to egg sensi-

Table 11.3 Frequency of positive reactions to foods in 82 patients with atopic dermatitis (after Gonzales de la Reguera et al., 1971)

Antigen	No positive	%
Milk	24	18.5
Egg	21	15.5
Fish	20	14.5
Wheat	13	9.5
Shell-fish	12	9.0
Fruits	11	8.1
Vegetables	11	8.1
Greens	10	7.5
Cacao	8	6.0
Meat	5	3.8

tivity Aas (1966), in a very extensive study, performed inhalation as well as oral provocation tests with a great many allergen extracts in 825 children with urticaria and asthma; 41 children (5 per cent) showed flare-ups of their urticaria on challenges with hen's eggs. Also Davies and Pepys (1976) have found specific IgE serum antibodies to egg-white and egg-yolk components in their patients.

Fish allergy

In 1937 De Besche called attention to fish allergy as a frequent cause of asthma in Norway. Actually, the first detailed report on atopic food allergy regarded fish. It came from Prausnitz and Küstner (1921). Both investigators were allergic. Prausnitz was a hay fever patient and Küstner, his assistant, was known to have been allergic to fish since the age of 6. He developed severe symptoms after eating the merest traces of marine or fresh-water fish. Consumption of cooked or baked fish lead to the following symptoms:

'After half an hour, itching of the scalp, neck, lower abdomen, dry sensation in the throat; soon afterwards swelling and congestion of the conjunctivae, severe congestion and secretion of the respiratory mucous membranes. The skin of the entire body, especially the face, becomes highly hyperaemic and all over the skin of the body there appear numerous wheals, 1–2 cm large, which itch very much and show a marked tendency to confluence. After about 2 h heavy salivation starts and is followed by vomiting after which the symptoms very gradually fade away. After 10 to 12 h all the symptoms have disappeared; only a feeling of debility persists for a day or so.'

About 40 years later Aas started a systematic clinical study of hypersensitivity to fish among Norwegian people and indeed a high incidence of fish allergy among atopic individuals was observed (Aas, 1966). The study included 1410 children below 15 years of age who were referred to the Allergy Clinic of the University Hospital in Oslo from all parts of Norway because of ailments with known or suspected allergic aetiology. A total of 825 children were found to have asthma and/or urticaria. Fish-provoked asthma in 50 (16 per cent) of these children and in 76 (9 per cent), exposure to fish resulted in urticaria; all fish-allergic children showed strong positive skin reactions to a fish extract. The majority of these children had multivalent allergies and were also hypersensitive to inhalants (house dust, danders, pollen, fungi) and other foods, such as eggs, cow's milk, nuts and peas.

IN-VITRO TESTS FOR ATOPIC ALLERGY

Numerous in-vitro procedures have been proposed as aids in the diagnosis of atopic food allergy: measurement of antibodies by Ouchterlony techniques, passive haemagglutination, or by passive cutaneous anaphylaxis in guinea-pigs (Peterson and Good, 1963); cytotoxicity tests (Bryan and Bryan, 1969); lymphocyte stimulation tests (May and Alberto, 1972a and b); measurement of specific IgE by RAST (Aas and Lundkvist, 1973; Davies and Pepys, 1976; Gillespie, Nakajima and Gleich, 1976) and histamine release from human basophils or rat mast cells (May et al., 1972; Haddad and Korotzer, 1972). Most of these methods are poor indicators of Type I immediate hypersensitivity in that they fail to detect specific IgE antibody. Only the latter two methods are useful to demonstrate the presence of atopic allergy to a particular compound.

May et al. (1972) studied 12 individuals with allergy to egg. All of them showed positive skin reactions, but in only 6 (50 per cent) did ovalbumin, the major egg protein (which as a rule also contains traces of ovomucoid, the potent egg allergen), release histamine from their basophils. In controls the histamine release test was negative. Similar results were obtained in patients with milk, wheat and soybean allergies.

Table 11.4 records the findings of Haddad et al. (1972). They found a good correlation between skin reactions and the rat mast cell degranulation test. In this test the number of mast cells, passively sensitized with IgE of the patient's serum, are measured which degranulate after contact with the allergen. In a subsequent publication Schur, Hyde and Wypych (1974) studied 13 egg-sensitive patients. In these patients a significant relationship between specific IgE levels to egg allergen, skin tests and clinical symptoms were observed. No relationship could be demonstrated, however, between egg-white sensitivity and atopic eczema. Also Aas et al. (1973) studied 56 children with a clinical allergy to cod. Using the RAST technique, specific IgE to cod allergen could be demonstrated; in sera of children tolerant to fish no anti-cod IgE was detected. More recently a good correlation between results of skin tests, clinical symptoms and specific IgE antibodies (RAST technique) to various food constituents has also been found by Hoffman and Haddad (1974), Gillespie, Makajima and Gleich (1976) and Davies and Pepys (1976).

A remarkable case of food allergy has been described by MacLaren, Ho and Lopapa (1972). The patient (a man of 43 years old) had a positive family history of atopy on both sides. As a child he could tolerate only breast milk and rice cereals. Cow's milk produced severe eczema; later he developed asthma and became allergic to other foods like nuts and fish. Eating minute amounts of walnuts immediately produced severe symptoms, with nausea, urticaria and asthmatic attacks. Skin testing and in-vitro tests (rat mast cell degranulation tests) indicated that he had an atopic hypersensitivity to milk, eggs, nuts and fish (Table 11.5). Skin tests with walnut, coconut, peanut and pecan produced a severe anaphylactic (shock) reaction.

PROPERTIES OF ATOPIC ALLERGENS FROM FOODS

During the last 10 years attempts have been made to characterize the compounds in foods responsible for symptoms in atopic individuals. So far, the atopic allergens present in cow's milk, hen's eggs, tomatoes and fish (cod) have been identified (Bleumink, 1970; Elsayed and Aas, 1970, 1971; Elsayed, Aas and

Table 11.4 Summary of findings in patients with immediate hypersensitivity reactions to foods – correlation with result of skin tests and rat mast cell degranulation tests (RMCDT) (after Haddad et al., 1972)

Antigen	No. subjects	Symptoms	Skin test +	−	ND	RMCDT +	−
Milk	4	Urticaria, rhinitis, angioedema, asthma, shock	4	0		4	0
Egg	6	Urticaria, shock eczema	5	0	1	6	0
Shellfish	8	Urticaria, angioedema	5	1	2	8	0
Fish	9	Urticaria, angioedema	6	1	2	9	0
Walnut	7	Urticaria, angioedema	7	0		7	0
Peanut	4	Urticaria, angioedema	3	1		4	0
Chocolate	3	Urticaria	3	0		2	1

ND = not done

Table 11.5 Clinical symptoms, skin tests and rat mast cell degranulation tests (RMCDT) in a patient with severe food sensitivity (after MacLaren et al., 1972)

Food	Clinical symptoms	Skin test results	RMCDT (% degranulation)
Milk	Vomiting and diarrhoea during infancy	4+	65
Egg	Urticaria in childhood, rare recurrence now	4+	72
Walnut	Severe asthma, urticaria, vomiting	Not done	89
Almond	Not known	Anaphylactic reaction	90
Coconut	Asthma, urticaria	Anaphylactic reaction	78
Pecan	Not known	Anaphylactic reaction	89
Peanut	Asthma, urticaria	Anaphylactic reaction	65
Cashew nut	Not known	Not done	92
Hazelnut	Not known	Not done	81
Codfish	Asthma, urticaria	4+	96
Halibut	Asthma, urticaria	4+	86
Salmon	None	1+	16
Shrimp	None	Neg.	8
Lobster	None	Neg.	4
Crab	None	Neg.	6
Controls			2–6

Christensen, 1971). These studies have shown that for a given food a relatively large fraction is unimportant in human atopic food allergy, and that this fraction can be separated from the strongly allergenic components. The most important data concerning the major allergenic components have been collected in Table 11.6.

It may be observed that the quantities of active material which may be isolated from a standard amount of the various foodstuffs differ considerably. It is noteworthy that the two foodstuffs against which severe reactions are relatively common (fish and egg) appear to contain relatively large amounts of active material. The skin reactivity of these two allergens is also much higher that that of modified β-lactoglobulin and many inhalant allergens (Berrens, 1971; Bleumink, 1970). A remarkable point is that the molecular weights of the active components appear to be of the same order of magnitude, ranging from 14 500 for the allergenic fraction of cod to 36 000 for the active β-lactoglobulin fraction of cow's milk.

The molecular weights of inhalant allergens so far identified also fall in the same range (Bleumink, 1970; Berrens, 1971; Stanworth, 1973); apparently, therefore, allergenic activity is narrowly restricted to glycoproteins with a molecular weight of approximately 15 000–35 000.

In addition, the active protein fractions are stable against heat treatments and some of these are resistant to proteolytic enzymes (Bleumink, 1970; Wüthrich and Schwarz-Speck, 1970). The active principles from tomatoes and fish are, for example, not inactivated by heating solutions of the allergen; the allergen in egg is still active after boiling and bovine β-lactoglobulin

is one of the most stable milk proteins. Furthermore, the tomato allergen is stable towards the action of trypsin and chymotrypsin, whereas Prausnitz and Küstner (1921) presented evidence that incubation of the active fraction from fish (haddock) with trypsin or pepsin did not lead to a marked decrease of activity. Ovomucoid, the skin reactive fraction in egg, inhibits the proteolytic activity of trypsin; moreover, egg white also contains a chymotrypsin inhibitor (ovoinhibitor). Finally the active allergenic fraction from pasteurized milk is only slightly susceptible to proteolytic enzymes.

These findings imply that after oral ingestion the skin reactive components of foodstuffs will have a very good chance of reaching the circulation unaltered, even after heat processing of the foods in question. Actually, normal food processing and household handling will not lead to inactivation of the atopic allergens present in milk, egg and fish. On the contrary, further analysis has revealed that pasteurization, spray-drying and cooking of milk give rise to a marked *increase* of specific activity as assayed by intracutaneous tests in susceptible individuals (Bleumink, 1970). Model experiments have shown that this increase in activity is due to non-enzymatic browning (Maillard) reactions between ε-amino-groups of lysine in the protein molecule and reducing sugars such as lactose and glucose (Bleumink, 1970).

During Maillard reactions N-substituted 1-amino-2-deoxy-ketose residues are formed. Figure 11.1 records the skin reactivities of β-lactoglobulin preparations modified by non-enzymatic browning reactions, as a function of the number of lysine groups which have been made to react with lactose molecules. Native β-lacto-

Table 11.6 Properties of skin reactive components of some foods[a]

Food	Active component	Mg of component isolated from 100 g	Skin reactivity[b] (μg)	Mol. weight	Carb. content %	Stability during heating at 100°	Resistance against the action of trypsin and chymotrypsin	Remarks
Fish (cod)	Sarcoplasmic protein	200	0.001	14 500	1.5	+ +	?	
Tomatoes	Glycoprotein fraction	2.5	0.15	20 000–30 000	– 29	+ +	+ +	Produced during storage and ripening of the fruits
Egg (white)	Ovomucoid fraction	225	0.0025	31 500	24	+ +	+ +	Ovomucoid inhibits the proteolytic act of trypsin
Cow's milk	β-Lactoglobulin modified	100	0.10	36 000	0.2	+	+[c]	Not present in breast milk

[a] For isolation and chemical characterization see Bleumink (1970)

[b] Minimum amount of material eliciting (1+) positive skin reaction; wheal and erythema reactions similar to the skin reactivity observed after injection of 3 μg of histamine-HCl in normal individuals.

[c] Native β-lactoglobulin is only slightly susceptible to enzymes. Incorporation of lactose residues increases the resistance towards trypsin.

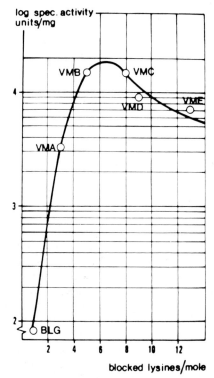

Fig. 11.1 Semilogarithmic plot of specific skin reactivity of a number of lactulose-β-lactoglobulin conjugates as a function of the number of ε-amino groups which have been made to react with sugar. Skin reactivity is expressed as the reciprocal of the minimum amount in milligrams, eliciting a one plus reaction in intracutaneous assays. BLG=native β-lactoglobulins, VMA-VME: preparations with increasing amount of 1-amino-1-deoxy-2-ketose residues. (After Bleumink, 1970.)

globulin has a low skin reactivity while the modified preparations have activities more than 1000 times as great. Similarly, pasteurized milk and instant milk products were found to have high skin reactivities whereas fresh cow's milk showed threshold activity only. It is important to note that many inhalant allergens, and the tomato allergen, have also been found to incorporate 1-deoxy-ketose sugar side chains (attached at the sugar carbon C1) to the ε-amino groups of lysine residues in the peptide chain of protein or glycoprotein carrier molecules (Berrens, 1971). Degradation of these groups, for example by ultraviolet irradiation, leads to a marked decrease of activity (Berrens, Henocq and Radermecker, 1973b).

The above findings cannot be interpreted to mean, however, that the particular 1-amino-1-deoxy-2-ketose residues are antigenically active in a strict immunological sense. Studies of Berrens and his co-workers (Berrens and van Rijswijk-Verbeek, 1973a; Berrens et al., 1973b; Berrens and van Liempt, 1974) suggest that in atopic hypersensitivity at least two separate

mechanisms may play a role. Firstly, the reaction of allergenic molecules with specific IgE antibody may lead to the release of histamine from basophils and mast cells. Secondly, a non-immunological reaction of allergenic molecules with complement may occur without the involvement of IgE. Thus, atopic individuals may differ in the susceptibility of their complement system to activation with inhalant allergens, such as house dust and human dander (Berrens et al., 1973a). In atopic individuals this suggested lability of their complement system could, for example, allow the release of C3a and C5a (anaphylatoxins) which in turn trigger histamine release. Furthermore it has been suggested that the complement activation capacity of proteins is directly related to the number of 1-amino-1-deoxy-2-ketose residues present in the molecules (Berrens et al., 1974). Incorporation of lactose residues in β-lactoglobulin molecules leads to a protein with a markedly increased complement activation capability (Berrens et al., 1974). In atopic hypersensitivity reactions with allergens which do not incorporate these groups (cod, egg and pollens), an IgE-mediated mechanism is probably dominant. In reactions with milk allergen (modified β-lactoglobulin) and many inhalant allergens (except pollen) both mechanisms may be operative. Skin tests and other in-vivo methods cannot discriminate between these two mechanisms. They would both lead to an immediate release of histamine, either via C3a and C5a or via IgE on basophils and mast cells.

OTHER HUMORAL REACTIONS TO FOODSTUFFS

ANTIBODY FORMATION TO FOOD CONSTITUENTS

Normal individuals

The presence in human serum of antibodies to food proteins, especially to milk, wheat and egg, has been a subject of fluctuating interest for many years. Lippard, Schloss and Johnson demonstrated in 1936 that almost all children fed on cow's milk developed precipitating antibodies to milk proteins. Subsequent research corroborated this early observation. Gunther, Aschaffenburg, Matthews, Parish and Coombs (1960), for example, found that 98 per cent of 286 normal infants between 2 weeks and 2 years of age had detectable antibodies to milk protein. Also, Peterson et al. (1963) demonstrated the presence of circulating antibodies to milk proteins in 67 per cent of 288 infants and children tested, whereas Rothberg and Farr (1965a) were able to detect specific antibodies to bovine serum albumin (BSA) in the sera of 74 per cent of 535 normal children; in 41 per cent of the sera, anti-α-lactalbumin activity could also be demonstrated.

From an experimental point of view Rothberg and

Farr (1965b) could stimulate antibody production in adult rabbits by feeding them milk. Four of 6 rabbits produced antibody against BSA and α-lactalbumin (ALA). Anti-BSA was first detected in some sera 14 days after the initiation of milk feeding and antibody to ALA was present on the 35th day. Only very small amounts of antigen were found capable of initiating antibody production (Rothberg, Kraft and Farr, 1967). During follow-up studies the latter authors fed 25 adult male rabbits BSA; the average daily consumption was approximately 275 mg of protein. After 5 days the mean concentration of native BSA in the serum (as determined immunologically) was found to be 0.05 μg of protein per ml. Virtually all animals had developed detectable antibody 14 days after the start of protein feeding. Worthy of special notice was the observation of Rothberg *et al.* (1967) that the immune specificities of rabbit antibodies produced to orally administered BSA were similar to those of antibodies produced after parenteral immunization.

Returning to the human situation, comprehensive studies have indicated that several factors may influence the antibody production to dietary protein. Schloss and Worthen (1916) and Anderson and Schloss (1923) drew attention to this point in presenting evidence that young infants more readily form precipitating antibody to food proteins. Much later, Rothberg *et al.* (1965a) showed that circulating antibody to BSA may be detected more frequently among children under 16 (75 per cent) than among individuals 16–40 years of age (25 per cent), or among older age groups (8 per cent). Matsumura, Kuroume, Mitomo and Kobayashi (1966) estimated the concentration of antibodies to milk and egg proteins in the sera of several age groups of children. They found that the average concentration of food protein antibody rises sharply in infancy, reaching a maximum at 1–3 years and falling gradually thereafter (Gunther *et al.*, 1960; Lippard *et al.*, 1936).

With respect to the immunoglobulin class of the antibody produced, Kletter, Gery, Freier and Davies (1971a) showed the peak response of IgG-class antibodies to milk is reached at 3 months of age; IgA-class antibodies develop more slowly and reach a peak incidence and highest mean titre at 7 months. Studies performed by other groups have also made clear that the incidence and the titre of detectable antibody to food constituents decreases with increasing age (Bleumink, Young, de Maat-Bleeker and Stoop, 1968; Gunther, Check, Mathews and Coombs, 1962; Bürgin-Wolff and Berger, 1963; Gold and Godek, 1961). The decrease in mean titre of IgG- and IgA-class antibodies after the age of 1 year, and the reduced incidence of anti-food IgE antibodies in adults, have been attributed to changes in the permeability of the intestine to protein, and more adequate proteolysis with increasing age. Soothill,

Stokes, Turner, Norman and Taylor (1976) have presented evidence to suggest that transient IgA deficiency in infancy may predispose to atopy. The authors allege that because of inadequate IgA production IgE synthesis may be enhanced.

Patients with gastrointestinal disease

In patients with gastrointestinal diseases the concentration of circulating antibody to dietary proteins is often very high. Wright and Truelove (1965) found, for example, high levels of antibodies to milk protein, wheat-gluten and ovalbumin in the sera of patients with ulcerative colitis (as compared to normal controls). Also Taylor and Truelove (1961a) determined the antibody titre to casein, α-lactalbumin and β-lactoglobulin in the sera of 75 patients with ulcerative colitis and 90 control persons; a higher percentage of anti-milk activity was found in the patient group. On the other hand, Dudek, Spiro and Thayer (1965), and Sewell, Cooke, Cox and Meynell (1963) did not find an increased incidence or higher concentration of milk antibodies in ulcerative colitis patients as compared to matched controls. In the sera of patients with coeliac disease and idiopathic steatorrhoea elevated concentrations of antibodies to wheat and milk protein fractions are usually detected (Alarçon-Segovia, Herskovic, Wakin, Green and Scudamore, 1964; Berger and Savary-Piot, 1964; Berglund, 1965; Davidson, 1961; Immonen, 1965; Lalande, Halpern, Ky, Frésal and Rey, 1967; Taylor, Thomson, Truelove and Wright, 1961b). Moreover, Berger *et al.* (1964) demonstrated that in patients with coeliac disease, antibodies to gliadin and cow's milk protein were present not only in the sera but also in the stools (coproantibodies). The latter antibodies are mainly of the IgA class (Kletter, Freier, Davies and Gery, 1971b). Taylor *et al.* (1961a, b, 1964) determined the antibody concentration to casein, α-lactalbumin, β-lactoglobulin and wheat-gluten fraction III, in 277 patients with various gastrointestinal disorders and in a group of matched controls (402 persons). The results have been collected in Table 11.7. It may be observed from this table that patients with severe aphthous ulceration, coeliac disease, idiopathic steatorrhoea or ulcerative colitis are liable to show high concentrations of antibodies to wheat and cow's milk protein. However, in pernicious anaemia and in pancreatic steatorrhoea there is no striking difference from the control subjects in the levels of circulating antibodies to dietary antigens.

The significance of high antibody titres in many patients with gastrointestinal disease is unknown. One possibility is that they represent an epiphenomenon consequent to damage of the intestinal wall, allowing antigens to enter the mucosa. Moreover, it is reasonable to assume that antibody formation to food proteins, especially in infancy, may also follow aspiration. This

Table 11.7 Correlation between gastrointestinal disease and detectable antibodies to dietary proteins[a] (after Taylor et al., 1964)

Disease	Number of patients	Protein component[a]			
		Casein	α-Lactalbumin	β-Lactoglobulin	Gluten fraction III
Aphthous ulcer	36	+ +	+	+	+
Pernicious anaemia	50	−	−	+	+
Duodenal ulcer	24	−	−	−	+
Coeliac disease	17	+ +	+ +	+ +	+ +
Idiopathic steatorrhoea	42	+ +	+ +	+ +	+ +
Regional enteritis	33	−	−	−	−
Ulcerative colitis	75	+ +	−	+ +	+

[a] A minus sign indicates no significant differences from the findings in the control group, a plus sign indicates a difference significant at the 5% level and a double plus indicates a difference significant at the 1% level.

could lead to direct contact of protein material with the respiratory mucous membrane followed by absorption of increased quantities of intact (not digested) protein molecules (Hill, 1964; Nelson, 1964). Children with (recurrent) respiratory infections or with various swallowing difficulties frequently experience vomiting, resulting in aspiration of food constituents. These children often have elevated concentrations of detectable antibody to milk proteins (Crawford, Roane, Hanissian and Triplett, 1965; Handelman and Nelson, 1964; Nelson, 1964; Peterson et al., 1963). Model experiments have indicated that animals develop milk precipitins more readily from aspirated milk proteins than from ingested ones (Handelman et al., 1964). Moreover, it has been shown that protein molecules introduced into the pulmonary alveoli of dogs are absorbed into the circulatory system antigenically intact and in reasonable quantities (Bensch, Dominguez and Liebow, 1967; Schultz, Grismer, Wada and Grande, 1964).

SYSTEMIC ANAPHYLAXIS

Observations in animals and in man reveal that high concentrations of circulating antibodies to dietary proteins may lead to severe shock reactions following re-exposure to the antigen. Thus guinea-pigs or rabbits injected with cow's milk, wheat or egg proteins develop high titres of circulating antibodies against the particular antigens. Some of these animals may die rapidly with anaphylactic shock if a further injection of the antigen is given or after oral administration of the foodstuffs (Ratner, Dworetzky, Oguri and Aschheim, 1958a, b, c; Smith, Peel and Barrow, 1961). In humans severe shock reactions sometimes may be observed after ingestion of foods, especially of milk, egg, fish, nuts and shellfish.

The descriptions of these reactions resemble those of animal anaphylaxis and range from prostration, circulatory failure and pulmonary congestion to complete and immediate collapse (Collins-Williams, 1955; Freedman, 1961; Mortimer, 1961; Rubin, Shapiro, Muehlbauer and Grolnick, 1965; Stanfield, 1959; Vendel, 1948); a few millilitres of milk may suffice for the provocation of these symptoms (Freedman, 1961; Hill, 1964). Although these reactions are rare they constitute a highly significant risk for the patient. In a group of 89 children studied by Goldman et al. (1963), in which the diagnosis of milk allergy was established by repeated oral challenges with milk or purified milk protein, 8 patients (9 per cent) showed shock reactions. Only a small amount of milk was needed to produce sudden alarming symptoms with profound weakness and signs of shock, sometimes associated with vomiting, diarrhoea and urticaria. The symptoms also appeared after oral challenges with small quantities of purified cow's milk proteins (casein, β-lactoglobulin, α-lactalbumin). It must be emphasized in this connection that shock reactions may be caused both by Type I and Type III allergic reactions. Golbert, Paterson and Pruzansky (1969) reported on 15 cases of systemic reactions to ingested antigens, including 12 with food hypersensitivity and 3 with drug allergy. All had acute, potentially fatal reactions with syncope (in 4), cyanosis (in 8), dyspnoea (in 14), abdominal distress (in 6); angioedema and urticaria occurred in all. Most of the patients had other atopic diseases and many of them had appreciable but not necessarily unusually high titres of reaginic antibody against the antigens which caused anaphylaxis.

GASTROINTESTINAL SYMPTOMS

The diagnosis of food sensitivity often rests upon the clinical documentation of symptoms after repeated challenges following periods when the patient is symptom-free on a diet in which the suspected food is eliminated (provocation and elimination methods). Symptoms may occur immediately after provocation, or may be delayed;

Table 11.8 Correlation of tests with food allergy (after Galant *et al.*, 1973)

Test		Allergic responses		Controls
		Immediate	Delayed onset	
Skin test with allergens	Subjects	10/14 (71%)	3/23 (13%)	0/6 (0%)
	Allergens	11/15 (73%)	3/35 (9%)	0/12 (0%)
Histamine release with allergens	Subjects	10/14 (71%)	9/23 (39%)	5/21 (24%)
	Allergens	11/15 (73%)	9/35 (26%)	6/43 (14%)
Specific antibodies (radioimmunodiffusion)				
IgE	Subjects	6/11 (55%)	10/21 (48%)	0/15 (0%)
	Allergens	6/13 (46%)	10/35 (29%)	0/56 (0%)
IgG	Subjects	7/11 (64%)	17/21 (81%)	8/15 (53%)
	Allergens	9/13 (69%)	21/35 (60%)	13/56 (23%)
Foods involved		Egg, milk, peanut, halibut, walnut	Chocolate, milk, egg, peanut	–
Symptoms after provocation		Asthma, urticaria, angioneurotic oedema	Asthma, rhinitis, pallor, fatigue, stomach ache, vomiting, diarrhoea, headache	–

a division is therefore sometimes made between *immediate-onset* food sensitivity (within 1–5 h) and *delayed-onset* sensitivity (5 h or longer) (Galant, Bullock and Frick, 1973).

Food sensitivities of immediate onset usually fulfil the criteria of a Type I atopic hypersensitivity reaction. As a rule in these cases the diagnosis is relatively simple and a good correlation is usually found between the history and the results of provocation methods, skin testing and *in-vitro* parameters (Galant *et al.*, 1973; Haddad *et al.*, 1972). In contrast, food sensitivities of delayed onset present many more problems. Here there is often a considerable overlap of immunological reactions and toxic intolerance phenomena (for example, in gluten-induced reactions and in lactose intolerance). Also, Galant *et al.* (1973) have shown that a high percentage of delayed-onset sensitivities may on certain criteria be considered as Type I reactions. They found, for example, that in 9 out of 23 patients with symptoms of delayed onset, significant histamine release occurred (Table 11.8). Nevertheless, 5 of 21 asymptomatic, non-atopic controls showed similar histamine release. Further, it has been postulated that in some of the patients with delayed-onset symptoms (in which no clue has been found for intolerance or atopic reactions), Arthus-type phenomena may be involved in the elicitation of the disease. This would involve IgG or IgM antibody and complement consumption and the reactions would typically occur 6 or more hours after challenge. Relevant to this point, several cases of food sensitivities

have been described (Freier, 1973; Parish, 1971; Matthews and Soothill, 1970; Sandberg and Bernstein, 1972) which fulfil the criteria of Arthus-type reactions: a delayed time of onset after provocation, high levels of specific IgG antibody and evidence of complement consumption (decrease in plasma C3 levels).

Several other syndromes have been described in which it has been assumed that immunoglobulins of the IgG class have a pathological role; in Table 11.9 some examples have been collected. In the recorded cases milk has been found to elicit the symptoms, elimination has led to an improvement, and in many instances high levels of antibodies were found (for details see Bleumink, 1970, and Freier, 1973). As yet, direct evidence is lacking that Arthus reactions play a prominent role in the pathogenesis of the Heiner syndrome, cot death and of several gastrointestinal diseases including coeliac disease. It is reasonable to assume, however, that in some individual cases of coeliac disease or milk sensitivity Type III reactions lead to clinical symptoms or to aggravation or perpetuation of the disease (Davidson and Burnstine, 1956; Fallström, Winberg and Anderson, 1965; Kuitunen, Visakorpi and Hallman, 1965; Kuitunen, Visakorpi, Savilahti and Pelkonen, 1975; Fontaine and Navarro, 1975; Shiner, Ballard and Smith, 1975). Thus, in coeliac disease, IgG antibodies to milk and gluten are demonstrable, also complement consumption has sometimes been found to occur after gluten challenge. However, other findings are also compatible with the involvement of lymphocyte-dependent antibody (Ezeoke,

Table 11.9 Examples of Type III allergic reactions to foods

Symptoms	Antibodies to dietary antigens[a] demonstrated	Response on elimination (recovery)	Response on provocation[b] (eliciting symptoms)	Accompanying symptoms	Laboratory findings	References
1. Anaphylactic shock	++	+	+	Vomiting, diarrhoea, urticaria, circulatory failure, pulmonary congestion, collapse		Freedman (1961); Goldman, Anderson, Sellars, Saperstein, Kniker and Halpern (1963a); Mortimer (1961); Stanfield (1959); Vendel (1948); Golbert, Patterson and Pruzansky (1969)
2. Heiner syndrome (milk precipitin disease)	++	+	+	Pulmonary haemosiderosis, intermittent wheezing, anaemia, failure to thrive, diarrhoea	Eosinophilia, elevated IgE, iron deficiency	Anderson, Weiss, Rebuck, Cabal and Sweet (1974); Boat, Polman and Whitman (1975); Heiner and Sears (1960, 1962); Hill (1964); Holland, Hong, Davis and West (1962)
3. Gastrointestinal symptoms: allergic gastroenteropathy	+	+	+	Oedema, anaemia, growth retardation, asthma, rhinitis	Hypoproteinemia, eosinophilia of peripheral blood, gastrointestinal protein loss	Ament (1972); Waldman, Wochner, Laster and Gordon (1967)
milk-induced hypochromic microcytic anaemia	+	+	+	Gastrointestinal bleeding, nasal pruritis, eczema	Blood in stools and vomiting, elevated serum alkaline phosphatase	Kravis, Donsky and Lecks (1967); Wilson, Heiner and Lahey (1964)
milk-induced steatorrhoea	++	+	+	Diarrhoea, failure to thrive	Increased IgA, partial villous atrophy in most cases	Davidson and Burnstine (1956); Kuitunen, Visakorpi and Hallman (1965); Kuitunen, Visakorpi, Savilahti and Pelkonen (1975); Lalande, Halpern, Ky, Frézal and Rey (1967)
recurrent vomiting, diarrhoea	+	+	+	Failure to thrive	No villous atrophy, no lactase deficiency	Fontaine and Navarro (1975); Gerrard, Lubos, Hardy, Holmlund and Webster (1967); Goldman, Anderson, Sellars, Saperstein, Kniker and Halpern (1963a); Goldman, Sellars, Halpern, Anderson, Furlow and Johnson (1963b); Kilby, Walker Smith and Wood (1975); Kuitunen, Visakorpi, Savilahti and Pelkonen (1975); Matsumura, Kuroumi and Susuki (1967); Shiner, Ballard and Smith (1975); Wilken-Jensen (1965)

[a] It cannot be excluded that the antibodies are only the result and not the cause of the observed symptoms.

[b] The allergenic activity resides in the protein fraction of the foods; in milk: the whey proteins, particularly the γ-globulins and bovine serum albumin; in egg: ovalbumin; in wheat: gluten.

Ferguson, Fakhri, Hekkens and Hobbs, 1974), or a defect in T-lymphocyte function (Asquith, 1974). Recently evidence has been presented which suggests that in gastrointestinal ulcer, Arthus reactions with food constituents might be involved (Siegel, 1974). Similarly, Pock-Steen (1973) has advanced the hypothesis that gluten, milk and other dietary proteins may play a role in some chronic dyspepsias by exerting an antigenic stimulus on the small-intestinal mucosa and thus inducing a state of hypersensitivity towards these foods. These assumptions need further evaluation. Finally, with respect to food antibodies, Davies, Johnson, Rees, Elwood and Abernethy (1974) found that compared with controls, a higher proportion of patients with myocardial infarction had circulating antibodies to milk and egg but not to gluten. The differences were very striking in the patients who died within some months of infarction.

DELAYED TYPE FOOD ALLERGY

MODEL STUDIES

Cell-mediated immune (CMI) reactions (also called delayed or Type IV reactions) are initiated essentially by T-lymphocytes which respond to antigens deposited at a local site, for example the skin or the gastrointestinal mucous membrane. CMI reactions are thought to play a prominent role in contact dermatitis, in tumour surveillance and homograft rejection. In contact dermatitis, as a rule, low molecular weight substances are involved. Model studies suggest that delayed-type allergic reactions to low molecular weight food constituents might also occur. Bicks and his co-workers (Bicks et al., 1967a; Bicks, Azar and Rosenberg, 1967b) have reported on their model studies regarding delayed hypersensitivity reactions in the intestinal tract of animals. The stimulus to their studies was the observation of Bicks and Rosenberg (1964) and Rosenberg and Fisher (1964) that guinea-pigs epicutaneously sensitized with 2,4-dinitrochlorobenzene (DNCB) showed colonic lesions when DNCB was applied to the mucosal surface with an inert adhesive paste. Bicks et al. (1967a) presented evidence to support the theory that the colonic lesions were a manifestation of a delayed hypersensitivity state. The morphological lesions were associated histologically with a cellular infiltration, and sometimes an active inflammatory reaction occurred. Moreover, the animals showed d-xylose malabsorption. Likewise, morphological lesions associated with d-xylose malabsorption have also been observed in the small intestine of miniature swines by a DNCB contactant reaction (Bicks et al., 1967b). Noteworthy is the observation that guinea-pigs and swine may also be sensitized to DNCB via the oral route by prolonged primary contact of the chemical with the mucosa of the colon (Bicks et al., 1967a). The orally sensitized animals were shown to be skin sensitive to DNCB as demonstrated by the development of contact dermatitis on skin challenge tests; repeated contact of the chemical with the intestinal mucosa was observed to lead specifically to delayed-type colonic reactions. The morphological lesions were characterized by chronic inflammatory cells in the supporting connective tissue, perivascular cuffing and vascular congestion (Bicks and Rosenberg, 1969a).

SUBSTANCES INVOLVED

In man, delayed-type allergic phenomena may be involved in the elicitation of symptoms after oral contact with low molecular weight substances in foods. Jansen (1959), for example, described a case of hypersensitivity to quinine, where sensitization, presumably, had taken place by skin contact. The patient experienced an immediate shock reaction some 30 min after the consumption of quinine in tonic water, and a delayed exacerbation of his eczema the following day. Similar cases have been described by Belkin (1967), Lockey (1971), Levantine and Almeyda (1974). Certain allergic manifestations can also follow the ingestion of milk (and some other foodstuffs) which are not due to cow's milk constituents, but to contaminants such as penicillin and sulfa drugs. Thus, small traces of penicillin, sometimes found in milk of penicillin-treated cows, may provoke allergic reactions (shock and dermatitis) in individuals previously sensitized to this antibiotic by skin contact or drug therapy (Welch, 1957; Vickers, Bagratuni and Alexander, 1958; Collins-Williams, 1962; Wicher, Reisman and Arbesman, 1969). Similarly, benzoates added to many foodstuffs as preservatives may give rise to exacerbations of eczema in individuals which have a delayed hypersensitivity to compounds of comparable chemical structure present in cosmetics, pharmaceuticals and topically applied medicaments (Fisher, 1967). This is an example of cross sensitization frequently found in contact allergy. For example, persons who have become hypersensitive to para-aminobenzoic acid (used in many anti-sunburn lotions) may also show delayed allergic reactions and dermatitis on contact with para-hydroxybenzoic esters (nipa-esters), p-hydroxybenzoic acid, benzoic acid and benzoates present in cosmetics, foodstuffs, soaps, soft drinks and medicaments. The following compounds have been reported to have caused skin reactions such as erythema, eczema, purpura and urticaria after ingestion in previously sensitized persons: azo dyes, garlic, onion, lemon, orange peel, cinnamon, oil of laurel, p-hydroxybenzoate and quinine (Hjorth and Fregert, 1972). Traces of metal, dissolved by cooking acid or salty food in stainless steel, may result in the persistence of dermatitis from metals such as chromium, nickel and cobalt. Primary sensitization in these cases has taken place by skin contact.

Adverse reactions following the ingestion of flavours (menthol, salicylates) butylated-hydroxyanisole and butylated-hydroxytoluene, cyclamates, saccharin and the azo dye tartrazine are in all probability not allergic (Feingold, 1968; Lockey, 1971; Juhlin, Michaëlsson and Zitterström, 1972; Levantine and Almeyda, 1974; Miller, White and Schwartz, 1974). It has been shown that aspirin is an important eliciting factor in a considerable percentage of patients with chronic urticaria and asthma (Chafee and Settipane, 1974; Doeglas, 1975); besides the latter, the symptoms noticed are angioneurotic oedema, eye symptoms (increased tear secretion and burning), nasal congestion, swelling of the throat and hoarseness and dyspnoea. In individual patients, tachycardia, fever and purpura may occur. Many of the aspirin-sensitive patients are also intolerant of tartrazine, benzoates and the analgesics indomethacin and paracetamol (Samter and Beers, 1967; Michaëlsson and Juhlin, 1973; Doeglas, 1975; Stenius and Lemola, 1976). It has been suggested that the effect of all of these substances might be attributable to their inhibitive effect on the synthesis of the prostaglandins PGE2 and PGF2.

UNRESPONSIVE STATE

In the guinea-pig the development of contact sensitivity, which usually occurs when certain chemicals are placed on the skin, can be prevented by prior feeding of the same sensitizer. This immunological tolerance was first reported by Chase (1946) – the so-called Chase–Sulzberger phenomenon – and has subsequently been demonstrated by many others. An unresponsive state can also be induced in man by prior application of DNCB to the buccal mucosa (Lowney, 1971). Also experiments in adult male volunteers have shown that 20 mg or more of DNCB given by mouth in capsule form may induce an unresponsive state (Lowney, 1973). In this respect it is interesting that the Indians already knew that chewing of poison ivy (a very strong sensitizer) prevented the development of contact dermatitis to *Rhus toxicodendron*, a frequently occurring weed in North America (Agrup, 1970).

NON-IMMUNOLOGICAL HYPERSENSITIVITY REACTIONS

HISTAMINE LIBERATORS

On provocation some foods may lead to symptoms closely resembling allergic symptoms. For example, strawberries produce urticaria in many individuals and shellfish may give rise to shock and skin disorders (Winkelman, 1957; Paton, 1959).

These phenomena have been thought to be of an immunological nature, but further investigations suggest that the particular symptoms are caused by substances which appear to release histamine from mast cells and circulating basophils without the involvement of IgE. In rare cases the consumption of foodstuffs, which have been stored for rather long periods of time may give rise to symptoms which are probably attributable to histamine intoxication. Doeglas, Huisman and Nater (1967) reported on a case of a young man, 20 years of age, who developed dermal symptoms, headache and a fall in blood pressure after eating a certain brand of old Gouda cheese. Chemical analysis revealed the presence of high quantities of histamine (85 mg 100 g cheese), presumably formed by a salt-resistant *Lactobacillus*. In addition Boyer, Depierre, Tissier and Jacob (1956) described an epidemic outbreak of histamine intoxication in the summer of 1955 in 400 out of 2000 individuals who had eaten tunny fish transported over a long distance during very warm weather. The fish contained 69–400 mg histamine per 100 g of muscle tissue; the histamine may have resulted from decarboxylation of histamine by bacteria.

COMPLEMENT ACTIVATION

During the last few years some evidence has been presented to show that food constituents may activate the complement system without the involvement of antibodies. Lipopolysaccharides (endotoxins) are suspect. Recently Berrens and his co-workers (1973a, 1974) have suggested that proteins incorporating 1-amino-1-deoxy-2-ketose residues may activate the complement system via C3 without the involvement of antibodies. The complement-activating capacity appears to be related to the number of deoxy-ketose residues present in the molecules (Berrens *et al.*, 1973a, 1974.) These groups are formed by non-enzymatic browning (Maillard) reactions between ε-amino groups in the protein molecules and reducing sugars (Fig. 11.2).

Non-enzymatic browning is a fairly common reaction in all foodstuffs containing proteins and reducing sugars and it may occur during storage (internal browning in fruits and nuts), industrial processing (roasting, pasteurization, sterilization, evaporation and spray-drying) and household handling (Bleumink, 1967, 1970; Cole, 1967; Ellis, 1959). For example, all commercially available milk products and infant formulas contain relatively large amounts of 'browned' proteins whereas fresh cow's milk and breast milk do not (Bleumink, 1970). Hence it is possible that a number of cases of adverse reactions observed after provocation with milk formulas, boiled egg and nuts might result from direct activation of the complement system. Moreover, complement consumption sometimes found in coeliac and 'milk-sensitive' patients after provocation (Mathews *et al.*, 1970) may also be attributable to direct activation of complement by browned proteins present in the foodstuffs used.

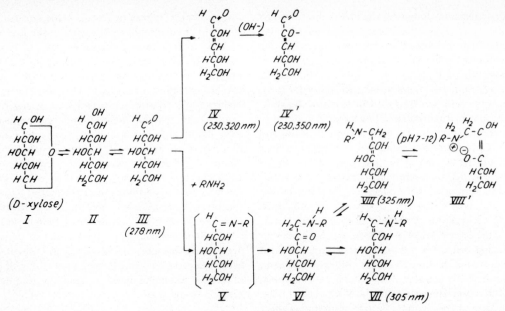

Fig. 11.2 Reaction scheme of non-enzymatic browning of reducing sugar (*D*-xylose, for example) with protein (R-NH2). (After Bleumink 1967.) IV = 3-deoxy-pentosulose; IV¹ = anion of IV; V = Schiff base; VI = 1-amino-1-deoxy-2-ketose (AMADORI compound); VII = 1.2 enol of VI; VIII = 2.3 enediol of VI, VIII¹ = (pseudo)-isoxazoline ring of VIII. (305 nm) indicates the absorption maximum in uv spectrum.

Thus other mechanisms than IgG-mediated ractions cannot be excluded in these cases.

Hexulose-(pentulose)-protein conjugates have also been found to inhibit the proteolytic activity of trypsin, chymotrypsin and carboxypeptidase-B (Berrens, 1971). The inhibitory activity appears to correlate with the degree of browning of the substances (Berrens, 1971). Aminopeptidase-B is involved in the conversion of kallidin-10 into bradykinin, both so-called kinins which are vasoactive and stimulate smooth muscle; they are released in inflammatory processes and are usually rapidly inactivated enzymatically. If, however, amino-peptidase-B is inhibited an overflow of kallidin-10 will occur, thus leading to an intensification of the primary response. Also active kinins are probably released in local inflammatory processes in the gastrointestinal tract. It is possible therefore that small amounts of ingested proteins (incorporating N-substituted-1-amino-1-deoxy-2-ketose residues) will lead, by virtue of their capacity to inhibit aminopeptidase-B, to an intensification of the primary response, giving rise to increased dilatation of the blood vessels and contraction of smooth muscles, and thus to aggravation and perpetuation of the gastrointestinal disease.

LYMPHOCYTE STIMULATION BY LECTINS

Finally some foods also contain proteins capable of activating (T-) lymphocytes non-specifically. These substances (called phytohaemagglutinins, blastomitogens,

lectins or plantagglutinins) are present, for example in soybean, wheat and edible legumes (Naspitz and Richter, 1968; Sharon and Lis, 1972; Yachnin and Svenson, 1972). Most intensively investigated are the haemagglutinins derived from *Phaseolus vulgaris*. Although the mitogenic substances (blastogenic or leucoagglutinins) are now considered to be distinct from the erythro-(haem)agglutinins the two properties occur in the same extracts of plant materials.

Recently, bovine β-lactoglobulin (a major protein in milk) has also been found to possess blastogenic activity (Asquith, Housley and Cooke, 1970). Also *in-vitro* experiments have shown that proteins from egg, wheat, milk and soybean stimulate lymphocytes (to form blasts) from allergic and non-allergic individuals (May *et al.*, 1972a). *In-vivo* stimulation also occurs (May *et al.*, 1972b). The mitogens investigated thus far proved relatively labile to heat treatment and have molecular weights between 26 000 and 400 000. A point of special notice is that these particular foods contain protease inhibitors as well (Birk, 1968). This could promote inadequate proteolysis of the foods so that the lectins had relatively greater chance of reaching the gastrointestinal mucosa unaltered. Finally, soybean (used as substitute for milk in milk-sensitive patients), peas, beans and lentils sometimes produce adverse reactions in man (Perlman, 1966); stimulation of lymphocytes may be one of the underlying mechanisms leading to inflammatory responses.

CONCLUSION

There are numerous reports in the literature on food allergy, but most studies are concerned with the description of clinical symptoms and with methods for diagnosis and therapy. In the past many diseases were claimed by enthusiastic clinicians to be due to food allergy, but subsequent investigation has raised serious doubts as to their real association.

Recent work, which has included biochemical and immunological testing, has indicated that food allergy is relatively rare. Nevertheless it does occur and allergic reactions caused by foods may be divided into three categories. Type I, atopic or anaphylactic reactions which are observed in atopic individuals and which overlap with inhalant hypersensitivities; children seem particularly to be at risk. Type III, or Arthus phenomena leading to delayed onset symptoms after consumption of milk, egg and possibly certain cereals. Symptoms attributable to Type IV reactions and elicited by food constituents are probably rare.

REFERENCES

Aas, K. (1966) Studies of hypersensitivity to fish. A clinical study. *International Archives of Allergy and Applied Immunology*, 29, 346–363.

Aas, K. & Lundkvist, U. (1973) The radioallergosorbent test with a purified allergen from codfish. *Clinical Allergy*, 3, 255–261.

Agrup, G. (1970) Contact dermatitis. XII. Unresponsiveness to contact sensitizers in man. *British Journal of Dermatology*, 83, 516–517.

Alarcón-Segovia, D., Herskovic, T., Wakin, K. G., Green, P. A. & Scudamore, H. H. (1964) Presence of circulating antibodies to gluten and milk fractions in patients with non-tropical sprue. *American Journal of Medicine*, 36, 485–499.

Ament, M. E. (1972) Malabsorption syndromes in infancy and childhood. *Journal of Paediatrics*, 81, 685–697.

Anderson, A. F. & Schloss, O. M. (1923) Allergy to cow's milk in infants with nutritional disorders. *American Journal of Diseases of Children*, 26, 451–474.

Anderson, J. A., Weiss, L., Rebuck, J. W., Cabal, L. A. & Sweet, L. C. (1974) Hyperreactivity to cow's milk in an infant with LE and tart cell phenomena. *Journal of Paediatrics*, 84, 59–67.

Asquith, P. (1974) Cell-mediated immunity in coeliac disease. In *Coeliac Disease. Proceedings of the Second International Coeliac Symposium*, ed. Hekkens, with J. M. & Peña, A. S., pp. 242–260. Leiden: Stenfert Kroese.

Asquith, P., Housley, J. & Cooke, W. T. (1970) Lymphocyte stimulation by bovine β-lactoglobulin. *Nature*, 228, 462–464.

Bachman, K. D. & Dees, S. C. (1957) Milk allergy. II. Observations on incidence and symptoms of allergy to milk in allergic infants. *Paediatrics*, 20, 400–407.

Belkin, G. A. (1967) Cocktail purpura, an unusual case of quinine sensitivity. *Annals of Internal Medicine*, 66, 583.

Bensch, K. G., Dominguez, E. & Liebow, A. A. (1967) Absorption of intact protein molecules across the pulmonary air-tissue barrier. *Science*, 157, 1204–1206.

Berger, von E. & Savary-Piot, A. (1964) Nachweis von Nahrungsmittel-Antikörpern im Stuhl bzw. im Gastrointestinaltractus bei Allergikern gegen Kuhmilch, bei Cöliakie-Patienten und Nicht-Allergikern. *Schweizerische Medizinische Wochenschrift*, 94, 480–484.

Berglund, G. (1965) The presence of circulating antibodies to milk and gluten in some patients with coeliaci. *Acta Paediatrica Scandinavica*, Suppl. 159, 106–107.

Berrens, L. (1971) *The Chemistry of Atopic Allergens*. Basel: Karger.

Berrens, L. & Van Liempt, P. M. J. (1974) Synthetic protein-sugar conjugates as models for the complement-inactivating property of atopic allergens. *Clinical and Experimental Immunology*, 17, 703–707.

Berrens, L. & Van Rijswijk-Verbeek, J. (1973a) Inactivation of complement (C3) in human serum by atopic allergens. *International Archives of Allergy and Applied Immunology*, 45, 30–39.

Berrens, L., Hénocq, E. & Radermecker, M. (1973b) Photo-inactivated allergens. I. Preparation, physicochemical and biological properties. *Clinical Allergy*, 3, 449–459.

de Besche (1937) An asthma bronchiale in man provoked by cat, dog and different other animals. *Acta Medica Scandinavica*, 92, 237–255.

Bicks, R. O. & Rosenberg, E. W. (1964) A chronic delayed hypersensitivity reaction in the guinea-pig colon. *Gastroenterology*, 46, 543–549.

Bicks, R. O. & Rosenberg, E. W. (1969a) Delayed hypersensitivity contact reactions in the gut. *Southern Medical Journal*, 62, 830–832.

Bicks, R. O., Azar, M. M. & Rosenberg, E. W. (1967b) Delayed hypersensitivity reactions in the intestinal tract. II. Small intestinal lesions associated with xylose malabsorption. *Gastroenterology*, 53, 437–443.

Bicks, R. O., Azar, M. M., Rosenberg, E. W., Dunham, W. G. & Luther, J. (1967a) Delayed hypersensitivity reactions in the intestinal tract. I. Studies of 2,4-dinitrochlorobenzene-caused guinea-pig and swine colon lesions. *Gastroenterology*, 53, 422–436.

Bicks, R. O., Azar, M. M., Bale, G. F., Rosenberg, E. W. & Goldenberg, J. (1969b) Delayed hypersensitivity reactions in the intestinal tract. III. Pig stomach gastritis and parietal cell antibodies. *American Journal of Digestive Diseases*, 14, 385–393.

Birk, Y. (1968) Chemistry and nutritional significance of protease inhibitors from plant sources. *Annals of the New York Academy of Science*, 146, 388–399.

Bleumink, E. (1967) Isolation and chemical characterization of some atopic food allergens. Thesis, Utrecht.

Bleumink, E. (1970) Food allergy, the chemical nature of the substances eliciting symptoms. *World Review of Nutrition and Dietetics*, 12, 505–570.

Bleumink, E., Maat-Bleeker, F. de, Young, E., en Stoop, J. W. (1968) Koemelk-allergie bij jonge kinderen. *Nederlands Tijdschrift voor Geneeskunde*, 112, 2029–2034.

Boat, T. T., Polman, S. H., Whitman, V., Kleinerman, J. I., Stein, R. C. & Doershuk, C. F. (1975) Hyperreactivity to cow's milk in young children with pulmonary hemosiderosis and corpulmonale secondary to nasopharyngeal obstruction. *Journal of Paediatrics*, 87, 723.

Boyer, J., Depierre, F., Tissier, M. & Jacob, J. (1956) Intoxications histaminiques collectives par le thon. *Presse Medicale*, **64**, 1003–1004.

Bryan, W. T. K. & Bryan, M. P. (1969) Cytotoxic reactions in the diagnosis of food allergy. *Laryngoscope*, **79**, 1453–1472.

Bürgin-Wolff, A. & Berger, E. (1963) The formation of antibodies to various proteins of cow's milk in infants, children, adults and pregnant women. *Experientia*, **19**, 22–23.

Chafee, F. H. & Settipane, G. A. (1974) Aspirin intolerance I. Frequency in an allergic population. *Journal of Allergy and Clinical Immunology*, **53**, 193–199.

Chase, M. W. (1946) Inhibition of experimental drug allergy by prior feeding of the sensitizing agent. *Proceedings of the Society for Experimental and Biological Chemistry*, **61**, 257–259.

Cole, S. J. (1967) The Maillard reaction in food products; carbon dioxide production. *Journal of Food Science*, **32**, 245–250.

Collins-Williams, C. (1955) Acute allergic reactions to cow's milk. *Annals of Allergy*, **13**, 415–421.

Collins-Williams, C. (1962) Cow's milk allergy in infants and children. *International Archives of Allergy and Applied Immunology*, **20**, 38–59.

Crawford, L. V., Roane, J., Hanissian, A. & Triplett, F. (1965) Milk antibodies. *Southern Medical Journal*, **58**, 1140–1142.

Davidson, L. (1961) Milk proteins in ulcerative colitis. *British Medical Journal*, **ii**, 1358.

Davidson, M. & Burnstine, R. (1956) Steatorrhea related to a factor in cow's milk. *Quarterly Review of Paediatrics*, **11**, 151.

Davies, D. F., Johnson, A. P., Rees, B. W. G., Elwood, P. C. & Abernethy, M. (1974) Food antibodies and myocardial infarction. *Lancet*, **i**, 1012–1014.

Davies, R. & Pepys, J. (1976) Egg allergy, influenza vaccine and immunoglobulin E antibody. *Journal of Allergy and Clinical Immunology*, **57**, 373–383.

Doeglas, H. M. G. (1975) Reactions to aspirin and food additives in patients with chronic urticaria, including the physical urticarias. *British Journal of Dermatology*, **93**, 135–144.

Doeglas, H. M. G., Huisman, J. & Nater, J. P. (1967) Een geval van histamine-intoxicatie door het eten van kaas. *Nederlands Tijdschrift voor Geneeskunde*, **111**, 1526–1529.

Dudek, B., Spiro, H. M. & Thayer, W. R. (1965) A study of ulcerative colitis and circulating antibodies to milk proteins. *Gastroenterology*, **49**, 544–547.

Ellis, J. P. (1959) The Maillard reaction. *Advances in Carbohydrate Chemistry*, **14**, 63–134.)

Elsayed, S. &. Aas, K. (1970) Characterization of a major allergen (cod); chemical composition and immunological properties. *International Archives of Allergy and Immunology*, **38**, 536–548.

Elsayed, S. & Aas, K. (1971) Isolation of purified allergen (cod) by isoelectric focusing. *International Archives of Allergy and Applied Immunology*, **40**, 428–438.

Elsayed, S., Aas, K. & Christensen, T. (1971) Partial characterization of homogeneous allergens (cod). *International Archives of Allergy and Applied Immunology*, **40**, 439–447.

Ezeoke, A., Ferguson, N., Fakhri, O., Hekkens, W. Th. J. M. & Hobbs, J. R. (1974) Antibodies in the sera of coeliac patients which can coopt K cells to attack gluten-labelled targets. In *Coeliac Disease. Proceedings of the Second International Symposium*, ed. Hekkens, W. Th. J. M. & Peña, A. S., pp. 176–186. Leiden: Stenfert Kroese.

Fallström, S. P., Winberg, J. & Andersen, H. J. (1965) Cow's milk induced malabsorption as a precursor of gluten intolerance. *Acta Paediatrica Scandinavica*, **54**, 101–115.

Feinberg, S. M., Durham, O. C. & Dragstedt, C. A. (1946) *Allergy in Practice*, pp. 306–328. Chicago: Year Book.

Feingold, B. F. (1968) Recognition of food additives as a cause of symptoms of allergy. *Annals of Allergy*, **26**, 309–313.

Fisher, A. A. (1967) *Contact Dermatitis*. Philadelphia: Lea and Febiger.

Fisherman, E. W. & Cohen, G. N. (1973) Chemical intolerance to butylated-hydroxyanisole (BHA), butylated-hydroxytoluene (BHT) and vascular response as an indicator and monitor of drug intolerance. *Annals of Allergy*, **31**, 126–133.

Fontaine, J. L. & Navarro, J. (1975) Small intestinal biopsy in cow's milk protein allergy in infancy. *Archives of Diseases of Childhood*, **50**, 357.

Freedman, S. S. (1961) Milk allergy in infantile atopic eczema. *American Journal of Diseases of Children*, **102**, 106–111.

Freier, S. (1973) Paediatric gastrointestinal allergy. *Clinical Allergy*, Suppl. **3**, 597–618.

Galant, S. P., Bullock, J. & Frick, O. L. (1973) An immunological approach to the diagnosis of food sensitivity. *Clinical Allergy*, **3**, 363–372.

Gerrard, J. W., Lubos, M. C., Hardy, L. W., Holmlund, B. A. & Webster, D. (1967) Milk allergy: clinical picture and familial incidence. *Canadian Medical Association Journal*, **97**, 780–785.

Gerrard, J. W., MacKenzie, J. W. A., Goluboff, N., Garson, J. Z. & Maningas, C. S. (1973) Cow's milk allergy: prevalence and manifestations in an unselected series of newborns. *Acta Paediatrica Scandinavica*, Suppl. 234, 2–21.

Gillespie, D. N., Nakajima, S. & Gleich, G. J. (1976) Detection of allergy to nuts by radioallergosorbent test. *Journal of Allergy and Clinical Immunology*, **57**, 302–309.

Golbert, T. M., Patterson, R. & Pruzansky, J. J. (1969) Systemic allergic reactions to ingested antigens. *Journal of Allergy*, **44**, 96–107.

Gold, E. & Godek, G. (1961) Antibodies to milk in serum of normal infants and infants who died suddenly and unexpectedly. *American Journal of Diseases of Children*, **102**, 542.

Goldman, A. S., Anderson, D. W., Sellars, W. A., Saperstein, S., Kniker, W. T. & Halpern, S. R. (1963a) Milk allergy. I. Oral challenge with milk and isolated milk proteins in allergic children. *Paediatrics*, **32**, 425–443.

Goldman, A. S., Sellars, W. A., Halpern, S. R., Anderson, D. W., Furlow, T. E. & Johnson, C. H. (1963b) Milk allergy. II. Skin testing of allergic and normal children with purified milk proteins. *Paediatrics*, **32**, 572–579.

González de la Reguera, I., Iñigo, J. F. & Oehling, A. (1971) The importance of food sensitization in atopic dermatitis. *Dermatologica*, **143**, 288–291.

Gunther, M., Cheek, E., Matthews, R. H. & Coombs, R. R. A. (1962) Immune responses in infants to cow's milk proteins taken by mouth. *International Archives and Applied Immunology*, **21**, 257–278.

Gunther, M., Aschaffenburg, R., Matthews, R. H., Parish, W. E. & Coombs, R. R. A. (1960) The level of antibodies to the proteins of cow's milk in the serum of normal infants. *Immunology*, **3**, 296–306.

Haddad, Z. H. & Korotzer, J. L. (1972) Immediate hypersensitivity reactions to food antigens. *Journal of Allergy and Clinical Immunology*, **49**, 210–218.

Handelman, N. I. & Nelson, T. L. (1964) Association of milk precipitins with esophageal lesions causing aspiration. *Paediatrics*, **34**, 699–703.

Hansen, K. (ed.) (1957) *Allergie*, pp. 213–219. Stuttgart: Thieme.

Harris, M. C. & Shure, N. (1957) *Practical Allergy*, pp. 133–145, 205–221. London: Butterworth.

Hedström, V. (1958) Food allergy in bronchial asthma. *Acta Allergologica*, **12**, 153–185.

Heiner, D. C. & Sears, J. W. (1960) Chronic respiratory disease associated with multiple circulating precipitins to cow's milk. *American Journal of Diseases of Children*, **100**, 500–501.

Heiner, D. C., Sears, J. W. & Kniker, W. T. (1962) Multiple precipitins to cow's milk in chronic respiratory disease. *American Journal of Diseases of Children*, **103**, 634–654.

Hellerström, S. & Rajka, G. (1967) Clinical aspects of atopic dermatitis. *Acta Dermato-Venereologica*, **47**, 75–82.

Hill, L. W. (1964) Some advances in pediatric allergy in the last ten years. *Paediatric Clinics of North America*, **11**, 17–31.

Hjorth, N. & Fregert, S. (1972) Contact dermatitis. In *Textbook of Dermatology*, 2nd edn, ed. Rook, A., Wilkinson, D. S. & Ebling, F. J. G., pp. 305–385. Oxford: Blackwell.

Hoffman, D. R. & Haddad, L. H. (1974) Diagnosis of IgE-mediated reactions to food antigens by radioimmunoassay. *Journal of Allergy and Clinical Immunology*, **54**, 165–173.

Holland, N. H., Hong, R., Davis, N. C. & West, C. D. (1962) Significance of precipitating antibodies to milk proteins in the serum of infants and children. *Journal of Paediatrics*, **61**, 181–195.

Horesh, A. J. (1972) Buckwheat sensitivity in children. *Annals of Allergy*, **30**, 685–689.

Immonen, P. (1965) Precipitins to cow's milk and wheat proteins in gastrointestinal disorders. *Acta Paediatrica Scandinavica*, Suppl. **159**, 104–105.

Jacobson, E. D., Hibbs, S. & Faloon, W. W. (1962) Effect of adrenal steroids and of gluten upon malabsorption induced by neomycin. *American Journal of Clinical Nutrition*, **10**, 325–331.

Jansen, L. H. (1959) Het gelijktijdig bestaan van verschillende vormen van allergie. *Nederlands Tijdschrift voor Geneeskunde*, **103**, 1713–1716.

Juhlin, L., Michaëlsson, G. & Zetterström, O. (1972) Urticaria and asthma induced by food- and drug-additives in patients with aspirin hypersensitivity. *Journal of Allergy and Clinical Immunology*, **50**, 92–98.

Kaufman, H. S. & Frick, O. L. (1976) Immunological development in infants of allergic parents. *Clinical Allergy*, **6**, 321–327.

Kilby, A., Walker Smith, J. A. & Wood, C. B. S. (1975) Small intestinal mucosa in cow's milk allergy. *Lancet*, **i**, 531.

Kletter, B., Gery, I., Freier, S. & Davies, A. M. (1971a) Immune responses of normal infants to cow milk. I. Antibody type and kinetics of production. *International Archives of Allergy and Applied Immunology*, **40**, 656–666.

Kletter, B., Freier, S., Davies, A. M. & Gery, I. (1971b) The significance of coproantibodies to cow's milk proteins. *Acta Paediatrica Scandinavica*, **60**, 173–180.

Kravis, L. P., Donsky, G. & Lecks, H. I. (1967) Upper and lower gastrointestinal tract bleeding induced by whole cow's milk in an atopic infant. *Paediatrics*, **40**, 661–665.

Kuitunen, P., Visakorpi, J. K. & Hallman, N. (1965) Histopathology of duodenal mucosa in malabsorption syndrome induced by cow's milk. *Annales Paediatrici*, **205**, 54–63.

Kuitunen, P., Visakorpi, J. K., Savilahti, E. & Pelkonen, P. (1975) Malabsorption syndrome with cow's milk intolerance; clinical findings and course in 54 cases. *Archives of Diseases of Childhood*, **50**, 351–356.

Lalande, J. A., Halpern, B. N., Ky, N. T., Frézal, J. et Rey, J. (1967) Problèmes immunologiques dans la maladie coéliaque et l'intolérance au lait de vache chez l'enfant. *Revue Française d'Allergologie*, **7**, 65.

Lehmus, V. & Roine, K. (1958) Food allergy in children with asthma and eczema. *Acta Allergologica*, **12**, 186–198.

Levantine, A. & Almeyda, J. (1974) Cutaneous reactions to food and drug additives. *British Journal of Dermatology*, **91**, 359–362.

Lippard, V. W., Schloss, O. M. & Johnson, P. A. (1936) Immune reactions induced in infants by intestinal absorption of incompletely digested cow's milk protein. *American Journal of Diseases of Children*, **51**, 562–574.

Lockey, S. D. (1971) Reactions to hidden agents in foods, beverages and drugs. *Annals of Allergy*, **29**, 461–466.

Lowney, E. D. (1971) Tolerance of dinitrochlorobenzene, a contact sensitizer, in man. *Journal of Allergy and Clinical Immunology*, **48**, 28–35.

Lowney, E. D. (1973) Suppression of contact sensitization in man by prior feeding of antigen. *Journal of Investigative Dermatology*, **61**, 90–93.

MacLaren, W. R., Ho, F. C. & Lopapa, A. (1972) The rat mast cell degranulation test as applied to a case of severe food allergy. *Annals of Allergy*, **30**, 41–44.

Matsumura, T., Kuroume, T. & Suzuki, M. (1967) BDB haemagglutination applied to food allergy in children. *International Archives of Allergy and Applied Immunology*, **31**, 217–229.

Matsumura, T., Kuroume, T., Mitomo, A. & Kobayashi, K. (1966) Age differences of BDB haemagglutinating antibody titres against milk and egg allergens. *International Archives of Allergy and Applied Immunology*, **30**, 341–350.

Matthews, T. S. and Soothill, J. F. (1970) Complement activation after milk feeding in children with cow's milk allergy. *Lancet*, **ii**, 893–895.

May, C. D. & Alberto, R. (1972a) *In-vitro* responses of leucocytes to food proteins in allergic and normal children: lymphocyte stimulation and histamine release. *Clinical Allergy*, **2**, 335–344.

May, C. D. & Alberto, R. (1972b) *In-vivo* stimulation of peripheral lymphocytes to proliferation after oral challenge of children allergic to foods. *International Archives of Allergy and Applied Immunology*, **48**, 525–532.

Michaëlsson, G. & Juhlin, L. (1973) Urticaria induced by preservatives and dye additives in foods and drugs. *British Journal of Dermatology*, **88**, 525–532.

Miller, R., White, L. W. & Schwartz, H. J. (1974) A case of episodic urticaria due to saccharin ingestion. *Journal of Allergy and Clinical Immunology*, **53**, 240–242.

Morrison Smith, J. (1973) Skin tests and atopic allergy in children. *Clinical Allergy*, **3**, 269–275.

Mortimer, E. Z. (1961) Anaphylaxis following ingestion of soybean. *Journal of Paediatrics*, **58**, 90–92.

Naspitz, Ch. K. & Richter, M. (1968) The action of

phytohemagglutinin *in vivo* and *in vitro*: a review. *Progress in Allergy*, **12**, 1–85.

Nelson, T. L. (1964) Spontaneously occurring milk antibodies in mongoloids. *American Journal of Diseases of Children*, **108**, 494–498.

Osváth, P. & Markus, V. (1968) Diagnostic value of thrombopenia and eosinophilia after food ingestion in children with milk and egg allergy. *Acta Paediatrica of the Academy of Science (Hung.)*, **9**, 279.

Osváth, P., Márton, H. & Lehotzky, H. (1973) Study of the frequency of cow's milk sensitivity in the families of milk-allergic and asthmatic children. *Acta Allergologica*, **28**, 101–107.

Parish, W. E. (1971) Detection of reaginic and short-term sensitizing anaphylactic or anaphylactoid antibodies to milk of allergic and normal persons. *Clinical Allergy*, **1**, 369–380.

Paton, W. D. M. (1959) Lobsters, lymph and histamine-liberation. *International Archives of Allergy and Applied Immunology*, **15**, 35–46.

Perlman, F. (1966) Food allergy and vegetable proteins. *Food Technology*, **58**, 1438–1445.

Peterson, R. D. A. & Good, R. A. (1963) Antibodies to cow's milk proteins – their presence and significance. *Paediatrics*, **31**, 209–221.

Pock-Steen, O. Ch. (1973) The role of gluten, milk and other dietary proteins in chronic or intermittent dyspepsia. *Clinical Allergy*, **3**, 373–383.

Prausnitz, C. & Küstner, H. (1921) Studien über die Veberempfindlichkeit. Zentralblatt für Bakteriologie. *Parasitenkunde und Infektions krankheiten*, **86**, 160–169.

Ratner, B. & Untracht, S. (1952) Egg allergy in children. *American Journal of Diseases of Children*, **83**, 309–316.

Ratner, B., Dworetzky, M., Oguri, S. & Aschheim, L. (1958a) Studies on the allergenicity of cow's milk. I. The allergenic properties of alpha-casein, beta-lactoglobulin and alpha-lactalbumin. *Pediatrics*, **22**, 449–452.

Ratner, B., Dworetzky, M., Oguri, S. & Aschheim, L. (1958b) Studies on the allergenicity of cow's milk. II. Effect of heat treatment on the allergenicity of milk and protein fractions from milk as tested in guinea pigs by parenteral sensitization and challenge. *Paediatrics*, **22**, 648–652.

Ratner, B., Dworetzky, M., Oguri, S. & Aschheim, L. (1958c) Studies on the allergenicity of cow's milk. III. Effect of heat treatment on the allergenicity of milk and protein fractions from milk as tested in guinea-pigs by sensitization and challenge by the oral route. *Paediatrics*, **22**, 653–658.

Rosenberg, E. W. & Fischer, R. W. (1964) DNCB allergy in the guinea pig colon. *Archives of Dermatology (Chicago)*, **89**, 99–103.

Rothberg, R. M. & Farr, R. S. (1965a) Anti-bovine serum albumin and anti-alpha-lactalbumin in the serum of children and adults. *Paediatrics*, **35**, 571–588.

Rothberg, R. M. & Farr, R. S. (1965b) Antibodies in rabbits fed milk and their similarities to antibodies in some human sera. *Journal of Allergy*, **36**, 450–462.

Rothberg, R. M., Kraft, S. C. & Farr, R. S. (1967) Similarities between rabbit antibodies produced following ingestion of bovine serum albumin and following parenteral immunization. *Journal of Immunology*, **98**, 386–395.

Rubin, J. M., Shapiro, J., Muehlbauer, P. & Grolnick, M. (1965) Shock reaction following ingestion of mango. *Journal of the American Medical Association*, **193**, 397–398.

Samter, M. & Beers, R. F., Jr (1967) Concerning the nature of intolerance to aspirin. *Journal of Allergy and Clinical Immunology*, **40**, 281–293.

Sandberg, D. H. & Bernstein, C. W. (1972) Alteration of plasma C3-complement component following challenge with food antigens in the sensitive patient. *Paediatric Research*, **6**, 383.

Schloss, O. M. & Worthen, T. W. (1916) The permeability of the gastroenteric tract of infants to undigested protein. *American Journal of Diseases of Children*, **11**, 342–360.

Schultz, A. L., Grismer, J. T., Wada, S. & Grande, F. (1964) Absorption of albumin from alveoli of perfused dog lung. *American Journal of Physiology*, **207**, 1300–1304.

Schur, S., Hyde, J. S. & Wypych, J. I. (1974) Egg-white sensitivity and atopic eczema. *Journal of Allergy and Clinical Immunology*, **53**, 88.

Sedlis, E., Prose, P. H. & Holt, L. E. (1966) Infantile eczema. *Postgraduate Medicine*, **40**, 63–72.

Sewell, P., Cooke, W. T., Cox, E. V. & Meynell, M. J. (1963) Milk intolerance in gastrointestinal disorders. *Lancet*, **ii**, 1132–1135.

Sharon, N. & Lis, H. (1972) Lectins: cell-agglutinating and sugar-specific proteins. *Science*, **177**, 949–959.

Sherman, W. B. (1959) Atopic hypersensitivity. *Medical Clinics of North America*, **49**, 1597–1612.

Shiner, M., Ballard, J. & Smith, M. E. (1975) The small intestinal mucosa in cow's milk allergy. *Lancet*, **i**, 136–140.

Siegel, J. (1974) Gastrointestinal ulcer – Arthus reaction! *Annals of Allergy*, **32**, 127–130.

Smith, H. G., Peel, M. & Barrow, G. I. (1961) Anaphylaxis in guinea-pigs following routine milk inoculation. *Monthly Bulletin of Ministry of Health-Laboratory Service*, **20**, 189–196.

Soothill, J. F., Stokes, C. R., Turner, M. W., Norman, A. P. & Taylor, B. (1976) Predisposing factors and the development of reagenic allergy in infancy. *Clinical Allergy*, **6**, 305–319.

Stanfield, J. P. (1959) A review of cow's milk allergy in infancy. *Acta Paediatrica Scandinavica*, **48**, 85–99.

Stanworth, D. R. (1973) *Immediate Hypersensitivity*. Amsterdam: North-Holland.

Stenius, B. S. M. & Lemola, M. (1976) Hypersensitivity to acetylsalicylic acid (ASA) and tartrazine in patients with asthma. *Clinical Allergy*, **6**, 119–129.

Stifler, W. C. (1965) Some challenge studies with foods. *Journal of Paediatrics*, **66**, 235–241.

Taylor, K. B. & Truelove, S. C. (1961a) Circulating antibodies to milk proteins in ulcerative colitis. *British Medical Journal*, **ii**, 924–929.

Taylor, K. B., Truelove, S. C. & Wright, R. (1964) Serologic reactions to gluten and cow's milk proteins in gastrointestinal disease. *Gastroenterology*, **46**, 99–106.

Taylor, K. B., Thomson, D. L., Truelove, S. C. & Wright, R. (1961b) An immunological study of coeliac disease and idiopathic steatorrhoea. Serological reactions to gluten and milk proteins. *British Medical Journal*, **ii**, 1727–1731.

Tomasi, T. B., Jr & Katz, L. (1971) Human antibodies against bovine immunoglobulin M in IgA-deficient sera. *Clinical and Experimental Immunology*, **9**, 3–10.

Vendel, S. (1948) Cow's milk idiosyncrasy in infants. *Acta Paediatrica Scandinavica*, Suppl. V, **35**, 2–37.

Vickers, H. R., Bagratuni, L. & Alexander, S. (1958) Dermatitis caused by penicillin in milk. *Lancet*, **i**, 351–352.

Waldmann, T. A., Wochner, R. D., Laster, L. & Gordon,

R. S. (1967) Allergic gastroenteropathy, a cause of excessive gastrointestinal protein loss. *New England Journal of Medicine*, **276**, 761–769.

Welch, H. (1957) Severe reactions to antibiotics, a nationwide survey. *Antibiotic Medicine and Clinical Therapy*, **4**, 800–813.

Wicher, K., Reisman, R. E. & Arbesman, C. E. (1969) Allergic reaction to penicillin present in milk. *Journal of the American Medical Association*, **208**, 143–145.

Wilken-Jensen, K. (1958) Food allergy in theory and practice. *Acta Allergologica*, **12**, 142–152.

Wilken-Jensen, K. (1965) Cow's milk allergy, from a clinical point of view. *Acta Paediatrica Scandinavica*, Suppl. 159, 101–104.

Wilson, J. F., Heiner, D. C. & Lahey, M. E. (1964) Milk-induced gastrointestinal bleeding in infants with hypochromic microcytic anemia. *Journal of the American Medical Association*, **189**, 568–572.

Winkelman, R. K. (1957) Chronic urticaria. *Mayo Clinic Proceedings*, **32**, 329.

Wright, R. & Truelove, S. C. (1965) Circulating antibodies to dietary proteins in ulcerative colitis. *British Medical Journal*, **ii**, 142–144.

Wüthrich, B. & Schwarz-Speck, M. (1970) Milch- und Hühnerei-Eiweiss-Allergie: Ausfall der Hautteste mit Gesamtextrakten und mit Hydrolysaten. *Dermatologica*, **141**, 102–112.

Yachnin, S. & Svenson, R. H. (1972) The immunological and physicochemical properties of mitogenic proteins derived from *Phaseolus vulgaris*. *Immunology*, **22**, 871–883.

Young, E. (1965) Overgevoeligheid voor voedingsmiddelen. *Nederlands Tijdschrift voor Geneeskunde*, **109**, 1853–1857.

12. Bacterial and viral infections of the gastrointestinal tract

D. B. L. McClelland

INTRODUCTION

The mucous membranes of the body are the major routes of entry for microbial infections, and infections which are localized in, or invade via, the gastrointestinal tract are exceedingly important causes of morbidity and mortality in humans and in animals. The practical value of effective manipulation of mucosal defense mechanisms is illustrated by the success of oral polio vaccination. Over the past few years, knowledge of immune mechanisms acting in the intestine has increased enormously so that we are now well placed to follow the principles of oral immunization which were stated by Besredka in 1927: 'Follow the route which the virus takes in its penetration into the body.' However, the relationships between the gastrointestinal tract and its pathogens cannot be easily divorced from the relationship of the host to its normal intestinal microflora, so that the strict definition of what constitutes an 'infection' in the gastrointestinal tract may be difficult.

INFECTION OR SYMBIOSIS?

Metchnikoff was one of the first to consider the disturbing implication of man's lifelong coexistence with the huge numbers of unpleasant organisms within. 'As soon as he is born, man becomes the habitat of a very rich microbial flora. The skin, the mucous membranes ... the intestines and the genital organs offer a feeding ground for bacteria and inferior fungi of all kinds. For long it was thought that in healthy individuals all these microorganisms were inoffensive and sometimes even useful. It was supposed that when an infective malady was set up a specific pathogenic microorganism was added to this benign flora. Exact bacteriological researches have, however, demonstrated ... that the normal vegetation in healthy persons often includes representatives of noxious species of bacteria' (Metchnikoff, 1905).

Seventy years later, the immunological relationship of host to pathogen in the intestine is better understood, but many fascinating questions about the nature of the usually peaceful coexistence of the animal host and its normal enteric flora remain unanswered. A major property of the immunological system is the ability to recognize with great specificity and to attack 'non-self' organisms or substances, yet this system has evolved alongside the development of powerful and specific systems which allow totally separate organisms – such as man and *E. coli* or bacteroids – to maintain close symbiotic relationships. The immunological system of the gastrointestinal mucosa must have evolved the ability to distinguish not merely between self and non-self antigens, but between 'acceptable' and 'non-acceptable' microorganisms within the intestine, so that it preserves the ability to mount a defensive response against pathogens, and avoids the production of an inappropriate response against the normal microbial flora. As discussed below, and in Chapter 1, the mucosal immune system has distinctive features which permit it to meet these requirements.

Specific adaptive immunological mechanisms play a part in controlling normal and abnormal microbial flora in the intestine, but many other non-immunological factors are also involved which may be highly specific (Savage, 1972; Jones and Rutter, 1972). Although this chapter is mainly about specific immunological mechanisms it would be misleading to consider these in isolation from the other factors, some of which are considered in the next section.

To summarize:

1. The existence in the gastrointestinal tract of a normal microflora which itself contains potential pathogens makes it difficult to define 'infection' in the intestine.

2. The immune system of the intestine must function effectively against pathogens while the symbiotic relationship with the normal flora is preserved.

3. Non-immunological factors are of great importance in determining the intestinal microflora.

THE INTESTINAL MICROFLORA AND FACTORS MAINTAINING ITS STABILITY

The numbers of bacteria to be found at different levels of the normal human gastrointestinal tract are shown in Figure 12.1. The upper small intestine contains a rather scanty aerobic and anaerobic bacterial flora (Dickman, Chapelka and Schaedler, 1976). In the distal ileum, the total counts may rise to 1×10^8/ml, consisting mainly of anaerobic bacteroides and Gram-negative

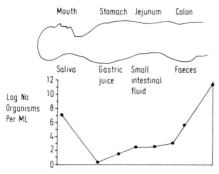

Fig. 12.1 Total bacterial counts in different regions of the gastrointestinal tract in a normal individual.

aerobes such as *E. coli*. The total counts in the distal large bowel reach those in stool (1×10^{11} per gram) and the proportion of anaerobes is increased, outnumbering

Table 12.1 Factors involved in interbacterial antagonism in the intestine

Altered pH
Altered redox potential
Competition for essential nutrients
Antimicrobial products – bacteriocins
　　　　　　　　　　　　　　 – volatile organic acids
Bile salt deconjugation
Competition for epithelial binding sites

the aerobic organisms by perhaps 10 000 to 1 (Drasar, Shiner and McLeod, 1969; Cregan and Hayward, 1953; Shiner, Waters, Allan and Gray, 1963; Gorbach, 1971; Drasar and Hill, 1974). Less information is available about the normal viral population of the intestine, but ECHO, polio, Coxsackie or adeno viruses can be isolated from up to 31 per cent of healthy controls

Table 12.2 Local host factors influencing the intestinal flora

Diet
Gastric acid secretion
Intestinal motility
Anatomical disturbance
Bile salt concentrations
pH
Redox potential
Host inhibitory factors in intestinal secretions:
　　lactoferrin
　　lysozyme
　　antibody
Antimicrobial factors active at the epithelial surface or in the lamina propria:
　　antibody
　　complement (?)
　　mediators of immediate-type hypersensitivity (?)
　　cell-mediated immune responses
　　interferon (?)
Interactions of host cell surface structures with bacterial surface structures

(Cramblett, Azimi and Haynes, 1971) and modern methods including immune electron-microscopy are revealing increasing numbers of viruses and virus-like particles in the faeces of patients and controls (Flewett and Boxall, 1976).

The microflora of the intestine is influenced both by the interactions of the various members of the flora with each other, and by their interactions with the host (Tables 12.1 and 12.2 and Fig. 12.2). The outcome of these relationships in the normal animal is a stable microecological system in which different types of micro-organisms are associated selectively with different parts of the intestine (Savage, 1972).

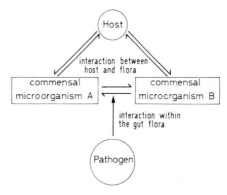

Fig. 12.2 The normal bacterial flora of the intestine is determined by complex interactions of bacteria with each other and with the host's defence mechanisms. A pathogen must be able to disturb these relationships to establish itself and produce disease.

INTERACTIONS BETWEEN MICROORGANISMS IN THE INTESTINE

Studies carried out *in vitro* have indicated that some bacteria can produce a variety of metabolites or anti-biotic-like substances which can inhibit the growth of other species (Florey, 1946; Donaldson 1964). An example is the production of bacteriocins (Nomura, 1967) which are specific antimicrobials of limited spectrum which appear to influence the ability of a particular strain to survive in the intestine (Branche, Young, Robinet and Massey, 1963). Other inhibitory effects may be due to the lowering of the Redox potential in the lumen (Paine, 1958), altering pH (Torrey and Kahn, 1923) or modification of bile salts to produce factors inhibitory for other organisms (Floch, Binder, Filburn and Gershengoren, 1972).

The complexity of the relationships between members of the normal bacterial flora has been emphasized by Freter (1974a). The ecological interactions are dependent on the environment in which they are tested and while specialized experimental techniques such as continuous flow culture systems may mimic certain features of the intestinal environment, the definition of appropriate conditions for testing microbial interactions remains a serious problem.

NON-IMMUNOLOGICAL HOST FACTORS INFLUENCING THE INTESTINAL FLORA

The composition of the intestinal flora is determined by the interaction of the microbial factors already discussed with many aspects of the host's physiology, some of which are mentioned in Table 12.2 (reviewed by Donaldson, 1964; Gorbach, 1971; Tannock and Savage, 1974).

Diet

There are many reports of alterations in bowel flora as a result of changes in diet which are frequently grossly unphysiological (Donaldson, 1964). The most dramatic and probably the most important example is the effect on the bowel flora in the neonate which is produced by substituting artificial feeds for human milk (*vide infra*).

Gastric secretion

Gastric acid secretion has a major influence on the intestinal flora, and it has been clearly shown that both achlorhydria (Sherwood, Goldstein, Haurani and Wirts, 1964) and hypochlorhydria (Giannella, Broitman and Zamchek, 1972; Heading *et al.*, 1974) are associated with increased numbers of bacteria in the proximal small bowel. Cash *et al.* (1974) have shown that the infectious dose of *Vibrio cholerae* is reduced by a factor of 1×10^4 in normal volunteers after feeding 2 g of sodium bicarbonate. The role of other antimicrobial mechanisms in the stomach has received little attention, but other factors such as gastric juice immunoglobulins and lysozyme (McClelland, Finlayson, Samson, Nairn and Shearman, 1971; Lai A Fat, McClelland and van Furth, 1976) may be of particular importance during postprandial periods when the gastric pH rises and the acid barrier may be less effective.

Intestinal motility

The importance of intestinal motility in controlling flora was suggested by the observations of Dixon and Paulley (1963) who showed that if the normal rapid transit of bacteria was slowed by the use of the ganglion-blocking drug mecamylamine there was a substantial increase in the number of coliforms in the rat small intestine. A more recent study (Summers and Kent, 1970) showed similar though smaller changes. Clinical evidence of the importance of normal intestinal motility in resisting pathogen invasion was provided by DuPont and Hornick (1973) who demonstrated that the use of diphenoxylate in the treatment of shigellosis prolongs the fever and nullifies the benefit of antibiotic treatment.

The effectiveness of bacterial clearance by intestinal motility may be influenced by other factors. Early observations by Florey (1933) showed that villous movement in the small bowel appeared to assist the mucous coating of particles such as bacteria, on the surface of the mucosa. Antibody in intestinal secretions may assist this mechanism both by agglutinating bacteria (McClelland, Samson, Parkin and Shearman, 1972) and inhibiting bacterial adherence to the mucosa (Williams and Gibbons, 1972).

Anatomical alterations

Anatomical alterations causing stasis such as surgical bypass procedures or non-surgical abnormalities such as diverticula of the small intestine can produce striking disturbances in flora (Tabaqchali, 1970).

Non-immunological factors in secretions

Bacterial overgrowth may be associated with abnormalities in metabolism of bile salts which may themselves influence bacterial flora (Floch *et al.*, 1972). Lactoferrin and lysozyme are both present in intestinal secretions (Schulze and Heremans, 1966; Tourville, Adler, Bienenstock and Tomasi, 1969) and their interaction with secretory antibody is discussed below. Although the lumen of the intestine is regularly described as being an anti-complementary milieu (Glynn, 1974), the possibility remains that complement may be involved in reactions occurring in microenvironments in or near the mucosa and this view is supported by the fact that some complement components are synthesized by the intestinal mucosa (Colten, Gordon, Borsos and Rapp, 1968; Lai A Fat *et al.*, 1976).

HOST CELL SURFACE INTERACTIONS WITH BACTERIAL SURFACE STRUCTURES

Savage (1972) has shown that in rodents there are clearly defined surface populations of microorganisms which associate very constantly with the epithelium of certain parts of the intestine and stomach. These apparently specific surface interactions may have a counterpart in the pig, in which the susceptibility to *E. coli* enteritis appears to depend on the animal's possession of an intestinal epithelial surface which permits adhesion of pathogenic organisms, all of which carry the surface antigen designated K88. This may be the first example of a genetic basis for susceptibility or resistance to enteric infection in a mammal (Rutter, Burrows, Sellwood and Gibbons, 1975). A similar association has been described for the K99 antigen of *E. coli* in the calf (Guineé, Jansen and Agterberg, 1976).

ADAPTIVE IMMUNITY TO MICROORGANISMS IN THE INTESTINE

Immunoglobulins in secretions

The origins, structure, properties and functional characteristics of secretory immunoglobulins are discussed in Chapter 1. However, certain aspects of the secretory immune system are particularly relevant to intestinal infection.

Antibody activity associated with secreted immunoglobulins

Technical problems associated with demonstrating antibody activity in intestinal secretions (Shearman, Parkin and McClelland, 1972) make it essential to interpret studies of secretory antibody with some caution. A wide range of antimicrobial antibody activities has been demonstrated by a variety of techniques which do not necessarily reflect the biological function of the antibody in the intestine. The more recent studies which distinguish the immunoglobulin class of the antibody activity emphasize that this is mainly associated with IgA (Table 12.3).

Table 12.3 Antimicrobial antibody activities in human intestinal secretions which have been associated with secretory IgA

Organism	Reference
E. coli	(1), (2), (3), (13)
Klebsiella	(2)
Serratia	(2)
Vibrio cholera	(4), (5)
Shigella	(6), (14)
Polio virus/polio vaccine	(7), (8), (9)
ECHO virus	(10)
Coxsackie virus	(10), (11)
Candida albicans	(12)

(1) Tourville et al. (1968).
(2) McClelland et al. (1972).
(3) McNeish et al. (1974).
(4) Northrup and Hossain (1970).
(5) Waldman et al. (1972).
(6) Reed & Williams (1971).
(7) Berger et al. (1967).
(8) Keller et al. (1968).
(9) Ogra et al. (1968).
(10) Ogra (1971).
(11) Ogra and Karzon (1970).
(12) Chilgren et al. (1967).
(13) Michael, Ringenback and Hottenstein, 1971.
(14) Mel, Terzin and Vukšić (1965b).

Antibody activity may be found in the absence of any attempt to immunize ('natural antibody'); it may also follow known infection, or attempts at immunization by a variety of routes. The distinction between 'natural' and 'immune' antibody in the intestine is artificial since in conventional animals or normal humans the intestine is exposed from birth to a massive microbial antigenic stimulus. The finding of secretory IgA agglutinins to a wide variety of commensal intestinal bacteria in normal humans confirms the ability to produce a local immuno-logical response to the normal flora (McClelland et al., 1972).

Inflammation and secretion immunoglobulins

The predominant class of immunoglobulin in the normal small and large intestine is IgA; with inflammation the situation may be different in respect to both locally produced and serum-derived immunoglobulin.

The term 'pathotopic potentiation' was used by Fazekas de St Groth, Donnelley and Graham (1951) to describe the influx of immune factors from the circulation to a site of inflammation. Local immediate-type hypersensitivity reactions could cause this response, since the necessary equipment appears to be present in the mucosa. There are mucosal IgE-containing cells, and IgE can be detected in secretions (Brown, Borthistle and Chen, 1975). The lymphocyte-like cells in the epithelium which contain histamine granules (Rudzik and Bienenstock, 1974) could fulfil the function of mast cells.

Serum-derived antibody may interact with antigens in the intestine to produce harmful consequences. Such a mechanism is recognized in the respiratory tract in neonatal pneumonitis caused by respiratory syncytial virus which appears to be due in part to an immune complex reaction between virus and passively acquired maternal antibody (Chanock et al., 1967). It has been proposed that similar immune complex-mediated tissue damage may contribute to the mucosal lesions of inflammatory bowel disease (Monteiro et al., 1971) and mucosal damage by an Arthus-type reaction has been demonstrated experimentally (Ferguson and MacDonald, 1975). However, at present little is known about the part such mechanisms play in human intestinal infections.

The distribution of the immunoglobulin class of plasma cells in the lamina propria is also altered in inflammation. In ulcerative colitis there is a marked increase in IgG-containing cells (Söltoft, Binder and Gudmand-Hoyër, 1973; Brandtzaeg, Baklien, Fausa and Hoel, 1974). These changes are mirrored by the finding that, in rectal biopsies from active ulcerative colitis, the mucosa synthesizes strikingly increased amounts of IgG in vitro (McClelland, Lai A Fat and van Furth, 1976). In gastric biopsies from patients with biliary gastritis, IgG synthesis is greatly increased (McClelland et al., 1976) as is the proportion of IgG to IgA immunocytes (McClelland, Samson and Shearman, unpublished). Little information is available about changes in numbers or class of the intestinal immunocytes in man in response to infection, but a recent study has demonstrated an increase in mucosal IgA synthesis in vitro following viral (Norwalk agent) gastroenteritis (Agus, Falchuk, Sessoms, Wyatt and Dolin, 1974).

These few examples indicate the need to consider mucosal immunoglobulin synthesis and transport in pathological as well as in normal conditions, and the need for further studies of the immunological aspects of mucosal inflammation in gastrointestinal infections.

Function of secretion antibody in relation to infection
Despite the extensive information about the origins and structure of the secretory IgA molecule, surprisingly little is known about its physiological functions, and many of the functions attributed to secretory IgA are the subject of dispute (Table 12.4). It is essential to be

Table 12.4 Functions of IgA antibody

Viral neutralization
Bacterial agglutination
Inhibition of bacterial motility
Bacterial killing (with co-factors)
Alteration of bacterial growth
Anti-toxin activity
Inhibition of bacterial adherence to mucosal surfaces
Opsonization (?)
Complement fixation (?)
Binding to mucin (?)
Non-antibody binding of proteins (antitrypsins)
Inhibition of bacterial enzymes
Inhibition of antigen uptake

aware of the technical difficulties in producing pure IgA preparations for biological testing (Steele, Chaicumpa and Rowley, 1974) and it is also important, in assessing the role of secretory antibody *in vivo*, to consider the possible role of other events, such as a local cell-mediated immune response or a systemic antibody response occurring at the same time as the secretory antibody response.

Bacterial killing and virus neutralization
Many studies have shown virus neutralization and protective effects in association with secretory IgA antibodies (Tomasi and Grey; 1973; Waldman and Ganguly, 1974) while other studies have demonstrated antibacterial activities (Table 12.3). IgA is efficient in bacterial agglutination because of the multiple valency conferred by its dimeric structure (Ishizaka, Ishizaka, Lee and Fudenberg, 1965). It inhibits the motility of organisms *in vitro* (Samson, Shearman and McClelland, unpublished). Bacterial killing by IgA has been the subject of conflicting reports since Adinolfi, Glynn, Lindsay and Milne (1966) showed that IgA antibody from human colostrum could lyse *E. coli* in the presence of complement and physiological concentrations of lysozyme. This finding has been confirmed by Burdon (1973) and Hill and Porter (1974), but other studies in a rabbit system have not shown a secretory IgA-mediated bactericidal action (Eddie, Schulkind and Robbins, 1971;

Steele *et al.*, 1974). These conflicting findings may be due to differences in technique, such as concentrations of lysozyme or the nature of the antigen employed, or to species differences.

Brandtzaeg, Fjellanger and Gjeruldsen (1968) found that streptococci coated by salivary IgA showed an altered growth pattern with increased chain formation. The division rates of many enteric bacteria are very much slower *in vivo* than in artificial culture systems (Gorbach, 1971), and growth-inhibiting effects of IgA antibody may be partially responsible for this.

Antitoxin activity
Antibody activity to cholera toxin has been shown in association with the 11s IgA-antibody fraction from rabbit intestinal homogenates by Kaur, McGhee and Burrows (1972). Human colostrum contains an inhibitor of *E. coli* and cholera enterotoxin which is probably secretory IgA (Stoliar *et al.*, 1976). Inhibition of the binding of cholera toxin to mucosal epithelium has been demonstrated (Fubara and Freter, 1973).

Adherence inhibition
Certain pathogenic bacteria must adhere to the mucosal epithelium to exert their effects (Table 12.5). Freter (1969) demonstrated the inhibition of adherence of cholera vibrios to mucosa by antibody. Also antibody inhibits the adherence of enteropathogenic *E. coli* to the intestinal mucosa in pigs (Jones and Rutter, 1972; Wilson and Hohmann, 1974) and human salivary IgA antibody can inhibit the adherence of streptococci to human oral epithelium (Williams and Gibbons, 1972).

The mechanisms of this adherence-inhibiting effect of antibody has not been fully elucidated, but its possible significance has been reviewed by Gibbons (1974). The mechanism may be due to the masking of surface structures such as the K-antigens of enteropathogenic *E. coli* which are involved in bacterial adherence (Ch. 14). Also, Genco, Evans and Taubman (1974) have shown that rat salivary antibody (mainly IgA) can modify streptococcal adherence by selectively inhibiting the synthesis of bacterial surface polysaccharides required for adherence. Alteration of mucosal adherence is probably an important factor in the immunological protection against some types of bacterial pathogen and may in addition play a role in controlling the ecology of the normal intestinal flora. It should be pointed out, however, that non-antibody factors in secretions may also play a major role in altering bacterial adherence (Ørstavik, 1974; Gibbons, 1974).

Antigen exclusion
Antibody in secretions may block or reduce the ability of the mucosa to take up an antigen present in the intestinal lumen. This property may be particularly im-

Table 12.5 Ways in which bacterial pathogens may associate with the intestinal mucosa to produce disease (adapted from Savage, 1972)

Mode of association	Example of disease	Organisms	Site	Reference
Bacteria attach to mucosa without penetration, induce disease by multiplying and producing exotoxin	Cholera	*Vibrio cholera*	SI	(1)
	E. coli enteritis	Enterotoxin-producing *E. coli*	SI	(2)
Bacteria attach to and penetrate the mucosa but do not reach the subepithelial tissues, induce disease by multiplying in and damaging epithelial cells, may also produce exotoxin	Bacillary dysentery	Shigella spp.	LI	(3)
	E. coli enteritis	Invasive strains of *E. coli*	LI	(4)
Bacteria attach to and penetrate mucosa to reach subepithelial tissues, multiply in submucosa and may spread systemically, may grow intracellularly in mononuclear phagocytes	Salmonella enteritis	Salmonella spp.	SI	(5)
	Typhoid fever	*Salmonella typhi*	SI and LI	(6), (7)

SI = Small intestine. LI = Large intestine.

(1) Finkelstein (1970).
(2) Smith (1972).
(3) Takeuchi, Formal and Sprinz (1968).
(4) Staley *et al.* (1970a, b).

(5) Takeuchi and Sprinz (1967).
(6) Sprinz *et al.* (1966).
(7) Carter and Collins (1974).

portant in determining the effectiveness of attempts to orally immunize (Ch. 1).

Opsonization

There have been conflicting reports on the ability of secretory IgA antibodies to enhance bacterial phagocytosis. Wernet, Breu, Knop and Rowley (1971) found apparent opsonization of *E. coli* by rabbit and pig colostral IgA using the *in-vivo* uptake of bacteria by mouse peritoneal cells as an indicator. It is difficult to interpret these findings, since the results could be due to intracellular or extracellular bacterial killing, or to adherence of bacteria within the peritoneal cavity as well as being due to phagocytosis. Also, the IgA preparations used were contaminated with other immunoglobulin classes. The last criticism also applies to the experiments of Girard and de Kalbermatten (1970) who used human intestinal fluid as a source of opsonins. Kaplan, Dalmasso and Woodson (1972) found a complement-dependent opsonizing effect of human secretory IgA on the phagocytosis of red cells by polymorphs, but Zipursky, Brown and Bienenstock (1973), in similar experiments, showed that the apparent complement-dependent opsonization by secretory IgA was due to IgM contamination which could be removed by a solid phase immunoabsorbent. Several other reports support this latter observation (Eddie *et al.*, 1971; Huber, Douglas, Huber and Goldberg, 1971). Aggregated secretory IgA appears to be cytophilic for human neutrophils (Spiegelberg, Lawrence and Henson, 1974), but the biological significance of this findings is not clear.

Complement activation

Although aggregated secretory IgA can activate complement via the alternate pathway, the only study of complement activation by secretory IgA combined with antigen did not show alternate pathway activation (Colten and Bienenstock, 1974). This finding does not entirely exclude the possibility that secretory IgA combined with other antigens could be active.

Mucosal cell-mediated immune responses

There is little direct evidence that cell-mediated immune (CMI) responses occurring locally in the gastrointestinal mucosa play a part in the defence against microbial infections. However, a variety of indirect evidence suggests that such responses may occur and may be important in some situations.

The lymphoid cells of the mucosa and lamina propria together with the gut-associated lymphoid tissues contain the cell types necessary to mount a CMI response (Ch. 1) and the recirculation of T-lymphoblasts to the intestine (Sprent and Miller, 1972; Guy-Grand, Griscelli and Vassalli, 1975) provides a mechanism for placing sensitized cells in the appropriate locations. In animal models, delayed hypersensitivity reactions can be produced in small intestinal tissue in response to tuberculoprotein or *Nippostrongylus brasiliensis*, leading to a histological picture of crypt hypertrophy and villous atrophy (Ferguson and McDonald, 1974). The fact that these changes do not occur in thymectomized animals (Ferguson and Jarrett, 1975) strongly suggests that the lesions are T-cell mediated, although interpretation is complicated by the fact that T-cell function appears to be required for normal development of the IgA system in mice (Crewther and Warner, 1972), fowl (Perey and Bienenstock, 1973), rabbits (Clough, Mims and Strober, 1971) and probably also in man (McFarlin, Strober and Waldman, 1972).

Further evidence that CMI responses to microbial

antigens can occur at secretory surfaces comes from studies of the respiratory tract. In experimental animals there is good evidence of respiratory tract CMI to agents including rubella virus (Morag, Ogra and Beutner, 1974), *M. tuberculosis*, influenza vaccine and pseudomonas lipopolysaccharide. Furthermore, in human volunteers, leucocytes obtained in bronchial washings respond to influenza, mumps and *M. tuberculosis* in the macrophage migration inhibition test (reviewed by Waldman and Ganguly, 1974).

In man intestinal biopsies from patients with untreated coeliac disease, when exposed to gluten *in vitro*, produce a macrophage-migration inhibiting factor which may be a product of gluten-sensitized T-lymphocytes in the mucosa (Ferguson, MacDonald, McClure and Holden, 1975). There are no comparable published studies involving intestinal responses to microbial antigens, but the histological appearance of the mucosa in certain infections suggests that a delayed-hypersensitivity reaction is implicated. Sprinz *et al.* (1966) studied the changes in jejunal histology in human volunteers who were infected by mouth with *Salmonella typhosa*. There was a marked cellular infiltration, mainly confined to the crypt regions of the mucosa and consisting of mononuclear phagocytes, lymphocytes and plasma cells which occurred at a very early stage of the infection before there was any evidence of a systemic immune response.

Other mucosal responses involving leucocytes

A mucosal polymorph response to infection was experimentally demonstrated by Florey (1933) who showed that the presence of a pathogenic bacterium in the guinea-pig intestine rapidly elicited a large exudation of phagocytic cells (polymorphs and a few mononuclear cells) into the lumen. These cells could be seen apparently migrating through the epithelium, and many polymorphs containing phagocytosed bacteria were seen in the lamina propria.

The emigration of polymorphs into the lumen may be increased as a result of maturation of the intestinal coliform flora (Yong, 1971). It is also possible to induce emigration of polymorphs by an apparently immunologically specific mechanism, namely, by feeding bovine serum albumin to guinea-pigs immunized systemically with this antigen (Bellamy and Neilsen, 1974). In these experiments the polymorph exudation was not accompanied by any evidence of mucosal damage, but in a comparable study in which passive immunization preceded antigen feeding, a severe local Arthus-type reaction was induced (Ferguson *et al.*, 1975).

The population of leucocytes in the intestine may be influenced by the production of chemotactic substances by bacteria. Keller *et al.* (1973) have demonstrated that culture filtrates of *E. coli* contain chemotactic activity

for polymorphs and mononuclear phagocytes. The role of these factors in the mucosal response to bacteria is not clear, but they may contribute to the appearance of large numbers of leucocytes in faeces, which is a well-recognized finding in Shigella, *E. coli* and Salmonella infections (Willmore and Shearman, 1918; Harris, Du Pont and Hornick, 1972). On the basis of these several observations it seems likely that the traffic of polymorphs and monocytes into the lumen of the intestine has more significance than the mere 'cell graveyard' function which has been suggested (Teir and Rytömaa, 1966).

INTERACTIONS OF IMMUNOLOGICAL AND
NON-IMMUNOLOGICAL MECHANISMS CONTROLLING THE
INTESTINAL FLORA

The composition of the intestinal bacterial flora at a given time is determined by the interactions of host factors (adaptive responses and non-adaptive responses) with bacterial factors (interbacterial antagonisms and adaptive responses).

The interaction of host adaptive responses and bacterial antagonism is illustrated by experiments in which germ-free mice, some immunized with cholera vaccine, were infected with cholera vibrios. Immunized animals had lower bacterial counts in the caecum than the control animals. However, when animals were provided with an 'antagonistic' bacterial flora consisting of normal intestinal bacteria prior to infection with cholera vibrios, two additional observations were made. Firstly, total vibrio counts were lower than in the mono-contaminated animals, regardless of immunization. Secondly, the reduction in vibrio counts in immunized animals was very much greater in the presence of the 'antagonistic' flora (Shedlofsky and Freter, 1974).

A second type of interaction is illustrated by experiments in which changes occur in the antigenicity of intestinal bacteria. Sack and Miller (1969) showed successive alterations in the vibrio serotypes in mono-contaminated animals, and Shedlofsky and Freter (1974) showed a similar change occurring 2 to 3 weeks after their animals had been contaminated with the vibrio, at the time when production of antibody could first be detected in the intestine. It seems likely, therefore, that one effect of antibody in the intestine may be to exert a selective pressure favouring the appearance of mutants which are antigenically different or deficient and which may gain a transient ecological advantage, perhaps because of the absence of a specific adherence-inhibitory antibody. A mechanism of this type may underlie the dynastic succession of *E. coli* serotypes which occurs in the human intestine (Emslie-Smith, 1965; Robinet, 1962).

Other examples of interactions of immunological and non-immunological control mechanisms include the cooperation of antibody, lysozyme and lactoferrin, the possible role of agglutinating antibody in altering transit of bacteria due to intestinal motility, and the influence of digestive enzymes on immunoglobulins in secretions (Fubara and Freter, 1972).

BACTERIAL INFECTIONS AND IMMUNE DEFICIENCIES

One critical test of the relative importance of immunological and non-immunological mechanisms in homeostasis of intestinal flora is to examine the disturbances of intestinal microbial flora in immunologically deficient individuals. Patients with selective IgA deficiency may be clinically healthy, as were two of the earliest reported cases (Rockey, Hanson, Heremans and Kunkel, 1964), or when recurrent infections occur, these are usually respiratory and not gastrointestinal (Amman and Hong, 1971). Patients with panhypogamma-globulinaemia are also susceptible to recurrent chest infections. They commonly also have small intestinal infection with *Giardia lamblia* (Hermans, Huizenga, Hoffman, Brown and Markowitz, 1966) but do not appear unduly susceptible to infections with gastrointestinal bacterial pathogens (Rosen, 1974). Furthermore, studies of the bacterial flora in hypogamma-globulinaemic subjects have shown only modest increases in anaerobic organisms (which in some cases relate at least in part to diminished gastric acid output), and no striking elevation in numbers of aerobic bacteria (Parkin *et al.*, 1972; Brown, Butterfield, Savage and Tada, 1972). However, it may be more informative to study the numbers of bacteria which are closely associated with the mucosa, by culturing mucosal biopsies, as has been suggested by Webster (1975), since this method has been of value in demonstrating abnormalities in tropical sprue (Tomkins, Draser and James, 1975). *G. lamblia* infestation is common in these patients and appears to be related to deficiency of mucosal antibody, though direct evidence is lacking.

Children with thymic aplasia who survive beyond infancy are susceptible to a wide selection of bacterial, viral and fungal infections which often prove fatal (Rosen, 1974; Gelfand, Biggar and Orange, 1974). Children with severe combined immunodeficiency are highly susceptible to all kinds of viral, fungal, bacterial and protozoal infections, and often have loose, diarrhoeal stools which grow pathogenic enterobacteria (Rosen and Janeway, 1966; Rosen, 1974).

Clinical observations suggest therefore that so far as protection from gastrointestinal infection is concerned, antibody-mediated immune mechanisms may be more dispensable than cell-mediated immunity, and that in the presence of severe defects in cell-mediated immunity, non-immunological mechanisms are not sufficient to maintain a normal intestinal microflora.

MUCOSAL IMMUNIZATION

Although mucosal immunization is discussed in Chapter 1, certain aspects are particularly relevant to immunization against microbial agents.

Handling of antigens at the mucosal surface

Large molecules can be taken up by the intestinal mucosa (Fig. 12.3) by a mechanism which appears closely related anatomically to the route of secretion of IgA (Tourville, Adler, Bienenstock and Tomasi, 1969). In addition, the mucosa overlying the Peyer's patches appears to be adapted for the uptake of large molecules and even intact microorganisms (Bockman and Cooper, 1973; Hess, Cottier, Sordat, Joel and Chanana, 1973). Antigen uptake may be inhibited by the presence of specific antibody (Fig. 12.3), either locally produced IgA, or IgG (André, Lambert, Bazin and Heremans, 1974; Walker and Isselbacher, 1974). Antigen which traverses the mucosal epithelium may sensitize precursors of mucosal antibody-forming cells. This probably occurs within the Peyer's patches which then release sensitized precursors of IgA-antibody producing cells which recirculate to the intestinal lamina propria (Pierce and Gowans, 1975). This 'loop' provides the possibility of a negative feedback signal to control the uptake of further antigen by the mucosa.

Antigen which crosses the epithelium may be retained within the mucosa or mucosal lymphoid tissues, or may reach the portal or lymphatic vessels. Thus BSA or ovalbumin does not localize in the Peyer's patches or the mucosa (Bienenstock and Dolezel, 1971; Hunter, 1972), but DNCB appears to be retained in the mucosa (Silverman and Pomeranz, 1972) as does flagellin (Hunter, 1972).

If antigen is transported through the mucosa or Peyer's patch, its subsequent fate may be determined by its physical or antigenic properties (Hunter, 1972) and by the presence or absence of circulating antibody to it. If there is sufficient circulating antibody to form antibody-excess complexes, these are taken up by the liver and rendered non-immunogenic, whereas in antigen excess the antigen reaches the spleen and evokes antibody production (Thomas and Parrot, 1974). This is a second possible site for a negative feedback signal.

A further important consideration is the possibility of inducing tolerance to antigen administered via the intestine. This occurs with small doses of haptens (Chase, 1945) and sheep red cells given by certain regimes (André, Bazin and Heremans, 1973). The mechanism of tolerance induction is uncertain but may relate to the site of localization of absorbed antigen in liver or spleen. This in turn is probably a consequence of events occurring at the mucosal level which determine the further distribution of antigen.

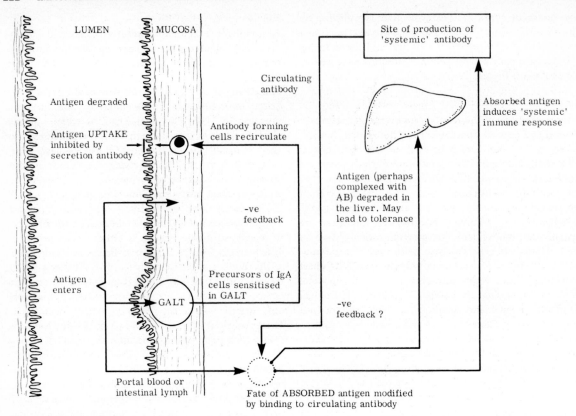

Fig. 12.3 Pathways involved in the mucosal antibody response, showing sites at which the response to antigen presented to the mucosal surface may be modified by changes in the immune status of the individual.

Local or systemic immunization

Immunization given by the mucosal route may induce both a mucosal immune response and a systemic antibody response. The latter may be due to absorption of antigen which reaches sites of systemic antibody production, or to the seeding from the Peyer's patches of sensitized IgG- or IgM-antibody forming cells which localize in extraintestinal lymphoid tissues (Craig and Cebra, 1971). Conversely, parenteral immunization with some antigens may induce the production of antibody at mucosal surfaces or parenteral 'priming' may lead to enhanced responses to subsequent mucosal boosting (Ogra *et al.*, 1974).

Responses to mucosal immunization have mostly been studied by assessment of humoral antibody responses. As discussed below, these responses may be an inadequate indicator of mucosal immunity. The induction of cell-mediated immunity is also important in the protection against some infections (Collins and Carter, 1974) and it is possible in some circumstances to achieve a state of cellular hypersensitivity by oral administration of a non-replicating antigen such as schistosome egg antigen (Perrotto, Hang, Isselbacher and Warren, 1974). Furthermore, there may be other, at present uncharacterized, responses to mucosal im-

munization underlying the apparently non-specific protection against bacterial infection described by Raettig (1976).

Antigens for mucosal immunization

The preceding section emphasized the complexity of the factors which underlie the selection of an agent which will lead to effective enhancement of immunity at a mucosal surface. The existence of negative feedback signals at several levels, plus the possibility of inducing tolerance via the mucosal route, suggests there may be intrinsic difficulties in utilizing this route for immunization. Detailed studies are needed of the local processing and fate of bacterial and viral preparations considered as possible immunogens.

Practical requirements

A useful oral immunogen must clearly be effective in inducing immunity as determined by the final arbiter of epidemiological testing in the field. It should not require complex administration schedules requiring repeated dosage or frequent boosters. Ideally it should be capable of protecting against a range of agents endemic in an area and it should be stable, preferably without refrigeration. Live vaccines must fulfil stringent safety requirements with no risk of reversion to wild-type strains (for example, see below – cholera).

Design of oral bacterial vaccines

Production of live vaccines depends on developing modified organisms which are stably avirulent. Avirulence because of poor growth within the host may be a result of temperature sensitivity, antibiotic dependence or biochemical deficiency (WHO, 1972). Loss of pathogenic mechanisms may also lead to avirulence, as in the case of Shigella variants with impaired cell penetration (Schneider and Formal, 1963) or strains of cholera vibrio with absent or inactive toxin production (Finkelstein, 1976, Table 12.6).

Table 12.6 Factors in the design of a cholera vaccine

Routes of administration
Parenteral
Oral
Combined

Nature of immunogen
Non-replicating: toxin modified by gluteraldehyde or formaldehyde
                killed bacteria
                bacterial antigen
Replicating: mutant strain producing no toxin, B region of toxin only, or B region plus inactive A region

Target of the host immune response
Enterotoxin: B Region (binding)
            A Region (adenylcyclase stimulator)
Vibrio: adherence determinants
       replication within the intestine

Extracts from bacteria which have been studied as potential immunogens include the 'core antigen' of the Enterobacteriaceae (Lüderitz, 1970) and the lipid 'A' core of *Salmonella minnesota* (Galanos, Lüderitz and Westphal, 1971); the latter evokes antibodies against antigenically distinct pathogenic enterobacteriacae such as pathogenic *E. coli* strains. An *E. coli* antigen extractable by desoxycholate (Ocklitz, Mochmann, Schmidt and Hering, 1967) is at present under study, and vaccines based on ribosomal extracts of salmonellae, which are highly effective in animal models (Venneman and Bigley, 1969), require evaluation in man. The cholera enterotoxin has been extensively studied as an immunogen (*vide infra*).

Replicating or non-replicating antigen

It might be expected that killed vaccines would be less effective than live replicating vaccines because of rapid loss of antigen by transit through the intestine. Practical experience suggests that this is true of both viral and bacterial vaccines, as illustrated below in the section dealing with individual infections. It is, however, worth mentioning that the combination of parenteral inactivated vaccine with mucosally administered booster doses of live vaccine may be very effective in evoking both local and systemic antibody responses.

Site of expression of immunity

A further consideration in planning oral immunization is the site in the body where the expression of local immunity is required. The studies of Ogra and Karzon (1969) indicated that a replicating viral antigen only elicited secretory antibody production at the site of vaccination, and not in other parts of the intestine. However, it now seems clear that oral immunization may induce the production of secretory antibody not only in the intestine but elsewhere, for example in the mammary gland. This has been shown for bacterial antigens (Allardyce *et al.*, 1974; Goldblum *et al.*, 1975), haptens (Montgomery, Rosner and Cohn, 1974) and viral antigens (Ogra *et al.*, 1974a). The possibility of inducing the production of specific colostrum and milk antibodies against enteric pathogens by immunizing women of child-bearing age should be considered as a further likely benefit of oral immunization.

Assessment of responses to local immunization

The assessment of the effectiveness of oral immunization techniques must be based on appropriate criteria (Joo, 1976; Felsenfeld, 1976). Many early studies examined serum antibody responses only; these may be of little or no relevance as a measure of protection. Satisfactory techniques of measuring antibody levels in secretions and specific antibody synthesis in mucosal biopsies are required, but it is difficult to design assays based on the relevant protective functions of antibody until it is more certain what these functions may be. Simple tests of bacterial agglutination or antigen binding may not be adequate and the assessment of the induction of cell-mediated immunity in the intestine may also be necessary. Final assessment must depend on adequate epidemiological proof of protection.

MICROBIAL FACTORS DETERMINING PATHOGENICITY

Mechanisms of pathogenicity

The ability of an organism to act as a pathogen is determined by its capacity to enter the host, normally by surviving on or penetrating the mucus membranes, and by its ability to multiply *in vivo* and cause damage to the host. An understanding of these mechanisms of pathogenicity is essential in studying the operation of host defence mechanisms, and ways in which they may be modified. Table 12.5 illustrates various ways in which bacterial pathogens associate with the intestine to produce disease.

Influences on host immune system

The success or failure of a pathogen depends in part on the extent to which the organism may stimulate, inhibit, resist or evade host defence mechanisms (Smith, 1972). Bacteria and viruses may stimulate host immune responses by acting as foreign antigens. In addition, bacterial products such as lipopolysaccharides may act as non-specific stimulators of the immune system; lymphocyte stimulation by bacterial products has been studied in detail in animal systems (Greaves and Janossy, 1972) and similar effects occur in humans (Oppenheim and Perry, 1965; Ivanyi and Lehner, 1974). Bacteria may also stimulate host defences non-immunologically by mechanisms such as the production of factors which are chemotactic for polymorphs and monocytes (Keller, Hess and Cottier, 1973).

In contrast to these examples of stimulation of host immune responses, microorganisms may also exert immunosuppressant effects. A variety of bacterial products, including enterobacterial endotoxin and cholera enterotoxin, may act as immunosuppressants under some experimental circumstances, although most of these products may, under different conditions, act as adjuvants. Schwab (1975) emphasizes the numerous points within the immune response at which such bacterial products may affect cell interactions. It seems certain that products of the high concentrations of bacteria in the gastrointestinal tract must play an important role in regulating the functions of the mucosal immune system.

Evasion of host immune responses by means of antigenic variation is widely practised by protozoans. The evolution of bacterial antigens within the gastrointestinal tract has been mentioned above as being probably a response to selective pressures exerted by intestinal antibody; this mechanism may well be important in maintaining the pathogenicity of organisms which cause enteric infections in endemic areas.

GASTROINTESTINAL IMMUNOLOGY OF SPECIFIC INFECTIONS

This section deals principally with disease affecting the gastrointestinal tract itself, but the intestinal tract mucosa is an important route of entry for agents which cause disease at sites remote from the intestine, with or without a phase of proliferation in the intestinal tract. Gastrointestinal immunology also has a bearing on systemic disorders in which the route of infection may not be via the intestine, as for example in bacterial meningitis in which host immunity may be altered by immune responses to intestinal microbial antigens cross reacting with the meningitis-producing organisms.

Diarrhoea is one of the commonest symptoms of gastrointestinal disease, and is most commonly caused by an infective agent. Many cases of diarrhoeal disease are due to well-recognized 'traditional' enteric pathogens, but until very recently, no microbial cause could be found for the majority of cases of gastroenteritis (Cramblett et al., 1971; Gorbach, 1971). This situation is now resolving for two reasons. New virological techniques and the recognition of previously unidentified viral pathogens, such as the rota- and corona viruses (reviewed by Flewett et al., 1976), provide an explanation for many cases of diarrhoea disease in infants and young children (British Medical Journal, 1975). Secondly, the role of enterotoxin producing E. coli in human disease has been extensively explored and it is becoming increasingly clear that these organisms are important pathogens in children and adults, and in animals (Sack, 1976). Although knowledge of the immunology of both the newly discovered enteric viruses and of enterotoxigenic E. coli is limited, especially in humans, these agents are discussed in some detail as this is clearly an area in which rapid advances in mucosal immunization should be made.

BACTERIAL INFECTIONS

E. coli

E. coli enteritis is an important cause of infant morbidity and mortality (Drachman, 1974), and it is increasingly being recognized as an important cause of adult diarrhoeal disease (Lancet, 1975). E. coli enteric disease is of great importance in veterinary practice, and many of the basic studies have been made in domestic animals.

Pathogenesis

Although certain serotypes designated 'enteropathogenic' have been clearly associated with outbreaks of diarrhoeal disease for many years, the pathogenesis of E. coli diarrhoea was not understood. It is now known that certain E. coli produce a heat-labile enterotoxin which closely resembles cholera toxin, both in its biochemical action of stimulating adenylcyclase activity in the epithelial cells (Sack et al., 1971; Carpenter, 1972), and in its antigenic properties, since there are immunological cross-reactions between the two toxins (Nalin, et al., 1974). A second heat-stable toxin of E. coli is also implicated in the causation of diarrhoea.

The ability to produce enterotoxin is not related to the classical enteropathogenic serotypes, although the number of serotypes in which toxin production occurs appears to be restricted (Lancet, 1975); toxin production is controlled by a plasmid (Smith and Halls, 1968; Gyles, So and Falkow, 1974). Pathogenicity is not solely determined by toxin production. Some strains invade the mucosa to produce a dysenteric syndrome with systemic illness, bloody diarrhoea and a severe ulcerating proctitis (Du Pont *et al.*, 1971*a*). For all strains it appears that adherence to the intestinal mucosal surface is an essential prerequisite of pathogenicity (Taylor, Maltby and Payne, 1958; Drucker, Yeivin and Sacks, 1967).

The factors determining mucosal adherence have been thoroughly studied in relation to *E. coli* pathogenic for pigs. An essential requirement for bacterial pathogenicity in certain strains of pig appears to be possession of the *E. coli* surface antigen K88 (Jones and Rutter, 1972) which permits adherence, proliferation, and enterotoxin production. Animals which are susceptible to K88 *E. coli* disease appear to possess a mucosal receptor site for the organism. The possession of this receptor site appears to be inherited as a Mendelian dominant, and animals in whom the bacteria do not adhere are not susceptible to infection by K88-bearing *E. coli* (Rutter *et al.*, 1975).

Further evidence of the specificity of the interaction between *E. coli* and the epithelial surface is provided by the observation that while porcine *E. coli* pathogens bearing the K88 antigen do not adhere to human intestinal epithelium (Wilson and Hohmann, 1974), human *E. coli* pathogens do adhere to human mucosa (McNeish, Turner, Fleming and Evans, 1975).

Immunity

Passively transferred immunity. In animals it is well established that immunoglobulins which are passively transferred in colostrum protect the neonate against both local intestinal and systematically invasive *E. coli* infection (Ch. 14; Logan, Stenhouse and Ormrod, 1974). Human infants who are fed colostrum and breast milk appear to have a reduced incidence of enteric infections (Robinson, 1951). Milk IgA antibody directed against *E. coli* (McClelland *et al.*, 1972) and *E. coli* enterotoxins (Stoliar *et al.*, 1976) may well play a part in this protection, although there are no experiments comparable to those of Logan *et al.* (1974) to examine the influence of immunoglobulins in the absence of other factors. Although the relative importance of antibacterial and anti-enterotoxin antibody has not been evaluated, experiments with *E. coli* diarrhoea in pigs show that antibody directed against the specific K88 surface antigen (which is required for adherence) can both block the adherence of the organisms to the mucosa and protect against infection (Rutter and Jones, 1973). Production of this protective antibody in maternal colostrum and milk can be induced by immunization (Rutter *et al.*, 1975), suggesting a very effective approach to prophylaxis.

Active immunity and immunization. Immunization against *E. coli* infection has been attempted in several animal species. Felsenfeld and colleagues have used streptomycin-dependent mutant organisms for oral immunization of primates and achieved protection (Felsenfeld, Wolf, Greer and Brannon, 1972) which appears to correlate with increased levels of immunoglobulin and antibody in intestinal fluid (Felsenfeld, 1976).

Porter and colleagues have shown that protection against *E. coli* enteritis in young pigs and calves can be produced by oral immunization using a crude *E. coli* antigen given with the food (Porter, Kenworthy and Thompson, 1975). This regime of prolonged feeding of killed bacteria produces local mucosal antibody responses to the antigen fed (Porter, Kenworthy, Noakes and Allen, 1974).

In humans effective protection by immunization against *E. coli* enteritis has not been reported, although a trial of an oral vaccine has been undertaken (WHO, 1972). The human intestine is certainly capable of producing an IgA-antibody response both to *E. coli* of the normal intestinal bacterial flora (McClelland *et al.*, 1972) and to pathogenic *E. coli*. McNeish, Gaze and Evans (1974) showed the appearance of specific agglutinins in intestinal fluid following *E. coli* enteritis in infants. The antibody was initially IgM (and exclusively IgM in the youngest infants) and IgA antibody appeared later only at the height of the response.

The protective activity of antibody remains to be demonstrated in most of these situations, and the relative importance of antibody to bacterial structural antigens and anti-enterotoxin is not clear. However, the experiments in the piglet model, already described, strongly suggest that the ability of antibody to block adherence of *E. coli* may have an important protective function.

The development of practical immunization against *E. coli* enteritis is likely to pose interesting problems. Many serotypes have been associated with clinical disease, and the list is constantly added to. Production of type-specific immunity would probably be of limited value for this reason alone. However, there is no evidence that the somatic serotype has *per se* any relationship to pathogenicity. Two properties appear to be essential for pathogenicity, regardless of somatic serotype, namely the production of toxin, and the ability to adhere to mucosa. These properties are subject to much less variability within the pathogens of a given species, making immunization a more feasible prospect. Immunization against the heat-labile enterotoxin is also a possibility, since this does not vary with the serotype of the organism. (Attempts to produce antitoxin immunity are discussed further in the section on cholera.)

The choice of killed versus attenuated organisms for oral *E. coli* immunization has not been resolved. There is, however, a strong suggestion that a killed vaccine is effective in the veterinary situation where it is possible to administer the vaccine repeatedly over long periods with the feed. Killed vaccines are much less likely to be effective in human clinical practice where the number of doses will be strictly limited, and the prolonged effect of a live vaccine will be required.

Shigella

The genus Shigella includes four main subgroups, *S. dysenteriae (shiga)*, *S. flexneri*, *S. boydii* and *S. sonnei*. *S. sonnei* and *S. flexneri* are the commonest disease-producing strains in many areas (Reller, Gangarosa and Brachman, 1970), but the frequency of *Shigella shiga* isolation has increased in the United States (Centre for Disease Control, 1972) following the Central American pandemic.

Pathogenesis

Host responses to infection. A very small number of bacterial cells of a virulent strain can cause infection (Levine *et al.*, 1973) which may be the reason why so many outbreaks occur in institutions or are water-borne (Drachman, 1974). Clinically, Shigella gastroenteritis usually begins abruptly with diarrhoea and fever. Blood and leucocytes in the stool are not seen as commonly as suggested in classical descriptions (Rosenstein, 1964). However, experimental infections in volunteers challenged with *S. flexneri* 2a (DuPont *et al.*, 1969) or *S. dysenteriae* I (Levine *et al.*, 1973) are severe, with passage of stools containing blood and mucus, and proctoscopic evidence of proctitis, with haemorrhage, oedema and polymorph infiltration (Levine *et al.*, 1973).

Mucosal invasion. Although virulent strains of Shigella produce an enterotoxin (Rout, Formal, Giannella and Dammin, 1975), the important characteristic determining pathogenicity appears to be the ability to invade the mucosa. *In-vitro* studies have demonstrated the ability of virulent *Shigellae* to invade cells in tissue culture (Ogawa, Yoshikura, Nakamura and Nakaya, 1967; Ogawa, Nakamura and Nakaya, 1968), and both animal studies (Gemski, Takeuchi, Washington and Formal, 1972) and experiments in human volunteers (Levine *et al.*, 1973) have clearly shown that invasive strains are pathogenic regardless of their toxin-producing ability, while toxin-producing non-invasive mutants do not produce disease.

Immunity

Shigella infection confers a degree of protection against subsequent reinfection with the same strain (Honjo *et al.*, 1967; DuPont *et al.*, 1969). The mechanism of this immunity is unknown. It does not correlate with levels of serum antibody (DuPont *et al.*, 1972), but immunity may be related to locally produced antibody. Since the pioneering studies of Davies (1922) showing the appearance of specific anti-Shigella agglutinins in stool and mucus of dysentery patients, there have been many demonstrations of Shigella 'copro-antibody' and its lack of relation to serum antibody. However, there

is no good evidence that mucosal immunity to Shigella is antibody-mediated (Reed and Williams, 1971) and the role of other mucosal immune mechanisms deserves more study.

Oral immunization against Shigella infection has been widely studied. Besredka (1927), during the First World War, successfully used oral Shigella immunization on a large scale. Much more recently Mel and his associates demonstrated the effectiveness of an orally administered streptomycin-dependent mutant strain in immunizing mice (Mel, Terzin and Vukšić, 1965a) and monkeys (Mel, Cvjetanović and Felsenfeld, 1970) against virulent *S. flexneri* serotypes. In a long series of clinical trials involving the administration of live vaccines to 20 000 adults and 10 000 schoolchildren the following points emerged: (1) protection against reinfection with vaccine strains ranges between 85 and 100 per cent in follow-up periods of up to 6 months (Fig. 12.4),

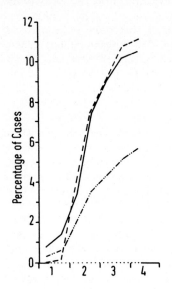

.... Sh. flexneri 2a dysentery; vaccinated group
—·—·— Sh. flexneri 2a dysentery; unvaccinated group
——— Other Shigella dysentery ; vaccinated group
— — — Other Shigella dysentery ; unvaccinated group

Fig. 12.4 The effect of oral immunization against shigellosis. The subjects who were immunized against *Shigella flexneri* 2a showed complete protection against infection with that organism, but their morbidity due to other types of Shigella dysentery was the same as that in the control group. (Reproduced from Mel *et al.*, 1965b.)

(2) post-immunization reactions are rare in adults and, although more common in children, are not serious, (3) no resistant strains have been identified in stools from immunized subjects, despite evidence of *in-vitro* conversion, and (4) the duration of immunity and the effectiveness of single booster doses is still under review (Mel, Papo, Terzin and Vukšić, 1965; Mel, Terzin and

Vukšić, 1965b; Mel, Gangarosa, Radovanović, Arsić and Litvinjenko, 1971).

Du Pont *et al.* (1972) have described two other immunizing strains of Shigella (a streptomycin-dependent mutant and a Shigella–*E. coli* hybrid) which have been safely given to volunteers. The level of immunity to challenge in these studies approximated to that following recovery from natural infection. Nevertheless, the protection achieved was less striking than that obtained by Mel and his associates, possibly because the latter studies, performed in an area of endemic Shigella infection, involved many subjects with some degree of pre-existing immunity from previous exposure.

Salmonella

The genus Salmonella contains approximately 1600 serotypes, although a relatively small number account for most isolations in human disease. Salmonella infection in man may produce a range of clinical illnesses from a silent intestinal carrier state, through gastro-enteritis in which infection is restricted to the intestine, to classical enteric fever in which the organism invades via the intestine to produce septicaemia. In enteric fever septicaemia is followed by a period of proliferation in the liver and spleen culminating in a secondary bacteraemia in which organisms are deposited to produce foci of infection at almost any site in the body (Hook, 1974). Enteric fever in man is classically caused by *S. typhi.*, but many other types can cause this syndrome (Dickenson and Pickens, 1978).

Pathogenesis

Invasion and proliferation. The initial steps of bacterial invasion are described in some detail since it is these early events which are most likely to be influenced by the intestinal immune system. An essential step in the pathogenesis of salmonella infection by the oral route is bacterial invasion of the intestinal mucosa (Table 12.5). Strains which are non-invasive do not cause disease when fed to animals or inoculated into the ligated ileal loop of a rabbit (Giannella, Formal, Dammin and Collins, 1973). Also the results of an *in-vitro* test of the ability of Salmonella to invade Hela cells in tissue culture correlate well with those obtained in experimental intestinal infections in animals (Giannella, Washington, Gemski and Formal, 1973).

The bacterial properties which determine the ability to penetrate the mucosa are not fully understood, but one factor which may be important is the possession by some strains of the Vi antigen, which is similar in many respects to the K antigens of *E. coli* (Glynn, 1972) The Vi antigen may have adherence or endocytosis-promoting qualities for epithelial cells and interfere with serum opsonic or bactericidal mechanisms. There is no doubt that the possession of the Vi antigen is associated with pathogenicity of Salmonella in animals (Felix and Pitt, 1934). Although its importance in human disease has been controversial, Hornick *et al.* (1970a) have shown that the Vi antigen is associated with greater pathogenicity in man.

Orskov and Moltke (1928) carried out an early study to determine the route of invasion of Salmonella ingested by mice but were unable to define the precise site of entry. Ozawa, Goto, Ito and Shibata (1973) concluded that the main site of entry involved the caecum and large intestine, while other groups have demonstrated very early systemic spread of infection, implying absorption in the small intestine. The situation in the mouse has been clarified by Carter and Collins (1974). *Salmonella enteritidis* given intragastrically moved rapidly through the small bowel and after 1 hour only 1 per cent of the challenge dose could be detected in the entire intestine. There was no evidence of bacteraemia. The primary site of infection was clearly shown to be the distal ileum, and possibly to a lesser extent the caecum. The bacteria appeared to concentrate in Peyer's patches in the distal ileum, and by 48 h the lymph nodes draining this area had become infected. Cultures of intestinal wall adjacent to the Peyer's patches contained very few viable organisms, demonstrating that the infection appeared strictly confined to the patch itself. The authors concluded that lymph from a particular area of mucosa probably drains through the regional Peyer's patch and thence to the mesenteric node, and that the invading salmonellae also follow this route. In the orally challenged chimpanzee, salmonellae readily penetrate the intestine, but appear to be arrested in the mesenteric nodes (Gaines, Sprinz, Tully and Tigertt, 1968) while jejunal biopsy studies in man suggest that the organism may enter via the upper small intestine (Sprinz *et al.*, 1966).

Influence of indigenous flora. The study of Carter *et al.* (1974) showed that only a few of the ingested organisms need survive in the intestine to produce a fatal infection. In the clinical situation, the ability of salmonellae to proliferate in the intestine is probably an important factor determining pathogenicity (Hornick *et al.*, 1970a). One factor which influences this is the antagonistic effect of the indigenous flora. This was well shown by Meynell and Subbaiah (1963), who used a genetic marker technique to measure the division rate, excretion rate and death rate of *S. typhimurium* given intragastrically to mice. In normal mice, bacteria multiplied slowly if at all in the intestine and were rapidly eliminated. In streptomycin-treated animals, the organisms grew as rapidly in the intestine as in culture medium.

Immunity

Host responses to infection. At an early stage in invasive Salmonella infection in man, macrophages, lymphocytes and plasma cells are concentrated in the lamina propria of the small intestine, with some histological features suggestive of a cell-mediated immune response. These changes can be observed before septicaemia occurs and before antibody becomes detectable in the serum (Sprinz et al., 1966). It is not clear that there is phagocytosis of the bacteria in the intestinal wall at this stage; in any case this would not be an effective way of removing the organisms, since salmonellae are capable of surviving and dividing within macrophages (Blanden, Mackaness and Collins, 1966). At subsequent stages of infection, studied in rodents, there is extensive necrosis and cell depletion of lymphatic organs, especially the thymus, parathymic nodes and spleen, indicating that the organism interferes profoundly with the animal's immunological defences (Stuart and Collee, 1967).

Serum antibody responses do not correlate particularly well with protection while the role of secretion antibody is not clear. The capacity of Salmonella for intracellular proliferation suggests that immunity depends at least in part on the induction of a cell-mediated immune response in which T-cell cooperation with macrophages kills the intracellular organisms (Mackaness, 1971; Collins and Carter, 1974).

Immunization. Animal studies with *S. typhimurium* (Germanier, 1972) and *S. enteritidis* (Collins and Carter, 1972) show that live attenuated vaccines are much more effective than killed vaccines, especially when given orally. Of the attenuated strains tested in mice, the only one conferring immunity similar to that following infection with a virulent organism appears to be the Gal E mutant discussed below (Germanier, 1970). Given parenterally, preparations of salmonella antigens may produce good protection in mice (Wong, Feeley, Northrup and Forlines, 1974), but by the intestinal route, killed vaccines seem to achieve at best a delay in the spread of bacteria from intestine to liver and spleen (Collins and Carter, 1972).

Natural infection in man appears to produce a moderate degree of immunity, although the relevant information is not wholly satisfactory (Marmion, Naylor and Stewart, 1953). In volunteers who were infected and subsequently rechallenged with the same strain, a substantial degree of immunity was acquired, only 25 per cent of previously infected individuals being susceptible to reinfection (Hornick et al., 1970b).

The effectiveness of parenteral vaccines has been clarified in large-scale WHO-supported trials. A significant degree of protection (80–90 per cent) lasting 3 years or more is conferred by inactivated whole vaccines (Cvjetanović and Uemuru, 1965). A similar degree of protection was shown in volunteer studies when a challenge dose of 1×10^5 organisms was used, although larger doses overcame the protection (Hornick et al., 1970b). There is no relationship between the clinical

effectiveness of these vaccines and any of the animal protection tests, or any of the serological responses in vaccines (Hornick et al., 1970b).

Killed oral vaccines have been tested extensively in the field and in volunteer studies. In volunteers large doses of killed vaccine gave protection and reduced the incidence of positive stool cultures following challenge (Du Pont et al., 1971b), suggesting some influence on intestinal immunity. In contrast, despite some encouraging initial results, the reports of recent field studies are uniformly disappointing. Chuttani (1976) reviewed the results of three successive trials in India involving almost 20 000 vaccinees and a similar number of controls. In all three trials the attack rate in vaccinees did not differ significantly from that in the controls.

Live oral vaccines offer a more encouraging prospect. Streptomycin-dependent mutants have, in one volunteer study, shown significant protection and a striking reduction of positive stool cultures (Hornick et al., 1970b). However, a more recent vaccine strain appears to be even more effective. This mutant is deficient in the enzyme UDP–galactose–epimerase which prevents synthesis of the complete cell-wall lipopolysaccharide. *In vivo*, supplied with exogenous galactose, the cell wall can be synthesized normally. The organism remains avirulent, however, because phosphorylated galactose accumulates within the bacterial cell and causes lysis (Germanier and Fürer, 1975). Volunteers were orally immunized with this organism in eight doses over a 1-month period. There were no adverse reactions and live organisms were rarely and only transiently detected in the stools. Six weeks after immunization the subjects were challenged with 1×10^5 virulent organisms, a dose sufficient to cause clinical illness in 25–50 per cent of normal subjects. The results of challenges are summarized in Table 12.7. Seven per cent of vaccinees

Table 12.7 Results of oral immunization of volunteers with Ty21a *Salmonelli typhi* mutant. Subjects were challenged with 1×10^5 virulent organisms 6 weeks after immunization. The number of subjects developing typhoid fever, and the duration of excretion of the pathogen, are shown for the vaccinated and control groups (Hornick et al., 1976)

Oral immunization with live attenuated S. typhi		
Clinical results of challenge		
	Number of subjects	*% ill*	*% protection*
Vaccinated	28	7	87
Control	43	53	
Bacteriological results of challenge		
% of subjects with positive stool cultures		
	In first 3 days	*After 3 days*
Vaccinated	39	11
Control	41	60

developed typhoid fever as against 53 per cent of controls, a protective rate of 87 per cent. Prolonged shedding of virulent organisms was also greatly reduced in the vaccinees (Hornick *et al.*, 1976).

In this study, as in previous investigations, no correlation was found between protection and serum antibody titres to any antigenic determinant of the pathogen. Studies of antibody responses in the secretions of these subjects have not been reported, and no information is available about tests of cell-mediated immunity. These findings encourage real hopes of a practical oral typhoid vaccine, although further extensive evaluation is required.

Cholera

In 1971, 171 000 cases of cholera were reported in 42 countries, and this figure probably represents an underestimate, since there are economic disincentives to reporting. Although current methods of cholera vaccination do confer statistically detectable degrees of protection for limited periods of time, it is clear that these measures are not adequate to contain the spread of the disease. Furthermore, in endemic areas, current immunization practices are doomed to failure on logistical grounds alone, since staff resources for case finding and inoculation are totally inadequate (Sommer and Mosley, 1973). The most important factors in controlling this disease are public health measures dependent on overall socioeconomic development. But in the absence of these advances, more effective methods of prophylaxis are essential, and the development of improved methods of immunization has attracted a major research effort in recent years. (For extensive recent reviews of cholera pathogenesis, epidemiology and immunology see Barua and Burrows, 1974, and Finkelstein, 1975.)

Pathogenesis

The cholera vibrio, as well as related organisms (the 'non-agglutinable' (NAG) vibrios, and *E. coli*), produce an enterotoxin which acts by stimulating the activity of adenyl cyclase in the intestinal epithelial cells. This leads to massive hyper-secretion, causing a rapid fluid and electrolyte depletion. The vibrios are localized entirely within the lumen and invasion of the mucosa does not occur. The localized nature of the infection emphasizes the importance of defence mechanisms which act at the mucosal surface and the need to develop effective means of enhancing these defences.

The enterotoxin. The toxin is a polymer of 84 000 Daltons' molecular weight consisting of two regions, the A region which activates adenyl cyclase, and the B region (termed choleragenoid) which is responsible for binding the entire molecule to the cell surface, probably by binding to the GM ganglioside (van Heyningen, 1976). (This binding is not specific to the intestinal epithelium;

most cell types will bind cholera toxin in the same way, with adenyl cyclase stimulation.) The binding B region is immunogenic, and antibodies to this region block the action of the toxin (Finkelstein, 1975). There are major similarities between the enterotoxins of *Vibrio cholerae*, *E. coli* and NAG, and the blocking effects of antibodies cross-react.

Mucosal attachment of vibrios. Although toxin production is the major pathogenic mechanism of the vibrio, it cannot affect the host unless the organism attaches to the mucosa and multiplies there in a manner very similar to that previously described for porcine *E. coli* enteropathogens. Germ-free mice are susceptible to the intestinal effects of oral cholera toxin, but despite this, they can be colonized with heavy intestinal populations of vibrios with no clinical effect, probably because the organisms do not attach to the mucosa (Sack and Miller, 1969). The process of vibrio attachment to the intestinal mucosa was examined by Schrank and Verwey (1976) in rabbit intestinal loops, using frozen sections in an attempt to demonstrate the mucous layer without drying and fixation artefacts. They claim to show that in animals who were not immunized, the vibrios penetrated the mucous layer in the intervillous spaces at the same time as fluid accumulation began. Jones, Abrams and Freter (1976) demonstrated that binding of the vibrios to brush border preparations of intestinal epithelial cells occurs and is temperature sensitive and dependent on divalent cations. Vibrios appeared to be able to traverse the intestinal mucus *in vitro*. Nelson, Clements and Finkelstein (1976) have also explored the time, course and morphology of vibrio attachment in the rabbit intestine, using scanning and transmission electron-microscopy. Vibrios appeared to lie closely on the microvillus surface throughout the length of the villus, and in the adult intestinal loops, few organisms were seen until 4 h after exposure. There then appeared to be a rapid proliferation with huge numbers of adherent organisms. By 12–16 h after exposure, few organisms remained. Suggestive evidence was obtained that vibrios were removed in association with secreted mucus, by a mechanism reminiscent of that described by Florey (1933).

Non-immunological factors in resistance to cholera. Vibrios are sensitive to acid; in volunteer studies the dose of vibrios required to produce diarrhoea was 1×10^8 organisms. When administered with an antacid the infecting dose fell to 1×10^4 organisms (Cash *et al.*, 1974a). The practical importance of gastric acid in resistance was demonstrated in the recent Naples outbreak when 20 per cent of the male patients had a history of gastric resection (de Lorenzo *et al.*, 1973).

Immunity in cholera (Table 12.8)

The main battle between host defences and the vibrio must take place within the intestine, at the mucosal

Table 12.8 Immunity to cholera in man

Stimulus to immunity	Protection acquired	Duration	References
Natural infection in endemic area	Reinfection frequent		Woodward (1971)
Experimental infection of volunteers	100%	Up to 1 year	Cash et al. (1974)
Parenteral toxoid	'Probably minimal'		Verwey (quoted by Finkelstein, 1976)
Parenteral whole cell or antigen preparations	50% or less; poor in children	3–6 months	Benenson et al. (1968); Finkelstein (1976)
Oral vaccination with atoxic mutant	60%	Not known	Woodward et al. (1976)

surface. Circulating antibody against either the vibrio or its toxin is unlikely to be important other than as a marker of events which occur at the site of infection.

It should be possible to induce immunity to cholera, since normal volunteers in whom cholera was induced experimentally were almost totally protected against the clinical effects of rechallenge with the homologous organism 4–12 months later. These individuals were not resistant to heterologous challenge, suggesting that bacterial surface structures, rather than the common enterotoxin, were the target of the immune response (Cash et al., 1974b). These findings do not support the field observations made by Woodward (1971), who found that the risk of reinfection is only slightly less than the risk of a first infection. The patients studied by Woodward, however, were in an endemic area, and not therefore comparable with the volunteers who had no previous exposure to the disease. The moderate effectiveness of parenteral cholera vaccines containing killed vibrios or somatic antigens also suggests that antibacterial immunity can be induced in man. In contrast effective immunity mediated by antitoxin can be induced in animals but not, so far, in man (see below).

Targets for immunological defences in cholera (Table 12.8) (i) antitoxin immunity. The cholera enterotoxin acts at the cell surface and is probably localized exclusively on the surface of the microvilli (Peterson, Lo Spalluto and Finkelstein, 1972). It is possible that small amounts of enterotoxin may penetrate into the submucosa, as suggested by Kao, Sprinz and Burrows (1972), and this may account for the appearance of circulating antibody to toxin following infection. The site at which lymphoid cells are sensitized to produce antibody to toxin or toxoid given by the intestinal route is not certain; Pierce and Gowans (1975) showed that a secondary response, with the appearance of many intestinal mucosal cells producing antibody to cholera toxin, can be readily evoked by feeding the toxoid, provided the animals had previously been primed by an intraperitoneal dose of the antigen. To induce the appearance of mucosal antibody-forming cells by oral immunization alone required prolonged administration of large amounts of antigen. These findings suggest that contact between toxoid and the receptive cells is inefficient in the unsensitized animal. It is not clear whether the good secondary response to oral antigen reflects a high sensitivity to small amounts of absorbed antigen, or whether the ability of antigen to reach responsive lymphoid cells is altered in the primed animal.

The binding of toxin to the microvilli can be blocked by antibody (Walker, Field and Isselbacher, 1974), and the in-vivo effects of toxin can be neutralized by antibody applied before, or at the same time as, the toxin (Mosley and Ahmed, 1969). Parenteral immunization with pure toxoid provides protection in rabbits (Finkelstein, 1970). Fujita and Finkelstein (1972) compared the effectiveness of different routes of immunization on resistance to challenge by various routes, and showed that while parenteral immunization provided protection against toxin given parenterally, the most effective protection against toxin given orally was provided by oral immunization using a high molecular weight, heat-aggregated inactive polymer of the toxin. In this study, oral immunization evoked antibody responses in the serum, but it is significant that the protection against challenge persisted after circulating antibody became undetectable.

The protective role of antibody to toxin has not been clearly shown in man. The evidence, reviewed by Finkelstein (1975), is often clouded by the use of impure toxin preparations which also evoke antibody to other antigens. Preliminary results of a current assessment of gluteraldehyde-inactivated toxoid suggest that the protection obtained is minimal (Verwey, quoted by Finkelstein, 1976).

(ii) Inhibition of vibrio attachment. The evidence reviewed above stresses the need for vibrios to associate closely with the mucosa to multiply and affect the host. Freter's work (reviewed by Freter, 1974a), has shown that anti-vibrio antibody in the lumen of the intestine reduces the number of vibrios which adhere, although the total number of organisms is not altered. The study of Schrank and Verwey (1976) suggested an altered anatomical distribution of vibrios in actively or passively immunized animals, with reduced penetration to the intervillous spaces, and a tendency to clump and remain in the lumen. An analogy with the effects of antibody to the adherence determinant of pathogenic *E. coli* is suggested, but no specific adherence factor has yet been identified in the vibrio.

(iii) Inhibition of vibrio multiplication. The early studies of Freter (reviewed by Watanabe, 1974) demonstrated antibody in stools in patients following either natural infection, parenteral immunization, or oral immunization. More recently, IgG, IgA and IgM class antibacterial antibody has been shown in stool and duodenal fluid of cholera patients by immunodiffusion or radioactive antiglobulin methods (Northrup and Hossain, 1970; Waldman *et al.*, 1971).

The possible modes of action of antibacterial antibody in the intestine have been discussed in an earlier section: Waldman *et al.* (1971) found vibriocidal activity in the intestinal secretion of choleric patients which appeared to be associated with IgA. This observation is partially supported by the work of Freter (1970) who demonstrated that vibrios adsorbed to the epithelial surface are killed by an antibody-dependent mechanism which was blocked by metabolic inhibitors.

Immunization. *Parenteral cholera vaccines in man.* Many early field trials of parenteral vaccines gave a misleading impression that these vaccines conferred protection (Cvjetanović and Uemura, 1965; Cvjetanović, 1965), but most of these trials were inadequately controlled. Subsequently, well-controlled trials with a variety of vaccines have been conducted in Bangladesh, India and the Philippines. These are reviewed by Benenson, Mosley, Fahimuddin and Oseasohn (1968) and Finkelstein (1975). The principal points which emerge are as follows (Table 12.8). Protection is only of moderate degree, and is especially poor in children who constitute the major at-risk population. Previous immunization does not appear to modify the disease. Vaccination appears to be most effective in endemic areas, probably because it boosts pre-existing immunity. Protection is correlated with serum titres of vibriocidal antibody.

Oral cholera vaccines. Although animal studies have shown that oral administration of killed vaccines can induce some degree of immunity (above) there are several reasons to seek a suitable live attenuated strain for use in man (Table 12.8). By multiplying in the intestine, the magnitude and duration of the stimulation are increased, and induction of local immune responses should be more effective. Excretion of the vaccine strain might be expected to permit dissemination in endemic areas with poor sanitation. A mutant could be selected to produce an inactive toxin, and could therefore elicit immune responses directed both at the toxin and at surface determinants of the organism (Table 12.8). Two possible by-products of such a vaccine are (1) 'immunity' cross-reacting with enterotoxins produced by unrelated organisms such as *E. coli*, and (2) induction of antitoxin and/or antibacterial antibody production by the mammary gland, conferring protection on children who are breast fed. Although the perfect vaccine strain has not been developed, trials of a mutant which produces no toxin are encouraging. Given to volunteers in doses of 1×10^{10} organisms, there were no side effects, and after 1–4 doses, there was significant protection against challenge with virulent vibrios. Thirty per cent of the vaccinees and 83 per cent of controls became ill following challenge and the severity of illness was reduced in vaccinees (Woodward *et al.*, 1976). Unfortunately there is some evidence that this strain may revert to a virulent one. In earlier studies by Cash *et al.* (1974c) a strain was tested which grew inadequately in the vaccinees. It produced neither serological response nor protection, indicating the need for adequate intestinal replication of the vaccine strain. Sanyal and Mukerjee (1969) have also reported a live attenuated vaccine which is said to elicit good titres of antibody in the faeces in volunteer studies, but this strain again gave no evidence of adequate multiplication in the intestine, and has not been shown to be an effective vaccine.

CROSS-REACTIONS BETWEEN ENTERIC BACTERIA AND SYSTEMIC PATHOGENS. A NEW APPROACH TO IMMUNIZATION USING THE ENTERIC ROUTE

The normal individual has circulating antibodies to members of the enteric bacterial flora. If these antibodies are directed against antigens which are present on pathogenic organisms, they may confer some degree of protection. Recent studies demonstrate cross-reacting antigen between *E. coli*, *Haemophilus influenzae* and meningococcus (Robbins *et al.*, 1972). It may be possible to exploit these cross reactions to produce immunity.

Schneerson and Robbins (1975) showed that if adults were fed *E. coli* with the antigenic type 075:K100:H5, there was an increase in the serum antibody titre against the capsular antigen of the *H. influenzae* type b. This is due to the close similarity between the K100 antigen of *E. coli* and the *Haemophilus* capsular antigen. This method may well be effective in immunizing young infants against meningitis before their own (natural) antibodies appear, and the procedure is effective in baby rabbits (Myerowitz, Handzel, Schneerson and Robbins, 1973). This approach to immunization, using live, non-pathogenic, cross-reacting organisms given orally, has exciting possibilities.

Viruses and virus-like particles are commonly detectable in the gastrointestinal tract (Flewett and Boxall, 1976) and may not be associated with clinical illness. Pathogenic viruses may relate to the gastrointestinal tract in three broad ways : (1) infection localized to the intestine, (2) infection in which there is both intestinal proliferation and systemic spread, and (3) infections in which the intestinal mucosa is used mainly as a portal of entry for a virus whose effects are purely extraintestinal. This section is restricted to the role of antiviral immunity within the intestine itself.

Virus infections restricted to the gastrointestinal tract

Recent studies of intestinal viruses have done much to explain the high proportion of cases of diarrhoeal disease in both animals and humans for which no bacteriological cause could be found in earlier studies (Cramblett et al., 1971; Connor and Barrett-Connor, 1967). Mebus and colleagues first studied the aetiology of diarrhoeal disease in calves and showed its transmissible nature. Mebus, Stair, Underdahl and Twiehaus (1971) showed that it was due to a reovirus-like agent (Fernelius, Ritchie, Classick, Norman and Mebus, 1972). Flewett, Bryden, Davies, Woode, Bridger and Derrick (1973) found similar particles in the faeces of children suffering from acute gastroenteritis, and there has subsequently been a large number of reports of the association of these particles, now termed rota viruses, with childhood diarrhoeal disease (British Medical Journal, 1975). Morphologically similar viruses have also been associated with diarrhoeal disease in many other animal species. There appears to be a high degree of antigenic similarity between the inner capsid layer of all of these viruses (Woode et al., 1976) with varying degrees of cross-reaction between the outer coat antigens. The possession of such common antigens is already of value in the development of diagnostic reagents, and may have important implications for the production of vaccines against these agents.

A second group, the coronaviruses, are associated with transmissible gastroenteritis in pigs (Mebus, Stair, Rhodes and Twiehaus, 1973) and several other morphological types have been associated with human diarrhoeal disease. These include the 'Norwalk' agent (Dolin et al., 1972; Kapikian et al., 1972), and the 'Hawaii' agent (Wyatt et al., 1974; Schreiber, Blacklow and Trier, 1974). Recently Madely and Cosgrove (1975) have described very large numbers of small viruses in the faeces of patients with gastroenteritis. This may be yet another causative agent, although the causal relationship remains to be established.

Studies in which volunteers have been challenged with the Norwalk and Hawaii agent have provided information about the histopathological changes induced by these agents (Schreiber, Blacklow and Trier, 1973; Schreiber, Blacklow and Trier, 1974). The experimentally induced gastroenteritis was indistinguishable with the two different agents. The volunteers who became ill developed histological changes in the small-intestinal mucosa characterized by (1) a reduction in the crypt–villus ratio, (2) evidence of damage to the epithelial cells, and (3) infiltration of the lamina propria with polymorphonuclear and mononuclear cells.

Immunity to viruses causing gastroenteritis

Active immunity

Neonatal calves are very susceptible to challenge with both corona- and reovirus-like diarrhoea agents. Mebus, Torres-Medina, Twiehaus and Bass (1976) described the results of immunizing colostrum-deprived calves orally with attenuated virus of each type, and a mixed vaccine. A high degree of protection was achieved even when the animals were challenged with virulent virus 2–3 days after immunization, at a time before any antibody was detectable in the intestinal secretions. Antibody appeared in the secretion at 9–10 days following immunization and was mainly IgM and IgA. The nature of the protection which preceded antibody appearance was not explained; no production of interferon-like activity was detected. Human studies with the Norwalk agent indicated that clinical infection gave protection against a challenge with a filtrate containing virulent virus (Wyatt et al., 1974). The prospects for immunization are therefore excellent in veterinary practice where these diseases have major economic importance. The problems of growing the human virus have not yet been overcome (Flewett and Boxall, 1976).

Passive immunity

Maternal colostrum is of great importance in the protection of neonatal calves and pigs from viral gastroenteritis, and the protective ability of the colostrum appears to be highly correlated with its content of specific IgA antibody (Saif, Bohl and Gupta, 1972). The role of human colostrum and milk in protection against viral gastroenteritis is still not clear, although colostral IgA antibody to rotavirus has been demonstrated (Sommerville, R., personal communication).

Immunity to viruses which enter via the mucosa

Enteroviruses such as polio undergo primary multiplication in the lymphoid tissues of the alimentary tract and then spread via the blood to other organs, as well as undergoing re-excretion to the intestinal lumen. The mucosal immunology of polio has been particularly well studied as a result of the great success of oral polio immunization with live attenuated (Sabin) vaccine. Many other viruses, for example mumps and rubella, also enter via the mucosa and are susceptible to alterations in local mucosal immunity. As with bacterial antigens, the nature of the mucosal response is determined by the nature of the viral antigen, the route and site of administration and the duration of exposure. The experiments mentioned below illustrate these points.

Comparison of live and killed vaccines

In studies with polio vaccine it was shown that while comparable serum antibody responses could be elicited following either killed vaccine given parenterally or a live vaccine given orally, only the live vaccine elicited an antibody response in nasopharyngeal secretions (Ogra, Karzon, Righthand and MacGillivray, 1968). If the killed vaccine was administered intranasally, there was a prompt antibody response in the secretions, but this was of short duration (3 months) in contrast to the long-continued secretion antibody response following live vaccine (Ogra and Karzon, 1969).

The influence of site of immunization with live polio vaccine was studied in infants with double-barrelled colostomies. Live vaccine given into the distal colon elicited a serum antibody response, and a secretion antibody response which was maximal in the immunized distal colon, minimal in the non-immunized colon, and absent in the nasopharynx. The response to inactivated vaccine given into the distal colon was localized entirely to the distal colon. Viral replication was prevented in the sites which had been immunized. In children immunized via the distal colon, the nasopharynx was colonized on challenge with live vaccine, but the previously immunized colon was not. Production of mucosal colonization was not dependent on the presence of serum antibody, since the nasopharynx was resistant to recolonization following immunization with a dose of killed vaccine which did not elicit antibody in the serum (Ogra and Karzon, 1969). These studies emphasize the superiority of the immunity elicited by the live vaccine, which provokes both local and systemic responses of long duration, and also suggest a potential problem in the use of killed vaccines which may prevent a response to subsequent immunization with live vaccine by preventing replication of the vaccine strain.

The findings indicate that with the antibody-detection methods used, secretion antibody is principally localized to the site of immunization, even in the presence of a systemic response. The failure to detect a more widespread mucosal antibody response may reflect a lack of sensitivity in the methods used. In support of this view, Ogra (1974c) has reported that oral immunization with polio vaccine results in the appearance of secretory IgA antipolio antibody in mammary secretions.

Different live vaccines against the same virus may vary widely in the type of immune response they elicit. Plotkin, Farquhar and Ogra (1974) compared two live attenuated rubella vaccines termed RA-27/3 and HPV-77. The HPV-77 vaccine had been found unsatisfactory in preventing reinfection, and this correlated with the absence of an antibody response in nasal secretions. In contrast, the RA-27/3 vaccine, whether administered subcutaneously or intranasally, produced antibody responses in both secretions and serum, and gave good protection against reinfection, comparable to that which follows natural infection with rubella. These data suggest that in addition to the type of antigen used (replicating or non-replicating) other characteristics of the virus vaccine strain are important in influencing the nature of the immune response.

Mechanisms of antiviral immunity at mucosal surfaces

The studies described show a strong correlation between the presence of antibody in secretions and resistance to viral replication at a mucosal surface. It cannot be concluded, however, that antibody is the only effector mechanism at work. This is emphasized by the studies of Mebus et al. (1976), referred to above, which showed that immunity to calf gastroenteritis virus preceded by several days the appearance of specific antibody in the secretions. Experiments demonstrating the antiviral effects of passively administered colostrum-containing antibody would support an antiviral role of antibody, but are not conclusive, since many other factors in colostrum may well be involved (Goldman and Smith, 1973).

Cell-mediated immune mechanisms may also play an important part in the antiviral defence of mucous surfaces. Following rubella or mumps vaccination, or mumps infection, there is a cell-mediated immune response in mucosal-associated lymphoid tissues which can be detected by the production of antigen-specific migration inhibitory factor (MIF), and by *in-vitro* transformation of lymphocytes exposed to antigen (Ogra, Chiba, Beutner, and Morag, 1976). The cellular responses broadly parallel the appearance of specific antibody. For example, following intranasal immunization of guinea-pigs with rubella vaccine, cellular responses occur in the bronchial lymphocytes but not in spleen cells. Subcutaneous administration of the vaccine is followed by the appearance of cellular responses in spleen cells but not in bronchial lymphocytes. The separation of responses between splenic and mucosal sites suggests that the appearance of cellular reactivity at mucosal sites is independent of the responses at systemic sites. Similar data were obtained in children who underwent tonsillectomy following rubella vaccination or infection. Natural infection or immunization with RA 27/3 vaccine was followed by cellular responsiveness in both peripheral blood lymphocytes and tonsillar lymphocytes. In contrast, there was little or no tonsillar lymphocyte response after immunization with HPV-77 vaccine.

These and similar observations with mumps virus suggest that the mechanisms underlying the appearance of cell-mediated responsiveness at the mucosal surface are very similar to those which determine secretory antibody production. The relative importance of cell-mediated and antibody-mediated mechanisms in protection is not known.

VIRAL INFECTIONS IN IMMUNODEFICIENCIES

Further evidence for the importance of antibody in immunity against enteric viruses comes from studies of hypogammaglobulinaemic subjects. In the British Medical Research Council Study, hypogammaglobulinaemic patients were found to be at least eight times more susceptible to paralytic polio than the normal population (Medical Research Council, 1971). The patients who developed paralytic polio had no evidence of impaired cell-mediated immunity and this has been the experience of other groups (Chang, Weinstein and MacMahon, 1966; Schur et al., 1970).

It should be pointed out, however, that only 2 of the 30 patients in the MRC trial who received oral polio vaccine showed prolonged excretion of the vaccine virus. One of these was a child with severe combined immunodeficiency and the other a woman with selective IgA deficiency. The lack of prolonged excretion in the other 28 subjects suggests that *local* viral proliferation was inhibited by an antibody-independent mechanism.

In patients with isolated IgA deficiency, Ogra, Coppola, MacGillivray and Dzierba (1974) have shown that there is a local mucosal antibody response to inactivated polio vaccine given intranasally. The locally detected antibodies are of IgG and IgM class and they appear in the absence of detectable serum antibody. The level of nasopharyngeal IgG antibody appeared to be the factor which determined the outcome of local challenge with live virus. This study shows that secretory IgA can be replaced by IgG and IgM antibodies which are apparently locally produced and may protect against virus reinfection of the mucosa.

NUTRITION AND INFECTIONS OF THE GASTROINTESTINAL TRACT

Diarrhoeal disease remains an important cause of morbidity and mortality in the developed countries. In underdeveloped countries, infectious disease of the gastrointestinal tract, particularly diarrhoeal disease among children is a very major source of mortality (Gordon, Chitkara and Wyon, 1963; Gordon, Singh and Wyon, 1965; Morley, 1973).

'Acute diarrhoeal disease is an outstanding feature of life in the less developed regions, from the arctic to the tropics. Repeated attacks occur during and immediately after weaning. Malnutrition is especially common at that time. The two conditions are so inter-related that the illness is appropriately termed weanling diarrhoea. Not only is the condition world-wide, it is unsurpassed as an illustration of synergistic interaction between malnutrition and infection: costly in the disability it causes, in the deaths that follow and in immediate and long-term after effects' (Gordon and Scrimshaw, 1970).

CAUSES OF INTESTINAL INFECTIONS IN MALNUTRITION

As in temperate climates, many episodes of diarrhoea cannot be associated with recognized pathogenic organisms, and a study by James, Drasar and Miller (1972) failed to show any evidence of bacterial overgrowth in the small bowel of children with acute onset weanling diarrhoea. Malnourished children with chronic diarrhoea, however, have increased numbers of bacteria in the jejunum (Heyworth and Brown, 1975). The frequency of disease in the apparent absence of pathogenic organisms points to an imbalance between host and flora in which a microflora which would normally be 'commensal' behaves as if it were 'parasitic'.

MALNUTRITION AND SUSCEPTIBILITY TO INFECTION

The association between malnutrition and increased susceptibility to infection is suggested by many accounts of striking increases in the incidence and the severity of infectious disease in populations which have suffered a sudden decline in nutritional standards (reviewed by Gontzea, 1974). This effect of malnutrition may be due to changes in several aspects of immune function, and the nature of the immunological lesion may be markedly influenced by the type of nutritional deficiency (Good and Jose, 1975). These varying influences of different patterns of nutritional deficiency probably account for the very variable immune defects described in clinical reports of patients studied in different areas. There are few reports of altered mucosal immunity in subnutrition, but Sirisinha et al. (1975) have found decreased concentrations of IgA in the secretions of children with protein calorie malnutrition.

Completing the vicious circle linking malnutrition and infection are the gastrointestinal consequences of infection such as anorexia, dehydration and persisting post-infective malabsorption (Harrison et al., 1976). The nitrogen losses associated with acute infection are not readily replaced in the presence of malabsorption and inadequate diet, and common therapeutic responses

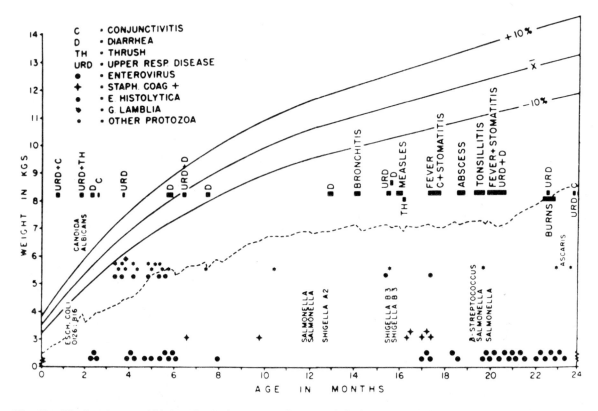

Fig. 12.5 The first 2 years of life in a developing country. Recurrent infections, particularly of the gastrointestinal tract, interact with subnutrition. Weight gain may be adequate in the early months of breast feeding, but slows drastically as weaning commences. (From data of Mata *et al.*, 1967. Reproduced from Gordon and Scrimshaw, 1970.)

tend to aggravate both caloric deprivation and dehydration (Morley, 1973).

The synergism between nutrition and infection is well illustrated by Fig. 12.5 which summarizes the clinical history of a South American peasant child, typical of the population studied by Mata, Urrutia and Gordon (1967) in which frequent episodes of diarrhoeal disease, gut parasitization and other infections are the norm.

BREAST FEEDING AND INTESTINAL INFECTIONS IN THE INFANT

The importance of this aspect of the study of gastro-intestinal diseases has been summed up by Morley (1973). 'Breast feeding is essential in the rural homes of developing countries. In the past in the U.K. and now in Asia and Africa doctors appreciate that if a child is not breast-fed it will die.' Breast milk has nutritional, immunological and microbiological properties profoundly different from those of artificial feeds.

Breast-fed infants have a gastrointestinal flora quite different from that of bottle-fed babies, consisting largely of bifidobacteria and only later developing flora typical of the adult (Smith and Crabb, 1961). Infections of the intestine (and other sites) cause much less morbidity and mortality in breast-fed infants (Robinson, 1951).

Table 12.9 Factors in human milk which influence the intestinal flora of the infant

A. Nutritional aspects which may affect the flora:

Composition differs widely from cows milk, e.g.
less calcium and phosphorus
less protein
higher lactose content
lower buffering capacity

B. Factors known to have effects on microorganisms:

Lactobacillus bifidus growth factors
Anti-staphylococcal factor
Immunoglobulins IgG, IgA and IgM
C3, C4, C3 proactivator
Lysozyme
Lactoferrin
Lactoperoxidase
Macrophages, polymorphs and lymphocytes

Some of the factors in human milk which influence the intestinal flora are summarized in Table 12.9. Compared with cow's milk or formulae, human milk has a high concentration of lactose, lower concentrations of protein, phosphate and salt, and a lower buffering capacity. Bullen and Willis (1971) have shown that these factors can influence the infant's intestinal flora. In addition, human milk contains factors which promote the growth of bifidobacteria and inhibit staphylococci (Gyorgy, 1971). Lysozyme, lactoferrin and immunoglobulin in milk can interact to kill bacteria and inhibit their growth (Adinolfi et al., 1966; Bullen, Rogers and Leigh, 1972; Hill and Porter, 1974) and normal colostrum and milk contains IgA antibodies against many viruses and bacteria (reviewed by Goldman and Smith, 1973). Colostrum also contains numerous mononuclear phagocytes, as well as lymphocytes and polymorphs (Smith and Goldman, 1968; McClelland, Gigi and Michie, unpublished) and these cells may have a protective role in the neonate.

The antibody specificity of colostral and milk immunoglobulin may be determined by intestinal antigenic stimuli. For example, mothers who suffered from Salmonella gastroenteritis in early pregnancy produced specific homologous anti-Salmonella IgA antibodies in the milk some 5 months later (Allardyce et al., 1974). This mechanism could allow the mother to provide the child with specific passive immunity to organisms which are prevalent in its local surroundings.

A full discussion of the role of colostrum and milk as the source of passive immunity for the infant is beyond the scope of this chapter. This does not detract from the fact that the transfer of immunity from mother to infant via colostrum and milk is probably, in quantitative terms, one of the most important aspects of gastrointestinal tract immunity to infection.

SUMMARY

Infections of the gastrointestinal tract cannot be considered in isolation from the microbial flora which normally populates the intestine. Specific immunological responses play a part in the homeostasis of the normal flora and the control of intestinal infection, but other non-immunological factors are also important. There have been great advances in the understanding of intestinal immunity, but many aspects of the function of secretory antibodies are not yet fully understood, nor are the factors which control mucosal immune responses to infective agents. Effector mechanisms involving mucosal cell-mediated immune responses may play an important part in immunity to intestinal infections, but further experimental evidence of this is required.

The better understanding of immunological responses to intestinal infections presents a tremendous challenge to immunologists because of the quantitative importance of these infections in most parts of the world.

In this chapter the role of intestinal immunity, and immunization, are discussed in relation to diseases of the intestine caused by E. coli, Shigella, Salmonella and Vibrio cholerae. Gastrointestinal immunity to virus infection is described with particular reference to viral gastroenteritis and polio. The important relationships between nutrition, gastrointestinal diseases and immunity are briefly reviewed, and the importance of breast feeding in intestinal immunity is emphasized.

REFERENCES

Adinolfi, M., Glynn, A. A., Lindsay, M. & Milne, C. M. (1966) Serological properties of γ-A antibodies to Escherichia coli present in human colostrum. Immunology, 10, 517–526.

Agus, S. G., Falchuk, Z. M., Sessoms, C. S., Wyatt, R. G. & Dolin, R. (1974) Increased jejunal IgA synthesis in vitro during acute infectious non-bacterial gastroenteritis. American Journal of Digestive Diseases, 19, 127–131.

Allardyce, R. A., Shearman, D. J. C., McClelland, D. B. L., Marwick, K., Simpson, A. J. & Laidlaw, R. B. (1974) Appearance of specific colostrum antibodies after clinical infection with Salmonella typhimurium. British Medical Journal, iii, 307–309.

Ammann, A. J. & Hong, R. (1971) Selective IgA deficiency: presentation of 30 cases and a review of the literature. Medicine, 50, 223–236.

André, C., Bazin, H. & Heremans, J. F. (1973) Influence of repeated administration of antigen by the oral route on specific antibody-producing cells in the mouse spleen. Digestion, 9, 166–175.

André, C., Lambert, R., Bazin, H. & Heremans, J. F. (1974) Interference of oral immunisation with the intestinal absorption of heterologous albumin. European Journal of Immunology, 4, 701–704.

Barua, D. & Burrows, W. (editors) (1974) Cholera. Philadelphia: Saunders.

Bellamy, J. E. C. & Nielsen, N. O. (1974) Immune-mediated emigration of neutrophils into the lumen of the small intestine. Infection and Immunity, 9, 615–619.

Benenson, A. S., Mosley, W. H., Fahimuddin, M. & Oseasohn, R. O. (1968) Cholera vaccine field trials in East Pakistan. 2. Effectiveness in the field. Bulletin of World Health Organisation, 38, 359–372.

Berger, R., Ainbender, E., Hodes, H. L., Zepp, H. D. & Hevisy, M. M. (1967) Demonstration of IgA polioantibody in saliva, duodenal fluid and urine. Nature, 214, 420–422.

Besredka, A. (1927) Local Immunisation, p. 181. Baltimore: Williams & Wilkins.

Bienenstock, J. & Dolezel, J. (1971) Immune response of the hamster to oral and parenteral immunisation. Cellular Immunology, 2, 326–334.

Blanden, R. V., Mackaness, G. B. & Collins, F. M. (1966) Mechanisms of acquired resistance in mouse typhoid. Journal of Experimental Medicine, 124, 585–600.

Bockman, D. E. & Cooper, M. D. (1973) Pinocytosis by epithelium associated with lymphoid follicles in the bursa of Fabricius, appendix, and Peyer's patches. An electron microscopic study. *American Journal of Anatomy*, **136**, 455–478.

Branche, W. C., Young, V. M., Robinet, H. G. & Massey, E. D. (1963) Effect of colicine production on *Escherichia coli* in the normal human intestine. *Proceedings of the Society for Experimental Biology and Medicine*, **114**, 198–201.

Brandtzaeg, P., Fjellanger, I. & Gjeruldsen, S. T. (1968) Adsorption of immunoglobulin A onto oral bacteria *in vivo*. *Journal of Bacteriology*, **96**, 242–249.

Brandtzaeg, P., Baklien, K., Fausa, O. & Hoel, P. S. (1974) Immunohistochemical characterisation of local immunoglobulin formation in ulcerative colitis. *Gastroenterology*, **66**, 1123–1136.

British Medical Journal editorial (1975) Viruses of infantile gastroenteritis. *British Medical Journal*, **iii**, 555–556.

Brown, W. R., Borthistle, B. K. & Chen, S.-T. (1975) Immunoglobulin E (IgE) and IgE containing cells in human gastrointestinal fluids and tissues. *Clinical and Experimental Immunology*, **20**, 227–237.

Brown, W. R., Butterfield, D., Savage, D. & Tada, T. (1972) Clinical, microbiological and immunological studies in patients with immunoglobulin deficiencies and gastrointestinal disorders. *Gut*, **13**, 441–449.

Bullen, C. L. & Willis, A. T. (1971) Resistance of the breast-fed infant to gastroenteritis. *British Medical Journal*, **iii**, 338–343.

Bullen, J. J., Rogers, H. J. & Leigh, L. (1972) Iron-binding proteins in milk and resistance to *Escherichia coli* infection in infants. *British Medical Journal*, **i**, 69–75.

Burdon, D. W. (1973) The bactericidal action of immunoglobulin A. *Journal of Medical Microbiology*, **6**, 131–139.

Carpenter, C. C. J. (1972) Cholera and other enterotoxin-related diarrheal diseases. *Journal of Infectious Diseases*, **126**, 551–564.

Carter, P. B. & Collins, F. M. (1974) The route of enteric infection in normal mice. *Journal of Experimental Medicine*, **139**, 1189–1203.

Cash, R. A., Music, S. I., Libonati, J. P., Schwartz, A. R. & Hornick, R. B. (1974c) Live oral cholera vaccine: evaluation of the clinical effectiveness of two strains in humans. *Infection and Immunity*, **10**, 762–764.

Cash, R. A., Music, S. I., Libonati, J. P., Craig, J. P., Pierce, N. F. & Hornick, R. B. (1974b) Response of man to infection with *Vibrio cholerae*. II. Protection from illness afforded by previous disease and vaccine. *Journal of Infectious Diseases*, **130**, 325–333.

Cash, R. A., Music, S. I., Libonati, J. P., Snyder, M. J., Wenzel, R. P. & Hornick, R. B. (1974a) Response of man to infection with *Vibrio cholerae*. I. Clinical, serologic and bacteriologic responses to a known inoculum. *Journal of Infectious Diseases*, **129**, 45–52.

Centre for Disease Control (1972) Cases of Shigas' bacillus infection. *Shigella surveillance*, **30**, 4–8.

Chang, T.-W., Weinstein, L. & MacMahon, H. E. (1966) Paralytic poliomyelitis in a child with hypogammaglobulinemia: probable implication of type 1 vaccine strain. *Paediatrics*, **37**, 630–636.

Chanock, R. M., Smith, C. B., Friedenwald, W. T., Parrot, R. H., *et al.* (1967) Vaccines against viral and rickettsial diseases of man. *Pan American Health Organization Scientific Publication*, **147**, 53.

Chase, M. W. (1945) Inhibition of experimental drug allergy by prior feeding of the sensitising agent. *Proceedings of the Society for Experimental Biology and Medicine*, **61**, 257–259.

Chilgren, R. A., Quie, P. G., Meuwissen, H. J. & Hong, R. (1967) Chronic mucocutaneous candidiasis, deficiency of delayed hypersensitivity and selective local antibody defect. *Lancet*, **ii**, 688–693.

Chuttani, C. S. (1976) Controlled trials of three different oral killed typhoid vaccines in India. 14th Congress of the International Association of Biological Standardisation. Douglas, Isle of Man, 1975. *Developments in Biological Standardisation*, **33**, 98–101. Basel: Karger.

Clough, J. D., Mims, L. H. & Strober, W. (1971) Deficient IgA antibody responses to arsanilic acid bovine serum (BSA) in neonatally thymectomised rabbits. *Journal of Immunology*, **106**, 1624–1629.

Collins, F. M. & Carter, P. B. (1972) Comparative immunogenicity of heat-killed and living oral Salmonella vaccines. *Infection and Immunity*, **6**, 451–458.

Collins, F. M. & Carter, P. B. (1974) Cellular immunity in enteric disease. *American Journal of Clinical Nutrition*, **27**, 1424–1433.

Colten, H. & Bienenstock, J. (1974) Lack of C_3 activation through classical or alternate pathways by human secretory IgA anti blood group A antibody. In *The Immunological A system*, ed. Mestecky, J. & Lawton, A. R., pp. 305–308. New York: Plenum Press.

Colten, H. R., Gordon, J. M., Borsos, T. & Rapp, H. J. (1968) Synthesis of the first component of human complement *in vitro*. *Journal of Experimental Medicine*, **128**, 595–604.

Connor, J. D. & Barrett-Connor, E. (1967) Infectious diarrhoeas. *Pediatric Clinics of North America*, **14**, No. 1, 197–221.

Craig, S. W. & Cebra, J. J. (1971) Peyer's patches – an enriched source of precursors of IgA-producing immunocytes in the rabbit. *Journal of Experimental Medicine*, **134**, 188–200.

Cramblett, H. G., Azimi, P. & Haynes, R. E. (1971) The etiology of infectious diarrhoea in infancy, with special reference to enteropathogenic *E. coli*. *Annals of the New York Academy of Sciences*, **176**, 80–92.

Cregan, J. & Hayward, N. J. (1953) The bacterial content of the healthy human small intestine. *British Medical Journal*, **i**, 1356–1359.

Crewther, P. & Warner, N. L. (1972) Serum immunoglobulins and antibodies in congenitally athymic (nude) mice. *Australian Journal of Experimental Biology and Medical Science*, **50**, 625–635.

Cvjetanović, B. (1965) Earlier field studies on the effectiveness of cholera vaccines. In Proceedings of the cholera research symposium, Jan. 24–29, 1965, Honolulu, Hawaii. *US Public Health Service publication*, **1328**, pp. 355–361. Washington: US Government Printing Office.

Cvjetanović, B. & Uemura, K. (1965) The present status of field and laboratory studies of typhoid and paratyphoid vaccines. *Bulletin of the World Health Organisation*, **32**, 29–36.

Davies, A. (1922) An investigation into the serological properties of dysentery stools. *Lancet*, **ii**, 1009–1012.

Dickenson, R. J. & Pickens, S. (1978) Morbidity and mortality in Salmonella food poisoning. A review of 47 in-patient cases. *Scottish Medical Journal*, **23**, 23–26.

Dickman, M. O., Chappelka, A. R. & Schaedler, R. W. (1976) The microbial ecology of the upper small bowel. *American Journal of Gastroenterology*, **65**, 57–62.

Dixon, J. M. S. & Paulley, J. W. (1963) Bacteriological and

histological studies of the small intestine of rats treated with mecamylamine. *Gut*, **4**, 169–173.

Dolin, R., Blacklow, N. R., Du Pont, H., Buscho, R. F., Wyatt, R. G., Kasel, J. A., Hornick, R. & Chanock, R. M. (1972) Biological properties of Norwalk agent of acute infectious non-bacterial gastroenteritis. *Proceedings of the Society for Experimental Biology and Medicine*, **140**, 578–583.

Donaldson, R. M. (1964) Normal bacterial populations of the intestine and their relation to intestinal function (1). *New England Journal of Medicine*, **270**, 938–945.

Drachman, R. H. (1974) Acute infectious gastroenteritis. *Paediatric Clinics of North America*, **21**, 3, 711–737.

Drasar, B. S. & Hill, M. J. (1974) *Human Intestinal Flora*, Ch. 2. London: Academic Press.

Drasar, B. S., Shiner, M. & McCleod, G. M. (1969) Studies on the intestinal flora. I. The bacterial flora of the gastrointestinal tract in healthy and achlorhydric persons. *Gastroenterology*, **56**, 71–79.

Drucker, M. M., Yeivin, R. & Sacks, T. G. (1967) Pathogenesis of *Escherichia coli* enteritis in the ligated rabbit gut. *Israel Journal of Medical Science*, **3**, 445–452.

Du Pont, H. L. & Hornick, R. B. Adverse effects of Lomotil therapy in shigellosis. *Journal of the American Medical Association*, **226**, 1525–1528.

Du Pont, H. L., Hornick, R. B., Dawkins, A. T., Snyder, M. J. & Formal, S. B. (1969) The response of man to virulent *Shigella flexneri* 2a. *Journal of Infectious Diseases*, **119**, 296–299.

Du Pont, H. L., Hornick, R. B., Snyder, M. J., Dawkins, A. T., Heiner, G. G. & Woodward, T. E. (1971b) Studies of immunity in typhoid fever. Protection induced by killed oral antigens or by primary infection. *Bulletin of the World Health Organisation*, **44**, 667–672.

Du Pont, H. L., Hornick, R. B., Snyder, M. J., Libonati, J. P., Formal, S. B. & Gangarosa, E. J. (1972) Immunity in shigellosis. II. Protection induced by oral live vaccine or primary infection. *Journal of Infectious Diseases*, **125**, 12–16.

Du Pont, H. L., Formal, S. B., Hornick, R. B., Snyder, M. J., Libonati, J. P., Sheahan, D. G., Labrec, E. H. & Kalas, J. P. (1971a) Pathogenesis of *Escherichia coli* diarrhea. *New England Journal of Medicine*, **285**, 1–9.

Eddie, D. S., Schulkind, M. L. & Robbins, J. B. (1971) The isolation and biologic activities of purified secretory IgA and IgG anti-*Salmonella typhimurium* 'O' antibodies from rabbit intestinal fluid and colostrum. *Journal of Immunology*, **106**, 181–190.

Emslie-Smith, A. M. (1965) Observations on strains of *E. coli* exhibiting ecological dynasticism in the faecal flora of man. *Ernahrungsforschung*, **10**, 302–307.

Fazekas, D. E., St Groth, S., Donnelley, M. & Graham, D. M. (1951) Studies in experimental immunology of influenza. VIII. Pathotopic Adjuvants. *Australian Journal of Experimental Biology and Medical Science*, **29**, 323–337.

Felix, A. & Pitt, R. M. (1934) Virulence of *B. typhosus* and resistance to O antibody. *Journal of Pathology and Bacteriology*, **38**, 409–420.

Felsenfeld, O. (1976) Standardisation of *Escherichia coli* oral vaccines. 14th Congress of the International Association of Biological Standardisation, Douglas, Isle of Man, 1975. *Developments in Biological Standardisation*, **33**, 113–117. Basel: Karger.

Felsenfeld, O., Wolf, R. H., Greer, W. E. & Brannon, R. B. (1972) Oral immunization with polyvalent streptomycin-dependent *Escherichia coli* vaccine. *Applied Microbiology*, **14**, 444–448.

Ferguson, A. & Jarrett, E. E. (1975) Hypersensitivity reactions in the small intestine. I. Thymus dependence of experimental partial villous atrophy. *Gut*, **16**, 114–117.

Ferguson, A. & MacDonald, T. T. (1974) Tissue damage mediated by lymphocytes in local small intestinal immune reactions (Abstract). *Gut*, **15**, 834.

Ferguson, A. & MacDonald, T. T. (1975) Effects of local hypersensitivity reactions on small intestinal morphology. *Behring Institute Mitteilungen*, **57**, (in press).

Ferguson, A., MacDonald, T. T., McClure, J. P. & Holden, R. J. (1975) Cell-mediated immunity to gliadin within the small-intestinal mucosa in coeliac disease. *Lancet*, **i**, 895–897.

Fernelius, A. L., Ritchie, A. E., Classick, L. G., Norman, J. O. & Mebus, C. A. (1972) Cell culture adaptation and propagation of a reovirus like agent of calf diarrhoea from a field outbreak in Nebraska. *Archiv. für die gesamte Virusforschung*, **37**, 114–130.

Finkelstein, R. A. (1970) Antitoxic immunity in experimental cholera: observations with purified antigens and the ligated ileal loop model. *Infection and Immunity*, **1**, 464–467.

Finkelstein, R. A. (1970) Properties of cholera exo-enterotoxin (choleragen) and its natural toxoid (choleragenoid). *Toxicon*, **10**, 441–450.

Finkelstein, R. A. (1975) Immunology of cholera. *Current Topics in Microbiology and Immunology*, **69**, 137–196.

Finkelstein, R. A. (1976) Possibilities of immunisation against cholera and related enterotoxic enteropathies. 14th Congress of the International Association of Biological Standardisation, Douglas, Isle of Man, 1975. *Developments in Biological Standardisation*, **33**, 102–107. Basel: Karger.

Flewett, T. H. & Boxall, E. (1976) The search for viruses in the gastrointestinal tract. *Clinics in Gastroenterology*, **5**, 2, 359–385.

Flewett, T. H., Bryden, A. S., Davies, H., Woode, G. N., Bridger, J. C. & Derrick, J. M. (1974) Relation between viruses from acute gastroenteritis of children and new newborn calves. *Lancet*, **ii**, 61–63.

Floch, M. H., Binder, H. J., Filburn, B. & Gershengoren, W. (1972) The effect of bile acids on intestinal microflora. *American Journal of Clinical Nutrition*, **25**, 1418–1426.

Florey, H. W. (1933) Observations on the functions of mucus and the early stages of bacterial invasion of the intestinal mucosa. *Journal of Pathology and Bacteriology*, **37**, 283–289.

Florey, H. W. (1946) The use of micro-organisms for therapeutic purposes. *Yale Journal of Biology and Medicine*, **19**, 101–117.

Freter, R. (1969) Studies of the mechanism of action of intestinal antibody in experimental cholera. *Texas Reports on Biology and Medicine*, **27**, (Suppl. 1), 299–316.

Freter, R. (1970) Mechanism of action of intestinal antibody in experimental cholera. II. Antibody mediated antibacterial reaction at the mucosal surface. *Infection and Immunity*, **2**, 556–562.

Freter, R. (1974a) Gut associated immunity to cholera. In *Cholera*, ed. Barua, D. & Burrows, W., Ch. 18. Philadelphia: Saunders.

Freter, R. (1974b) Interactions between mechanisms controlling the intestinal microflora. *American Journal of Clinical Nutrition*, **27**, 1409–1416.

Fubara, E. & Freter, R. (1972) Availability of locally synthesised and systemic antibodies in the intestine. *Infection and Immunity*, **6**, 965–981.

Fubara, E. S. & Freter, R. (1972) Source and protective

function of coproantibodies in intestinal disease. *American Journal of Clinical Nutrition*, 25, 1357–1363.

Fubara, E. S. & Freter, R. (1973) Protection against enteric bacterial infection by secretory IgA antibodies. *Journal of Immunology*, 111, 395–403.

Fujita, K. & Finkelstein, R. A. (1972) Antitoxic immunity in experimental cholera: comparison of immunity induced perorally and parenterally in mice. *Journal of Infectious Diseases*, 125, 647–655.

Gaines, S., Sprinz, H., Tully, J. G. & Tigertt, W. D. (1968) Studies on infection and immunity in experimental typhoid fever. VII. The distribution of *Salmonella typhi* in chimpanzee tissue following oral challenge, and the relationship between the numbers of bacilli and morphologic lesions. *Journal of Infectious Diseases*, 118, 293–306.

Galanos, C., Lüderitz, O. & Westphal, O. (1971) Preparation and properties of antisera against the lipid-A component of bacterial lipopolysaccharides. *European Journal of Biochemistry*, 24, 116–122.

Gelfand, E. W., Biggar, W. D. & Orange, R. P. (1974) Immune deficiency. Evaluation, diagnosis and therapy. *Pediatric Clinics of North America*, 21, 4, 745–776.

Gemski, P., Jr., Takeuchi, A., Washington, O. & Formal, S. B. (1972) Shigellosis due to *Shigella dysenteriae*. I. Relative importance of mucosal invasion versus toxin production in pathogenesis. *Journal of Infectious Diseases*, 126, 523–530.

Genco, R. J., Evans, R. T. & Taubman, M. A. (1974) Specificity of antibodies to *Streptococcus mutans*: significance in inhibition of adherence. In *The Immunoglobulin A System*, ed. Mestecky, J. & Lawton, A. R., pp. 327–336. New York: Plenum Press.

Germanier, J. (1970) Immunity in experimental salmonellosis. I. Protection induced by rough mutants of *Salmonella typhimurium*. *Infection and Immunity*, 2, 309–315.

Germanier, J. (1972) Immunity in experimental salmonellosis. III. Comparative immunisation with viable and heat inactivated cells of *Salmonella typhimurium*. *Infection and Immunity*, 5, 792–797.

Germanier, J. & Fürer, E. (1975) Isolation and characterisation of *S. typhi* gal E mutant Ty21a. A candidate strain for live oral typhoid vaccine. *Journal of Infectious Diseases*, 131, 553–558.

Giannella, R. A., Broitman, S. A. & Zamchek, N. (1972) Gastric acid barrier to ingested microorganisms in man: studies *in vivo* and *in vitro*. *Gut*, 13, 251–256.

Giannella, R. A., Formal, S. B., Dammin, G. J. & Collins, H. (1973) Pathogenesis of salmonellosis: studies of fluid secretion, mucosal invasion, and morphologic reaction in the rabbit ileum. *Journal of Clinical Investigation*, 52, 441–453.

Giannella, R. A., Washington, O., Gemski, P. & Formal, S. B. (1973) Invasion of HeLa cells by *Salmonella typhimurium*: A model for study of invasiveness of Salmonella. *Journal of Infectious Diseases*, 128, 69–75.

Gibbons, R. J. (1974) Bacterial adherence to mucosal surfaces and its inhibition by secretory antibodies. In *The Immunoglobulin A System*, ed. Mestecky, J. & Lawton, A. R., pp. 315–325. New York: Plenum Press.

Girard, J. P. & De Kalbermatten, A. (1970) Les immunoglobulines dans les sécrétions duodéno-pancréatiques et la bile. *Schweizerische Medizinische Wochenschrift*, 100, 336–338.

Glynn, A. A. (1972) Bacterial factors inhibiting host defence mechanisms. In *Microbial Pathogenicity in Man*

and Animals, ed. Smith, H. & Pearce, J. H. London: Cambridge University Press.

Glynn, A. A. (1974) Antibodies in infection. In *Progress in Immunology*, II, ed. Brent, L. & Holborrow, J., Vol. 4. Amsterdam: North Holland Publishing.

Goldblum, R. M., Ahlstedt, S., Carlsson, B., Hanson, L. A., Jodal, U., Lidin-Janson, G. & Sohl-Akerlund, A. (1975) Antibody forming cells in human colostrum after oral immunisation. *Nature*, 257, 797–799.

Goldman, A. S. & Smith, C. W. (1973) Host resistance factors in human milk. *Journal of Pediatrics*, 82, 1082–1090.

Gontzea, I. (1974) *Nutrition and Anti-Infectious Defence*. Basel: Karger.

Good, R. A. & Jose, D. (1975) *Immunodeficiency secondary to nutritional deprivation: Clinical and laboratory observations, Immunodeficiency in animals and man*. In *Birth Defects: Original Articles*, ed. Bergsma, D., Series II, pp. 291–322. Massachusetts: Sinauer.

Gorbach, S. L. (1971) Progress in gastroenterology: intestinal microflora. *Gastroenterology*, 60, 1110–1129.

Gorbach, S. L. & Khurana, C. H. (1972) Toxigenic *Escherichia coli*. A cause of infantile diarrhea in Chicago. *New England Journal of Medicine*, 287, 791–795.

Gordon, J. E. & Scrimshaw, N. S. (1970) Infectious disease in the malnourished. *Medical Clinics of North America*, 54, 6, 1495–1508.

Gordon, J. E., Chitkara, I. O. & Wyon, J. B. (1963) Weanling diarrhea. *American Journal of Medical Sciences*, 245, 345–377.

Gordon, J. E., Singh, S. & Wyon, J. B. (1965) Causes of death at different ages by sex, and by season, in a rural population of the Punjab 1957–1959 – A field study. *Indian Journal of Medical Research*, 53, 906–916.

Greaves, M. & Janossy, G. (1972) Elicitation of selective T and B lymphocyte responses by cell surface binding ligands. *Transplantation Reviews*, 11, 87–130.

Guineé, P. A. M., Jansen, W. M. & Agterberg, C. M. (1976) Detection of the K99 antigen by means of agglutination and immunoelectrophoresis in *Escherichia coli* isolated from calves and its correlation with enterotoxigenicity. *Infection and Immunity*, 13, 1369–1377.

Guy-Grand, D., Griscelli, C. & Vassalli, P. (1974) The gut-associated lymphoid system: nature and properties of the large dividing cells. *European Journal of Immunology*, 4, 435–443.

Gyles, C., So, M. & Falkow, S. (1974) The enterotoxin plasmids of *Escherichia coli*. *Journal of Infectious Diseases*, 130, 40–49.

György, P. (1971) The uniqueness of human milk – biochemical aspects. *American Journal of Clinical Nutrition*, 24, 970–975.

Harris, J. C., Du Pont, H. L. & Hornick, R. B. (1972) Fecal leukocytes in diarrheal illness. *Annals of Internal Medicine*, 76, 697–703.

Harrison, M., Kilby, A., Walker Smith, J. A., France, W. E., Wood, B. S. (1976) Cow's milk intolerance, a possible association with gastroenteritis, lactose intolerance and IgA deficiency. *British Medical Journal*, i, 1501–1504.

Heading, R. C., Parkin, D. M., Barnetson, R. St C., McClelland, D. B. L. & Shearman, D. J. C. (1974) Small-intestinal bacterial flora in dermatitis herpetiformis. *American Journal of Digestive Diseases*, 19, 704–708.

Hermans, P. E., Huizenga, K. A., Hoffman, H. N., Brown, A. L. & Markowitz, H. (1966) Dysgammaglobulinemia associated with nodular hyperplasia of the small intestine. *American Journal of Medicine*, **40**, 78–89.

Hess, M. W., Cottier, H., Sordat, B., Joel, D. D. & Chanana, A. D. (1973) The intestinal barrier to bacterial invasion. In *'Non-Specific' Factors Influencing Host Resistance*, ed. Braun, W. & Ungar, J., pp. 447–451. Basel: Karger.

van Heyningen, S. (1976) The subunits of cholera toxin: structure, stoichiometry and function. *Journal of Infectious Diseases*, **133**, Suppl. S5–S13.

Heyworth, B. & Brown, J. (1975) Jejunal microflora in malnourished Gambian children. *Archives of Diseases in Childhood*, **50**, 27–33.

Hill, I. R. & Porter, P. (1974) Studies of bactericidal activity to *Escherichia coli* of porcine serum and colostral immunoglobulins and the role of lysozyme with secretory IgA. *Immunology*, **26**, 1239–1250.

Honjo, S., Takasaka, M., Fujiwara, T., Kaneko, M., Imaizumi, K., Ogawa, H., Mise, K., Nakamura, A. & Nakaya, R. (1967) Shigellosis in Cynomolgus monkeys (*Macaca irus*). V. resistence acquired by the repetition of experimental oral infection with *Shigella flexneri* 2A and fluctuation of serum agglutinin titer. *Japanese Journal of Medical Science and Biology*, **20**, 341–348.

Hook, E. W. (1974) Salmonella infections. In *Harrison's Principles of Internal Medicine*, 7th edn., Ch. 136. Tokyo: McGraw Hill Koganisha.

Hornick, R. B., Greisman, S. E., Woodward, T. E., Du Pont, H. L., Dawkins, A. T. & Snyder, M. J. (1970a) Typhoid fever: Pathogenesis and immunologic control. I. *New England Journal of Medicine*, **283**, 686–691.

Hornick, R. B., Greisman, S. E., Woodward, T. E., Du Pont, H. L., Dawkins, A. T. & Snyder, M. J. (1970b) Typhoid fever: pathogenesis and immunologic control. II. *New England Journal of Medicine*, **283**, 739–746.

Hornick, R. B., Du Pont, H. L., Levine, M. M., Gilman, R. H., Woodward, W. E., Snyder, M. J. & Woodward, T. E. (1976) Efficacy of a live oral typhoid vaccine in human volunteers. 14th Congress of the International Association of Biological Standardisation, Douglas, Isle of Man, 1975. *Developments in Biological Standardisation*, **33**, 89–92. Basel: Karger.

Huber, H., Douglas, S. D., Huber, C. & Goldberg, L. S. (1971) Human monocyte receptor sites. Failure of IgA to demonstrate cytophilia. *International Archives of Allergy and Applied Immunology*, **41**, 262–267.

Hunter, R. L. (1972) Antigen trapping in the lamina propria and production of IgA antibody. *Journal of the Reticuloendothelial Society*, **11**, 245–252.

Ishizaka, K., Ishizaka, T., Lee, E. H. & Fudenberg, H. (1965) Immunochemical properties of human γA isohemagglutinin. I. Comparisons with γG- and γM-globulin antibodies. *Journal of Immunology*, **95**, 197–208.

Ivanyi, L. & Lehner, T. (1974) Stimulation of human lymphocytes by B-cell mitogens. *Clinical & Experimental Immunology*, **18**, 347–356.

James, W. P. T., Drasar, B. S. & Miller, C. (1972) Physiological mechanism and pathogenesis of weanling diarrhea. *American Journal of Clinical Nutrition*, **25**, 564–571.

Jones, G. W., Abrams, G. D. & Freter, R. (1976) Adhesive property of *Vibrio cholerae*: adhesion to isolated rabbit brush border membranes and haemagglutinating activity. *Infection and Immunity*, **14**, 232–239.

Jones, G. W. & Rutter, J. M. (1972) Role of the K88 antigen in the pathogenesis of neonatal diarrhea caused by *Escherichia coli* in piglets. *Infection and Immunity*, **6**, 918–927.

Joo, I. (1971) Present status and perspectives of vaccination against typhoid fever. In *International Conference on the Application of Vaccines Against Viral, Rickettsial and Bacterial Diseases of Man*, pp. 329–341. Washington: Pan American Health Organisation.

Joo, I. (1976) Antigenicity testing of inactivated (*E. coli*) oral enteric bacterial vaccines for human use. 14th Congress of the International Association of Biological Standardisation, Douglas, Isle of Man, 1975. *Developments in Biological Standardisation*, **33**, 75–79. Basel: Karger.

Kapikian, A. Z., Wyatt, R. G., Dolin, R., Thornhill, T. S., Kalica, A. R. & Chanock, R. M. (1972) Visualisation by immune electron microscopy of a 27 n.m. particle associated with acute infectious nonbacterial gastroenteritis. *Journal of Virology*, **10**, 1075–1081.

Kantor, H. S., Tao, P. & Wisdom, C. (1974) Action of *Escherichia coli* enterotoxin: on Adenylate cyclase behaviour of intestinal epithelial cells in culture. *Infection and Immunity*, **9**, 1003–1010.

Kao, V. C. Y., Sprinz, H. & Burrows, W. (1972) Localization of cholera toxin in rabbit intestine. An immunohistochemical study. *Laboratory Investigation*, **26**, 148–153.

Kaplan, M. E., Dalmasso, A. P. & Woodson, M. (1972) Complement-dependent opsonization of incompatible erythrocytes by human secretory IgA. *Journal of Immunology*, **108**, 275–278.

Kaur, J., McGhee, J. R. & Burrows, W. (1972) Immunity to cholera: the occurrence and nature of antibody-active immunoglobulins in the lower ileum of the rabbit. *Journal of Immunology*, **108**, 387–395.

Keller, R. & Dwyer, J. E. (1968) Neutralisation of poliovirus by IgA coproantibodies. *Journal of Immunology*, **107**, 192–202.

Keller, H. U., Hess, M. W. & Cottier, H. (1973) Influence of *E. coli* culture filtrates on the migration of leucocytes including lymphocytes. In *'Non-specific' Factors Influencing Host Resistance*, pp. 190–195. Basel: Karger.

Lai A Fat, R. F. M., McClelland, D. B. L. & Van Furth, R. (1976a) *In vitro* synthesis of immunoglobulins, secretory component, complement and lysozyme by human gastrointestinal tissues. I. Normal tissues. *Clinical and Experimental Immunology*, **23**, 9–19.

Lancet (editorial) (1975) *E. coli* enteritis. *Lancet*, **ii**, 1131–1132.

Lerner, A. M. (1974) Enteric viruses. Coxsackie viruses, echoviruses, reoviruses. In *Harrison's Textbook of Medicine*, 7th edn, Ch. 190. Tokyo: McGraw Hill Koganisha.

Levine, M. M., Du Pont, H. L., Formal, S. B., Hornick, R. B., Takeuchi, A., Gangarosa, E. J., Snyder, M. J. & Libonati, J. P. (1973) Pathogenesis of *Shigella dysenteriae* 1 (Shiga) dysentery. *Journal of Infectious Diseases*, **127**, 261–270.

de Lorenzo, F., Soscia, M., Manzillo, G., Balesterici, G. G. (1973) Epidemic of cholera El Tor in Naples 1973. *Lancet*, **i**, 669.

Logan, E. F., Stenhouse, A. & Ormrod, D. J. (1974) The role of colostral immunoglobulins in intestinal immunity to conbacillosis in the calf. *Research in Veterinary Science*, **17**, 280.

Lüderitz, O. (1970) Recent results on the biochemistry of the cell wall lipopolysaccharide of Salmonella bacteria. *Angewandte Chemie*, International Edition, **9**, 649–663.

Mackaness, G. B. (1971) Resistance to intracellular infection. *Journal of Infectious Diseases*, **123**, 439–444.

McClelland, D. B. L., Lai A Fat, R. F. M. & van Furth, R. (1976) *In vitro* synthesis of immunoglobulin, secretory component, complement and lysozyme by human gastrointestinal tissues. II. Pathological tissues. *Clinical and Experimental Immunology*, 23, 20–27.

McClelland, D. B. L., Samson, R. R., Parkin, D. M. & Shearman, D. J. C. (1972) Bacterial agglutination studies with secretory IgA prepared from human gastrointestinal secretions and colostrum. *Gut*, 13, 450–458.

McClelland, D. B. L., Finlayson, N. D. C., Samson, R. R., Nairn, I. M. & Shearman, D. J. C. (1971) Quantitation of immunoglobulins in gastric juice by electro-immunodiffusion. *Gastroenterology*, 60, 509–514.

McFarlin, D. E., Strober, W. & Waldmann, T. A. (1972) Ataxia-telangiectasia. *Medicine*, 51, 281–314.

McNeish, A. S., Gaze, H. & Evans, N. (1974) Agglutinating antibodies in the duodenal secretions of infants with enteropathic *E. coli* gastroenteritis (Abstract). *Gut*, 15, 834.

McNeish, A. S., Turner, P., Fleming, T. & Evans, N. (1975) Mucosal adherence of human enteropathogenic *E. coli*. *Lancet*, ii, 946–948.

Madley, C. R. & Cosgrove, B. P. (1975) Viruses in infantile gastroenteritis. *Lancet*, ii, 124.

Marmion, D. E., Naylor, G. R. E. & Stewart, I. O. (1953) Second attacks of typhoid fever. *Journal of Hygiene*, 51, 260–267.

Mata, L. J., Urrutia, J. J. & Gordon, J. E. (1967) Diarrhoeal disease in a cohort of Guatemalan village children observed from birth to age two years. *Tropical and Geographical Medicine*, 19, 247–257.

Mebus, C. A., Stair, E. L., Rhodes, M. B. & Twiehaus, M. J. (1973) Neonatal calf diarrhoea: propagation, attenuation and characteristics of a corona virus like agent. *American Journal of Veterinary Research*, 34, 145–150.

Mebus, C. A., Stair, E. L., Underdahl, N. R. & Twiehaus, M. J. (1971) Pathology of neonatal calf diarrhoea induced by a reo-like virus. *Veterinary Pathology*, 8, 490–505.

Mebus, C. A., Torres-Medina, A., Twiehaus, M. J. & Bass, E. P. (1976) Immune response to orally administered calf reovirus like agent and corona virus vaccine. 14th Congress of the International Association of Biological Standardisation, Douglas, Isle of Man, 1975. *Developments in Biological Standardisation*, 33, 396–403. Basel: Karger.

Medical Research Council (1971) Hypogammaglobulinaemia in the United Kingdom. *MRC Special Report Series*, 310. London: HMSO.

Mel, D. M., Cvjetanović, B. & Felsenfeld, O. (1970) Studies on vaccination against bacillary dysentery. 5. Studies in *Erythrocebus patas*. *Bulletin of the World Health Organisation*, 43, 431–437.

Mel, D. M., Terzin, A. L., Vukšić, L. (1965a) Studies on vaccination against bacillary dysentery. 1. Immunization of mice against experimental Shigella infection. *Bulletin of the World Health Organisation*, 32, 633–636.

Mel, D. M., Terzin, A. L. & Vukšić, L. (1965b) Studies on vaccination against bacillary dysentery. 3. Effective oral immunization against *Shigella flexneri* 2a in a field trial. *Bulletin of the World Health Organisation*, 32, 647–655.

Mel, D. M., Papo, R. G., Terzin, A. L. & Vukšić, L. (1965) Safety tests and reactogenicity studies on a live dysentery vaccine intended for field trials. *Bulletin of the World Health Organisation*, 32, 637–645.

Mel, D. M., Gangarosa, E. J., Radovanović, M. L., Arsić, B. L. & Litvinjenko, S. (1971) Studies on vaccination against bacillary dysentery. 6. Protection of children by oral immunization with streptomycin-dependent Shigella strains. *Bulletin of the World Health Organisation*, 45, 457–464.

Metchnikoff, E. (1905) *Immunity in Infective Disease*, tr. Binnie, F. G. London: Cambridge University Press.

Meynell, G. G. & Subbaiah, T. V. (1963) Antibacterial mechanisms of the mouse gut. 1. Kinetics of infection by *Salmonella typhi-murium* in normal and streptomycin-treated mice studied with abortive transductants. *British Journal of Experimental Pathology*, 44, 197–208.

Michael, J. G., Ringenback, R. & Hottenstein, S. (1971) The antimicrobial activity of human colostral antibody in the newborn. *Journal of Infectious Diseases*, 124, 445–448.

Monteiro, E., Fossey, T., Shiner, M., Drasar, B. S. & Allison, A. J. (1971) Antibacterial antibodies in rectal and colonic mucosa in ulcerative colitis. *Lancet*, i, 249–251.

Montgomery, P. C., Rosner, B. R. & Cohn, J. (1974) The secretory antibody response. Anti-DNP antibodies induced by Dinitrophenylated Type III pneumococcus. *Immunological Communications*, 3, 143–156.

Morag, A., Beutner, K. R., Morag, B. & Ogra, P. L. (1974) Development and characteristics of *in vitro* correlates of cellular immunity to rubella virus in the systemic and mucosal sites in guinea-pigs. *Journal of Immunology*, 113, 1703–1709.

Morley, D. (1973) *Paediatric Priorities in the Developing World*, Ch. 6. London: Butterworth.

Mosley, W. H. (1969) Vaccines and somatic antigens. The role of immunity in cholera. A review of epidemiological and serological studies. *Texas Reports on Biology and Medicine*, 27, (Suppl. 1), 227–241.

Mosley, W. H. & Ahmed, A. (1969) Active and passive immunisation in the adult rabbit ileal loop as an assay for the production of antitoxin by cholera vaccines. *Journal of Bacteriology*, 100, 547–549.

Myerowitz, R. L., Handzel, Z. T., Schneerson, R. & Robbins, J. B. (1973) Induction of *Haemophilus influenzae* type b capsular antibody in neonatal rabbits by gastrointestinal colonisation with cross-reacting *Escherichia coli*. *Infection and Immunity*, 7, 137–140.

Nalin, D. R., Al-Mahmud, A., Curlin, G., Ahmed, A. & Peterson, J. (1974) Cholera toxoid boosts serum *Escherichia coli* antitoxin in humans. *Infection and Immunity*, 10, 747–749.

Nelson, E. T., Clements, J. D., Finkelstein, R. A. (1976) *Vibrio cholerae*. Adherence and colonisation in experimental cholera: Electron microscopic studies. *Infection and Immunity*, 14, 527–547.

Nomura, M. (1967) Colicins and related bacteriocins. *Annual Review of Microbiology*, 21, 257–284.

Northrup, R. S. & Hossain, S. A. (1970) Immunoglobulins and antibody activity in the intestine and serum in cholera. II. Measurement of antibody activity in jejunal aspirates and sera of cholera patients by radioimmunodiffusion. *Journal of Infectious Diseases*, 121, (Suppl.), S142–S146.

Ocklitz, H. W., Mochmann, H., Schmidt, E. F. & Hering, L. (1967) Oral immunisation of mice with a soluble protective antigen obtained from entero pathogenic serotypes of *Escherichia coli*. *Nature*, 214, 1053–1054.

Ogawa, H., Nakamura, A. & Nakaya, R. (1968) Cinemicrographic study of tissue cell cultures infected with *Shigella flexneri*. *Japanese Journal of Medical Science and Biology*, 21, 259–273.

Ogawa, H., Yoshikura, H., Nakamura, A. & Nakaya, R. (1967) Susceptibility of cell cultures from various mammalian tissues to the infection by Shigella. *Japanese*

Journal of Medical Science and Biology, **20**, 329–339.

Ogra, P. L. (1971) The secretory immunoglobulin system of the gastrointestinal tract. In *The Secretory Immunoglobulin System*, ed. Dayton, H., Small, P. A., Chanock, R. M., Kaufman, H. E. & Tomasi, T. B., pp. 259–273. Maryland: U.S. Department of Health Education Welfare; National Institute of Child Health and Development.

Ogra, P. L. (1974c) Discussion. In *The Immunoglobulin A System*, ed. Mestecky, T. & Lawton, A. R., p. 309. New York: Plenum Press.

Ogra, P. L. & Karzon, D. T. (1969) Distribution of poliovirus antibody in serum, nasopharynx and alimentary tract following segmental immunisation of lower alimentary tract with polio-vaccine. *Journal of Immunology*, **102**, 1423–1430.

Ogra, P. L. & Karzon, D. T. (1970) The role of immunoglobulins, in the mechanism of mucosal immunity to virus infection. *Pediatric Clinics of North America*, **17**, 2, 385–400.

Ogra, P. L., Chiba, Y., Beutner, K. R., Morag, A. (1976) Vaccination by non-parenteral routes: characteristics of immune response: 14th Congress of the International Association of Biological Standardisation, Douglas, Isle of Man, 1975. *Developments in Biological Standardisation*, **33**, 19–26. Basel: Karger.

Ogra, P. L., Coppola, P. R., MacGillivray, M. H. & Dzierba, J. L. (1974) Mechanism of mucosal immunity to viral infections in γA immunoglobulin-deficiency syndromes. *Proceedings of the Society for Experimental Biology and Medicine*, **145**, 811–816.

Ogra, P. L., Karzon, D. T., Righthand, F. & MacGillivray, M. (1968) Immunoglobulin response in serum and secretions after immunisation with live and inactivated poliovaccine and natural infection. *New England Journal of Medicine*, **279**, 893–900.

Ogra, P. L., Wallace, R. B., Umana, G., Ogra, S. S., Grant, D. K. & Morag, A. (1974) Implications of secretory immune system in viral infections. In *The Immunoglobulin A System*, ed. Mestecky, J. & Lawton, A. R., pp. 271–282. New York: Plenum Press.

Olson, G. B. & Wostmann, B. S. (1966) Lymphocytopoiesis, plasmacytopoiesis and cellular proliferation in nonantigenically stimulated germfree mice. *Journal of Immunology*, **97**, 267–274.

Oppenheim, J. J. & Perry, S. (1965) Effects of endotoxins on cultured leucocytes. *Proceedings of the Society for Experimental Biology and Medicine (New York)*, **118**, 1014–1019.

Orskov, J. & Moltke, O. (1928) Studien über den Infektions-mechanismus bei verschiedenen Paratyphus-infektionen aus wissen Mausen. *Immunitätsforschung und Experimentelle Therapie*, **59**, 357–405.

Ørstavik, D. S. (1974) Report of discussion. In *The Immunoglobulin A System*, ed. Mestecky, J. & Lawton, A. R., p. 353. New York: Plenum Press.

Ozawa, A., Goto, J., Ito, Y. & Shibata, H. (1973) Histopathological and biochemical responses of germfree and conventional mice with salmonella infection. In *Germfree Research, Biological Effect of Gnotobiotic Environments*, ed. Heneghan, J. B. New York: Academic Press.

Paine, T. F. (1958) The inhibitory actions of bacteria on Candida growth. *Antibiotics and Chemotherapy*, **8**, 273–281.

Parkin, D. M., McClelland, D. B. L., O'Moore, R. R., Percy-Robb, I. W., Grant, I. W. B. & Shearman, D. J. C. (1972) Intestinal flora and bile salt studies in hypogammaglobulinaemia. *Gut*, **13**, 182–188.

Perey, D. Y. E. & Bienenstock, J. (1973) Effects of bursectomy and thymectomy on ontogeny of fowl IgA, IgG and IgM. *Journal of Immunology*, **111**, 633–637.

Perrotto, J. L., Le Ming Hang, Isselbacher, K. J. & Warren, K. S. (1974) Systemic cellular hypersensitivity induced by an intestinally absorbed antigen. *Journal of Experimental Medicine*, **140**, 296–299.

Peterson, J. W., LoSpalluto, J. J. & Finkelstein, R. A. (1972) Localisation of cholera toxin *in vivo*. *Journal of Infectious Diseases*, **126**, 617–628.

Pierce, N. F. & Gowans, J. L. (1975) Cellular kinetics of the intestinal immune response to cholera toxoid in rats. *Journal of Experimental Medicine*, **142**, 1550–1563.

Plotkin, S. A., Farquhar, J. D. & Ogra, P. L. (1974) Immunological properties of RA27/3 Rubella virus vaccine. A comparison with strains presently licensed in the United States. *Journal of the American Medical Association*, **225**, 585–590.

Porter, P., Kenworthy, R. & Thompson, I. (1975) Oral immunisation and its significance in the prophylactic control of enteritis in the pre-ruminant calf. *Veterinary Record*, **97**, 24–28.

Porter, P., Kenworthy, R., Noakes, D. E. & Allen, W. D. (1974) Intestinal antibody secretion in the young pig in response to oral immunization with *Escherichia coli*. *Immunology*, **27**, 841–853.

Raettig, H. (1976) Non-specific immunity after local immunisation. 14th Congress of the International Association of Biological Standardisation, Douglas, Isle of Man, 1975. *Developments in Biological Standardisation*, **33**, 13–18. Basel: Karger.

Reed, W. P. & Williams, R. C. (1971). Intestinal immunoglobulins in Shigellosis. *Gastroenterology*, **61**, 35–45.

Reller, L. B., Gangarosa, E. J., Drachman, P. S. (1970) Shigellosis in the United States. Five-year review of nation-wide surveillance 1964–1968. *American Journal of Epidemiology*, **91**, 161–169.

Robbins, J. B., Myerowitz, R. L., Whisnant, J. K., Argaman, M., Schneerson, R., Handzel, Z. I. & Gotschlich, E. C. (1972) Enteric bacteria cross-reactive with *Neisseria meningitidis* Groups A and C and *Diplococcus pneumoniae* Types I and II. *Infection and Immunity*, **6**, 651–656.

Robinet, H. G. (1962) Relationship of host antibody to fluctuations of *Escherichia coli* serotypes in the human intestine. *Journal of Bacteriology*, **84**, 896–901.

Robinson, M. (1951) Infant morbidity and mortality. A study of 3266 infants. *Lancet*, **i**, 788–794.

Rockey, J. H., Hanson, L. A., Heremans, J. F. & Kunkel, H. G. (1964) Beta-2A aglobulinaemia in two healthy men. *Journal of Laboratory and Clinical Medicine*, **63**, 205–212.

Rosen, F. S. (1974) Primary immunodeficiency. *Paediatric Clinics of North America*, **21**, 3, 533–549.

Rosen, F. S. & Janeway, C. A. (1966) The gammaglobulins. III. The antibody deficiency syndromes. *New England Journal of Medicine*, **275**, 709–715.

Rosenstein, B. J. (1964) Shigella and Salmonella enteritis in infants and children. *Bulletin of the John Hopkins Hospital*, **115**, 407–415.

Rout, W. R., Formal, S. B. Giannella, R. A. & Dammin, G. J. (1975) Pathophysiology of Shigella diarrhea in the Rhesus monkey: intestinal transport, morphological and bacteriological studies. *Gastroenterology*, **68**, 270–278.

Rudzik, O. & Bienenstock, J. (1974) Isolation and characterisation of gut mucosal lymphocytes. *Laboratory Investigation*, **30**, 260–266.

Rutter, J. M. & Jones, G. W. (1973) Protection against enteric disease caused by *Escherichia coli* – a model for vaccination with a virulence determinant. *Nature*, 242, 531–532.

Rutter, J. M., Burrows, M. R., Sellwood, R. & Gibbons, R. A. (1975) A genetic basis for enteric disease caused by *E. coli*. *Nature*, 257, 135–136.

Sack, R. B. (1976) Enterotoxigenic *E. coli* – an emerging pathogen. *New England Journal of Medicine*, 295, 893–894.

Sack, R. B. & Miller, C. E. (1969) Progressive changes of vibrio serotypes in germ-free mice infected with *Vibrio cholerae*. *Journal of Bacteriology*, 99, 688–695.

Sack, R. B., Gorbach, S. L., Banwell, J. G., Jacobs, B., Chatterjee, B. D. & Mitra, R. C. (1971) Enterotoxigenic *Escherichia coli* isolated from patients with severe cholera-like disease. *Journal of Infectious Diseases*, 123, 378–385.

Saif, L. J., Bohl, E. M. & Gupta, R. K. (1972) Isolation of porcine immunoglobulins and determination of the immunoglobulin classes of transmissable gastroenteritis viral antibodies. *Interaction and Immunity*, 6, 600.

Sanyal, S. C. & Mukerjee, S. (1969) Live oral cholera vaccine: report of a trial on human volunteer subjects. *Bulletin of the World Health Organisation*, 40, 503–511.

Savage, D. C. (1972) Survival on mucosal epithelia, epithelial penetration and growth in tissues of pathogenic bacteria. In *Microbial Pathogenicity in Man and Animals*, ed. Smith, H. & Pearce, J. H. Cambridge University Press.

Savage, D. C. & McAllister, J. S. (1970) Microbial interactions at body surfaces and resistance to infectious diseases. In *Resistance to Infectious Disease*, ed. Dunlop, R. H. & Moon, H. W. Saskatoon: Modern Press.

Schneerson, R. & Robbins, J. B. (1975) Induction of serum *Haemophilus influenzae* type b capsular antibodies in adult volunteers fed cross-reacting *Escherichia coli* 075:K100:45. *New England Journal of Medicine*, 292, 1093–1096.

Schneider, H. & Formal, S. B. (1963) Spontaneous loss of guinea pig virulence in a strain of *Shigella flexneri* 2a. *Bacteriological Proceedings*, 63, 66.

Schrank, G. D. & Verwey, W. F. (1976) Distribution of cholera organisms in experimental *Vibrio cholerae* infections. Proposed mechanisms of pathogenesis and antibacterial immunity. *Infection and Immunity*, 13, 195–203.

Schreiber, D. S., Blacklow, N. R. & Trier, J. S. (1973) The mucosal lesion of the proximal small intestine in acute infectious non-bacterial gastroenteritis. *New England Journal of Medicine*, 288, 1318–1323.

Schrieber, D. S., Blacklow, N. R. & Trier, J. S. (1974) The small intestinal lesion induced by Hawaii agent acute infectious non-bacterial gastroenteritis. *Journal of Infectious Diseases*, 129, 705–708.

Schulze, H. E. & Heremans, J. F. (1966) The molecular biology of human proteins. *The Proteins of Digestive Secretions*. Vol. 1, Ch. 5. Amsterdam: Elsevier.

Scrimshaw, N. S., Taylor, C. E. & Gordon, J. E. (1968) Interactions of infection and nutrition. *World Health Organisation Monograph Series*.

Schur, P. H., Borel, H., Gelfand, E. W., Alper, C. A. & Rosen, F. S. (1970) Selective gamma-G globulin deficiencies in patients with recurrent pyogenic infections. *New England Journal of Medicine*, 283, 631–634.

Schwab, J. H. (1975) Immunosuppression by bacteria. In *The Immune System and Infectious Disease*. 4th International Convocation on Immunology, Buffalo, N.Y., 1974, ed. Neter, E. & Milgrom, F., pp. 64–75. Basel: Karger.

Shearman, D. J. C., Parkin, D. M. & McClelland, D. B. L.

(1972) The demonstration and function of antibodies in the gastrointestinal tract. *Gut*, 13, 483–499.

Shedlofsky, S. & Freter, R. (1974) Synergism between ecologic and immunologic control mechanisms of intestinal flora. *Journal of Infectious Diseases*, 129, 296–303.

Sherwood, W. C., Goldstein, F., Haurani, F. I. & Wirts, C. W. (1964) Studies of the small-intestinal bacterial flora and of intestinal absorption in pernicious-anaemia. *American Journal of Digestive Diseases*, 9, 416–425.

Shiner, M., Waters, T. E., Allan, J. D. & Gray, M. B. (1963) Culture studies of the gastrointestinal tract with a newly devised capsule. Results of tests *in vitro* and *in vivo*. *Gastroenterology*, 45, 625–632.

Silverman, A. S. & Pomeranz, J. R. (1972) Studies on the localisation of hapten in guinea-pigs fed picryl chloride. *International Archives of Allergy and Applied Immunology*, 42, 1–7.

Sirisinha, S., Suskind, R., Edelman, R., Asrapaka, C. & Olson, R. E. (1973) Secretory and serum IgA in children with protein-calorie malnutrition. In *The Immunoglobulin A System*, ed. Mestecky, J. & Lawton, A. R., pp. 389–398. New York: Plenum Press.

Smith, H. (1972) The little-known determinants of microbial pathogenicity. In *Microbial Pathogenicity in Man and Animals*, ed. Smith, H. & Pearce, J. H. London: Cambridge University Press.

Smith, H. W. & Crabb, W. E. (1961) The faecal bacterial flora of animals and man: its development in the young. *Journal of Pathology and Bacteriology*, 82, 53–66.

Smith, C. W. & Goldman, A. S. (1968) The cells of human colostrum. I. *In vitro* studies of morphology and functions. *Pediatric Research*, 2, 103–109.

Smith, H. W. & Halls, S. (1968) The transmissible nature of the genetic factor in *Escherichia coli* that controls enterotoxin production. *Journal of General Microbiology*, 52, 319–334.

Smith, N. W. & Sack, R. B. (1973) Immunologic cross-reactions of enterotoxins from *Escherichia coli* and *Vibrio cholerae*. *Journal of Infectious Diseases*, 127, 164–170.

Söltoft, J., Binder, V. & Gudmand-Hoyër, E. (1973) Intestinal immunoglobulins in ulcerative colitis. *Scandinavian Journal of Gastroenterology*, 8, 293–300.

Sommer, A. & Mosley, W. H. (1973) Ineffectiveness of cholera vaccination as an epidemic control measure. *Lancet*, i, 1232–1235.

Spiegelberg, H. L., Lawrence, D. A. & Henson, P. Cytophilic properties of IgA to human neutrophils. In *The Immunoglobulin A System*, ed. Mestecky, J. & Lawton, A. R. New York: Plenum Press.

Sprent, J. & Miller, J. F. A. P. (1972) Interaction of thymus lymphocytes with histoincompatible cells. II. Recirculating lymphocytes derived from antigen-activated thymus cells. *Cellular Immunology*, 3, 385–404.

Sprinz, H., Gangarosa, E. J., Williams, M., Hornick, R. B. & Woodward, T. E. (1966) Histopathology of the upper small intestine in typhoid fever – biopsy study of experimental disease in man. *American Journal of Digestive Diseases*, 11, 615–624.

Staley, T. E., Corley, L. D. & Jones, E. W. (1970a) Early pathogenesis of colitis in neonatal pigs monocontaminated with *Escherichia coli*. Fine structural changes in the colonic epithelium. *American Journal of Digestive Diseases*, 15, 923–935.

Staley, T. E., Corley, L. D. & Jones, E. W. (1970b) Early pathogenesis of colitis in neonatal pigs monocontaminated with *Escherichia coli*. Fine structural changes in the circulatory compartments of the lamina propria and submucosa. *American Journal of Digestive Diseases*, **15**, 937–951.

Steele, E. J., Chaicumpa, W., Rowley, D. (1974) Isolation and biological properties of three classes of rabbit antibody to *Vibrio cholerae*. *Journal of Infectious Diseases*, **130**, 93–103.

Stoliar, O. A., Pelley, R. P., Kaniecki-Green, E., Klaus, M. H. & Carpenter, C. C. J. (1976) Secretory IgA anti-enterotoxin in human breast milk. *Lancet*, **i**, 1258–1261.

Stuart, A. E. & Collee, J. G. (1967) Selective lymphoid depletion and generalised lymphoid depletion in mouse typhoid. *Journal of Pathology and Bacteriology*, **94**, 429–437.

Summers, R. W. & Kent, T. H. (1970) Effects of altered propulsion on rat small intestinal flora. *Gastroenterology*, **59**, 740–744.

Tabaqchali, S. (1970) The pathophysiological role of small intestinal bacterial flora. *Scandinavian Journal of Gastroenterology*, **6**, 139–163.

Takeuchi, A. & Sprinz, H. (1967) Electron microscope studies of experimental salmonella infection in the pre-conditioned guinea pig. II. Response of the intestinal mucosa to the invasion by *Salmonella typhimurium*. *American Journal of Pathology*, **51**, 137–161.

Takeuchi, A., Formal, S. B. & Sprinz, H. (1968) Experimental acute colitis in the rhesus monkey following peroral infection with *Shigella flexneri*. *American Journal of Pathology*, **52**, 503–529.

Tannock, G. W. & Savage, D. C. (1974) Influences of dietary and environmental stress on microbial populations in the murine gastrointestinal tract. *Infection and Immunity*, **9**, 591–598.

Taylor, J., Maltby, M. P. & Payne, J. M. (1958) Factors influencing the response of ligated-rabbit-gut segments to injected *Escherichia coli*. *Journal of Pathology and Bacteriology*, **76**, 491–499.

Teir, H. & Rytömaa, T. (1966) Elimination of granulocytes in the intestinal tract and its pathological consequences. In *Methods and Achievements in Experimental Pathology*, Vol. 1, pp. 639–676, ed. Bajusz, E. & Jasmin, G. Basel: Karger.

Thomas, H. C. & Parrott, D. M. V. (1974) The induction of tolerance to a soluble protein antigen by oral administration. *Immunology*, **27**, 631–639.

Thomas, H. C. & Vaez-Zadeh, F. (1974) A homeostatic mechanism for the removal of antigen from the portal circulation. *Immunology*, **26**, 375–382.

Tomasi, T. B. & Grey, H. M. (1973) Structure and function of immunoglobulin A. *Progress in Allergy*, **16**, 81–213.

Tomkins, A. M., Draser, B. S. & James, W. P. T. (1975) Bacterial colonisation of jejunal mucosa in acute tropical sprue. *Lancet*, **i**, 59–62.

Torrey, J. C. & Kahn, M. C. (1923) The inhibition of putrefactive spore-bearing anaerobes by *Bacterium acidophilus*. *Journal of Infectious Diseases*, **33**, 482–497.

Tourville, D. R., Bienenstock, J. & Tomasi, T. B. (1968) Natural antibodies of human serum, saliva and urine reactive with *Escherichia coli*. *Proceedings of the Society for Experimental Biology and Medicine*, **128**, 722–727.

Tourville, D. R., Adler, R. N., Bienenstock, J. & Tomasi, T. B. (1969) The human secretory immunoglobulin system: immunohistological localisation of γA secretory 'piece' and lactoferrin in normal human tissues. *Journal of Experimental Medicine*, **129**, 411–423.

Venneman, M. R. & Bigley, N. J. (1969) Isolation and partial characterization of an immunogenic moiety obtained from *Salmonella typhimurium*. *Journal of Bacteriology*, **100**, 140–148.

Waldman, R. H. & Ganguly, R. (1974) Immunity to infections on secretory surfaces. *Journal of Infectious Diseases*, **130**, 419–440.

Waldman, R. H. & Ganguly, R. (1975) The immune system and infectious disease. 4th International Convocation on Immunology, Buffalo, New York, ed. Neter, E. F. & Milgrom, F., pp. 334–346. Basel: Karger.

Waldman, R. H., Bencic, Z., Sakazaki, R., Sinha, R., Ganguly, R., Deb, B. C. & Mukerjee, S. (1971) Cholera immunology. I. Immunoglobulin levels in serum, fluid from the small intestine, and faeces from patients with cholera and non-choleraic diarrhoea during illness and convalescence. *Journal of Infectious Diseases*, **123**, 579–586.

Waldman, R. H., Bencic, Z., Sinha, R., Deb, B. C., Sakazaki, R., Tamura, K., Mukerjee, S. & Ganguli, R. (1972) Cholera immunology. II. Serum and intestinal secretion antibody response after naturally occurring cholera. *Journal of Infectious Diseases*, **126**, 401–407.

Walker, W. A., Isselbacher, K. J. & Bloch, K. J. (1972) Intestinal uptake of macromolecules: Effect of oral immunization. *Science*, **177**, 608–610.

Walker, W. A., Isselbacher, K. J. & Bloch, K. J. (1973) Intestinal uptake of macromolecules. II. Effect of parental immunization. *Journal of Immunology*, **111**, 221–226.

Walker, W. A. & Isselbacher, K. J. (1974) Uptake and transport of macromolecules by the intestine. Possible role in clinical disorders. *Gastroenterology*, **67**, 531–550.

Walker, W. A., Field, M. & Isselbacher, K. J. (1974) Specific binding of cholera toxin to isolated intestinal microvillous membranes. *Proceedings of the National Academy of Sciences (U.S.A.)*, **71**, 320–324.

Watanabe, Y. (1974) Antibacterial immunity in cholera. In *Cholera*, ed. Barua, D. & Burrows, W., Ch. 16. Philadelphia: Saunders.

Webster, A. D. B. (1975) The gut and immunodeficiency disorders. *Clinics in Gastroenterology*, **5**, 2, 323–340.

Wernet, P., Breu, H., Knop, J. & Rowley, D. (1971) Antibacterial action of specific IgA and transport of IgM, IgA and IgG from serum into the small intestine. *Journal of Infectious Diseases*, **124**, 223–226.

Willmore, J. G. & Shearman, C. H. (1918) On the differential diagnosis of dysenteries: the diagnostic value of the cell-exudate in the stools of acute amoebic and bacillary dysentery. *Lancet*, **ii**, 200–266.

Williams, R. C. & Gibbons, R. J. (1972) Inhibition of bacterial adherence by secretory immunoglobulin A: a mechanism of antigen disposal. *Science*, **177**, 697–699.

Wilson, M. R. & Hohmann, A. W. (1974) Immunity to *Escherichia coli* in pigs. Adhesion of enteropathogenic *Escherichia coli* to isolated intestinal epithelial cells. *Infection and Immunity*, **10**, 776–782.

Wong, K. H., Feeley, J. C., Northrup, R. S. & Forlines, M. E. (1974) Vi antigen from *Salmonella typhosa* and immunity against typhoid fever. I. Isolation and immunologic properties in animals. *Infection and Immunity*, **9**, 348–353.

Woode, G. N., Bridger, J. C., Jones, J. M., Flewett, T. H., Bryden, A. S., Davies, M. A. & White, G. B. B. (1976) Morphological and antigenic relationships between viruses (rotaviruses) from acute gastroenteritis of children, calves, piglets, mice and toads. *Infection and Immunity*, **14**, 804–810.

Woodward, W. E. (1971) Cholera reinfection in man. *Journal of Infectious Diseases*, **123**, 61–66.

Woodward, W. E., Gilman, R. H., Hornick, R. B., Libonati, J. P. & Cash, R. A. (1976) Efficacy of a live oral cholera vaccine in human volunteers. 14th Congress of the International Association for Biological Standardisation, Douglas, Isle of Man, 1975. *Developments in Biological Standardisation*, 33, 108–112. Basel: Karger.

World Health Organization (1972) Oral enteric bacterial vaccines. *WHO Technical Report Series*, 500.

Wyatt, R. G., Dolin, R., Blacklow, N. R., Dupont, H. L., Buscho, R. F., Thornhill, T. S., Kapikian, A. Z. & Chanock, R. M. (1974) Comparison of three agents of acute infectious non-bacterial gastroenteritis by cross-challenge in volunteers. *Journal of Infectious Diseases*, 129, 709–714.

Yong, C. W. (1971) M.Sc. Thesis, University of Saskatchewan, Saskatoon, quoted by Bellamy & Nielson, Immune-mediated emigration of neutrophils into the lumen of the small intestine. *Infection and Immunity*, 1974, 615–619.

Zipursky, A., Brown, E. J. & Bienenstock, J. (1973) Lack of opsonization potential of 11S human secretory IgA. *Proceedings of the Society for Experimental Biology and Medicine*, 142, 181–184.

13. Immunological aspects of infection with gastrointestinal parasites (protozoa and nematodes)

D. Catty and I. N. Ross

INTRODUCTION

Parasites, both protozoan and metazoan, have complex life cycles, often with many stages of development, and an attendant complex pathology in the host. As the process of infection moves from one stage to the next so the host becomes the involuntary recipient of mixtures of foreign metabolites and tissue components which give rise to prolonged periods of diverse antigen stimulation. Even with those parasites for which the lumen or tissues of the intestine serve as the only host environment, powerful parasitic antigens may, and usually do, find their way across the intestinal barrier into the blood or lymphatic circulation. In some cases parasites also undergo parenteral phases of development as a natural course of infection or reach the intestine following a migration through the body. Hence the origin of immune responses to gastrointestinal parasites are not usually restricted to local lymphoid tissues.

The special interest in the immunology of intestinal parasitic infestations stems from the fact that the induced immune response can, in the course of time, be marshalled to act in a collaborative fashion within the intestine and give the host the capacity to eject a resident infestation and/or to resist specifically and often vigorously the insult of a further challenge.

So far the great complexity of parasite–host interactions has allowed rather limited progress in our understanding of the pattern of immunological events which initiates control of the establishment, survival and pathogenicity of such infections. One of the major difficulties is that immune reactions inevitably take place against the background of many other pathological processes generated by the infection (e.g. tissue damage, disruption of secretory and absorptive functions of the intestine, the release of pharmacologically active molecules, etc.). In cases of natural infection other factors such as mixed parasitaemia and/or an associated malnutrition of the host have also to be taken into account. Nevertheless, in recent years significant advances have been made in the understanding of some of the principle mechanisms involved in host immunity to gastrointestinal parasites. These have come largely from studies on experimental infestations in laboratory animals in which a more analytical approach can be made and some of the problems avoided. Experimental infections therefore feature prominently in the record of achievements in this important field of investigation. However, as this chapter will make apparent, in many areas of special clinical importance knowledge is still fragmentary and much basic work still remains to be done.

PROTOZOAN INFESTATIONS

There are at least 21 protozoan species which are able to colonize man's alimentary canal. Their activities may range from the commensal to the parasitic and their effects may be minimal to strongly pathogenic (Table 13.1). Twelve of these species are normally considered to be pathogens, but several of this group are also found in apparently healthy individuals. It follows that the distinctions between a commensal and frankly pathogenic existence in the intestine concern factors as much associated with the immune status of the host as with the invasive and destructive properties of the parasite.

Table 13.1 Protozoan species causing disease of the human gastrointestinal tract on gaining access via the intestine or mouth

Species	Disease
Entamoeba histolytica	Dysentery, extraintestinal abscesses
Entamoeba coli	None
Entamoeba hartmanii	None
Entamoeba polecki	May be a cause of dysentery
Entamoeba gingivalis	Gingival infection
Endolimax nana	None
Iodamoeba butschlii	Diarrhoea
Dientamoeba fragilis	Diarrhoea
Trichomonas hominis	None
Trichomonas tenax	Oral disease
Giardia lamblia	Diarrhoea, steatorrhoea, malabsorption
Chilomastix mesnili	None
Retortamonas intestinalis	None
Enteromonas hominis	None
Isospora hominis	Diarrhoea
Isospora belli	Diarrhoea
Isospora nataliensis	None
Cryptosporidium	Diarrhoea, malabsorption, colitis
Balantidium coli	Diarrhoea, liver abscesses
Toxoplasma gondii	Encephalitis, blindness, acute lymphadenopathy
Sarcosporidium	Cystic invasion of muscles

This point is well emphasized in each of the protozoan infections chosen for review in this section. *Toxoplasmosis gondii* and Sarcosporidiosis are not considered here since they are essentially systemic parasitic infections which gain entry via the intestine.

AMOEBIASIS

Of the many species of amoebae known to colonize the intestine of man, *Entamoeba histolytica* is by far the most important pathogen. This species has a wide distribution in tropical and subtropical regions and affects approximately one-tenth of the world population (Ramamurti and Stickl, 1973). In susceptible hosts the parasites become established in the mucosal crypts of the appendix, caecum and ascending colon where they penetrate the submucosa and multiply to form ulcerative abscesses (Takeuchi and Phillips, 1976). Such abscesses lead to the symptoms of amoebic dysentery. Extra intestinal spread may occur to many organs, but most commonly to the liver via the portal vein. Reproduction occurs by binary fission of the trophozoites. The infective stage is the quadrinucleated cyst excreted into the faeces. Transmission may take place by food, flies or by water, in which cysts may remain viable for up to one month. Transmission may also occur venereally (Kean, 1976). Since infection may be asymptomatic the incubation period is not known exactly although dysentery may occur as early as 8 days after infection. Both dysentery and amoebic hepatic abscess (AHA) are more common in children under 5 years than in older age groups, and in men compared with women.

Humoral immunity

Amoebae are present at the periphery of the ulcers and their cytoplasm may extend to establish contact with healthy host cells. As Cox (1968) rightly points out, the periphery of the ulcers may therefore provide the conditions for released antigens to reach immunologically competent cells. As a result an antibody response may occur even if the infection does not spread via the lymphatics. This is evident from the high incidence of circulating antibody in cases where infection remains localized. As might be expected, however, greater titres of antiamoebic antibodies are produced in the invasive form of the disease. Analysis of the *E. histolytica* trophozoite has detected at least 7 water-soluble antigenic components (Khan and Meerovitch, 1970; Alam and Ahmad, 1974). The antigens that produce the IgG response to infection appear to be located on the surface of the trophozoite, probably in the glycocalyx, as detected by immunofluorescence and horseradish peroxidase labelling techniques (O'Shea, del Socorro, and Feria-Velasco, 1974; Feria-Velasco, O'Shea and del Socorro, 1974). Other immunoglobulins that may be

elevated in amoebiasis are IgM and IgE (Dasgupta, 1974); serum IgA levels remain normal.

The presence of asymptomatic cyst-passing individuals and the relapsing nature of some infections suggests that an element of immunological control can be exerted by the host upon the invasive capacity of the intestinal parasites. However, there is no convincing evidence that protection is conferred upon subjects cured of existing infection (Krupp, 1974) even though persistently high antibody titres are known to occur in the invasive disease (Krupp and Powell, 1971a). Also in cases of spontaneous recovery from experimental infections in man no protection is usually shown (Beaver, Jung, Sherman, Read and Robinson, 1956). Indeed the only evidence of a protective antibody response so far obtained has been in one study (Krupp and Powell, 1971a) where a group of patients were treated and then shown to suffer little reinfection. High antibody levels to many amoebic antigens were detected in these patients. In general it must be assumed that in the intestine of man an adaptive protective antibody response can only be induced as a result of long-term exposure to the parasite. Long-term exposure may be necessary because *E. histolytica* undergoes antigenic variation as a means of escape from successive immune responses. Biagi, Beltran and Ortega (1966) exposed amoebae to fluorescein-labelled antibody; these rounded up and became immobile. However, a proportion of the parasites internalized the immune complexes from their membranes and resumed amoeboid movements. Such amoebae then failed to bind further antibody and were not susceptible to immobilization; this would suggest that *E. histolytica* is able to modulate surface antigen. Antigenic variation might account for the general observation in amoebiasis in man that the presence of precipitating antibody responses of high titre and of immediate intradermal hypersensitivity (indicating the existence of IgE antibodies) does not prevent the development of acute infection (Maddison, 1965; Maddison, Kagan and Elsdon-Dew, 1968).

Although in the majority of cases antibody responses appear to have little protective activity, they have been used extensively in *in-vitro* studies, including in the diagnosis of infestation. Immunofluorescence has proved particularly useful as a reliable means of diagnosis (Jeanes, 1969). By this technique a marked fall in antibody titre has been found to occur between 20 days and 2 months after treatment (Ambrose-Thomas and Truong, 1969). Stamm, Ashley and Bell (1976) have found that levels rarely remain higher than 1:64 after one year, in the absence of recurrent infection.

The indirect haemagglutination (IHA) test as developed for amoebiasis (Kessel, Lewis, Ma and Kim, 1961; Kessel, Lewis, Pasquel and Turner, 1965) detects IgG antibodies (Maddison, Kagan and Norman, 1968) and is very sensitive, becoming positive a few weeks after infection. It has been found to be nearly 100 per cent positive in AHA and over 90 per cent positive in amoebic dysentery (Krupp and Powell, 1971b). Excluding those infants who have a positive IHA due to passive placental transfer of IgG antibody from an infected or previously infected mother (Jasso, Tejerina and Gutierez, 1974), children under the age of 5 years with amoebic dysentery may have low titres in this test (Miller and Scott, 1970; Gilman, Davis, Gan and Bolton, 1976). In general, although the IHA titre gradually falls following infection, high levels may still be detected for up to 3 years or longer in the absence of recurrent infection (Krupp and Powell, 1971b). This is probably due to the retention of amoebic antigens in the reticuloendothelial system for long periods (Krupp and Powell, 1971a). When interpreting the IHA results, it is therefore important to know in endemic areas the range of titres due to background exposure of the community to infection. Combination of this test with the pattern found on immunoelectrophoresis against amoebic antigens (Krupp and Powell, 1971a) does, however, help to distinguish between active infection and antibodies persisting after treatment.

A suggestion that at least two antibody systems are involved in the disease comes also from the observations of Maddison, Powell and Elsdon-Dew (1965) that removal from sera of haemagglutinins by absorption does not remove precipitating antibodies. In gel diffusion tests antibody can be detected 2 to 4 weeks after illness (Healy *et al.*, 1971), but many remain positive for some years after infection (Krupp and Powell, 1971b).

Until the question of the specificity of the protective antibody response has been clarified, it will be difficult to reconcile the above observations in man with those obtained in experimental animals and in *in-vitro* studies. As early as 1950 Swartzwelder and Müller had obtained some degree of protection from active infection in rats by immunization with lysates of the cultured parasite, and in dogs Swartzwelder and Avant (1952) found that a single infection induced a high degree of resistance to reinfection with homologous and heterologous pathogenic amoebae. This state of resistance could be transferred to normal dogs by serum alone. A partial protection against amoebic infection was conferred also in the hamster using passive transfer of human immune serum (Sepulvada, Tanimoto-Leki and de la Hoz, 1974). *In vitro*, immune serum has been shown to produce immobilization of trophozoites and denaturation of the amoebic membrane (Manzo, Castenda and Chevez, 1974), together with neutralization of virulence (Sepulvada, Tanimoto-Leki and de la Torre, 1974). Normal human serum has also been shown to have a mild cytopathogenic effect on amoebic trophozoites (Ortiz-Ortiz, Sepulvada and Chevez, 1974).

On the basis of these and other studies it would appear that protective humoral responses, even those not actually initiated from within the intestine, can nevertheless be induced to operate against a localized infection, provided the appropriate specificity is present. In some experiments in guinea-pigs, Krupp (1974) has shown that protective specificities are directed towards a high molecular weight (650 000) chromatographic fraction of a sonicated extract of amoebae. Three immunizing injections of this fraction in adjuvant gave complete protection to intracaecal challenge of parasites. Although it is not known whether this antigen, or group of antigens, is released into the intestinal tissues in the course of normal infection it is possible that chemically abbreviated infections, i.e. successfully treated cases, fail to provide an appropriate stimulus for protection. In these and in the other studies noted above, antibodies to only some amoebic antigens persisted for any appreciable length of time after chemotherapy.

Cellular immunity

The complex pathology of intestinal lesions in amoebiasis might also include an element of specific cell-mediated immunity. *In-vivo* and *in-vitro* tests have been performed to study this possibility. Delayed intradermal responses often occur in antigen-tested individuals who are known to be excretors of cysts (Maddison, Kagan and Elsdon-Dew, 1968). Savanat, Viriyanond and Nimitmongkol (1973) found that peripheral blood lymphocytes of 22 out of 24 cases of advanced amoebiasis gave a significant degree of specific stimulation in the presence of antigen *in vitro*. For each patient this response did not appear to be related to the number of precipitating antibody bands present to the same antigens, indicating that the cellular reactivity was not directly correlated with the humoral antibody response. Furthermore, in later studies it has been shown that antigen-stimulated lymphocyte transformation *in vitro* is only associated with cases of AHA, no significant response occurring in individuals with intestinal amoebiasis (Harris and Bray, 1976). Other studies confirm the regular appearance of antigen-sensitive lymphocytes in patients with AHA (e.g. Ortiz-Ortiz, Zamacona-Ravelo and Capin, 1974; Ortiz-Ortiz, Zamacona-Ravelo, Sepulvada and Capin, 1975). This observation may be explained if one postulates that cell-mediated immune mechanisms are only activated by the prolonged presence of large amounts of antigen, possibly in extraintestinal sites. Whether a cell-mediated immune response confers any protective immunity upon the host is unknown. Experimental evidence that thymus-derived antigen-sensitive T-cells may directly influence parasite survival in the intestine is very difficult to obtain. For instance it is well known that in man and in some laboratory animals systemic corticosteroid treatment can enhance the virulence of the parasite and exacerbate amoebic dysentery (Biagi and Beltran, 1969; Lewis and Antia, 1969; Kanani and Knight, 1969). As steroids are known to depress T-cell dependent cellular immunity, these observations could be interpreted as providing evidence for the protective rôle of cell-mediated reactions in amoebiasis. However, the immune suppressive effect of steroids may be as much an influence on thymus-dependent antibody responses as on a direct cell-mediated local inflammatory reaction.

The early stages of amoebiasis can be accompanied by an intrinsic form of immunosuppression which may enhance parasite survival in the host. An impairment of T-cell function has been reported by Solis *et al.* (1975), as indicated by a reduced number of peripheral T-rosetting cells in 9 out of 10 patients; Ortiz-Ortiz, Garmilla, Zamacona-Revelo and Sepulvada (1973) and Ortiz-Ortiz *et al.* (1975) have, in addition, shown a specifically reduced capacity of lymphocytes from amoebiasis patients to release macrophage migration-inhibition factor *in vitro*, a suppressed responsiveness which was reversible with treatment.

As the history of research into amoebiasis reveals, the experimental approach in laboratory animals provides excellent opportunities to study in detail the significance of host immune processes in this important disease.

GIARDIASIS

Giardia lamblia is a flagellate protozoan infecting the upper small intestine of man. Prevalence is said to be 7 per cent (Mahmoud and Warren, 1975), but infestation is more common in tropical areas, in the lower socio-economic classes (Kidney and Holland, 1967) and especially so in young children and in immunologically compromised individuals (Ament, Ochs and Davis, 1973; Webster, 1976). The active form of the parasite is the trophozoite which multiplies by binary fission and is found in the glandular crypts of the duodenal and jejunal mucosa. Infection occurs by ingestion of cysts which are formed in the lower ileum by secretion of a hyaline wall around the trophozoite (Petersen, 1972), before being passed in the faeces. Transmission may occur by the direct faecal-oral route, in food or in water where the cysts may remain viable for longer than 3 months (Rendtorff, 1954c); also the house fly may be an inefficient transmitter (Rendtorff, 1954b). Close proximity is important as a high incidence of infestation is found in the relatives of infected individuals (Willcox, 1975). Stool examination for cysts is an unreliable method of diagnosis (Kamath and Murugasu, 1974), the most satisfactory method being by small intestinal aspiration and/or biopsy to identify trophozoites. The 'Enterotest' capsule may be used (see Thomas, Goldsmid and Wicks, 1974) and a serological test is available which

detects serum IgG antibodies by indirect immunofluorescence (Ridley and Ridley, 1976).

In susceptible individuals symptoms of infection develop 1 to 3 weeks after ingestion of cysts. The multiplying parasites cause mucosal irritation, accompanied by excessive mucous secretion which leads to chronic or recurrent diarrhoea, steatorrhoea and dehydration. The development of a symptomatic infection is said to be dependent upon the number of cysts ingested (Rendtorff, 1954a), but this dose effect may be moderated by immunity since silent, asymptomatic 'carrier' infestations have been reported in adults, and in those developing symptoms the course of the disease may vary considerably. In some cases the infestation is self-limiting with a phase of mild diarrhoea and abdominal cramps but a spontaneous resolution in 1 to 4 weeks. In others a chronic infection causes a reversible malabsorption state that may include folic acid and vitamin B_{12} deficiency (Cowan and Campbell, 1973), milk intolerance (Hoskins, Winawar, Broitman, Gottlieb and Zamcheck, 1967), disaccharidase deficiency and a protein-losing enteropathy (Ament *et al.*, 1973). Acquired immunity is not universal in adults and epidemics of the disease do occur.

Although primarily an infection of the small intestine, Giardia may also be a cause of cholecystitis and biliary tract disease (Drenckhahn, 1943; McGowan, Nussbaum and Burroughs, 1948; Cortner, 1959), and evidence of pancreatic insufficiency during infection has been observed (Gupta and Mehta, 1973; Chawla *et al.*, 1975). Giardiasis is also alleged to cause large-bowel disease (Fairise and Jannin, 1913; De Muro, 1939; Kacker, 1973), but with insubstantial evidence, and also to result in a number of allergic manifestations (Bierman, 1972), including urticarial eruptions (Harris and Mitchell, 1949; Wilhelm, 1957; Webster, 1958) and uveitis (Carrol, Anast and Birch, 1961). Halstead and Sadun (1965) have postulated that the oral intake and subsequent digestion of muscle provides an appropriate environment for the liberation of parasite excretory allergens which could induce a condition of immediate hypersensitivity. The marked eosinophilic infiltration of the lamina propria in duodenal biopsies noted by these authors broadly supports the concept of an allergic condition within the tissues, although the nature of the inducing allergen(s) is not known. On this basis Halstead and Sadun (1965) have suggested that a parasite-induced allergy to one or more components of the host diet may be involved in the pathogenesis of Giardia infection.

The mucosal lesion in giardiasis may be patchy throughout the small intestine (Ament and Rubin, 1972) and intestinal biopsy may show a varied picture from normal appearance to a flat, but not atrophic, mucosa (Ridley and Ridley, 1976). Unlike coeliac disease there is no damage to the microvilli and the basement membrane remains intact. There is little tissue invasion by the trophozoites, as evidenced by their infrequent presence in the lamina propria and epithelial cells of the small intestine (Brandborg, Tankersley and Gottlieb, 1965; Morelki and Parker, 1967).

Humoral immunity

Although the picture of parasites localized to the lumen of the intestine is highly suggestive that their elimination in, for example, self-limiting infections, and in refractory hosts, operates at the mucosal level, the precise nature of the protective response is not known. However, the probable importance of the local secretory immune system is demonstrated by the high incidence of giardiasis, namely in 50–80 per cent of individuals with primary immunodeficiency syndromes affecting antibody-producing function (Ament et al., 1973; Webster, 1976). A strong association between giardiasis and the non-familial immunoglobulin-deficiency syndromes has also been reported by Ament and Rubin (1972), Brown, Butterfield, Savage and Tada (1972), Ajdukiewicz, Youngs and Bouchier (1972), and the infection has also been detected in cases of intestinal nodular lymphoid hyperplasia, hypogammaglobulinae-mic sprue, selective IgA deficiency (Hermans et al., 1966; Hoskins et al., 1967; Gryboski, Self, Clemett and Herskovic, 1968; Anderson, Pellegrino and Schaefer, 1970; Hughes, Cerda, Holtzapple and Brooks, 1971; Michaels, Humbert, Dubois, Stewart and Ellis, 1971; Johnson, Goldberg, Pops and Weiner, 1971; Ament et al., 1973; McClelland, Warwick and Sheerman, 1973), and in one case of infantile X-linked agammaglobu-linaemia (Ochs, Ament and Davis, 1972). Brown et al. (1972) considered that the susceptibility to Giardia may be due to the lack of secretory immunoglobulins, mainly of IgA, in the intestinal tissues, which leads primarily to bacterial colonization and the development of steator-rhoea, giardiasis being a secondary aggravation of an existing pathology. However, more recent observations by Jones and Brown (1974) have shown that the development of giardiasis is by no means dependent upon a predisposing immunoglobulin deficiency, and can be found in patients with normal serum concentrations of IgG, IgA, IgM and IgE and significantly elevated levels of intestinal IgG. Hence it seems reasonable to conclude that in spite of the known association between giardiasis and immunoglobulin deficiencies, the disease as seen in otherwise apparently healthy individuals is not aetio-logically related to unsuspected deficiencies of immuno-globulin synthesis or secretion.

In healthy individuals some observations on the mucosal immune response to infection have been made. There is an infiltrate of plasma cells in the lamina propria (which is not seen in B-cell-deficient infected patients), and in biopsies taken early in infection there is an increase in IgM-staining cells by fluorescence (Ridley and Ridley, 1976).

Cellular immunity

Ferguson, McClure and Townley (1976) have reported increased numbers of intraepithelial lymphocytes in biopsies of the small intestine of children with diarrhoea due to giardiasis, a finding also seen in coeliac disease but not in other infective diarrhoeas. This appears to be the only information in man concerning the influences of T-cells in the disease. However, in the experimental animal there is additional information. Giardia muris causes a significant mortality in congenitally athymic (nude) mice. These animals can be protected by thymic transplants (Boorman, Lina, Zurcha and Niewerkerk, 1973). In the nude mouse it remains to be determined whether the susceptibility to infection is due to the failure to synthesize antibody locally at the site of infection (e.g. IgA antibody which is T-cell dependent) or to a lack of the capacity to mount a T-cell-mediated response to parasite antigens in the local tissues. Intact mice have been shown to develop a long-term resistance to murine giardiasis (Roberts-Thomson, Grove, Stephens and Warren, 1976; Roberts-Thomson, Stevens, Mahmoud and Warren, 1977). Clearly much information can be gained from further studies on this useful experimental murine system.

COCCIDIOSIS

The coccidia are a group of intracellular parasites living mainly in epithelial cells during the endogenous stages of their complex life cycles. They show remarkable host specificity and some species are exclusively pathogens of the gastrointestinal tract of man. In this account of host responses to the coccidia of man, Toxoplasma gondii is omitted since, although it can now be regarded as a coccidian by virtue of its morphology and described complete life cycle (Hutchison, Dunachie, Siim and Work, 1970), it is essentially a parasite affecting the systemic tissues. The immunological aspects of this infection have recently been reviewed by Remington and Krahenbuhl (1976).

The pathogenic intestinal coccidia of man are Isospora belli, I. hominis and Cryptosporidium (Matsu-bayashi and Nozawa, 1948; Barksdale and Routh, 1948; Webster, 1957; Levine, 1962; Henderson, Gil-lespie, Kaplan and Steber, 1963; French, 1964; Brand-borg, Goldberg and Breidenbach, 1970). Infective sporozoites of these 3 species when ingested in food undergo schizogony in the epithelial cells of the small and large intestine. The parasites may be intracyto-plasmic, as in the case of Isospora spp., or attached to the microvillous border as in Cryptosporidium infec-tions. In general the damage to the mucosa causes only superficial lesions and in Isospora infections the disease is usually self-limiting with relatively mild symptoms of fever, intestinal colic and transient mucous diarrhoea. Ingestion of 2500–3000 cysts of *I. belli* is sufficient to cause symptoms after 8 hours. Spontaneous recovery may occur within a period of a few weeks to several months (Matsubayashi and Nozawa, 1948). Trier, Moxey, Schimmel and Robles (1974) have described the pathology of a case of chronic intestinal coccidiosis (*I. belli*). The patient had intermittent diarrhoea over 20 years with eosinophilia and malabsorption. The severe mucosal lesion, occurring at the duodeno-jejunal junction, showed shortened, rudimentary villi and hypertrophied crypts with coccidia in the villous epithelium and a mixed infiltrate in the lamina propria and between the epithelial cells. This consisted of eosinophils, polymorphs, small lymphocytes and plasma cells. The damage to the epithelial cells did not correlate with the presence of coccidia since many normal cells were invaded and yet damaged cells often contained no parasites.

Two cases of infection with *Cryptosporidium* have also been described; in one patient there was an acute self-limiting enterocolitis (Nime, Burek, Page, Holscher and Yardley, 1976) with parasites demonstrable in a rectal biopsy together with a chronic inflammatory cell infiltration of the lamina propria. The other case was a patient under immunosuppression with cyclophosphamide and steroids. Watery diarrhoea was found to be associated with the presence of the parasite in the jejunum, where increased numbers of lamina propria plasma cells, neutrophils and lymphocytes were observed.

Two other cases of coccidial infection in man have been reported recently which, as in many cases of giardiasis (see above), suggest an association between protozoan gastrointestinal disease and host immune deficiency. One infected patient presented with a lymphoma (Ohtaki *et al.*, 1976) and the other with alpha heavy-chain disease (Henry, Bird and Doe, 1974).

Virtually nothing is known of the immunology of intestinal coccidial infections in man, but the principles which underlie the development of resistance can most probably be derived from the detailed studies of related *Eimeria* infections of domestic animals, particularly those of poultry and cattle. The relative roles and interactions of humoral and cell-mediated immune responses to *Eimeria* spp. have been extensively explored by Rose (1971a, b; 1972; 1973; 1974a, b, c); Rose and Long (1971) and Rose, Long and Bradley (1975).

Resistance to experimental *Eimeria* infections is well recognized and can be measured by a reduction or absence of oocyst production, after one or more immunizing infections. Low-level infection with oocysts over a prolonged period confers the best resistance to subsequent infection (Joyner and Norton, 1973), and

does not depend upon premunition. Although the protective response is a form of local immunity operating against the invasive stages of the parasite, it can operate at sites distant to the source of initial stimulation, as indicated by studies using the paired caecum of the domestic fowl. In this host *Eimeria tenella* and probably *E. necatrix* contain protective antigens which, when they are presented in a series of challenge infections, induce an immunological blockade to invasion and development of the parasite at progressively earlier stages of the life cycle.

Humoral immunity

Antibodies appear to play a significant role in the protective immune response of the fowl. Although serum titres of precipitating antibodies may not reflect the refractory state of the host to challenge, this may be accounted for by stimulation of local antibody production by the 'immunizing' infections or by the presence of circulating protective antibodies of a non-precipitating type. Numerous antigenic components are present in *Eimeria* parasites (Rose, 1959) and these probably differ at different stages of the life cycle. In addition, immunogenicity of the antigens varies between different species and strains of *Eimeria* and the immunity produced is specific to the strain used for immunization (Rose, 1974b). Rose (1974c) obtained protection of chicks to *E. maxima* by injection of 'immune' globulin from infected birds. Oocyst production by a challenge infection given to the treated chicks was very much lower than in untreated chicks or chicks given normal globulin before challenge. The earlier studies by Rose and her colleagues had shown that selective suppression of immunoglobulin synthesis by neonatal surgical bursectomy of chick embryos followed by sub-lethal X-irradiation, or treatment of birds with antisera to the bursal cells, gave an increased production of oocysts by primary infection of *E. maxima*, or rendered immunized fowl as susceptible to infection as untreated controls. These results are fairly easy to interpret since suppression of bursal cell activity does not generally influence the activity of thymus-derived cells.

Cellular immunity

Experiments designed to test the role of cell-mediated immunity, dependent upon cells of thymus origin, are more difficult to perform and the results have been equivocal. For instance, the passive transfer of mesenteric lymph-node cells or thoracic-duct lymphocytes from *E. nieschulzi*-infected rats gives some protection to normal rats (Rommel and Heydorn, 1971), but this does not rule out the possibility that antibody-producing cells are the effective agents in the inoculum. As methods of selective suppression of cell-mediated immunity, neither thymectomy nor immunosuppressive chemotherapy has provided any conclusive results. Although some degree of increased susceptibility to infection has been noted following these procedures, this has often been restricted to primary infections. Furthermore, the results could also be explained on the basis of a partial or short-term suppression of T-cell dependent antibody responses.

Enhancement of macrophage function, as reflected by increased degradation of sporozoites by macrophages in immunized birds (Rose, 1974a), could be mediated by specific soluble T-cell products. Alternatively, however, it may be due to the opsonization of *Eimeria* sporozoites by serum antibody.

NEMATODE INFESTATIONS

Gastrointestinal nematode infestations are very widely distributed amongst vertebrate species. In man, hookworm disease (*Ancylostoma* spp., *Necator americanus*), trichinosis (*Trichinella spiralis*) and ascariasis (*Ascaris lumbricoides*) are examples of diseases which are still common in some parts of the world. Cattle and sheep suffer seasonally from a range of worms taken in from the pasture, including *Haemonchus contortus*, *Nematodirus* spp., *Trichostrongylus* spp., *Ostertagia* spp. and *Oesophogostomum* spp. Other domestic and laboratory animals likewise have their own particular infestations and some of these have proved to be especially useful for study.

In general the life cycle of nematodes begins with the egg and passes through four larval stages before reaching the adult, with growth and a moult of cuticle occurring between each larval stage. The infective form is either an embryonated egg or a larva (usually the third-stage larva). Many infections are taken in by the oral route and by a process of larval development within some region of the gastrointestinal tract give rise to adults. In the ascarid group, post-entry development involves a preliminary migration through the body to the lungs. Hookworm larvae, by contrast, enter via the skin but travel also to the lungs before reaching the intestine. Other variations in the life cycle are also represented. The life cycles of common parasites of medical importance have been reviewed by Sadun (1976).

It has long been known that acquired resistance develops to some species of adult nematodes resident in the gastrointestinal tract. This is not universal, however, even in cases where obvious immune responses have taken place in the host. Considering their essentially similar details of development and structure (apart from size), the nematodes' capacity to adapt to a wide range of microenvironments for larval and adult stages is most remarkable. The choice of location of moulting, feeding, growth, egg laying and other activities will obviously greatly influence the extent of tissue damage accumulated by the host and would also be expected to influence the quality and effectiveness of the hosts' immune defence mechanisms. Some infestations are terminated spontaneously after only a brief but productively successful encounter with the host. As a result of this experience, the host may be able to expel in an even more dramatic manner a second (challenge) infection. This happens, for instance, in *Nippostrongylus* in the rat (Sarles and Taliaferro, 1936). On the other hand, many parasites (e.g. hookworms in man) are not actively rejected in this way, although some control on the parasitic burden may be exerted; yet others (e.g. stomach worms of sheep) may be subjected to seasonal rejection episodes. Some adult infestations (e.g. *Ascaris* in man) may survive in the host for many years. Such variability in the outcome of infection has led to much speculation as to the relative protective activity of different forms of immune response, and their effects upon different stages of parasite development. The increase in interest in this important field of study has developed side by side with an impressive growth in experimentation since Culbertson (1941) first reviewed the problem. Ideas have changed significantly with advances in the understanding of the complex and collaborative nature of immune mechanisms. Previous reviews have been provided by Thorson (1970), Ogilvie and Jones (1973), Ogilvie and Love (1974), Larsh and Weatherly (1974), Ogilvie and Worms (1976) and Catty (1976). Real progress has been slow, but the last few years have seen some exciting results which throw new light on controversies of very long standing. Many of these results have come from systematic studies of a limited number of host–parasite systems, some of great economic importance such as *Haemonchus contortus* in the sheep, and others which have proved particularly amenable to analysis in controlled laboratory conditions, notably *Nippostrongylus brasiliensis* in the rat, *Trichinella spiralis* in the mouse and guinea-pig and *Trichostrongylus colubriformis* in the guinea-pig.

Apart from providing some entirely new principles concerning host–nematode relationships, these recent studies have confirmed and extended earlier observations that the outcome of many gastrointestinal infestations is a host response which changes the microenvironment of the parasites. This response is broadly of an inflammatory nature and results variously in a failure of developing larvae successfully to invade or colonize the tissues, in retarded development of larvae, in an alteration in the growth and fecundity of adults and, at its most extreme, in a change in the adult survival pattern which is sometimes dramatic as in the case of active adult rejection episodes. The immune effector mechanisms which are now thought to be responsible for these various influences upon the worms includes the direct effects of antibody upon the physiology of the parasites, locally induced anaphylactic reactions, and the activity of specifically sensitized lymphocytes. At the present time it is by no means clear how many of these mechanisms are operative in any single parasitic situation, since the relevant evidence for each is to a great extent restricted to a small number of test systems. The following account attempts to review briefly the nature of some important immune protective mechanisms against gastrointestinal nematodes.

LOCAL ANTIBODY PRODUCTION

The first important studies on local antibody production in the intestine were performed by Douvres (1962) who tested extracts of intestinal mucosa of cattle infected with *Oesophogostomum radiatum* against larvae cultivated *in vitro*. He showed the formation of immune precipitates at the body openings of living worms which were advancing through the third stage and into the third mould. Antibodies were seen in all extracts from singly or doubly infected (resistant) cattle, but not with identical extracts from helminth-free stock. Dobson (1966, 1967) detected antibodies in mucosal extracts and exudates from sheep infected with *O. columbianum*. Two precipitin lines against the worm antigens were present in extracts of resistant animals, but there were none in non-resistant or singly infected sheep. No precipitating antibodies could be shown in the serum of resistant hosts. This supported the view that these antibodies were locally produced and might initiate Arthus reactions and the formation of caseous nodules which wall-off this particular parasite from the surrounding tissues of the intestine. It was also shown that the presence of antibodies in the mucus of infected sheep enhanced the secretion's inhibitory activity upon the respiration of the

third-stage larvae. Other nematodes are known to induce the release of factors into the intestine which are either toxic or growth-inhibiting upon the worms (Frick and Ackert, 1948).

As for the nature and specificity of antibodies produced in the intestine, very few studies have been made. Crandall, Cebra and Crandall (1967), with fluorescent reagents, have described an increase in IgM-containing cells in the intestinal mucosa of *Trichinella spiralis*-infected rabbits, cells presumptively involved in a conventional early antibody response; increases in IgG cells occurred later. The proportion of cells staining for IgA remained consistently high throughout the course of infection and appeared to constitute a local mucosal antibody response since there were always few IgA cells in the spleen. Further studies by Crandall and Crandall (1972) in the mouse, again using this parasite, revealed a relative increase in IgM and IgG_1 cells in the mucosa in the second week of a primary infection, and after repeated infections IgG_1 cells increased in the spleen, mesenteric lymph nodes and Peyer's patches. IgG_1 and IgG_2 antibodies showed specificity for the stichosome cells of infected larvae which are the major source of metabolites with strong protective antigen activity (Despommier and Muller, 1970a, b). These results correspond closely to those obtained by Catty (1967, 1969) and Hankes (1968) in which the infected guinea-pig mucosa becomes infiltrated with antibody-producing cells specific to larval metabolites in the second week of infection (Fig. 13.1). Catty, Pritchard and Hankes (1978) have, in addition, traced the uptake of the parasite metabolite antigens from the intestinal lumen into villous interepithelial macrophages – an event which precedes antibody synthesis. They showed by fluorescent antibody that these antigens are transported by wander-

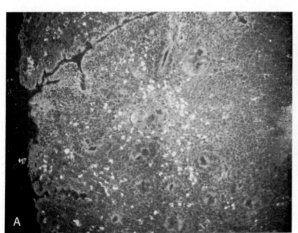
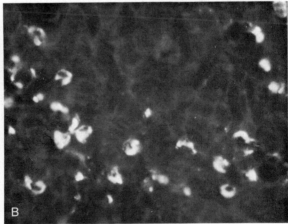

Fig. 13.1 A. Antibody-producing cells in the lamina propria of the jejunum in *Trichinella spiralis* infected guinea-pigs, 13 days after infection. The cells are labelled with FITC-conjugated metabolic antigens by a direct staining technique on frozen sections of intestine. B. Higher power section of (A) showing detail of some of the labelled plasma cells.

ing cells to the bases of villi and thence to Peyer's patches and the microvasculature of the small intestine.

THE SELF-CURE PHENOMENON

Although all forms of immune response can usually be identified as a result of nematode infection, except in the few examples cited above, their origins in the different lymphoid tissues and the kinetics of the responses in relation to antigen release have not been adequately studied. However, one outstanding feature of host responses is the universal development of immediate hypersensitivity (reviewed by Sadun, 1972; Zvaifler, 1976). The causative antibodies are produced entirely within the IgE (reagin) class of immunoglobulin in some hosts, including man, in reagin-like molecules in some other hosts, and also within IgG_1 molecules in animals such as the guinea-pig and the mouse. IgE antibodies are part of the spectrum of immunoglobulins which, across the species, are involved in the expression of allergic reactions associated with mucosal surfaces (Orange, Stechs</br>chulte and Austen, 1970; Ishizaka and Ishizaka, 1970). They have been identified in nematode and other helminth infections of man and a wide range of other hosts (e.g. Ogilvie, 1964, 1967; Zvaifler, Sadun and Becker, 1966; Ogilvie and Jones, 1969, 1971; Dobson, Morseth and Soulsby, 1971; Catty and Fraser, 1972). In many cases the levels of IgE immunoglobulin are very significantly elevated in the serum of infected human beings (Johannson, Mellbin and Vahlquist, 1968; Kojima, Yokogawa and Tada, 1972; Grove, Burston and Forbes, 1974; Radermecker, Bekhti, Poncelet and Salmon, 1974). There is continuing interest in the possible mechanisms by which infection of animals with nematodes induces synthesis of antiparasite IgE antibodies and potentiates IgE antibody responses to other antigens (e.g. Orr and Blair, 1969; Jarrett and Urquhart, 1971; Jarrett and Stewart, 1972, 1973; Jarrett, 1973).

It is clear from recent experiments by Jarrett, Haig, McDougall and McNulty (1976) and Bazin and Platteau (1976) that IgE antibody responses in rats can be induced to non-parasite protein antigens presented to the host orally; the form of presentation of the antigen seems therefore to be as much a predisposing factor in the induction of IgE antibody as the nature of parasitic antigens. Jarrett et al. (1976) obtained primary IgE responses in Hooded Lister rats after feeding 10 μg of egg albumin and secondary responses with a further 1 μg orally. From previous studies (Jarrett and Stewart, 1974) it is evident that induction of IgE antibody is critically dependent upon antigen dose, i.e. secondary responses can be actively inhibited by over-optimal stimulation. These authors argue that the larger the dose of antigen presented across the intestinal mucosal barrier the less likely it is that persistent IgE responses will

result and they suggest that the failure to respond with IgE antibody synthesis is the normal event in non-atopic individuals through the absorption of inhibitory levels of antigen. This is, however, difficult to reconcile with observations of IgE responses to parasites of the intestine where the amount of antigen presented to the host may be very large.

Studies of the distribution of IgE-producing cells in man and in experimentally infected rats have revealed a predominance at mucosal surfaces, including the intestine, and in local regional lymph nodes (Tada and Ishizaka, 1970). Ishizaka, Urban and Ishizaka (1976) have shown that in N. brasiliensis-infected rats the regional lymph nodes are the major source of serum IgE; the response to infection is detectable on the 8th day and, when reaching a maximum on the 14th day, about 20 per cent of the immunoglobulin-bearing (B-) cells in the mesenteric lymph nodes bear IgE on their surface. Rats with the same infection have also been studied by Mayrhofer, Bazin and Gowans (1976) who found that the lamina propria of the small intestine contains numerous mast cells staining, by fluorescent antibody, for IgE, both as membrane-bound and intracellular molecules. The intraepithelial mast cells, the 'globule leukocytes', also contain cytoplasmic IgE. The IgE antibody response to infection was found in this study also to be localized mainly to the draining regional mesenteric lymph nodes.

IgE antibody produced in close proximity to the intestine will be available to sensitize the mast cells of the intestinal mucosa, thus providing the conditions necessary for local anaphylactic sensitivity to the presence of parasite allergens. The sensitization of mast cells with IgE antibody, that gives rise to the allergies of the immediate type, has long been regarded by clinical allergists as a nuisance and of no potential benefit. However, to quote Dobson (1972), 'the persistence of any body system is a compelling argument for the survival advantage of the system. The formation of high levels of reaginic antibodies following so many metazoan parasite infections is indeed a compelling reason for rationalizing the anaphylactic reactions mediated by these antibodies with the protection of the host against invasions of the mucosae by parasites.'

The term 'self-cure' was used originally by Stoll (1929) to describe a phenomenon in sheep continuously exposed to the stomach nematode (Haemonchus contortus) from the pasture. During periods of high intake of infective larvae there sometimes occurs an elimination of a previously established worm population. Although with new knowledge this does not appear to be strictly a 'cure' mechanism, since the host is susceptible to the new intake of worms, the phenomenon shows all the characteristics of an immune response stimulated by an excessive antigen challenge from the newly acquired developing larvae operating against the previously established adults. The classic analysis by Stewart (1953, 1955) has provided convincing evidence that local anaphylactic reactions accompany such self-cure. Furthermore, Soulsby and Stewart (1959) showed that a powerful allergen, released from *H. contortus* larvae at the third moult, gave rise to the reaction.

The self-cure reaction, as exemplified above, is probably representative of many crisis situations in the host exposed continuously or repeatedly to infection, although its significance in the spontaneous termination of single controlled infections is less well explored and forms a subject of considerable controversy at the present time (see below). The phenomenon does, however, illustrate some well-established principles in the dynamics of nematode–host reactivity. It must be remembered that parasites have a long evolutionary history of coexistence with their hosts. No advantage is to be gained by any parasite whose invasiveness results in the hosts' early demise or alternatively in an effective and immediate rejection. In long-established parasite–host relationships we see the end result of progressive mutual adaptations to the benefit of both partners. Two factors seem to be of particular importance in this process of adaptation: the threshold level of antigen-release at which protective responses by the host are brought into play, and the probable restriction of the parasites' overall antigenicity to certain metabolites released at

some critical stages of development. These points are discussed in detail by Sprent (1959), Dineen, (1963a, b) and Donald, Dineen, Turner and Wagland (1964).

Histopathological studies of the infected intestine give broad-based support to the concept of local anaphylaxis. There is, for instance, a striking infiltration of mast cells or basophils into the tissues around the site of most infections, e.g. *Trichostrongylus colubriformis* in the guinea-pig (Rothwell, Pritchard and Love, 1974). Furthermore, the numbers of mast cells may increase dramatically with the onset of worm expulsion. This is most carefully described in the case of *N. brasiliensis* infection of the rat (Wells, 1962; Whur, 1966, 1967; Murray, Jarrett and Jennings, 1971; Murray, Miller, Sanford and Jarrett, 1971; Murray, 1972 – see Fig. 13.3). Some definite indication that intestinal mast cells may become sensitized with IgE antibody early in this infection comes from the observation by Wilson and Bloch (1968) that reagin-sensitized mast cells can be present in the rat peritoneum from the 10th day.

Rats, mice and guinea-pigs infected with *Trichinella spiralis* also show an equivalent rise in the number of mast cells and globule leucocytes in the intestinal mucosa close to the invading worms (Ruitenberg and Elgersma, 1976; Pritchard, 1977). In the rat and mouse the mast-cell response has been shown to be dependent upon the presence of T-cells; anti-thymocyte serum treatment of rats has an adverse effect upon mast-cell

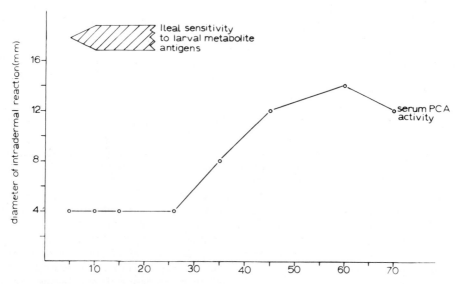

Fig. 13.2 Development of passive cutaneous anaphylaxis (PCA) reactivity, with time after infection, in the serum of guinea-pigs (mean of 16 animals) infected with 400 larvae of *Trichinella spiralis*, as measured by the sensitizing capacity of serum injected into the skin of normal guinea-pigs which are challenged with larval antigens intravenously 17 hours later. The activity of the passively sensitizing antibodies (anaphylactic antibodies) is measured by the size (diameter) of the PCA reaction developing within 30 minutes of antigen challenge. Reactions of less than 5 mm diameter are negative. Shown above is the general pattern of development of local anaphylactic sensitivity in the distal (infected) segment of the ileum of a comparable group of infected guinea-pigs. This sensitivity is determined by the Schultz–Dale reaction in which the intestinal segment is exposed *in vitro* to antigen; the resulting induced contraction of the tissue can be recorded. The figure is intended to show only the general trend of development of local intestinal sensitivity with time.

degranulation (attributable to a predicted, although not tested, decrease in IgE antibody level by this procedure) and in congenitally athymic (nude) mice intestinal mast-cell counts fail to increase as they do in thymus-intact infected littermates. In the guinea-pig the rise in inter-epithelial mast cells coincides with the development of an antigen-inducible anaphylactic response in the infected part of the intestine (by Schultz–Dale test) and the number of mast cells with deeply staining cyto-plasmic granules returns to normal at the time of worm expulsion (Pritchard, 1977), possibly as a result of a pan-mucosal degranulation episode. An interesting further observation in the infected nude mouse is that the adult female trichinae survive in the small intestine for sig-nificantly longer periods than in thymus-intact mice and they grow considerably larger. They also produce greater numbers of tissue-invasive larvae and they tend not to be shifted so rapidly down the length of the small bowel – these factors can be related to a reduced in-flammatory lesion in the local tissues (Catty and Swift, 1978).

Mixed cell inflammatory responses, too, almost in-variably accompany acute parasite-rejection episodes. The composition and timing of such reactions is not inconsistent with the expected results of high local amine concentrations released through extensive mast-cell degranulation. In particular, the local tissue (and circulating) eosinophilia is very characteristic (Hirsch, 1965). It is seen, for instance, in the intestine of rats infested with *Nippostrongylus* (Taliaferro and Sarles, 1939) and guinea pigs infested with *T. spiralis* (Catty, 1969). In the latter example early oedema and intense tissue eosinophilia precede the mixed inflammation, especially in animals superinfected and undergoing acute rejection. In studies on local antibody production in this infection (reviewed by Catty, 1976) the appearance of positive staining cells is found to coincide with the development of immediate hypersensitivity in the local intestinal tissue, as demonstrated by the Schultz–Dale reaction (Coulson, 1953; Ivey, 1965). The sensitivity is due to the production of anaphylactic antibodies which are probably produced locally in the intestinal tissues since reactions can be elicited before these antibodies appear in the serum (Fig. 13.2). In trichinosis of guinea pigs, therefore, evidence of several kinds points to both the presence and activity of immediate hypersensi-tivity in response to infection.

THE 'LEAK–LESION' HYPOTHESIS

In 1936 Sarles and Taliaferro demonstrated the passive transfer of acquired immunity to *Nippostrongylus* in the rat, using antiserum from infected donors, and many experiments have since been performed in this system to show that immune serum can routinely bring about expulsion of a population of transferred adult parasites.

Since no formal evidence is available to suggest that the protective antibodies that do exist in the serum are also actively secreted into the intestinal lumen during infec-tion, Urquhart, Mulligan, Eadie and Jennings (1965) and Barth, Jarrett and Urquhart (1966) have proposed that in infected rats the anaphylactic release of amines from mast cells gives rise to conditions in which a leak-age of protective serum antibodies occurs across the epi-thelial barrier into the intestine. The 'Leak–Lesion' hypothesis, as first proposed, had a threefold basis: the evidence of the universal production of reaginic anti-bodies in helminth infestations; an observed correlation

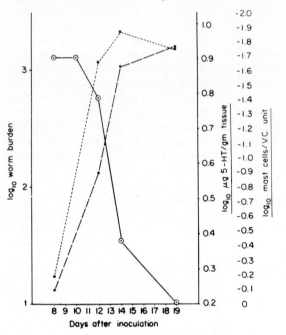

Fig. 13.3 Worm kinetics (⊙), 5-HT levels (●) and intestinal mast cell population (♦) in rats infected with 3000 *N. brasiliensis*. Associated with worm expulsion, there is a marked increase in mast cells and a corresponding rise in 5-HT levels in the bowel wall. (Reproduced from Murray, 1972, by courtesy of Academic Press.)

between local intestinal mast cells, eosinophils and hist-amine levels in rats during the expulsion phase (Wells, 1962; Whur, 1966, 1967); and lastly the demonstration by Barth *et al*. (1966) that infected rats sensitized also to ovalbumin could, under the influence of an ovalbumin-induced anaphylactic shock, displace the worms from the intestine, but only if immune serum was given before the shocking antigen. Subsequent work on the release of amines in the infected intestine, on the kinetics of mast-cell responses in the local tissues (Fig. 13.3), on the effects of amine inhibitors in prolonging infection and on the leakage of tracer-labelled macromolecules across the intestinal barrier (Fig. 13.4), has provided a body of evidence (reviewed extensively by Murray,

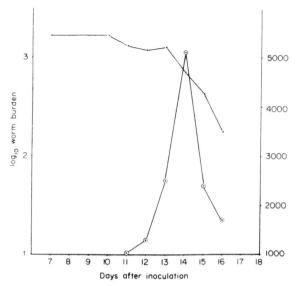

Fig. 13.4 Leak of plasma ([^{131}I] PVP) into the intestine of rats infected with 3000 *N. brasiliensis*. ⊙, calculated plasma in intestinal contents. ●, kinetics of worm burden from Figure 13.3. (Reproduced from Murray, 1972, by courtesy of Academic Press.)

1972) to substantiate the original hypothesis. In addition the role of amines in immunity to *Trichostrongylus colubriformis* in the guinea-pig has been investigated. In this infection too, treatment with amine inhibitors prolongs infection (Rothwell, Dineen and Love, 1971; Rothwell *et al.*, 1974). Furthermore, administration of amines early in infection leads to a rapid expulsion of the worms.

The concept of antibody leakage offers no explanation as to how serum antibodies (or for that matter locally produced and secreted antibodies) affect the worms sufficiently to dislodge them from the intestine in the manner proposed. Work from other sources has indicated that protective serum antibodies (i.e. from infected donor rats) are usually IgG$_1$, and complement is not required for their activity against the worms (Jones, Edwards and Ogilvie, 1970; Jones and Ogilvie, 1971). The presence of neither IgA nor IgE antibodies in sera is correlated with protective activity. This does not, of course, mean that antibodies other than serum IgG$_1$ may not be of crucial importance at the site of worm rejection (the role of protective IgE antibodies as mediators of specific anaphylaxis is the most significant element of the proposed mechanism), but other antibodies produced locally may also contribute to the induction of the mixed cell exudate which accompanies rejection and which may be the actual cause of parasite dislodgement. When considering all the available evidence with respect to the local changes in the intestine induced by nematode parasites, there are certain

reasons for believing that the leakage of serum antibody into sites of worm infestation may not in all cases be an essential component. The probable necessity to consider alternative mechanisms in worm expulsion is indicated particularly by the following observations:

1. Passive transfer of infected donor serum in most nematode infestations, including those in which acquired immunity clearly develops, does not provide passive immunity in a wide range of hosts tested. This implies either that a leakage of serum antibody with protective activity is not a general phenomenon in such situations or that the concept of protective serum antibodies is not generally applicable.

2. The acquired immune response which actively rejects one parasite species from the intestine may be shown to operate subsequently against another species with no demonstrable antigen cross-reactivity. This occurs, for example, in mice who have expelled *Ancylostoma caninum* and then challenged with *T. spiralis* (Cox, 1952; Goulson, 1958) and in rats who have expelled *Nippostrongylus* and are then challenged with *T. spiralis* (Louch, 1962). Such results clearly suggest that any direct effect of antibodies on the worms may not be the crucial factor in inducing an active rejection episode. Although raised specifically to one set of parasite antigens, the antibodies' main effects may be implemented through indirect and essentially non-specific mechanisms.

3. The maintenance *in vitro* of adult *Nippostrongylus* in immune serum has no demonstrable effect on their viability within the system (Mulligan, 1968; Ogilvie, 1973).

4. Although protective antibodies exist in the serum of *Nippostrongylus*-immune rats they seem unable to act alone in inducing expulsion of adults (Ogilvie and Jones, 1973); there is also a specific requirement for the activity of sensitized lymphocytes. The evidence for specific collaboration between antibodies and cells in the expulsion of this parasite is discussed in a later section.

CELL-MEDIATED IMMUNITY

Delayed hypersensitivity reactions can usually be elicited in nematode infections and *in-vitro* correlates of cell-mediated immunity have been demonstrated for some species infesting the gastrointestinal tract (see Soulsby, 1972). In recent years techniques for the transfer of specifically sensitized lymphoid cells between inbred animals have revealed a definite specific cellular involvement in the immunity developing in a few of these species. Some especially interesting work has been performed using a guinea-pig-adapted strain of the sheep nematode *Trichostrongylus colubriformis*. Wagland and Dineen (1965), Dineen and Wagland (1966), Dineen, Ronai and Wagland (1968) and Dineen, Wagland and Ronai (1968) have shown that in this system the transfer of lymphocytes from immune donors to non-immune recipients can induce a protection to challenge infection. The protection is better afforded by mesenteric lymph-node cells than by spleen cells, and when these are labelled with ^{51}Cr they can be seen to accumulate in the intestinal tissues surrounding the infection and here undergo a phenomenon of 'allergic death' when in close contact with the parasites. In more extensive studies Dobson and Soulsby (1974) have shown a rapid blasto-genesis of Peyer's patch lymphocytes in the first few days of infection. Cells are disseminated into the infected lamina propria and local mesenteric lymph nodes in a progressive manner during this period. Cell recruitment continues downwards as the parasites themselves are shifted into lower segments of the small intestine. There is also evidence of a fairly massive recruitment of splenic lymphocytes which converge on the infected area and the regional lymph nodes. In primary infections a release of antigen-sensitive cells into the circulation occurs in the first few days but disappears as immune elimination gets under way. In previously infected animals the delay in appearance of these cells is cor-related with an earlier rejection episode and is consistent with the view that an active recruitment of cells takes place in the intestine during rejection. Other details of the cellular response have been contributed by Dineen and Adams (1971) who have found that cells which initiate the rejection of *T. colubriformis* in the guinea-pig are thymus derived and form part of the long-lived recirculating pool of lymphocytes. In *N. brasilensis* infections of the rat there is a local enteropathy with villous atrophy and crypt hyperplasia. The development of this lesion has been shown to be thymus dependent (Ferguson and Jarrett, 1975) and would seem for this reason to be an immune-based reaction as opposed to a toxic response. However, since both humoral and cell-mediated immune responses to the parasite are thymus dependent the induced changes in intestinal structure cannot be certainly identified as being the result of a local T-cell-mediated response to parasite antigens (Ferguson, 1976).

Larsh and his colleagues (Larsh, Goulson and Weatherly, 1964a, b) have studied the role of lympho-cytes in immunity to *T. spiralis* in the mouse. Using lymph-node cells, and later (Larsh, Race, Goulson and Weatherly, 1966) peritoneal exudate cells, from infected donors they successfully transferred immunity to chal-lenged recipients who did not, by sensitive assays, produce any detectable antibody as a result of cell transfer. More recently the adoptive immune system has been shown to be inducible by immunizing donors with worm extract and transferable with spleen cells (Larsh, Goulson, Weatherly and Chaffee, 1969, 1970a, b). Cell populations carrying the capacity to transfer immunity give rise to macrophage migration inhibition

in vitro in the presence of parasite antigens (Cypess and Larsh, 1970; Cypess, Larsh and Pegram, 1971; Stefanski and Malczewski, 1972) and the donors of such cells show delayed dermal hypersensitivity to purified parasite antigens (Larsh and Weatherly, 1974).

In trichinosis a role of lymphocytes in immunity has been substantiated in studies in the rat and the guinea-pig. Gore, Burger and Sadun (1970) were able to protect recipient rats from infections by the transfer of lymphoid cells from hyperinfected donors, whilst failing to achieve any similar effect with large doses of immunoglobulin. The normal expulsion of adults from the intestine was prolonged in neonatally thymectomized rats and in those treated with anti-lymphocyte globulin. Catty (1976), in reviewing guinea-pig experiments similar to those per-formed in mice using donor peritoneal exudate cells, has pointed out that successful adoptive transfer of im-munity is not restricted to the times after donor infec-tion when these animals show delayed dermal sensitivity to released antigens. Cells derived from animals in the post-delayed hypersensitivity phase (from 3 weeks after infection) also transfer significant immunity to the recipients. This type of experiment takes account of one important consideration in all adoptive transfer tests using lymphoid cells; it is difficult to preclude the pos-sibility that transferred cells are not providing an essential antibody-generating component (B-cells or helper T-cells) of the immunity mechanism. Gore, Burger and Sadun (1974) have examined this point in detail by determining antibody responses produced by the lymphoid cells transferred from *Trichinella*-infected rats into recipients. They found that at the seventh day after infection, 31 per cent of the recipients of sensitized cells gave a homocytotropic antibody response in the serum. Control animals receiving normal cells or no cells showed no such response at that time.

Although it seems reasonable to conclude that specifi-cally sensitized lymphocytes, probably thymus derived, are involved in the initiation and maintenance of pro-tective immunity towards nematode infections of the intestine, the means by which these cells could express their immune capabilities, other than by facilitating anti-body production, is by no means clear. Ogilvie and Jones (1967) and Wilson, Jones and Leskowitz (1967) have shown that IgE antibody synthesis in *Nippostrongylus*-infected rats is dependent upon an intact thymus. Thus the capacity of the mucosa, including that of the intestine, to generate an immediate hypersensitivity will depend upon the successful cooperative effects of specifically sensitised T-cells. These may be needed in relatively large numbers within the infected part of the lamina propria for successful stimulation of IgE-synthesizing cells. From the known effects of helminths in inducing and potentiating IgE responses we can infer that helminth products have some special inductive capacity which may involve the recruitment of extraordinarily large numbers of thymus-derived lymphocytes to areas of local IgE synthesis. In addition, the recently described dependency of the mast-cell response upon an intact T-cell system (Ruitenberg and Elgersma, 1976 – see above) reinforces the view that T-cells may have several indirect influences upon the course of infections of the gastrointestinal tract. In the view of Larsh and Weatherly (1974), however, the local cell-mediated response is a primary effector mechanism which gives rise, through the release of lymphotoxin, to tissue injury. The non-specific consequence of this (they consider) is a panmucosal and submucosal allergic inflammation which may produce an unfavourable environment for parasite survival.

SPECIFIC COLLABORATION BETWEEN ANTIBODIES AND CELLS

(i) Effects of antibodies on parasites

Some of the earliest described effects of the immune response on nematodes refer to the microprecipitations that form around the orifices of nematode larvae and adults incubated in serum from infected animals. The location of precipitates at these sites provided the first indication that the important protective antigens are by-products of the excretion–secretion systems of the worms (ES antigens). Roth (1941) observed precipitates around the oral and genital orifices of *T. spiralis* larvae *in vitro*. Using fluorescent antibodies, Jackson (1960) showed that hyper-immune rabbit and rat sera combined with ES antigens at the oral and anal pores of living infective *Nippostrongylus* larvae, and with antigens lying internally to, and at the orifices of, the excretory and reproductive systems of living adults.

Mauss (1941), Thorson (1954a, b) and Mills and Kent (1965) have exposed infective larvae of some nematodes to immune sera and have in this way reduced their infectivity. This supports the original suggestion by Chandler (1932) that anti-helminth antibodies might interfere with the metabolism of worms. Thorson (1953, 1954b) found a lipolytic inhibitor of ES antigen in serum from rats immune to *Nippostrongylus* and on this basis suggested that part of the protective immunity to nematodes was due to antiparasite enzyme activity in antibodies of the host. In later work (1956a, b, 1963) Thorson identified proteolytic and lipolytic enzymes in the oesophagus of *Ancylostoma caninum* which were inactivated by immune dog serum. Several other similar effects have been shown with other parasite species, e.g. malic dehydrogenase from *Ascaris suum* (Rhodes, Marsh and Kelley, 1964; Rhodes *et al.*, 1965).

(ii) Antibodies and cells in immunity to *Nippostrongylus*

Parasite expulsion from the intestine is one obvious and extreme form of acquired immunity from infection, but immunity is also frequently expressed in a less dramatic manner as an inhibition of parasite development and/or of adult reproductive activity (Chandler, 1936; Thorson, 1956b; Campbell, 1955; Barth *et al.*, 1966). These are both gross effects and easily recognizable as immune mechanisms in which, by inference at least, antibodies to ES antigens may play a significant role. In *Nippostrongylus* infection of the rat, in which both inhibitory effects and an ultimate rejection of adults are observed, recent results of Ogilvie and her colleagues (reviewed by Ogilvie and Jones, 1973; Ogilvie and Love, 1974; Ogilvie and Worms, 1976) indicate that antibodies and cells may collaborate to bring about worm expulsion. They propose a two-step expulsion mechanism, the first depending upon the action of antibodies which damage the worms, and the second inducing the expulsion, depending upon sensitized lymphocytes. The worms affected by antibodies show an inability to take up trace-labelled inorganic ions, they have an altered pattern of enzyme secretion (Edwards, Burt and Ogilvie, 1971) and they show degenerative changes within the cytoplasm of their intestinal cells. All of these effects indicate a probable interference by antibody with worm metabolism, but they are not sufficient in themselves to bring about an expulsion. Nevertheless, they probably cause the observed stunting of adults and of the cessation of egg laying which precedes expulsion. The expulsion phase appears to be the result of a secondary active process since damaged worms are not expelled from either neonatal rats or irradiated rats even when the latter are given immune antiserum. The damaged worms can be expelled, however, by irradiated hosts treated with mesenteric lymph-node cells from uninfected syngeneic donors (Keller and Keist, 1972) and rats given sensitized lymphocytes from infected donors expel antibody-damaged worms much more rapidly than they do normal worms (Dineed, Ogilvie and Kelly, 1973).

The origin and nature of the antibodies which induce damage to *Nippostrongylus in vivo* have not been identified although the passive protective activities of IgG$_1$ serum antibodies have been implicated (Jones *et al.*, 1970). Moreover, the range of effects the antibodies have which allegedly render them susceptible to the actions of sensitized lymphocytes is not known. Antibodies to one important parasite enzyme, acetylcholinesterase, have, however, been identified in immune serum (Jones and Ogilvie, 1972). One cannot exclude the possibility that damage to worms is also induced by the effect of amines. It is known in other infections that amine inhibitors prolong the survival of adults in the intestine, e.g. *T. spiralis* (Campbell, Hartman and Cuckler, 1963) and *T. colubriformis* (Rothwell *et al.*, 1971, 1974).

At the present time the method of action of sensitized lymphocytes on *Nippostrongylus* expulsion is a matter of conjecture. Adults do not penetrate the intestinal mucosa but are seen deeply embedded within the crypts. Although an intense mixed inflammation, containing some lymphocytes, occurs in the lamina propria at the height of infection (prior to worm expulsion) there is no adherence of lymphocytes to the worms (Taliaferro and Sarles, 1939; Ogilvie and Jones, 1971). Their action must therefore be at a distance and could be the result of lymphokine release (Dineen et al., 1973), especially since the specific requirement for the cellular step in worm expulsion is thymus dependent (Keller and Keist, 1972). However, since thymus dependency in immune responses extends beyond the release of mediators by T-cells into a range of other activities, including co-operation in antibody synthesis, T-cell dependency in worm expulsion should not be taken to indicate necessarily that T-cell products have any direct action upon the worms.

CONCLUSIONS WITH RESPECT TO NEMATODE INFESTATIONS

As information accumulates on the nature of mammalian immune responses to gastrointestinal nematodes it is becoming apparent that a multiplicity of immune re-activities seems to be involved in the control of infestation. This is perhaps not surprising when one considers that the evolution of the specialized immune systems of highly evolved mammals has taken place in an environment which has provided a continuous challenge with antigenically and physiologically complex metazoan parasites and whose presence has no doubt played a part in the evolutionary process. Our current understanding does not allow us to detail the complete sequence of events taking place within the intestine or lymphoid tissues of the host which afford immunological control of any parasite. Studies of different systems have illuminated a number of immune mechanisms which undoubtedly are of importance, including local anaphylaxis, effects of antibody on worm metabolism and cell-mediated immunity. It is almost certainly true that the expression of immunity is the net result of the development of several forms of immune response which act collaboratively and locally to change the selected microenvironments of the worms. Since different species of worms differ considerably in their choice of environment within the intestine, and in the extent to which they invade the intestinal tissues, it would be unexpected if immune mechanisms were to be qualitatively and quantitatively the same in all situations and to have the same degree of success in removing the parasitic burden. Currently there is little or no convincing evidence against, and some evidence in support of, the hypothesis that expulsion of parasites from the intestine, when it does occur, is the result of an inflammatory response of multifactorial origin which, although induced specifically to the particular pattern of antigens released by the parasites, is essentially non-specific in its capacity to expel the worms.

REFERENCES

Ajdukiewicz, A. B., Youngs, G. R. & Bouchier, I. A. D. (1972) Nodular lymphoid hyperplasia with hypogammaglobulinaemia. *Gut*, **13**, 589–595.

Alam, M. & Ahmad, S. (1974) Immunogenicity of *Entamoeba histolytica* antigen fractions. *Transactions of the Royal Society of Tropical Medicine and Hygiene*, **68**, 370–373.

Ambrose-Thomas, P. & Truong, T. K. (1969) Le diagnostic sérologique de l'amibiase humaine par la technique des anticorps fluorescents. *Bulletin of the World Health Organisation*, **40**, 103–112.

Ament, M. E. & Rubin, C. E. (1972) Relation of giardiasis to abnormal intestinal structure and function in gastrointestinal immunodeficiency syndromes. *Gastroenterology*, **62**, 216–226.

Ament, M. E., Ochs, H. D. & Davis, S. D. (1973) The structure and function of the gastrointestinal tract in primary immunodeficiency syndromes: a study of 39 patients. *Medicine*, **52**, 227–248.

Anderson, F. L., Pellegrino, E. D. & Schaefer, J. W. (1970) Dysgammaglobulinaemia associated with malabsorption and tetany. *American Journal of Digestive Diseases*, **15**, 279–286.

Barksdale, W. L. & Routh, C. F. (1948) *Isospora hominis* infections among American personnel in the South West Pacific. *American Journal of Tropical Medicine and Hygiene*, **28**, 639–644.

Barth, E. E. E., Jarrett, W. F. H. & Urquhart, G. M. (1966) Studies on the mechanism of the self-cure reaction in rats infected with *Nippostrongylus brasiliensis*. *Immunology*, **10**, 459–464.

Bazin, H. & Platteau, B. (1976) Production of circulating reaginic (IgE) antibodies by oral administration of ovalbumin to rats. *Immunology*, **30**, 679–683.

Beaver, P. C., Jung, R. C., Sherman, H. J., Read, T. R. & Robinson, T. A. (1956) Experimental *Entamoeba histolytica* infections in man. *American Journal of Tropical Medicine and Hygiene*, **5**, 1000–1009.

Biagi, F. & Beltran, F. (1969) The challenge of amoebiasis: understanding pathogenic mechanisms. *International Review of Tropical Medicine*, **3**, 219–239.

Biagi, F. F., Beltran, H. F. & Ortega, P. S. (1966) Remobilisation of *Entamoeba histolytica* after exposure to immobilising antibodies. *Experimental Parasitology*, **18**, 87–91.

Bierman, S. M. (1972) Varicelliform eruption, vasculitis, spontaneous abortion, giardiasis and eosinophilia. *Archives of Dermatology*, **106**, 122–123.

Boorman, G. A., Lina, P. H. C., Zurcha, C. & Niewerkerk, H. T. M. (1973) Hexamita and Giardia as a cause of mortality in congenitally thymus-less (nude) mice. *Clinical and Experimental Immunology*, **15**, 623–627.

Brandborg, L. L., Goldberg, S. B. & Breidenbach, W. C. (1970) Human coccidiosis – a possible cause of malabsorption. The life cycle in small-bowel mucosal biopsies as a diagnostic feature. *New England Journal of Medicine*, **283**, 1306–1313.

Brandborg, L. L., Tankersley, C. & Gottlieb, S. (1965) Invasion of the small intestinal mucosa by *Giardiasis lamblia*. Fact or fiction? *Gastroenterology*, **48**, 808.

Brown, W. R., Butterfield, D., Savage, D. & Tada, T. (1972) Clinical, microbiological and immunological studies in patients with immunoglobulin deficiencies and gastrointestinal disorders. *Gut*, **13**, 441–449.

Campbell, C. H. (1955) The antigenic role of the excretions and secretions of *Trichinella spiralis* in the production of immunity in mice. *Journal of Parasitology*, **41**, 483–491.

Campbell, W. C., Hartman, R. K. & Cuckler, A. C. (1963) Induction of immunity to trichinosis in mice by means of chemically abbreviated infections. *Experimental Parasitology*, **14**, 29–36.

Carrol, M. E., Anast, B. P. & Birch, C. L. (1961) Giardiasis and uveitis. *Archives of Ophthalmology*, **65**, 775–778.

Catty, D. 'The immunology of experimental trichinosis in guinea-pigs.' Unpublished Ph.D. Thesis, University of Birmingham, 1967.

Catty, D. (1969) The immunology of nematode infections; trichinosis in guinea-pigs as a model. *Monographs in Allergy*, Vol. 5. Basel: Karger.

Catty, D. (1976) Immunity and acquired resistance to trichinosis. In *The Immunology of Parasitic Infections*, ed. Cohen, S. & Sadun, E. H. Oxford: Blackwell Scientific Publications.

Catty, D. & Fraser, K. F. (1972) Homocytotropic antibodies in the guinea-pig. Heterogeneity of antibodies induced by Trichinella infection. *International Archives of Allergy and Applied Immunology*, **43**, 371–382.

Catty, D. & Swift, K. (1978) Growth, Survival and Productivity of *Trichinella spiralis* in the Congenitally Athymic (Nude) Mouse. In preparation.

Catty, D., Pritchard, D. I. & Hankes, J. (1978) Antigen uptake by the small intestine of guinea pigs infected with *Trichinella spiralis*. *Proceedings of the Symposium Antigen Uptake by the Gut, Bangor, July 1975*. ed. Hemmings, W. A. M.T.P.: Lancaster. In press.

Chandler, A. C. (1932) Susceptibility and resistance to helminth infections. *Journal of Parasitology*, **18**, 135–152.

Chandler, A. C. (1936) Studies on nature of immunity to intestinal helminths. Renewal of growth and egg production in Nippostrongylus after transfer from immune to non-immune rats. *American Journal of Hygiene*, **23**, 46–54.

Chawla, L. S., Sehgal, A. K., Broor, S. L., Verma, R. S. & Chhittani, P. N. (1975) Tryptic activity in the duodenal aspirate following a standard test meal in giardiasis. *Scandinavian Journal of Gastroenterology*, **10**, 445–447.

Cortner, J. A. (1959) Giardiasis, a cause of coeliac syndrome. *American Journal of Diseases of Children*, **98**, 311–316.

Coulson, E. J. (1953) The Schultz–Dale technique. *Journal of Allergy*, **24**, 458–473.

Cowan, A. E. & Campbell, C. B. (1973) Giardiasis – a cause of vitamin B$_{12}$ malabsorption. *American Journal of Digestive Diseases*, **18**, 384–390.

Cox, F. E. G. (1968) Immunity to tissue protozoa. In *Immunity to Parasites*, ed. Taylor, A. E. R., pp. 5–23, 6th Symposium British Society for Parasitology. Oxford: Blackwell Scientific Publications.

Cox, H. W. (1952) The effect of concurrent infection with the dog hookworm *Ancylostoma caninum* on the natural and acquired resistance of mice to *Trichinella spiralis*. *Journal of the Elisha Mitchell Scientific Society*, **68**, 222–235.

Crandall, R. B. & Crandall, C. A. (1972) *Trichinella spiralis*: immunologic response to infection in mice. *Experimental Parasitology*, **31**, 378–398.

Crandall, R. B., Cebra, J. J. & Crandall, C. A. (1967) The relative proportions of IgG-, IgA- and IgM-containing cells in rabbit tissues during experimental trichinosis. *Immunology*, **12**, 147–158.

Culbertson, J. T. (1941) *Immunity against Animal Parasites*. New York: Columbia University Press.

Cypess, R. & Larsh, J. E. (1970) The macrophage inhibition assay (MIA) as an *in vitro* correlate of delayed hypersensitivity (DH) in mice sensitised to *Trichinella spiralis* antigen(s). Proceedings of the Second International Congress on Parasitology, Washington, D.C. *Journal of Parasitology*, **56**, 64–65.

Cypess, R., Larsh, J. E. & Pegram, C. (1971) Macrophage inhibition produced by guinea pig after sensitisation with a larval antigen of *Trichinella spiralis*. *Journal of Parasitology*, **57**, 103–106.

Dasgupta, A. (1974) Immunoglobulin in health and disease. III. Immunoglobulins in the sera of patients with amoebiasis. *Clinical and Experimental Immunology*, **16**, 163–168.

De Muro, P. (1939) Clinical aspects of giardiasis. *Acta Medica Scandinavia*, **99**, 78–116.

Despommier, D. D. & Muller, M. (1970a) The stichosome of *Trichinella spiralis*. 1. Its structure and function, part 1. *Journal of Parasitology*, **56**, 76–77.

Despommier, D. D. & Muller, M. (1970b) Functional antigens of *Trichinella spiralis*, part 1. *Journal of Parasitology*, **56**, 76.

Dineen, J. K. (1963a) Immunological aspects of parasitism. *Nature*, **197**, 268–269.

Dineen, J. K. (1963b) Antigenic relationship between host and parasite. *Nature*, **197**, 471–472.

Dineen, J. K. & Adams, D. B. (1971) The role of the recirculating thymus-dependent lymphocyte in resistance to *Trichostrongylus colubriformis* in the guinea-pig. *Immunology*, **20**, 109–113.

Dineen, J. K. & Wagland, B. M. (1966) The cellular transfer of immunity to *Trichostrongylus colubriformis* in an isogenic strain of guinea-pig. II. The relative susceptibility of the larval and adult stages of the parasite to immunological attack. *Immunology*, **11**, 47–57.

Dineen, J. K., Ogilvie, B. M. & Kelly, J. D. (1973) Expulsion of *Nippostrongylus brasiliensis* from the intestine of rats. Collaboration between humoral and cellular components of the immune response. *Immunology*, **24**, 467–475.

Dineen, J. K., Ronai, P. M. & Wagland, B. M. (1968) The cellular transfer of immunity to *Trichostrongylus colubriformis* in an isogenic strain of guinea-pig. IV. The localisation of immune lymphocytes in small intestine in infected and non-infected guinea pigs. *Immunology*, **15**, 671–679.

Dineen, J. K., Wagland, B. M. & Ronai, P. M. (1968) The cellular transfer of immunity to *Trichostrongylus colubriformis* in an isogenic strain of guinea-pig. III. The localisation and functional activity of immune lymph node cells following syngeneic and allogeneic transfer. *Immunology*, **15**, 335–341.

Dobson, C. (1966) Precipitating antibodies in extracts from the mucosa and tunica muscularis of the alimentary tract of sheep infected with *Oesophagostomum columbianum*. *Journal of Parasitology*, **52**, Research Note 5, 1037–1038.

Dobson, C. (1967) Changes in the protein content of the serum and intestinal mucus of sheep with reference to the

histology of the gut and immunological response to
Oesophagostonum columbianum infections. *Parasitology*, 57,
201–219.

Dobson, C. (1972) Immune response to gastrointestinal
helminths. In *Immunity to Animal Parasites* ed. Soulsby,
E. J. L., pp. 191–222. New York: Academic Press.

Dobson, C. & Soulsby, E. J. L. (1974) Lymphoid cell
kinetics in guinea pigs infected with *Trichostrongylus
colubriformis*. *Experimental Parasitology*, 35, 16–34.

Dobson, C., Morseth, D. J. & Soulsby, E. J. L. (1971)
Immunoglobulin E-type antibodies induced by *Ascaris
suum* infections in guinea pigs. *Journal of Immunology*,
106, 128–133.

Donald, A. D., Dineen, J. K., Turner, J. H. & Wagland,
B. M. (1964) The dynamics of the host–parasite
relationship. I. *Nematodirus spathiger* infection in sheep.
Parasitology, 54, 527–544.

Douvres, F. W. (1962) The *in vitro* cultivation of
Oesophogostonum radiatum, the nodular worm of cattle.
II. The use of this technique to study immune responses
of host tissue extracts against the developing nematode.
Journal of Parasitology, 48, 852–864.

Drenckhahn, C. H. (1943) Jaundice associated with *Giardia
lamblia* infestation. *Illinois Medical Journal*, 83, 119–121.

Edwards, A. J., Burt, J. S. & Ogilvie, B. M. (1971) The
effect of immunity upon some enzymes of the parasite
Nippostrongylus brasiliensis. *Parasitology*, 62, 339–347.

Fairise, C. & Jannin, L. (1913) Dysenterie chronique à
'Lamblia'. Etude parasitologique et anatomo-
pathologique. *Archives de Medicine Experimental*, 25,
525–551.

Ferguson, A. (1976) Coeliac disease and gastrointestinal food
allergy. In *Immunological Aspects of the Liver and
Gastrointestinal Tract*, ed. Ferguson, A. & MacSween,
R. N. M., Ch. 5, pp. 153–202. Lancaster: MTP Press.

Ferguson, A. & Jarrett, E. E. E. (1975) Hypersensitivity
reactions in the small intestine. I. Thymus dependence of
experimental 'partial villous atrophy'. *Gut*, 16, 114–117.

Ferguson, A., McClure, J. P. & Townley, R. R. W. (1976)
Intraepithelial lymphocyte counts in small intestinal
biopsies from children with diarrhoea. *Acta Paediatrica
Scandinavia*, 65, 541–546.

Feria-Velasco, A. & O'Shea del Socorro, M. (1974)
Ultramicroscopic demonstration of surface antigens in
trophozoites of *E. histolytica*. II. High resolution
cytochemical techniques. *Archivos de Investigaçion Medica
Mexico*, 5, 2, 315–324.

French, J. M. (1964) Steatorrhoea in a man infected with
coccidiosis (*Isospora belli*). *Gastroenterology*, 47,
642–648.

Frick, L. P. & Ackert, J. E. (1948) Further studies on
duodenal mucus as a factor in age resistance of chickens
to parasitism. *Journal of Parasitology*, 34, 192–206.

Gilman, R. H., Davis, C., Gan, E. & Bolton, M. (1976)
Seroepidemiology of amebiasis in the Orang Asli (Western
Malaysian Aborigine) and other Malaysians. *American
Journal of Tropical Medicine and Hygiene*, 25, 663–666.

Gore, R. W., Burger, H. J. & Sadun, E. H. (1970)
Mechanisms of immunity in rats infected with *Trichinella
spiralis*. *Journal of Parasitology*, 56, II, 1, 122.

Gore, R. W., Burger, H. J. & Sadun, E. H. (1974) Humoral
and cellular factors in the resistance of rats to *Trichinella
spiralis*. In *Trichinellosis: Proceedings of the Third
International Congress on Trichinosis*, ed. Kim, C. W.,
pp. 367–382. New York: Intext Publications.

Goulson, H. T. (1958) Studies on the influence of a prior
infection with *Ancylostoma carinum* on the establishment

and maintenance of *Trichinella spiralis* in mice. *Journal of
the Elisha Mitchell Scientific Society*, 74, 14–23.

Grove, D. I., Burston, T. O. & Forbes, I. J. (1974)
Immunoglobulin E and eosinophil levels in atopic and
non-atopic populations infested with hookworm. *Clinical
Allergy*, 4, 295–300.

Gryboski, J. D., Self, T. W., Clemett, A. & Herskovic, T.
(1968) Selective immunoglobulin A deficiency and
intestinal nodular lymphoid hyperplasia: correction of
diarrhoea with antibiotics and plasma. *Pediatrics*, 42,
833–840.

Gupta, R. K. & Mehta, S. (1973) Giardiasis in children. A
study of pancreatic functions. *Indian Journal of Medical
Research*, 61, 743–748.

Halstead, S. B. & Sadun, E. H. (1965) Alimentary
hypersensitivity induced by *Giardia lamblia*. Report of a
case of acute meat intolerance. *Annals of Internal Medicine*,
62, 564–569.

Hankes, J. J. 'Local immune responses in the resistance to
parasite infections.' Unpublished M.Sc. Thesis, University
of Birmingham, 1968.

Harris, R. H. & Mitchell, J. H. (1949) Chronic urticaria
due to *Giardia lamblia*. *Archives of Dermatology and
Syphology*, 59, 587–589.

Harris, W. C. & Bray, R. S. (1976) Cellular sensitivity in
amoebiasis – preliminary results of lymphocytic
transformation in response to specific antigen and to
mitogen in carrier and disease states. *Transactions of the
Royal Society of Tropical Medicine and Hygiene*, 70,
340–343.

Healy, G. R., Cahill, K. M., Elsdon-Dew, R., Juniper, K.
& Powell, S. J. (1971) The serology of amebiasis. *Bulletin
of the New York Academy of Medicine*, 47, 494–507.

Henderson, H. E., Gillespie, G. W., Kaplan, P. & Steber,
M. (1963) The human Isospora. *American Journal of
Hygiene*, 78, 302–309.

Henry, K., Bird, R. G. & Doe, W. F. (1974) Intestinal
coccidiosis in a patient with alpha-chain disease. *British
Medical Journal*, i, 542–543.

Hermans, P. E., Huizenga, K. A., Hoffman, H. N.,
Brown, A. L. & Markowitz, H. (1966)
Dysgammaglobulinaemia associated with nodular
lymphoid hyperplasia of the small intestine. *American
Journal of Medicine*, 40, 78–89.

Hirsch, J. G. (1965) In *The Inflammatory Process*, ed.
Zweifach, B. W., Grant, L. & McCluskey, R. T., p. 266.
New York: Academic Press.

Hoskins, L. C., Winawar, S. J., Broitman, S. A., Gottlieb,
L. S. & Zamchek, N. (1967) Clinical giardiasis and
intestinal malabsorption. *Gastroenterology*, 53, 265–279.

Hughes, W. S., Cerda, J. J., Holtzapple, P. & Brooks,
F. P. (1971) Primary hypogammaglobulinaemia and
malabsorption. *Annals of Internal Medicine*, 74,
903–910.

Hutchison, W. M., Dunachie, J. F., Siim, J. C. & Work,
K. (1970) Coccidian-like nature of *Toxoplasma gondii*.
British Medical Journal, i, 142–144.

Ishizaka, K. & Ishizaka, T. (1970) Biological function of
γE antibodies and mechanisms of reaginic hypersensitivity.
Clinical and Experimental Immunology, 6, 25–42.

Ishizaka, T., Urban, J. F. & Ishizaka, K. (1976) IgE
formation in the rat following infection with
Nippostrongylus brasiliensis. I. Proliferation and
differentiation of IgE-bearing cells. *Cellular Immunology*,
22, 248–261.

Ivey, M. H. (1965) Immediate hypersensitivity and
serological responses in guinea pigs infected with *Toxocara*

canis or *Trichinella spiralis. American Journal of Tropical Medicine and Hygiene*, **14**, 1044–1051.

Jackson, G. J. (1960) Fluorescent antibody studies of *Nippostrongylus muris* infections. *Journal of Infectious Diseases*, **106**, 20–36.

Jarrett, E. E. E. (1973) Reaginic antibodies and helminth infection. *Veterinary Record*, **93**, 480–483.

Jarrett, E. E. E. & Stewart, D. C. (1972) Potentiation of rat reaginic (IgE) antibody by helminth infection. Simultaneous potentiation of separate reagins. *Immunology*, **23**, 749–755.

Jarrett, E. E. E. & Stewart, D. C. (1973) Potentiation of rat reaginic (IgE) antibody by *Nippostrongylus brasiliensis* infection: effect of modification of life cycle of the parasite in the host. *Clinical and Experimental Immunology*, **15**, 79–85.

Jarrett, E. E. E. & Stewart, D. C. (1974) Rat IgE production. I. Effect of dose of antigen on primary and secondary reaginic antibody responses. *Immunology*, **27**, 365–381.

Jarrett, E. E. E. & Urquhart, G. M. (1971) The immune response to nematode infections. *International Reviews of Tropical Medicine*, **4**, 53–96.

Jarrett, E. E. E., Haig, D. M., McDougall, W. & McNulty, E. (1976) Rat IgE production. II. Primary and booster reaginic antibody responses following intradermal and oral immunization. *Immunology*, **30**, 671–677.

Jasso, L., Tejerina, J. & Gutierez, G. (1974) Persistence of maternal antibodies against *E. histolytica* in the newborn. *Archivos de Investigaçion Medica Mexico*, **5**, 2, 471–474.

Jeanes, A. L. (1969) Evaluation in clinical practice of the fluorescent amoebic antibody test. *Journal of Clinical Pathology*, **22**, 427–429.

Johansson, S. G. O., Mellbin, T. & Vahlquist, B. (1968) Immunoglobulin levels in Ethiopian pre-school children with special reference to high concentrations of Immunoglobulin E (IgND). *Lancet*, **i**, 1118–1121.

Johnson, B. L., Goldberg, L. S., Pops, M. A. & Weiner, M. (1971) Clinical and immunological studies in a case of nodular lymphoid hyperplasia of the small bowel. *Gastroenterology*, **61**, 369–374.

Jones, E. G. & Brown, W. R. (1974) Serum and intestinal fluid immunoglobulins in patients with giardiasis. *American Journal of Digestive Diseases*, **19**, 791–796.

Jones, V. E. & Ogilvie, B. M. (1971) Protective immunity to *Nippostrongylus brasiliensis*. The sequence of events which expels worms from the rat intestine. *Immunology*, **20**, 549–561.

Jones, V. E. & Ogilvie, B. M. (1972) Protective immunity to *Nippostrongylus brasiliensis* in the rat. III. Modulation of worm acetylcholinesterase by antibodies. *Immunology*, **22**, 119–129.

Jones, V. E., Edwards, A. J. & Ogilvie, B. M. (1970) The circulating immunoglobulins involved in protective immunity to the intestinal stage of *Nippostrongylus brasiliensis* in the rat. *Immunology*, **18**, 621–633.

Joyner, L. P. & Norton, C. C. (1973) The immunity arising from continuous low-level infection with *Eimeria tenella*. *Parasitology*, **67**, 333–340.

Kacker, P. P. (1973) A case of *Giardia lamblia* proctitis presenting in a V.D. clinic. *British Journal of Venereal Diseases*, **49**, 318–319.

Kamath, K. R. & Murugasu, R. (1974) A comparative study of four methods for detecting *Giardia lamblia* in children with diarrhoeal disease and malabsorption. *Gastroenterology*, **66**, 16–21.

Kanani, S. R. & Knight, R. (1969) Relapsing amoebic colitis

of 12 years standing exacerbated by corticosteroids. *British Medical Journal*, **ii**, 613–614.

Kean, B. H. (1976) Veneral amebiasis. *New York State Journal of Medicine*, **76**, 930–931.

Keller, R. & Keist, R. (1972) Protective immunity to *Nippostrongylus brasiliensis* in the rat. Central role of the lymphocyte in worm expulsion. *Immunology*, **22**, 767–773.

Kessel, J. F., Lewis, W. P., Ma, S. & Kim, H. (1961) Preliminary report on a hemagglutination test for Entamoeba. *Proceedings of the Society of Experimental Biology and Medicine, New York*, **106**, 409–413.

Kessell, J. F., Lewis, W. P., Pasquel, C. M. & Turner, J. A. (1965) Indirect hemagglutination and complement fixation tests in amoebiasis. *American Journal of Tropical Medicine and Hygiene*, **14**, 540–550.

Khan, Z. A. & Meerovitch, E. (1970) Studies on the purification of *Entamoeba histolytica* antigens by gel filtration. I. Some physicochemical properties of the isolated fractions. *Canadian Journal of Microbiology*, **16**, 485–492.

Kidney, W. & Holland, P. D. J. (1967) Giardiasis in children. *Journal of the Irish Medical Association*, **60**, 375–381.

Kojima, S., Yokogawa, M. & Tada, T. (1972) Raised levels of serum IgE in human helminthiases. *American Journal of Tropical Medicine and Hygiene*, **21**, 913–918.

Krupp, I. M. (1974) Protective immunity to amebic infection demonstrated in guinea pigs. *American Journal of Tropical Medicine and Hygiene*, **23**, 355–360.

Krupp, I. M. & Powell, S. J. (1971a) Antibody response to invasive amebiasis in Durban, South Africa. *American Journal of Tropical Medicine and Hygiene*, **20**, 414–420.

Krupp, I. M. & Powell, S. J. (1971b) Comparative study of the antibody response in amebiasis. Persistence after successful treatment. *American Journal of Tropical Medicine and Hygiene*, **20**, 421–424.

Larsh, J. E. & Weatherly, N. F. (1974) Cell-mediated immunity in certain parasitic infections. *Current Topics in Microbiology and Immunology*, **67**, 113–137.

Larsh, J. E., Goulson, H. T. & Weatherly, N. F. (1964a) Studies on delayed (cellular) hypersensitivity in mice infected with *Trichinella spiralis*. I. Transfer of lymph node cells. *Journal of the Elisha Mitchell Scientific Society*, **80**, 133–135.

Larsh, J. E., Goulson, H. T. & Weatherly, N. F. (1964b) Studies on delayed (cellular) hypersensitivity in mice infected with *Trichinella spiralis*. II. Transfer of peritoneal exudate cells. *Journal of Parasitology*, **50**, 496–498.

Larsh, J. E., Jr, Goulson, H. T., Weatherly, N. F. & Chaffee, E. F. (1969) Studies on delayed (cellular) hypersensitivity in mice infected with *Trichinella spiralis*. IV. Artificial sensitisation of donors. *Journal of Parasitology*, **55**, 726–729.

Larsh, J. E., Jr, Goulson, H. T., Weatherly, N. F. & Chaffee, E. F. (1970a) Studies on delayed (cellular) hypersensitivity in mice infected with *Trichinella spiralis*. V. Tests in recipients injected with donor spleen cells 1, 3, 7, 14 or 21 days before infection. *Journal of Parasitology*, **56**, 978–981.

Larsh, J. E., Jr, Goulson, H. T., Weatherly, N. F. & Chaffee, E. F. (1970b) Studies on delayed (cellular) hypersensitivity in mice infected with *Trichinella spiralis*. VI. Results in recipients injected with antiserum or 'freeze-thaw' spleen cells. *Journal of Parasitology*, **56**, 1206–1209.

Larsh, J. E., Jr, Race, G. J., Goulson, H. T. & Weatherly,

N. F. (1966) Studies on delayed (cellular) hypersensitivity in mice infected with *Trichinella spiralis*. III. Serologic and histopathologic findings in recipients given peritoneal exudate cells. *Journal of Parasitology*, **52**, 146–156.

Levine, N. D. (1963) Coccidiosis. *Annual Reviews in Microbiology*, **17**, 179–198.

Lewis, E. A. & Antia, A. U. (1969) Amoebic colitis: review of 295 cases. *Transactions of the Royal Society of Tropical Medicine and Hygiene*, **63**, 633–638.

Louch, C. D. (1962) Increased resistance to *Trichinella spiralis* in the laboratory rat following infection with *Nippostrongylus muris*. *Journal of Parasitology*, **48**, 24–26.

McClelland, D. B. L., Warwick, R. R. G. & Sheerman, D. J. C. (1973) IgA concentration. *American Journal of Digestive Diseases*, **18**, 347–348.

McGowan, J. M., Nussbaum, C. C. & Burroughs, E. W. (1948) Cholecystitis due to *Giardia lamblia* in a left-sided gall bladder. *Annals of Surgery*, **128**, 1032–1037.

Maddison, S. E. (1965) Characterisation of *Entamoeba histolytica* antigen–antibody reaction by gel diffusion. *Experimental Parasitology*, **16**, 224–235.

Maddison, S. E., Kagan, I. G. & Elsdon-Dew, R. (1968) Comparison of intradermal and serologic tests for the diagnosis of amebiasis. *American Journal of Tropical Medicine and Hygiene*, **17**, 540–547.

Maddison, S. E., Kagan, I. G. & Norman, L. (1968) Reactivity of human immunoglobulins in amebiasis. *Journal of Immunology*, **100**, 217–226.

Maddison, S. E., Powell, S. J. & Elsdon-Dew, R. (1965) Comparison of hemagglutinins and precipitins in amebiasis. *American Journal of Tropical Medicine and Hygiene*, **14**, 551–557.

Mahmoud, A. A. F. & Warren, K. S. (1975) Algorithms in the diagnosis and management of exotic disease. II. Giardiasis. *Journal of Infectious Diseases*, **131**, 621–624.

Manzo, N. T., Castenda, M. & Chevez, A. (1974) Ultramicroscopic study of membranolysis induced by immune serum in *E. histolytica*. *Archivos de Investigaçion Medica Mexico*, **5**, 2, 325–330.

Matsubayashi, H. & Nozawa, T. (1948) Experimental infection of *Isospora hominis* in man. *American Journal of Tropical Medicine and Hygiene*, **28**, 633–637.

Mauss, E. A. (1941) Serum fraction with which anti-trichinella (*Trichinella spiralis*) antibody is associated. *American Journal of Hygiene*, **34D**, 73–80.

Mayrhofer, G., Bazin, H. & Gowans, J. L. (1976) Nature of cells binding anti-IgE in rats immunised with *Nippostrongylus brasiliensis*: IgE synthesis in regional nodes and concentration in mucosal mast cells. *European Journal of Immunology*, **6**, 537–545.

Michaels, D. L., Go, S., Humbert, J. R., Dubois, R. S., Stewart, J. M. & Ellis, E. F. (1971) Intestinal nodular lymphoid hyperplasia, hypergammaglobulinaemia and haematologic abnormalities in a child with a ring 18 chromosome. *Journal of Pediatrics*, **79**, 80–88.

Miller, M. J. & Scott, F. (1970) The intradermal reaction in amebiasis. *Canadian Medical Association Journal*, **103**, 253–257.

Mills, C. K. & Kent, N. H. (1965) Excretions and secretions of *Trichinella spiralis* and their role in immunity. *Experimental Parasitology*, **16**, 300–310.

Morelki, R. & Parker, J. G. (1967) Ultrastructural studies of the human *Giardia lamblia* and subjacent jejunal mucosa in a subject with steatorrhoea. *Gastroenterology*, **52**, 151–164.

Mulligan, W. (1968) Immunity to intestinal helminths: the 'self-cure' reaction. In *Immunity to Parasites*, ed. Taylor,

A. E. R., pp. 51–54, 6th Symposium of the British Society for Parasitology. Oxford: Blackwell Scientific Publications.

Murray, M. (1972) Immediate hypersensitivity effector mechanisms. II. In vivo reactions. In *Immunity to Animal Parasites*, ed. Soulsby, E. J. L., pp. 155–190. New York: Academic Press.

Murray, M., Jarrett, W. F. H. & Jennings, F. W. (1971) Mast cells and macromolecular leak in intestinal immunological reactions. The influence of sex of rats infected with *Nippostrongylus brasiliensis*. *Immunology*, **21**, 17–31.

Murray, M., Miller, H. R. P., Sanford, J. & Jarrett, W. F. H. (1971) 5-hydroxytryptamine in intestinal immunological reactions. Its relationship to mast cell activity and worm expulsion in rats infected with *Nippostrongylus brasiliensis*. *International Archives of Allergy and Applied Immunology*, **40**, 236–247.

Nime, F. A., Burek, J. D., Page, D. L., Holscher, M. A. & Yardley, J. H. (1976) Acute enterocolitis in a human being infected with the protozoan Cryptosporidium. *Gastroenterology*, **70**, 592–598.

Ochs, H. D., Ament, M. E. & Davis, S. D. (1972) Giardiasis with malabsorption in X-linked agammaglobulinaemia. *New England Journal of Medicine*, **287**, 341–342.

Ogilvie, B. M. (1964) Reagin-like antibodies in animals immune to helminth parasites. *Nature*, **204**, 91.

Ogilvie, B. M. (1967) Reagin-like antibodies in rats infected with the nematode parasite *Nippostrongylus brasiliensis*. *Immunology*, **12**, 113–131.

Ogilvie, B. M. (1973) In *Parasites in the Immunised Host: Mechanisms of Survival*. *Discussion*, p. 91, CIBA Foundation Symposium 25 (New Series). Amsterdam: Elsevier.

Ogilvie, B. M. & Jones, V. E. (1967) Reaginic antibodies and immunity to *Nippostrongylus brasiliensis* in the rat. I. The effect of thymectomy, neonatal infections and splenectomy. *Parasitology*, **57**, 335–349.

Ogilvie, B. M. & Jones, V. E. (1969) Reaginic antibodies and helminth infections. In *Cellular and Humoral Mechanisms in Anaphylaxis and Allergy*, ed. Movat, H. Z., pp. 13–22. Basel: Karger.

Ogilvie, B. M. & Jones, V. E. (1971) Parasitological review. *Nippostrongylus brasiliensis*. A review of immunity and host–parasite relationship in the rat. *Experimental Parasitology*, **29**, 138–177.

Ogilvie, B. M. & Jones, V. E. (1973) Immunity in the parasitic relationship between helminths and hosts. *Progress in Allergy*, **17**, 93–144.

Ogilivie, B. M. & Love, R. J. (1974) Co-operation between antibodies and cells in immunity to a nematode parasite. *Transplantation Reviews*, **19**, 147–168.

Ogilvie, B. M. & Worms, M. J. (1976) Immunity to nematode parasites. In *Immunology of Parasitic Infections*, ed. Cohen, S. & Sadun, E. Oxford: Blackwell Scientific Publications.

Ohtaki, M., Michimata, Y., Susuki, T., Oikawa, K., Mikami, M., Onodera, S. & Yoshinaga, K. (1976) Malignant lymphoma initiated with malabsorption syndrome due to *Isospara belli* infection and lymphocytosis. *Tohoku Journal of Experimental Medicine*, **120**, 43–52.

Orange, R. P., Stechschulte, D. J. & Austen, K. F. (1970) Immunochemical and biologic properties of rat IgE. II. Capacity to mediate the immunologic release of histamine and slow-reacting substance of anaphylaxis (SRS-A). *Journal of Immunology*, **105**, 1087–1095.

Orr, T. S. & Blair, A. M. (1969) Potentiated reagin response to egg albumin and conalbumin in *Nippostrongylus brasiliensis* infected rats. *Life Science*, **8**, 1073–1077.

Ortiz-Ortiz, L., Sepulvada, B. & Chevez, A. (1974) New studies on normal and immune human serum action on trophozoites of *E. histolytica*. *Archivos de Investigaçion Medica Mexico*, **5**, 2, 337–342.

Ortiz-Ortiz, L., Zamacona-Ravelo, G. & Capin, N. R. (1974) Cellular hypersensitivity in Amoebiasis. III. *In vitro* effect of Concanavalin A and amoebic antigen on peripheral leukocytes from patients with amoebic liver abscess. *Archivos de Investigaçion Medica Mexico*, **5**, 2, 481–486.

Ortiz-Ortiz, L., Garmilla, C., Zamacona-Ravelo, G. & Sepulvada, B. (1973) Cellular hypersensitivity in amebiasis. II. A study of patients with acute amebic abscess of the liver. *Archivos de Investigaçion Medica Mexico*, **4**, 1, 191–196.

Ortiz-Ortiz, L., Zamacona-Ravelo, G., Sepulvada, B. & Capin, N. R. (1975) Cell-mediated immunity in patients with amoebic abscess of the liver. *Clinical Immunology and Immunopathology*, **4**, 127–134.

O'Shea del Socorro, M. & Feria-Velasco, A. (1974) Ultramicroscopic demonstration of surface antigens in trophozoites of *E. histolytica*. I. Immunofluorescence with human specific IgG. *Archivos de Investigaçion Medica Mexico*, **5**, 2, 307–314.

Petersen, H. (1972) Giardiasis (Lambliasis). *Scandinavian Journal of Gastroenterology*, **7**, 14, 1–44.

Pritchard, D. I. (1977) 'Immunity and acquired resistance to trichinosis.' Unpublished Ph.D. Thesis, University of Birmingham.

Radermecker, M., Bekhti, A., Poncelot, E. & Salmon, J. (1974) Serum IgE levels in protozoal and helminthic infections. *International Archives of Allergy and Applied Immunology*, **47**, 285–295.

Ramamurti, D. V. & Stickl, H. Amoebiasis and the *Entamoeba histolytica*. *Infection*, **1**, 92–97.

Remington, J. S. & Krahenbuhl, J. L. (1976) Immunology of Toxoplasma infection. In *Immunology of Parasitic Infections*, ed. Cohen, S. and Sadun, E., pp. 235–267. Oxford. Blackwell Scientific Publications.

Rendtorff, R. C. (1954a) The experimental transmission of human intestinal protozoan parasites. II. *Giardia lamblia* cysts given in capsules. *American Journal of Hygiene*, **59**, 209–220.

Rendtorff, R. C. (1954b) The experimental transmission of human intestinal protozoan parasites. III. Attempts to transmit *Endamoeba coli* and *Giardia lamblia* cysts by flies. *American Journal of Hygiene*, **60**, 320–326.

Rendtorff, R. C. (1954c) The experimental transmission of human intestinal protozoan parasites. IV. Attempts to transmit *Endamoeba coli* and *Giardia lamblia* by water. *American Journal of Hygiene*, **60**, 327–338.

Rhodes, M. B., Marsh, C. L. & Kelley, G. W., Jr, (1964) Studies in helminth enzymology. III. Malic dehydrogenases of *Ascaris suum*. *Experimental Parasitology*, **15**, 403–409.

Rhodes, M. B., Nayak, D. P., Kelley, G. W., Jr, & Marsh, C. L. (1965) Studies in helminth enzymology. IV. Immune responses to malic dehydrogenase from *Ascaris suum*. *Experimental Parasitology*, **16**, 373–381.

Ridley, M. J. & Ridley, D. S. (1976) Serum antibodies and jejunal histology in giardiasis associated with malabsorption. *Journal of Clinical Pathology*, **29**, 30–34.

Roberts-Thomson, I. C., Grove, D. I., Stevens, D. P. & Warren, K. S. (1976) Suppression of giardiasis during the intestinal phase of trichinosis in the mouse. *Gut*, **17**, 953–958.

Roberts-Thomson, I. C., Stevens, D. P., Mahmoud, A. A. F. & Warren, K. S. (1977) Acquired resistance to infection in an animal model of giardiasis. *Journal of Immunology*, **117**, 2036–2037.

Rommel, M. & Heydorn, A. O. (1971) Veisuche zur Uberragung der Immunität gegen *Eimeria*-Infektionen durch Lymphozyten. *Zeitschrift Parasitenkd*, **36**, 242–250.

Rose, M. E. (1959) Serological reactions in *Eimeria stiedae* infection of the rabbit. *Immunology*, **2**, 112–122.

Rose, M. E. (1971a) In *Poultry Diseases and World Economics*. 7th British Egg Marketing Board Symposium, pp. 93–108.

Rose, M. E. (1971b) Immunity to coccidiosis: protective effect of transferred serum in *Eimeria maxima* infections. *Parasitology*, **62**, 11–25.

Rose, M. E. (1972) Immune response to intracellular parasites. II. Coccidia. In *Immunity to Animal Parasites*, ed. Soulsby, E. J. L., pp. 365–388. New York: Academic Press.

Rose, M. E. (1973) In *The Coccidia*, pp. 295–341. Baltimore: University Park Press.

Rose, M. E. (1974a) Immune responses in infections with coccidia: macrophage activity. *Infection and Immunity*, **10**, 862–871.

Rose, M. E. (1974b) The early development of immunity to *Eimeria maxima* in comparison with that to *Eimeria tenella*. *Parasitology*, **68**, 35–45.

Rose, M. E. (1974c) Protective antibodies in infections with *Eimeria maxima*: the reduction of pathogenic effects *in vivo* and a comparison between oral and subcutaneous administration of antiserum. *Parasitology*, **68**, 285–292.

Rose, M. E. & Long, P. L. (1971) Immunity to coccidiosis: protective effects of transferred serum and cells investigated in chick embryos infected with *Eimeria tenella*. *Parasitology*, **63**, 299–313.

Rose, M. E., Long, P. L. & Bradley, J. W. A. (1975) Immune responses to infections with coccidia in chickens: gut hypersensitivity. *Parasitology*, **71**, 357–368.

Roth, H. (1941) The *in vitro* action of trichina larvae in immune serum – a new precipitin test in trichinosis. *Acta Pathologica et Microbiologica Scandinavia*, **18**, 160–167.

Rothwell, T. L. W., Dineen, J. K. & Love, R. J. (1971) The role of pharmacologically active amines in resistance to *Trichostrongylus colubriformis* in the guinea-pig. *Immunology*, **21**, 925–938.

Rothwell, T. L. W., Prichard, R. K. & Love, R. J. (1974) Studies on the role of histamine and 5-hydroxytryptamine in immunity against the nematode *Trichostrongylus colubriformis*. I. *In vivo* and *in vitro* effects of the amines. *International Archives of Allergy and Applied Immunology*, **46**, 1–13.

Ruitenberg, E. J. & Elgersma, A. (1976) Absence of intestinal mast cell response in congenitally athymic mice during *Trichinella spiralis* infection. *Nature*, **264**, 258–260.

Sadun, E. H. (1972) Homocytotropic antibody response to parasitic infections. In *Immunity to Animal Parasites* ed. Soulsby, E. J. L., pp. 97–129. New York: Academic Press.

Sadun, E. H. (1976) The life cycles of common parasites of medical importance. In *Immunology of Parasitic Infections*, ed. Cohen, S. & Sadun, E. H., pp. 469–480. Oxford: Blackwell Scientific Publications.

Sarles, M. P. & Taliaferro, W. H. (1936) The local points of defence and the passive transfer of acquired immunity to *Nippostrongylus muris* in rats. *Journal of Infectious Diseases*, 59, 207–220.

Savanat, T., Viriyanond, P. & Nimitmongkol, N. (1973) Blast transformation of lymphocytes in amebiasis. *American Journal of Tropical Medicine and Hygiene*, 22, 705–710.

Sepulvada, B., Tanimoto-Leki, M. & de la Hoz, C. P. R. (1974) Antiamebic passive immunity induction in hamster with immune serum injection. *Archivos de Investigaçion Medica Mexico*, 5, 2, 451–456.

Sepulvada, B., Tanimoto-Leki, M., & de la Torre, C. P. M. (1974) Virulence of *E. histolytica* culture neutralised with immune serum. *Archivos de Investigaçion Medica Mexico*, 5, 2, 447–450.

Solis, A. C., Feria, A. J. M., Martinez, J. M., Ortiz, L. A. T. & Sanchez, F. S. (1975) Immunological status of patients with amebic hepatic abscess. *Prensa Medica Mexicana*, 40, 275–281.

Soulsby, E. J. L. (1972) Cell mediated immunity responses in parasitic infections. In *Immunity to Animal Parasites*, ed. Soulsby, E. J. L., pp. 57–95. New York: Academic Press.

Soulsby, E. J. L. & Stewart, D. F. (1959) Serological studies of the self-cure reaction in sheep infected with *Haemonchus contortus*. *Australian Journal of Agricultural Research*, 11, 595.

Sprent, J. F. A. (1959) Parasitism, immunity and evolution. In *The Evolution of Living Organisms* ed. Leeper, G. S., pp. 149–165. Melbourne: Melbourne University Press.

Stamm, W. P., Ashley, M. J. & Bell, K. (1976) The value of amoebic serology in an area of low endemicity. *Transactions of the Royal Society of Tropical Medicine and Hygiene*, 70, 49–53.

Stefanski, W. & Malczewski, A. (1972) Specificity of migration inhibition test in parasitic invasions. II. Studies on *Trichinella spiralis*. *Bulletin de l'Académie Polonaise des Sciences*, Class II, Série des Sciences Biologique, 20, 261–262.

Stewart, D. F. (1953) Studies on resistance of sheep to infestation with *Haemonchus contortus* and *Trichostrongylus* spp. and on the immunological reactions of sheep exposed to infestation. V. The nature of the 'self-cure' phenomenon. *Australian Journal of Agricultural Research*, 4, 100–117.

Stewart, D. F. (1955) 'Self-cure' in nematode infestations of sheep. *Nature*, 176, 1273–1274.

Stoll, N. R. (1929) Studies with strongyloid nematode, *Haemonchus contortus*. Acquired resistance of hosts under natural reinfection conditions out-of-doors. *American Journal of Hygiene*, 10, 384–418.

Swartzwelder, J. C. & Avant, W. H. (1952) Immunity to amebic infection in dogs. *American Journal of Tropical Medicine and Hygiene*, 1, 567–575.

Swartzwelder, J. C. & Müller, G. R. (1950) A comparison of the infection rate and gross pathology of amebic infection in normal and antigen-injected rats. *American Journal of Tropical Medicine and Hygiene*, 30, 181–183.

Tada, T. & Ishizaka, K. (1970) Distribution of γE-forming cells in lymphoid tissues of the human and monkey. *Journal of Immunology*, 104, 377–387.

Takeuchi, A. & Phillips, B. P. (1976) Electron microscopic studies of experimental *Entamaeba histolytica* infection in the guinea pig. *Virchows Archives B. Cell Pathology*, 20, 1–13.

Taliaferro, W. H. & Sarles, M. P. (1939) The cellular reactions in the skin, lungs, and intestine of normal and immune rats after infection with *Nippostrongylus muris*. *Journal of Infectious Diseases*, 64, 157–192.

Thomas, G. E., Goldsmid, J. M. & Wicks, A. C. B. (1974) Use of the Enterotest duodenal capsule in the diagnosis of giardiases: a preliminary study. *South African Medical Journal*, 48, 2219–2220.

Thorson, R. E. (1953) Studies on the mechanism of immunity in the rat to the nematode *Nippostrongylus muris*. *American Journal of Hygiene*, 58, 1–15.

Thorson, R. E. (1954a) Effect of immune serum for rats on infective larvae of *Nippostrongylus muris*. *Experimental Parasitology*, 3, 9–15.

Thorson, R. E. (1954b) Absorption of protective antibodies from serum of rats immune to the nematode, *Nippostrongylus muris*. *Journal of Parasitology*, 40, 300–303.

Thorson, R. E. (1956a) Proteolytic activity in extracts of the esophagus of adults of *Ancylostoma caninum* and the effect of immune serum on this activity. *Journal of Parasitology*, 42, 21–25.

Thorson, R. E. (1956b) The stimulation of acquired immunity in dogs by injections of extracts of the esophagus of adult hookworms. *Journal of Parasitology*, 42, 501–504.

Thorson, R. E. (1963) Seminar on immunity to parasitic helminths. II. Physiology of immunity to helminth infections. *Experimental Parasitology*, 13, 3–12.

Thorson, R. E. (1970) Direct infection nematodes. In *Immunity to Parasitic Animals* ed. Jackson, G. J., Herman, R. & Singer, I., pp. 913–962. New York: Appleton-Century-Crofts.

Trier, J. S., Moxey, P. C., Schimmel, E. M. & Robles, E. (1974) Chronic intestinal coccidiosis in man: intestinal morphology and response to treatment. *Gastroenterology*, 66, 923–935.

Urquhart, G. M., Mulligan, W., Eadie, R. M. & Jennings, F. W. (1965) Immunological studies on *Nippostrongylus brasiliensis* infection in the rat: the role of local anaphylaxis. *Experimental Parasitology*, 17, 210–217.

Wagland, B. M. & Dineen, J. K. (1965) The cellular transfer of immunity to *Trichostrongylus colubriformis* in an isogenic strain of guinea pig. *Australian Journal of Experimental Biology and Medical Science*, 43, 429–438.

Webster, A. D. B. (1976) The gut and immunodeficiency disorders. *Clinics in Gastroenterology*, 5, 2, 323–340.

Webster, B. H. (1958) Human infection with *Giardia lamblia*. An analysis of 32 cases. *American Journal of Digestive Diseases*, 3, 64–71.

Webster, B. M. (1957) Human Isospariasis: a report of three cases with necropsy findings of one case. *American Journal of Tropical Medicine and Hygiene*, 6, 86–89.

Wells, P. D. (1962) Mast cell, eosinophil and histamine levels in *Nippostrongylus brasiliensis* – infected rats. *Experimental Parasitology*, 12, 82–101.

Whur, P. (1966) Relationship of globule leucocytes to gastrointestinal nematodes in the sheep, and *Nippostrongylus brasiliensis* and *Hymenolepis nana* infections in rats. *Journal of Comparative Pathology*, 76, 57–65.

Whur, P. (1967) Globule leucocyte response in hyperimmune rats infected with *Nippostrongylus brasiliensis*. *Journal of Comparative Pathology*, 77, 271–277.

Wilhelm, R. E. (1957) Urticaria associated with giardiasis lamblia. *Journal of Allergy*, 28, 351–353.

Willcox, M. (1975) Giardiasis in families. *British Medical Journal*, iii, 101.

Wilson, R. J. M. & Block, K. J. (1968) Homocytotropic antibody response in the rat infected with the nematode *Nippostrongylus brasiliensis*. II. Characteristics of the immune response. *Journal of Immunology*, **100**, 622–628.

Wilson, R. J. M., Jones, V. E. & Leskowitz, S. (1967) Thymectomy and anaphylactic antibody in rats infected with *Nippostrongylus brasiliensis*. *Nature*, **213**, 398–399.

Zvaifler, N. J. (1976) Immediate hypersensitivity (Type I) reactions. In *Immunology of Parasitic Infections*, ed. Cohen, S. & Sadun, E. H., pp. 409–430. Oxford: Blackwell Scientific Publications.

Zvaifler, N. J., Sadun, E. H. & Becker, E. L. (1966) Anaphylactic (reaginic) antibodies in helminthic infections. *Clinical Research*, **14**, 336.

14. Immunobiology of the alimentary tract in relation to oral immuno-prophylaxis against enteric infections in the piglet and calf

P. Porter

INTRODUCTION

The major incentives behind research into enteric diseases in farm animals are economic. Thus over the past 25 years approximately 20 per cent of pigs born in the United Kingdom and United States have died before reaching weaning age (cited by Moon, 1969). Gastrointestinal disorders are especially common with many deaths occurring from *Escherichia coli* (*E. coli*) infection (Sojka, 1973), and transmissible gastroenteritis (TGE). The latter has a mortality approaching 100 per cent in pigs under 7 days of age though older pigs are not seriously affected (Bohl, 1973). In older animals *E. coli* associated enteric syndromes cause major concern, producing poor animal nutrition rather than death.

The mechanisms of local immunity have received increasing attention because of their prospective role in vaccination against infectious agents that invade mucous surfaces. The intestinal mucosa is bathed throughout life by liberal supplies of immunoglobulins which are either of maternal origin or synthesized locally in the lamina propria. The maternal source is of major importance to those species which have an epitheliochorial placentation. This interposes several layers of epithelium between maternal and foetal circulations, so obstructing the transport of immunoglobulins. The porcine and bovine species along with other ruminants and equines fall into this category, and were it not for the transfer of specific antibodies to the neonatal offspring in the colostrum, death from rampant infection would usually be their fare in a conventional farm environment.

The purpose of this chapter is to describe concepts which are fundamental to an appreciation of immunity to enteric infection in young animals. The two species under consideration, the pig and the calf, show interesting differences in lactation, digestive physiology and nutrition; thus they provide a basis for interesting comparative studies in immunobiology of the alimentary tract.

PASSIVE AND ACTIVE IMMUNOGLOBULIN MECHANISMS IN THE ALIMENTARY TRACT

CLASSES OF IMMUNOGLOBULIN IN MAJOR FARM SPECIES

The isolation of specific immunoglobulins in mammals has been undertaken only in recent years. Vaerman,

Heremans and Van Kerckhoven (1969) exploited immunological cross-reactivity as a simple tool to establish the presence of IgA analogues in numerous species. In studies of the comparative antigenicity of γ-chains, Esteves and Binaghi (1972) were able to identify several determinants on the γ-chains, some of which were unique to the species concerned, whilst others were shared with other animals. In the avian species, however, IgG failed to show any similar antigenic determinants to those identified in the mammal. The current knowledge concerning the relationship between immunoglobulin classes in the major domestic species

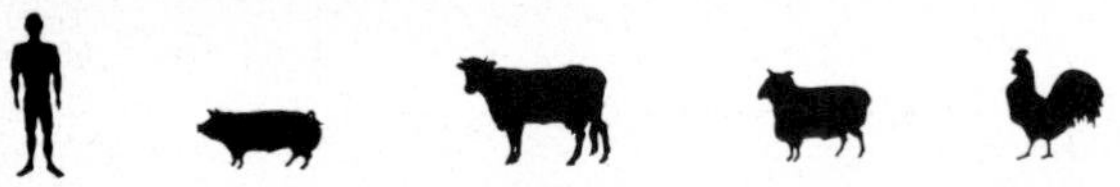

IgM	H	H	H	H
IgG	H	H	H	A
IgA	H	H	H	A
IgE	A	A	A	ND
IgD	ND	ND	ND	ND

H.   Homologous – cross reaction with human Ig heavy chains

A.   Analagous – similar physiochemical and biological parameters to human Ig's

ND   Not Demonstrated.

Fig. 14.1 Immunochemical and physicochemical characterization of immunoglobulin classes in farm domestic species.

and those identified in man is summarized in Figure 14.1.

With respect to secretory immunoglobulins, secretory IgA in the porcine and bovine species show structural similarities to human 11S IgA. There are numerous reports describing the isolation and molecular characteristics of secretory 11S IgA in the bovine (Mach, Pahud and Isliker, 1969; Porter and Noakes, 1970; Butler and Maxwell, 1972; Duncan, Wilkie and Winter, 1972) and also in the pig (Bourne, 1969; Porter, 1969a; Richardson and Kelleher, 1970; Porter, 1971a; Saif, Bohl and Gupta, 1972; Svendsen and Bienenstock, 1972). There is evidence of immunologic cross-reactivity with human α-chain, and furthermore the classic spur between precipitin lines in immunodiffusion of human 11S IgA and serum IgA characteristic of secretory component (Tomasi, Tan, Solomon and Prendergast, 1965; South *et al.*, 1966) has also been shown in the pig and cow. Thus in these respects there is total analogy with the human immunoglobulin. Finally, the molecular assembly, comprising secretory component, j-chains, α-chains and light chains, and the sites of localization of these constituent chains in the intestinal mucosa have been described for the pig (Allen and Porter, 1973a) and the calf (Porter, Noakes and Allen, 1972).

MATERNAL IMMUNOGLOBULINS AND PASSIVE IMMUNITY IN THE NEONATE

(i) Absorption and proteolysis of antibodies in the alimentary tract

Studies of blood serum from neonatal pigs and calves show no appreciable transmission of immunoglobulins from maternal to foetal circulations by any route other than intestinal absorption of suckled colostrum post partum. At birth the pig possesses a low molecular weight component belonging to the IgG class (Sterzl, Kostka, Řiha and Mandel, 1960) which is considered to be synthesized by the foetus (Prokešová, Kostka, Rejnek and Trávníček, 1970). The capacity to synthesize immunoglobulins is well developed in the last 3 to 4 weeks of foetal life (Binns, 1967) and this peculiar IgG in neonatal and germ-free serum might be associated with metabolic processes resulting in the release of immune receptors from lymphocyte membranes. The component is present in concentrations less than $50 \mu g/ml$ (Franěk, Řiha and Šterzl, 1961; Porter, 1969a) and although some antibacterial activity has been attributed to it (Porter and Hill, 1970), it is unlikely to play a significant role in neonatal defence compared with the levels of maternal antibody acquired from the colostrum.

The absorption of maternal immunoglobulins is of fundamental importance to survival. However, intestinal permeability to colostral antibodies in the pig and calf lasts only 24 to 36 hours. Most of the passive immunity is acquired during the first few hours of life and the efficiency of absorption, particularly in the pig, decreases very rapidly, having a half life of about 3 hours (Speer, Brown, Quinn and Catron, 1959). In the calf, the period of permeability may differ for each immunoglobulin class (Penhale *et al.*, 1973); thus IgG is absorbed for only 27 hours, IgA for 22 hours and IgM for 16 hours post partum.

The period of absorption may be curtailed by the onset of protein digestion (Hill, 1956; Deutsch and Smith, 1957; Chamberlain, Perry and Jones, 1965). However, this thesis may not be tenable since the absorption of polyvinyl pyrolidone (PVP) by the pig (Lecce, Matrone and Morgan, 1961) and calf (Hardy, 1969b) ceases at the same time as that of protein. Since PVP is not degraded by the digestive processes, it would seem that the reason for cessation of absorption of protein is not attributable simply to proteolysis.

Proteolytic activity in the gastrointestinal tract of the neonate must prejudice the absorption of antibody during the restricted period when this can take place. Immunoglobulin degradation in the alimentary tract of the pig can be extensive; far greater than in comparable studies of the calf (Hardy, 1969a). For example, the greater part of a saline solution of IgG administered to newborn pigs was split and after absorption the fragments were excreted in the urine. However, there is present in the colostrum of the sow high levels of a trypsin inhibitor which assists in the protection of antibodies against digestion. The colostral trypsin inhibitor is resistant to acid and pepsin and facilitates the absorption of antibodies in a biologically active form (Laskowski, Kassell and Hagerty, 1957). In the human species, where there is no transfer of immunoglobulin post partum, there are negligible levels of this component in the colostrum. If it is to be construed that lack of requirement for such a function can be correlated with virtual absence of the active component, then it is interesting that the level of the trypsin inhibitor in bovine colostrum is virtually one-tenth of that in pig colostrum. Nevertheless, only low levels of proteolytic enzyme activity are demonstrable in gastrointestinal secretions and tissue homogenates of the calf. Furthermore the pH of the abomasal contents is sufficiently high to restrict the extent of proteolysis due to pepsin and rennin (Pierce, 1962). Thus it is difficult to reconcile the view that trypsin inhibitor is important for the absorption of intact protein in the calf, but its importance in the young pig seems to be well established in that simultaneous peroral administration of the inhibitor substantially improves the absorption of intact antibody (Laskowski *et al.*, 1957; Nordbring and Olsson, 1958; Hardy, 1969a).

In studies of the changing pattern of protease development and decline of trypsin inhibitor in suckling piglets, Bainter (1973) reiterated the earlier concept that cessation of protein absorption was related to the start of protein digestion. Lecce (1966) suggested that cessation of macromolecular absorption, 'closure', was a function of the feeding regime; closure activity was associated with the amount of protein ingested and, surprisingly, also glucose. Piglets which ate more than 300 mEq of glucose showed accelerated 'closure' in the period 18 to 24 hours, suggesting that the pinocytotic capacity of the neonatal gut can be non-specifically stimulated with loss of available surface membrane for invagination. It is also significant that El Nageh (1970) found absorption in the calf to terminate because the population of epithelial cells present in the small intestine at birth were replaced by a first generation of new cells which were unable to absorb macromolecules. In summary, the views on 'closure' may be reconciled in that proteolytic mechanisms, exhaustion of pinocytotic capability, and cell replacement may all occur during a short period of time, with each having a significant role to play.

(ii) Local synthesis and transudation of immunoglobulins in mammary secretions

Approximately 80 per cent of the colostral immunoglobulin in the sow and the cow is accounted for by IgG. The selective transfer of IgG_1 to the bovine mammary secretions is apparently a unique characteristic of the ruminant species (Butler, 1969, 1971). In the sow, however, this immunophysiologic process is not operative (Porter, 1969a; Curtis and Bourne, 1971) and the major immunoglobulin class in the mammary secretions is IgG_2. The colostrum of both species is therefore mainly derived as a transudate from the serum and is not a true secretion. In the bovine it seems that at least during colostrum formation, IgA probably derives mainly from the mammary tissues (Porter, 1971b). The contribution of serum immunoglobulin to the colostrum in the sow has been evaluated using radio labelling techniques, and only 40 per cent of the IgA in colostrum derives as a transudate from the serum (Bourne and Curtis, 1973) and a substantial contribution must be made by local synthesis in the mammary tissues.

The failure of IgA to predominate in the colostrum of the pig and the cow, as it does in the human, is understandable in terms of the universal role of IgG for passive immunity. However, there are significantly contrasting features revealed in the change of immunoglobulin profile in the mammary secretions of these species as lactation progresses. In both species the total concentration of immunoglobulin falls dramatically during the first few days of lactation – a necessary economy in maternal immunoglobulins correlating with the closure in intestinal absorptive function in the suckling neonate. The physiologic requirement for transfer of maternal IgG is fulfilled within the first 24 to 36 hours. It is the rapid decline in IgG during this period which contributes most to the fall in total immunoglobulin content in the milk. In the pig, IgA emerges as the quantitatively dominant immunoglobulin in the milk (Fig. 14.2) whereas in the cow all the immunoglobulin classes decline to low levels and at no time is IgA quantitatively important (Porter, 1971b).

In the sow, almost 90 per cent of the IgA occurring in the milk and therefore most of the immunoglobulin after the first few days of lactation is synthesized locally (Bourne and Curtis, 1973). Yet in the bovine there is no evidence of plasmacytosis during lactation other than during the period of colostrum formation (Campbell, Porter and Petersen, 1950). This evidence has been

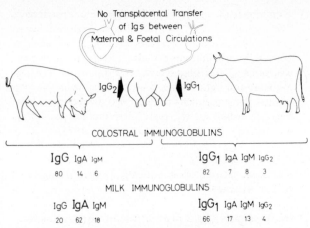

COLOSTRAL IMMUNOGLOBULINS

IgG	IgA	IgM		IgG_1	IgA	IgM	IgG_2
80	14	6		82	7	8	3

MILK IMMUNOGLOBULINS

IgG	IgA	IgM		IgG_1	IgA	IgM	IgG_2
20	62	18		66	17	13	4

Fig. 14.2 Contrasting characteristics of immunoglobulin profiles in porcine and bovine lactation showing the percentage composition of immunoglobulin classes in colostrum and milk.

supported by *in-vitro* studies of immunoglobulin synthesis using organ culture, demonstrating a state of IgA deficiency in the mammary gland, thereby accounting for the low concentration of immunoglobulin in milk throughout lactation (Butler *et al.*, 1971). This lactation anomaly appears to be a consistent feature of the ruminant species, being observed also in goats and sheep (Butler, 1974). In other herbivores such as the rabbit and horse, which rely on bacterial activity in the caecum for cellulose degradation, comparatively high levels of IgA are found in the milk (Vaerman, 1970).

(iii) Intestinal absorption of immunoglobulin classes by the neonate

Immunochemical studies of post-colostral piglet and calf serum show that IgG, IgA and IgM are absorbed from the colostrum ingested soon after birth. In many cases the immunoglobulin concentrations in neonatal serum during the first few days of life exceed the levels recorded in maternal serum. This is because the immunoglobulin levels in colostrum exceed those in the serum of the dam by as much as three- to four-fold. The pig shows some selectivity against the absorption of colostral secretory 11S IgA and the antibody function of this molecule is confined mainly to the lumen of the intestine (Porter, 1969b). In contrast the calf absorbs 11S IgA and the immunoglobulin profile of its serum becomes similar to that of the colostrum (Porter, 1972). The levels of passively acquired immunoglobulins in neonatal piglet and calf serum fall after 2 days of age. The pattern of decline is almost exponential, and half-lives of immunoglobulin classes can be calculated from assays of serum concentrations over a period of 2 to 3 weeks. In the pig precise measurements using immunoglobulins labelled with Iodine-125 have shown the mean half lives of IgM, IgA and IgG are 2.8, 2.7 and 9.1 days respectively (Curtis and Bourne, 1973).

The important protective role of maternal immunoglobulins is clearly evident in field studies with the calf where susceptibility to septicaemia caused by *E. coli* is correlated with a deficiency in absorption of maternal antibodies (Gay, Anderson, Fisher and McEwan, 1965). Logan and Penhale (1971) have evaluated the protective qualities of different immunoglobulin classes of the maternal colostrum by infection studies in neonatal calves following administration of IgG or IgM. They concluded that colostral IgM was the neonatal calf's most important survival factor.

LOCAL ALIMENTARY TRACT PROTECTION BY MATERNAL ANTIBODIES

(i) The significance of milk IgA in the pig

The importance of local antibody in the alimentary tract attributable to milk immunoglobulins is probably best demonstrated by changes which occur in serological titres of passive antibody during the first 2 weeks of life. The short half-life of passive immunity to bacterial antigens gives rise to an apparent critical antibody deficiency in the young pig during the period of 2 to 4 weeks of age (Miller *et al.*, 1962). At this time active response to common enteropathogens has failed to generate significant levels of circulating antibodies.

In sow colostrum, IgA accounts for approximately 14 per cent of the total immunoglobulin, and occurs in a molecular size range 6.4S to 18S with dimeric components in the 9S and 11S range predominating (Porter, 1969a). The low molecular weight forms which lack secretory component are probably derived from the serum by transudation across the mammary acinar epithelium (Bourne, 1973). It is these molecular classes of IgA which decline to negligible levels as lactation progresses and the total immunoglobulin profile changes. However, secretory 11S IgA, presumably synthesized in the mammary gland, is a major *E. coli* antibody in colostrum and also in milk. It contributes very little to circulatory passive immunity in the neonatal piglet and its main function appears to be the provision of local defence in the alimentary tract (Porter, 1969b; Hill and Porter, 1974).

The effectiveness of an antibody in local defence of the alimentary tract will be determined in some measure by its resistance to proteolytic degradation. An inhibitory function against enzymic cleavage of secretory IgA has been attributed to secretory component (Tomasi and Calvanico, 1968; Steward, 1971). Porcine colostral IgA shows considerably greater resistance to enzymic degradation than does IgG (Porter, 1973a). However, physiologic mechanisms probably contribute most to its effectiveness as an antibody in the intestine of the baby pig. Studies in fistulated pigs (Porter, Noakes and

Allen, 1970a) have shown that after a single feed IgA continues to pass along the intestine for more than 90 min, which is a greater period than the normal interval between suckling. Thus milk IgA provides an almost continuous coating of antibody for the small intestine. In this respect it is significant that highly effective passive immunity against enteric infections with TGE virus has been more closely associated with milk antibodies of the IgA class than those of the IgG class (Bohl, Gupta, Olquin and Saif, 1972). An antibody active at the local intestinal level is clearly more effective in this disease than a passive antibody circulating in the blood.

The specific protective function of milk IgA against enterobacterial infections has not been evaluated. Nevertheless, several experiments have demonstrated the protective benefits of oral antibodies. Thus orally administered antibodies from serum and milk exert a protective effect against enteropathogenic serotypes of *E. coli* in experimentally infected gnotobiotic pigs (Kohler and Bohl, 1966; Rejnek *et al.*, 1968; Miniats, Mitchell and Barnum, 1970; Wilson and Svendsen, 1971). These studies were conducted with piglets of an age when absorption of immunoglobulin no longer occurred, thereby ensuring that the observed protection would be attributable to the local activity of antibody in the lumen of the gut. In gnotobiotic pigs, 5 days old, Brandenburg and Wilson (1973) have also demonstrated the protective activity of IgG antibodies from milk. However, repeated administration of antibodies was required to maintain protection (Wilson, 1972b).

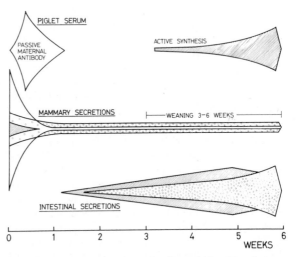

Fig. 14.3 Simple scheme showing interrelationship of serum antibodies, milk antibodies and intestinal antibodies contributing to protection of the piglet in early life.

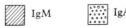 IgM   IgA

Comparisons have been made between oral and parenteral administration of antibodies (Owen, Bell, Williams and Oakes, 1961; Kohler, 1967); in general oral administration provides the most effective protection against infection. In the course of normal suckling a young pig ingests approximately 3g of immunoglobulin per day; in consequence a piglet at 7 days of age is probably obtaining, by mouth, an equivalent quantity of immunoglobulin to that contained in its entire blood circulation (Wilson, 1972a). Since these antibodies are directed at the main site of infection challenge, their local protective function must be important in the health and survival of the suckling animal.

Finally natural resistance to enteric infection in the young pig will be determined by the ability of the intestinal mucosa to actively take over the local protective function passively supplied in the milk; Figure 14.3 shows the way in which these changes take place in the first few weeks of life.

(ii) The significance of colostral IgA in the calf

A universal association of death with the absence, and survival with the presence, of incomplete antibodies in the serum of calves led Gay (1971) to postulate that titres of antibodies to *E. coli* might be correlated with resistance to infection. In addition Ingram and Malcomson (1970) demonstrated that such antibodies appeared in the sera of calves at an age when they became resistant to infection. Little is known about the immunoglobulin specificities related to these observations, but Logan and Penhale (1971) have tested colostral whey IgG and IgM fractions for protective efficiency against infective doses of *E. coli* in colostrum-deprived calves. IgM was significantly more effective than IgG; however, all the activity was not accounted for, since the recombined fractions were not comparable with the original colostrum.

The immunoglobulin profile and distribution of *E. coli* antibodies in post-colostral calf serum is very similar to that of the colostrum. In fact the young ruminant provides a unique example in which secretory 11S IgA is present in the blood in high concentrations. Thompson, Asquith and Cooke (1969) have demonstrated the presence of low levels of secretory IgA in the serum of patients with intestinal disease, which are probably attributable to the reabsorption of intestinal IgA from the lumen. In man intravenously injected 11S IgA disappears rapidly from the circulation (Butler, Rossen and Waldmann, 1967) and in the calf also the serum levels of passively acquired IgA decline rapidly with a half life of approximately 2 days. This is caused by loss into external secretions and the gastrointestinal tract is important in this respect (Porter, 1973d). The

low levels of immunoglobulin in bovine milk must contribute relatively little to local intestinal defence in the calf. Possibly this peculiar characteristic in the young ruminant, whereby colostral IgA is absorbed into the neonatal blood circulation and lost again into the alimentary tract, must compensate somewhat for the deficiencies in bovine milk. Probably this was the missing factor in the studies of Logan and Penhale (1971).

The transudation mechanism lasts effectively for a period of 7 to 10 days. Local synthesis of immunoglobulins within the tissues of the alimentary tract commences during this period and therefore under normal conditions a successful interrelationship between passive

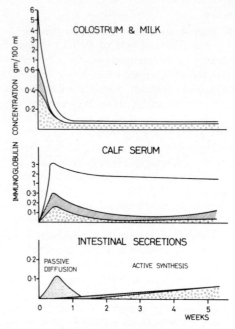

Fig. 14.4 Changing profiles of immunoglobulins in bovine mammary secretions, calf serum and intestinal secretions contributing to protection in the calf in early life.

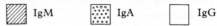

and active immune mechanisms must obtain. The changing patterns of immunoglobulin content of bovine mammary secretions, calf serum and intestinal secretions are related in Figure 14.4. This demonstrates the prospective continuum of humoral mechanisms utilized by the calf. Studies of antibody specificities attributable to different immunoglobulin classes in bovine colostrum and calf serum demonstrate that 11S IgA plays a significant role (Porter, 1972). Furthermore, immunity to *E. coli* challenge in neonatal calves has recently been correlated with the level of activity in the IgA and IgM class directed against capsular antigens (Wilson, 1973).

SYNTHESIS AND SECRETION OF IMMUNOGLOBULINS IN
THE INTESTINAL MUCOSA

(i) Ontogeny of the intestinal antibody system

The intestinal secretory immune system has been the focus of attention in numerous species (Vaerman, 1970). However, there is relatively little information concerning its development as a potential defence mechanism in the young mammal. Thus the reported studies for the human (Crabbé, Carbonara and Heremans, 1965; Rubin et al., 1965), rabbit (Crandall, Cebra and Crandall, 1967), rodents (Crabbé et al., 1969), primates (Felsenfeld, Greer, Kirtley and Jiricka, 1968) and dogs (Vaerman and Heremans, 1970) are concerned mainly with demonstrating that IgA is the predominant immunoglobulin contained in the lymphoid cells of the intestinal tissues. Although considerable emphasis has been placed on IgA because of its relative abundance in intestinal secretions, other immunoglobulins have been comparatively neglected. Furthermore, most studies have been conducted with animals at a stage of immunological maturity.

Immunohistological studies have defined a local secretory immune system mediated by an immunoglobulin analogous to human IgA, both in the pig (Porter and Allen, 1970; Vaerman, 1970; Atkins, Schofield and Reeders, 1971) and in the bovine (Porter, Noakes and Allen, 1972). In both species the secreted immunoglobulin has all the physiochemical properties of human 11S IgA with free as well as bound secretory component being detected in the secretions. In the newborn animal there are very few lymphoid cells in the lamina propria and the lymphoid follicles are poorly defined; this is true also of the germ-free animal. Subsequent to the generation of an intestinal microflora, these structures begin to develop and the lamina propria becomes infiltrated with lymphocytes and plasma cells. Many of the cells infiltrating the gastric mucosa of the young pig and calf produce IgM, and during the first few weeks of life these are numerically predominant to IgA cells at all levels of the intestine (Figs. 14.3 and 14.4). The potential contribution of IgM as an antibacterial antibody acting in concert with IgA in local defence is viewed as being important (Allen and Porter, 1970). Furthermore it is possible that IgM plays an initiating role in the onset of antibody response in the mammalian exocrine immune system, in much the same manner as it does in the systemic response to parenterally administered antigens (Allen and Porter, 1973b). The observation of Cebra (1969) gives support to this thesis in that rabbits infected with Trichinella showed a relative increase in intestinal IgM cells during a period 7 to 13 days post infection. Also in germ-free mice, the repeated injection of anti-μ-chain antiserum causes a decrease in numbers of IgM cells and also a virtual absence of IgA cells in the lamina propria of the gut, a finding consistent with IgM-producing cells being the precursors of IgA (Lawton, Asofsky, Hylton and Cooper, 1972). It is also significant that the exocrine role of IgA is taken over by IgM in cases of IgA deficiency (Stobo and Tomasi, 1966; Eidelman and Davis, 1968).

Peyer's patches have been a focus of attention in relation to their possible role as a bursa-equivalent in the mammal. Recent examination of embryonic development of the intestinal lymphoepithelial tissues in the pig provides some support for this hypothesis (Chapman, Johnson and Cooper, 1974). Lymphoid cells staining for IgM were seen in characteristic follicular distribution in Peyer's patches as early as 55 days gestation. This occurred before the development of immunocytes in other organs and it was unlikely that the thymus was implicated since immunoglobulin-staining cells were not evident in this organ till 10 to 15 days later. Thus lymphoid differentiation along plasma cell lines occurs in Peyer's patches of the foetal pig in absence of antigenic stimulus and before immunocytes are evident elsewhere, a fulfilment of at least some of the criteria of bursal function.

There is evidence that Peyer's patches may play an important role in seeding the lamina propria of the gastrointestinal tract with immunocytes. Cooper and Turner (1969) suggested that they may act as a source of IgM memory cells which migrate to other lymphoid tissues, and Craig and Cebra (1971) have shown that such cells have the potential to proliferate and differentiate into IgA-producing immunocytes in the lamina propria of the small intestine. Significantly Bienenstock and Dolezel (1971) failed to find any evidence of antigenic stimulation of Peyer's patches in hamsters after oral immunization. However, in gnotobiotic pigs, IgM cells were observed to develop in the Peyer's patch tissues in response to E. coli antigens (Porter, Kenworthy, Noakes and Allen, 1974). It remains to be determined whether such cells are committed antibody-forming cells or if they are potential precursors of cells in the lamina propria of the small intestine; yet from this point of view the recent observations of Uhr and Vitetta (1974) deserve emphasis; in studies of the synthesis and secretion of immunoglobulin in thoracic duct lymphocytes of young BALB/C mice, the predominant immunoglobulin on the surface of the cells was IgM, whereas the immunoglobulin synthesized and secreted was IgA. In contrast to normal mice, thoracic cells from germ-free mice synthesized and secreted substantial amounts of IgM, suggesting that in the absence of antigenic challenge the switching mechanism from IgM to IgA in these animals had not been activated.

(ii) Cellular localization, transport and function of intestinal immunoglobulin

Structural studies of porcine IgA (Porter, 1973a) and bovine IgA (Porter, 1973d) by reductive dissociation and polyacrylamide electrophoresis provide evidence of secretory component and also other low molecular weight electrophoretically fast polypeptide chains which appear to be the equivalent of the j-chain identified in secretory IgA by Halpern and Koshland (1970), and Mestecky, Zikan and Butler (1971). Immunofluorescent studies of the intestinal mucosa in the pig and calf have shown that secretory component is present in the crypt epithelium and intestinal mucins. Its synthesis and secretion proceed separately and independently from α-chain being detectable in the newborn in complete absence of α-chain (Allen and Porter, 1973a). The immunoglobulin is detected in immunocytes situated in the intercrypt stroma, in the epithelial cells and also in the mucus adhering to their apical surface, giving the appearance of a thin coat of bound antibody. IgM in the young pig and calf is transported into the secretions in a similar manner to IgA and there is no evidence of in-vivo complexing with secretory component. The interaction of IgA shows considerable specificity (Lawton, Asofsky and Mage, 1970; Mach, 1970; Brandtzaeg, 1971), possibly mediated by j-chain (Eskeland and Brandtzaeg, 1974). On the other hand IgM forms weak complexes and one might interpret from this that if secretory component is necessary for transport IgM would be poorly transmitted. However, in the calf intestine IgM is secreted in higher concentrations than IgA, at least during the preruminant stage (Porter, Noakes and Allen, 1972); and it appears without complexed secretory component.

The mechanism of transport of locally synthesized immunoglobulin across the epithelium to the intestinal lumen has recently been elucidated by immunoelectron microscopy (Allen, Smith and Porter, 1973). Many vesicles containing IgA were found in the apical cytoplasm of crypt epithelial cells and also in the intercellular spaces. The vesicles are probably taken into the epithelial cells by pinocytotic mechanisms and pass up through the cytoplasm to accumulate in the supranuclear region before being passed into the lumen. In recent studies of human tissues (Poger and Lamm, 1974; Brandtzaeg, 1974), histological localization of free and bound secretory component favour a model in which 11S IgA is assembled in the epithelial cell. The important biological function of secretory component is probably most concerned with its affinity for mucin; hence its role in the final stages of transport to the external surface will be that of binding the antibody in high local concentration, thus erecting a local barrier to infection. Intestinal secretions in the calf contain higher levels of IgM than IgA, mainly because IgM is less effectively bound in the mucin and therefore released more readily into the lumen. Its role on the mucosal surface may therefore be less effective; nevertheless it may make a significant contribution to the control of intestinal microflora by being free in the lumen.

CHARACTERISTICS OF THE ANTIBODY RESPONSE TO IMMUNIZATION VIA THE INTESTINAL MUCOSA

Studies of oral immunization have used faecal antibodies as an index of local intestinal response, but this provides no information about antibody activity in any specific region of the alimentary tract. Animals surgically prepared with Thiry-Vella loops have been used to study the secretory antibody response to bacterial antigens locally applied to the intestinal mucosa (Porter, Noakes and Allen, 1970b, 1972). The Thiry-Vella loop provides access to intestinal secretions without contamination from other sources such as saliva, bile and gastric secretions. Mucous secretion may be collected daily by attaching a polythene bag to the lower cannula or by irrigation with saline and collecting the washings. Biopsy specimens can be conveniently acquired, facilitating the fluorescent evaluation of sequential changes at a cellular level. The Thiry-Vella loop retains all the normal intestinal function having an intact blood and nerve supply; it retains absorptive and secretory function as well as peristaltic propulsion. This surgical preparation is therefore ideal in many respects for the study of long-term secretory antibody responses to antigens applied locally to the intestinal mucosa.

In considering the possible application of oral immunization to control enteric infections in young animals the main objective was to establish whether an adequate local immune response could be generated before the normal weaning period. In this context the successful studies in children given oral poliovirus at birth created an interesting precedent (Sabin et al., 1963, particularly since coproantibodies of the IgA class appeared within 3 weeks (Keller, Dwyer, Oh and D'Amodio, 1969). Similarly studies in fistulated baby pigs showed that antibodies in intestinal secretions could be stimulated in response to local application of heat-inactivated E. coli antigens within the first 3 weeks of life. The response was obtained in both surgically prepared and intact animals maintained on the sow (Porter et al., 1973), thus providing the basis of enhancing the competence of the young animal to cope with the challenge of enteropathogens after weaning.

Antibacterial agglutinins, mainly associated with IgA, appeared in the lumen within a few days of local antigenic challenge. However, intestinal antibody secretion did not persist at elevated levels for more than 3 to 4 weeks and a second dose of the same antigen induced an almost identical response with respect to intensity and duration (Porter, 1973c). In order to maintain consistent antibody secretion it was necessary to apply repeated doses. This apparent lack of memory in the secretory immune system in contrast to that normally associated with systemic immunity has also been registered in observations of the immune response to local intranasal administration of inactivated polio vaccine (Ogra and Karzon, 1969). Freter and Gangarosa (1963) had recorded essentially similar observations in relation to oral immunization with heat-killed *V. cholerae* in which repeated doses were necessary for the maintenance of detectable levels of coproantibody. Relevant to these observations, Mattioli and Tomasi (1973) have recorded that intestinal IgA plasma cells in mice have a half life of only 4.7 days, indicating that they do not play a significant role in long-term memory, and suggesting that the persistence of antibody production would depend on the recruitment of further immunocompetent cells.

There is little or no serological response to orally administered bacterial antigens in the young pig; and in the gnotobiotic pig, immunocytes containing IgA could not be detected in other tissues than the gastrointestinal tract (Porter *et al.*, 1974). One might infer from this that oral immunization gives rise to lymphoid cells restricted mainly to the lamina propria. Indeed available evidence would suggest that most immunoblasts generated in response to various antigenic stimuli are destined for the intestinal lamina propria (Hall and Smith, 1970). Griscelli, Vassalli and McCluskey (1969) have suggested that the presence of antigen in lymphoid tissue may be an essential factor in the 'homing' of antibody-forming cells to any particular tissue. Thus in orally immunized animals, with antigen being localized mainly in the gut, it might be anticipated that migrating cells would become established there.

Vaerman and Heremans (1970) calculated that most of the IgA in the mesenteric lymph of the dog was produced by plasma cells of the intestinal mucosa and that this was the major source of serum IgA. In germ-free mice oral immunization induced circulating antibodies exclusively of the IgA type (Crabbé *et al.*, 1969; Bazin, Levi and Doria, 1970). However, the serum IgA fraction is clearly seldom responsible for significant antibody activity, particularly as an antibacterial antibody (Cohen and Norins, 1968); otherwise it would have received equivalent attention to IgM and IgG in the definition of serological response. In numerous studies of locally induced immunity the secretory IgA antibody is readily detected whilst little or no activity was attributable to serum IgA. For example, the induction of local immunity in the rabbit mammary gland produces serum IgM and IgG antibodies and secretory IgA antibodies

in the milk (Genco and Taubman, 1969); similar observations are recorded for the sow (Bourne, 1973) and the cow (Wilson, Duncan, Heistand and Brown, 1972). Oral immunization frequently fails to produce serum antibody (Freter, 1962) and if serum antibodies do result they are seldom associated with serum IgA (Rothberg, Kraft and Farr, 1967; Kriebel, Kraft and Rothberg, 1969).

The germ-free pig produces an excellent model for studying the serological response to antigenic challenge via the intestinal mucosa since the animal can be reared without the complications of passively acquired maternal immunoglobulins. In this animal the main serological response to oral infection with *E. coli* was 7S IgG, and very little IgA was present in the serum (Porter and Kenworthy, 1970; Tlaskalová *et al.*, 1970). Hence antibody produced in the intestinal tissues is apparently destined almost entirely for local defence; the serological response in the IgG fraction can only reflect a reaction to antigen which has been carried to and processed at other sites.

Very few immunoglobulin-containing cells were detected in the intestinal tissues of germ-free pigs even in animals of 40 days of age, thus providing an excellent base line against which to assess the effects of local antigenic stimuli (Porter *et al.*, 1974). Repeated administration of heat-inactivated *E. coli* antigens produced an immunocyte response in the lamina propria which during the first few days was dominated by cells of the IgM class, and after 3 weeks, cells of the IgA class predominated. These cells were located in the region of the crypts, and both IgA and IgM immunoglobulins were observed in the apical cytoplasm of the epithelial cells. IgM-producing cells predominated in the Peyer's patches for at least 6 weeks, further indicating the significance of the immunoglobulin in the total response in cells of the intestinal lamina.

In the calf, also, there is evidence that IgM may normally play an important role in local intestinal defence. Immunofluorescent studies of intestinal tissues from young preruminant calves indicate the presence of two main populations of immunocytes synthesizing IgA and IgM; in intestinal secretions obtained from calves with Thiry-Vella loops the level of IgM frequently exceeded IgA (Porter *et al.*, 1972). Response of the intestinal mucosa to local antigenic stimuli with extracts of heat-inactivated Gram-negative bacteria produced antibody in the secretions over a period of 3 weeks (Allen and Porter, 1975). As previously observed in the pig, a second challenge with a similar antigenic dose produced an identical short-term response, indicating again the requirement for continuous stimuli to maintain a measurable level of antibody secretion.

Immunoglobulin-synthesizing cells infiltrated the intestinal tissues of the calf as early as 4 days of age and oral administration of bacterial antigens to colostrum-fed calves of this age produced a faecal antibody response, indicating that active intestinal secretion could be successfully interrelated with declining passive antibody.

MECHANISMS OF IMMUNITY AGAINST ENTERIC INFECTION

(i) BACTERIAL INHIBITION AND KILLING

Many biochemical and physiological factors are connected with establishing the balance of the bacterial population in the alimentary tract. The characteristic flora generated for each host species is more attributable to host factors than to immune mechanisms in the mucosal tissues. On the other hand many enteropathogens become involved in diarrhoea syndromes or cause them by interfering with the normal processes of nutrient absorption in the small intestine through elaboration of toxins. Immune mechanisms may only play a role in inhibition of such organisms provided the intestinal mucosa is alerted to the production and secretion of antibodies long before the organisms achieve pathogenic proportions in the lumen. This is the rationale behind oral immunization of the young animal before weaning.

The participation of secretory antibodies in controlling the pathogenic component of intestinal flora has not been fully evaluated. McClelland, Samson, Parkin and Shearman (1972) demonstrated that agglutination of a wide range of enteric organisms could be obtained with intestinal IgA. They postulated that agglutination may reduce the ability of an organism to colonize the intestine, possibly enhancing its clearance by intestinal peristalsis. Secretory IgA acts with lysozyme to lyse *E. coli* (Adinolfi, Glynn, Lindsay and Milne, 1966; Burdon, 1973; Hill and Porter, 1974) by activating the complement sequence presumably by the alternate pathway (Götze and Muller-Eberhard, 1971). IgM plays a significant role in the intestinal response of the young pig (Allen and Porter, 1973b) and calf (Porter *et al.*, 1972). There are adequate levels of lysozyme in intestinal secretions to effect bacteriolysis, but there is no evidence for a functional complement sequence, and *in-vitro* studies of antibacterial activity suggest that the most probable mechanism is bacteriostasis (Porter *et al.*, 1974).

IgA and IgM cells are more numerous in the lamina propria of the duodenum than in the jejunum and ileum (Allen and Porter, 1973b); this finding contrasts with the fact that, in the young pig, the population of enteric bacteria is much more abundant in the lower jejunum and ileum (Kenworthy and Crabb, 1963). However, Peyer's patches increase in number towards the distal small intestine and thus show a closer correlation with the increase in bacterial population towards that region. Studies in the rabbit demonstrate that Peyer's patches supply cells which have the potential to proliferate and differentiate into IgA-producing immunocytes which populate the intestinal mucosa (Craig and Cebra, 1971). It seems likely therefore that these mechanisms may combine to produce the major source of antibody secretion in the upper region of the small intestine. Hence, under such circumstances, secretory antibodies will not only play a part in local protection of the epithelial surface, but also would contribute to the control of the bacterial population in the lumen by traversing the whole of the alimentary tract aided by the normal peristaltic processes.

The intestinal mucosa contains all the elements required for cell-mediated immunity, including T-lymphocytes and an extensive system of macrophages which may also appear in secretions. Very little is known about the role of cell-mediated immune mechanisms in local defence; yet in the respiratory tract, sensitized lymphocytes appear in secretions following local immunization, and these are capable of releasing MIF on contact with the appropriate antigen (Waldman, Spencer and Johnson, 1972). Bellamy also (1973) has demonstrated the emigration of neutrophils into the lumen of the porcine small intestine; however, this was mediated by specific antibody and there was no evidence of T-cell involvement. It is interesting to speculate on the role of secretory IgA and IgM in this context, particularly in view of their demonstrated potentiality for opsonization of *E. coli* (Girard and Kalbermatten, 1971; Wernet, Breu, Knop and Rowley, 1971). Possibly secretory antibodies exhibit a dual role in facilitating the clearance of pathogenic bacteria in the lumen by phagocytosis.

(ii) BACTERIAL ADHESION

Peristaltic flow is a simple factor working against the establishment of microorganisms in the proximal regions of the small intestine. Adherence to the intestinal wall is considered to be an important prerequisite of many enteropathogens, enabling them to resist the flushing effect of peristalsis. Attachment of bacteria to the intestinal epithelium is known to be a preliminary to invasion with certain viruses and bacteria (Duguid, 1968). Several adhesive mechanisms have been identified in Enterobacteriaceae, the commonest being associated with the presence of filamentous surface appendages. Strains of *E. coli* isolated from piglets with diarrhoea often possess K88 antigens (Sojka, 1965) which, unlike other K antigens, are proteinaceous components forming fine filaments on the surface of the bacterium (Stirm, Ørskov, Ørskov and Birch-Andersen, 1967). The antigen is the product of an episomal gene which can be transferred (Ørskov and Ørskov, 1966).

Serotypes of *E. coli* which produce K88 also show adhesion to the intestinal mucosa of piglets (Arbuckle, 1970). From studies of transmission and elimination of the genetic elements responsible for synthesis of K88, Smith and Linggood (1970) concluded that the virulence of *E. coli* for piglets was associated with this factor. The potential protective function of antibodies was evident from the studies of Jones and Rutter (1972) who showed that adhesion of K88 positive *E. coli* to piglet intestinal tissue could be inhibited by antiserum. Furthermore, the colostrum of sows immunized with a crude preparation of K88 antigen conferred passive protection on neonatal piglets infected orally with the 0149:K99 (b), K88 ac(L):H10 serotype (Rutter and Jones, 1973).

It is also of interest that a common K antigen, designated K99, occurs in calf and lamb enteropathogenic strains and this, too, is controlled by a transmissible plasmid (Smith and Linggood, 1972). In studies with serotypes containing K99 and K88 antigens there was evidence of specificity for adhesion, K88 antigen being unable to bring about adhesion to calf and lamb intestine, and K99 being unable to bring about adhesion to pig intestine.

The use of these common antigens for immunization has attractive prospects, but it should be emphasized that there is by no means a universal dependence on such antigens for microbial pathogenicity (Gyles, Stevens and Craven, 1971). Colonization of the upper small intestine of the pig is not necessarily determined by the adhesive properties of K88 (Miniats and Gyles, 1972; Wilson and Hohmann, 1974) and this antigen is seldom identified in serotypes associated with post-weaning enteritis (Svendsen, Larson, Bille and Nielson, 1974), therefore other effector mechanisms must contribute.

In this respect pigs (White *et al.*, 1969) and calves (Smith, Hill and Sissons, 1970) show an inhibition in peristaltic flow in response to weaning from maternal milk. Furthermore, in gnotobiotic pigs during the first 24 hours of infection, intestinal stasis occurs, followed by a greatly increased volume of faeces (Kenworthy, 1974). The main factor promoting this effect may be attributable to the metabolic activity of the microflora resulting from the production of pharmacologically active amines (Porter and Kenworthy, 1969). Studies in conventionally weaned animals suggest that the site of production of such amines is important. In severely diarrhoeic animals, the small intestine was the main site of activity (Hill, Kenworthy and Porter, 1970a); the feeding of lactobacilli affected the catabolic activity and brought about a transfer from the small intestine to the colon during the diarrhoeic phase (Hill, Kenworthy and Porter, 1970b) with a consequent reduction in severity and duration of the symptoms. It remains to be determined whether or not local antibody mechanisms can mediate similar changes in microbial metabolism.

(iii) BACTERIAL TOXINS

The ability of *E. coli* to produce enterotoxin is considered to be a prime requirement of enteropathogenicity and has been identified with the presence of a transmissible plasmid (Smith and Halls, 1968). Several similarities exist between *E. coli* and *Vibrio cholerae* enterotoxins and their main function is the creation of a prolonged disturbance in fluid and electrolyte metabolism (reviewed by Kohler, 1972). Smith and Linggood (1971) suggested that adhesion of the bacterium presumably via K88 was an advantage in optimizing the effect of its toxin. In this respect Fubara and Freter (1973) consider that the protective function of secretory IgA antibodies in mice against enteric cholera infection was associated with inhibition of bacterial adsorption to the mucosa.

The role of immunity in neutralizing enterotoxicity of *E. coli* has been examined in several investigations. Recent studies of passive immunity indicate that antibodies may be produced in sow colostrum which neutralize enterotoxic activity in ligated intestinal loops (Wilson and Svendsen, 1971). However, in pigs surgically prepared with Thiry-Vella loops (Nagy, Penn and MacKenzie, 1974) there was no evidence to indicate the development of an antienterotoxic immunity following repeated inoculation of the loops with enteropathogenic strains of *E. coli*. These latter studies furnished evidence of an effective antibacterial mechanism, but this was thought to be bactericidal; the local nature of this reaction in the intestinal mucosa was evident from the fact that the activity was unaided by passively transferred antibodies. In this respect earlier studies on the control of post-weaning diarrhoea (Smith and Linggood, 1971) had similarly indicated that the protective function of immunity may be principally associated with bactericidal as opposed to antienterotoxic mechanisms. Further association of enterotoxin neutralization with antibacterial mechanisms derives from recent studies of oral immunization (Baljer, Chorherr, Sickel and Gieben, 1975); in the ligated intestine, test piglets vaccinated with heat-inactivated bacterial antigens resisted 100 to 1000 times greater doses of *E. coli* than control animals.

Taking the view that *E. coli* enterotoxins are poorly or not at all antigenic, it will be most appropriate to attack the problem via the antibacterial route. In this case, one is acting on the premise that if the bacterium is eliminated then so is the enterotoxin. For example, the bacterial proliferation which normally occurs in young pigs during the critical 2-week period post weaning is substantially reduced by oral immunization with heat-inactivated antigens, and in consequence so is the severity and duration of diarrhoea (Porter *et al.*, 1974).

The main effector mechanisms of mucosal antibodies in these circumstances seems to be bacterial agglutination and stasis. It is anticipated that these activities will not only inhibit bacterial multiplication at the mucosal surface but also interfere with adsorption by producing agglutinates of bacteria which might be readily disengaged by peristaltic flow. It is interesting that in the studies of Fubara and Freter (1973) the total counts of intestinal vibrio populations in experimentally infected germ-free mice were not affected; the protective effects of secretory IgA antibodies were entirely attributable to inhibition of bacterial adsorption. It is evident, therefore, that local antibody systems may not necessarily have to be directed against the toxins of an enteropathogen in order to inhibit its normal toxic action on the intestinal mucosa.

PROPHYLACTIC CONTROL OF POST-WEANING ENTERIC INFECTION IN THE PIG BY ORAL IMMUNIZATION

The predisposing factors in the pathogenesis of *E. coli* infection in the pig are complex, but there exists one certainty – that is, the protective function of maternal milk is withdrawn at weaning. This, together with the stress accompanying removal from the maternal environment, is usually sufficient to promote dramatic changes in the intestinal microflora; the period for 2 weeks after weaning is a critical one during which the young pig can show an alarming deterioration in health and performance. It is unlikely that any significance can be attached to serum immunoglobulin levels in relation to post-weaning enteric infections, since the organisms are not normally invasive and their damaging effects appear to be largely due to local toxic interaction with the tissues. A recent study supports this thesis since there was no correlation between serum immunoglobulin levels and incidence of *E. coli*-associated diarrhoea (Svendsen, Wilson and Ewert, 1972). Furthermore, earlier studies of parenteral vaccination (Miller *et al.*, 1962) failed to demonstrate any beneficial effects on post-weaning health and performance.

The small intestine is the most important site for absorption of nutrients and a temporary malabsorption syndrome is implicated in post-weaning diarrhoea (Kenworthy and Allen, 1966). Thus the maintenance of integrity and function of the small-intestinal epithelium is likely to be a very important contribution to post-weaning health. The role of IgA in protection of epithelial surfaces is now firmly established following the initial concepts of Heremans, Crabbé and Masson (1966) and Tomasi (1967). The primary objective in evaluating the prospects of exploiting local intestinal immune mechanisms for control of post-weaning enteric infection was to establish a successful interrelationship between active and passive antibody mechanisms. These have been discussed earlier in this text, and the changing antibody activities shown in Figure 14.3 demonstrate the relevance of intestinal antibody secretion to weaning.

As stated previously examination of fistulated animals showed that antibody function in the intestinal mucosa could be stimulated in the young pig before 3 weeks of age, but that did not persist after terminating daily antigenic challenge (Porter, 1973b). Dietary inclusion offered a satisfactory means of ensuring continuous challenge since the piglet would receive a dose of antigen with every feed. A practical problem which had to be met was that the feed intake of young pigs before weaning can be very variable. Hence heat-inactivated *E. coli* antigens were added as dietary supplements so that on average such piglets would consume approximately 10 to 30 times the minimum antigenic dose daily (Porter *et al.*, 1973).

Clinical studies were carried out in young pigs experimentally infected at weaning with a virulent enteropathogen, *E. coli* 0149. Intestinal colonization in orally immunized animals was delayed, clinical symptoms were reduced in intensity and duration, and generally there was a more rapid clearance of the infecting organisms than in control animals. Improved health was registered in terms of fewer deaths, better live-weight gains and food conversion ratios during the critical 2-week period post weaning (Porter *et al.*, 1974). Parenteral immunization provided no comparable benefits.

These observations were reproduced under normal conditions in conventional feeding trials affirming the value of the concept in its potential wider application. In a bacteriological survey of 42 litters of animals the

Table 14.1 Oral immunization by dietary supplementation with bacterial antigens: effect on piglet health and performance

Treatment	No. litters	No. pigs	Pigs scouring		Scour days		Pigs treated with antiobiotic		Weight gain (*lb*)	Feed conversion
			Total no.	% in each litter	No./litter	%/litter	Total no.	%/litter		
Antigen	12	110	49	49·1 ± 29·9	12·1 ± 8·9	3·7 ± 2·1	36	37·6	4·44 ± 1·40	1·44 ± 0·08
Control	12	94	66	73·1 ± 28·1[a]	15·1 ± 10·6	7·1 ± 5·2	63	79·4[a]	3·71 ± 1·39	1·73 ± 0·27

[a] Significant at P = 0·05.

levels of post-weaning bacterial growth in antigen-fed animals were substantially reduced compared with controls. In a detailed study of 24 litters fewer antigen-fed animals showed clinical symptoms and there was a significant reduction in the requirement for antibiotic therapy as well as a significant improvement in nutritional performance (Table 14.1).

More extensive trials comprising 124 litters of pigs were carried out in which antigen-fed pigs, particularly smaller animals, showed a significant weight advantage

LOCAL INTESTINAL PROTECTION BY MILK ANTIBODIES

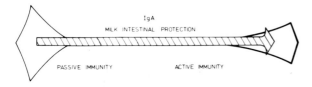

EARLY WEANING AND THE PROTECTION GAP

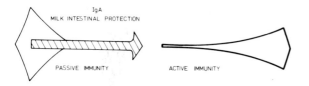

INTESTINAL IgA SYNTHESIS AND SECRETION

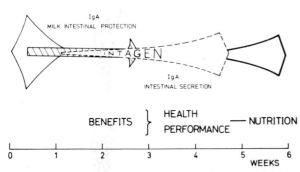

Fig. 14.5 Interrelationship of passive and active immune mechanisms showing the role of oral immunization in providing a continuum of antibody function in the alimentary tract post weaning. 'Intagen' is a sterile *E. coli* vaccine in a premix supplement developed for inclusion in animal feeds. It comprises antigens of recognized porcine enteropathogens.

over controls during the 2-week period post weaning. In litters with individual weights below average at weaning, the antigen-fed group showed a significantly greater gain of 1.4 lb per pig ($p < 0.01$) in the first 2 weeks

after weaning and 2.1 lb per pig ($p < 0.05$) in the 4-week period post weaning (Porter *et al.*, 1973). Preliminary investigations in other laboratories have substantiated these observations (Balger, 1974, 1975; Svendsen *et al.*, 1974). Thus enhanced immunocompetence due to oral immunization is generally reflected by improved health and performance. The simple features of this concept are outlined in Figure 14.5, showing the continuum of antibody function which can be marshalled to the benefit of the young animal at weaning.

PROPHYLACTIC CONTROL OF ENTERIC INFECTION IN THE EARLY WEANED CALF BY ORAL IMMUNIZATION

(i) AETIOLOGY OF ENTERIC INFECTION

It is commonly agreed that systemic infection with *E. coli* in the newborn calf is a consequence of colostrum deprivation or passive antibody inadequacy (Sojka, 1971). In contrast, the evidence in early weaned calves suggests that most cases of diarrhoea are not infectious in origin (Smith and Crabb, 1956; Smith, 1962) and the bacterial component of the alimentary tract may differ very little from that of healthy calves. Nevertheless this does not discount the fact that bacteria may aggravate the primary condition; indeed the administration of antibiotics is usually beneficial (Dalton, Fisher and McIntyre, 1960).

Relevant to this point the nutritive, physiological and clinical consequences of feeding reconstituted dried milk to calves was recorded in studies over a period of 5 years at the National Institute for Research in Dairying at Shinfield. It was observed that in units under continuous use, a significant deterioration in health and performance occurred in successive batches of calves reared in the units (Roy *et al.*, 1955). Furthermore, Wood (1955) recorded that under these conditions there was a build up of infection attributable to certain strains of *E. coli* which were associated with increased mortality.

Ingram and Lovell (1960) commented that in relation to *E. coli* infections, an attack upon the infection itself was less logical than the giving of some help to the host. They considered the disease to be largely due to a breakdown in a host–parasite relationship which might be an amicable one if man did not interfere. The natural resistance of the calf is evident from the studies of McEwen (1950) who routinely failed to establish infection by dosing normal calves with *E. coli* isolated from dead animals. Thus combining the views of Ingram and Lovell (1960) and that of Smith (1962) it seemed reasonable to pursue investigations into the health of a calf rather than the pathogenesis of a disease. From this standpoint we chose to examine the immunobiological mechanisms responsible for protection of the calf in early life.

(ii) INTESTINAL ANTIBODIES AND NATURAL
RESISTANCE TO INFECTION

In all herbivorous animals a part of the alimentary tract develops in early live with the specific purpose of providing a compartment for retention and microbial fermentation of the fibrous parts of the diet. In the bovine species this specialized digestive function is provided by a complex forestomach consisting of 4 compartments: rumen, reticulum, omasum and abomasum. The cellulolytic activity of the microflora in the forestomach of the ruminant provides numerous metabolites essential for nutrition (Annison and Lewis, 1959). However, the function of the remainder of the alimentary tract is unlikely to differ from that of the monogastric species. Furthermore these compartments of the alimentary tract take some weeks to develop in the young animal and therefore it is probable that the immunobiological mechanisms common to monogastric animals might be equally effective in the calf. Nonetheless some confusion existed in the literature as to the nature of the principal immunoglobulin involved, with IgG_1 (Curtain, Clark and Dufty, 1971) or IgA (Porter and Noakes, 1970; Mach and Pahud, 1971), both having been implicated.

Immunochemical studies of intestinal secretion from fistulated calves and immunofluorescent histological studies of biopsy specimens of intestinal tissues confirmed the presence of a secretory IgA system characteristic of that described in other species (Porter *et al.*, 1972). Free and bound secretory component and 11S IgA were demonstrated and the immunofluorescent localization of the component chains in the intestinal tissues was similar to that described in man and the pig. The IgG_1 was not at any time quantitatively important in intestinal secretions even though it was the major serum immunoglobulin. These observations gained support from an *in-vitro* examination of synthesis by bovine tissues in which IgA levels detected by radio immunoassay techniques were pronounced in tissues from ileum, duodenum and colon (Butler *et al.*, 1972). The distribution of immunoglobulins in bovine serum, mammary secretion and other external secretions is shown in a simple semiquantitative form in Figure 14.6 in order to clarify the special immunobiological features of the ruminant.

In considering the balance of the host–pathogen relationship it was conceivable that a young animal would be resistant to infection provided that it had the means of maintaining membrane integrity. The enteric flora provides a major antigenic challenge throughout life; from birth it is mainly responsible for generating immune reactions in the alimentary tract as well as stimulating rumen development and function. Enteropathogenic organisms are a normal but quantitatively minor component of the intestinal microflora; their

ability to proliferate must be suppressed and their invasiveness obstructed to maintain a successful balance.

The role of colostrum in protection of the neonate has already been considered, and attention drawn to the interesting phenomenon in the suckling calf whereby 11S IgA anti-*E. coli* antibodies are absorbed into the blood circulation and thereafter released into the external secretions including the alimentary tract. Clearly passive local immunity of this type is limited in duration, and active synthesis and secretion in the alimentary tract must interrelate to successfully maintain the young animal against bacterial challenge.

In such circumstances, it will be appreciated that the earliest onset of active antibody synthesis and secretion

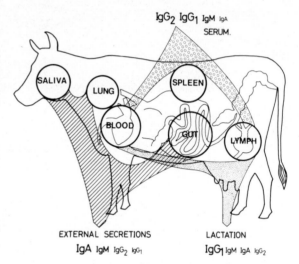

Fig. 14.6 Comparative proportions of immunoglobulins in bovine serum, mammary secretions and other external secretions.

in the intestinal mucosa of the young calf may be crucial to the young animal's survival. In histological studies of intestinal tissues from young fistulated animals, immunocytes synthesizing IgM and IgA were observed to be infiltrating the lamina propria as early as 4 days of age (Allen and Porter, 1975). Calves orally dosed with bacterial antigens at 5 days of age responded quickly with the secretion of antibodies, demonstrating that intestinal synthesis could suitably interrelate with declining passive maternal antibodies to provide a continuum of local antibody function in the alimentary tract of the calf. Immunization via the intestinal mucosa gave rise to secretory antibodies residing predominantly in the IgM and IgA classes with bacteriostatic or bacteriolytic function. Their localization on and in the intestinal mucosa provided the basis of an antibody interface between host and environment.

Table 14.2 Effect of oral immunization with bacterial antigens on calf health and performance

Treatment	No. calves	Calves scouring		Treatment		Weight gain (kg)		
		No. animals	No. days	Medicament	Antibiotic	0–3 wks	3–5 wks	0–5 wks
Antigen	96	27[a]	50[a]	25[a]	11[a]	7·00[b]	7·48	14·48[b]
Control	96	50	142	52	31	5·72	7·31	13·04

[a]$P = 0·01$.
[b]$P = 0·05$.

(iii) ORAL IMMUNIZATION AND ITS EFFECTS ON HEALTH AND PERFORMANCE

In previous studies in the pig (Porter et al., 1973) we elected to evaluate the beneficial effects of oral immunization in terms of such parameters as clinical symptoms, requirement for medication, and nutritional performance. The post-weaned pig provided a natural model for investigating enteric infection, obviating the need to adopt the use of the intraperitoneal route advocated by Mochmann et al. (1971) which is quite divorced from potential control by intestinal immunoglobulins. Similarly Roy and his colleagues (1955) had identified a valuable test model in the calf reared on reconstituted milk diets in an environment created by continuous occupancy.

Our prime concern was to obtain an improvement in animal health and performance in the presence of a normal bacterial challenge. Therefore we selected the model system of Roy et al. (1955) to establish whether or not oral immunization produced any beneficial effects. Strains of E. coli and Salmonellae most commonly encountered in enteric disorders of calves (Sojka, 1965) were chosen to prepare a vaccine for inclusion into diets replacing calves' milk, thus providing a convenient means of repeated dosage with every feed. The inclusion levels were calculated according to dose requirements and known feed intakes (Porter, Kenworthy and Thomson, 1975).

Two identical adjacent units with common services were constructed for the trial. The rooms were separated by a brick wall and there was strict attention to hygiene, using a disinfectant foot bath in the adjoining corridor and separate utensils and clothing. Occupation of the units was continuous by straggering the intakes of calves which were purchased in batches of 12. These were blocked in pairs according to weight and divided between the two rooms so that each batch half filled the available accommodation. The next batch filled the accommodation and subsequent batches occupied the positions vacated by previous animals. The length of occupancy of each intake was 5 weeks; the trial lasted 12 months and 16 batches of animals passed through the accommodation.

Animals in one unit were fed on the control diet and the others were fed on the same diet incorporating the bacterial antigens. The objectives of administering the vaccine were to prime the natural developing intestinal antibody system to enable the young animal to cope more competently with the anticipated challenge of its environment. In each batch of animals throughout the trial it was an almost consistent feature that the incidence of diarrhoea in the orally immunized group was considerably lower than in the controls. Consistent with the observations of Roy et al. (1955) most of the health problems occurred during the first 3 weeks of each calf's occupancy. In total, the incidence of diarrhoea, its duration in affected animals, the requirement for treatment with either medicaments or antibiotics (Table 14.2), were all significantly reduced. In consequence there were significant improvements in appetite and weight gain, and the overall deterioration in performance shown in the control groups was almost abolished.

CONCLUSION

Progress in the development and use of oral enteric bacterial vaccines was reviewed in 1972 by a WHO study group (WHO, 1972) who concluded that there was not enough well-substantiated basic information about immunization via the intestinal mucosa. The value of the young pig as a potential experimental model for E. coli-associated enteritis was highlighted. In this context it is worth noting that the parameters of health used in the studies reviewed here were not considered. Furthermore, it is significant that the majority of investigators have been concerned with evaluating oral immunization in mature subjects. In the young weaned animal, the benefits of enteric immunity may be more dramatically evident for it is growing rapidly at this time and elimination of a growth check over the critical post-weaning period will register significantly along with other health parameters.

The reduced requirement for therapeutic intervention has more than an economic appeal; there is less danger of carcass residues and moreover a much reduced likelihood of drug-resistant pathogens being excreted in the farm environment. Furthermore, there is evidence of a decrease in the total excretion of enteropathogens during these critical stress periods and long-term benefits in terms of farm health patterns should accrue.

Finally, it is the natural aspect of the concept which deserves emphasis: that in the young animal the intestinal immune system can be primed to combat the anticipated challenge of an infectious agent, which is a great opportunist when the host's resistance is undermined by stress. The findings to date provide encouraging evidence that oral immunization is capable of making a significant impact on the ever-present problem of clinical and sub-clinical infection, thereby helping to ease a major difficulty in intensive animal rearing systems.

REFERENCES

Adinolfi, M., Glynn, A. A., Lindsay, M. & Milne, C. M. (1966) Serological properties of IgA antibodies to *Escherichia coli* present in human colostrum. *Immunology*, **10**, 517–526.

Allen, W. D. & Porter, P. (1970) The demonstration of immunoglobulins in porcine intestinal tissue by immunofluorescence with observations on the effect of fixation. *Immunology*, **18**, 799–806.

Allen, W. D. & Porter, P. (1973a) Localization by immunofluorescence of secretory component and IgA in the intestinal mucosa of the young pig. *Immunology*, **24**, 365–374.

Allen, W. D. & Porter, P. (1973b) The relative distribution of IgM and IgA cells in intestinal mucosa and lymphoid tissues of the young unweaned pig and their significance in ontogenesis of secretory immunity. *Immunology*, **24**, 493–501.

Allen, W. D. & Porter, P. (1975) The localization of immunoglobulins in intestinal mucosa and the production of secretory antibodies in response to intralumenal administration of bacterial antigens in the preruminant calf. *Clinical and Experimental Immunology*, **21**, 407–418.

Allen, W. D., Smith, C. G. & Porter, P. (1973) Localization of intracellular immunoglobulin A in porcine intestinal mucosa using enzyme-labelled antibody. *Immunology*, **25**, 55–70.

Annison, E. F. & Lewis, D. (1959) *Metabolism in the Rumen*. Methuen's Monographs on Biochemical Subjects. London: Methuen.

Arbuckle, J. B. R. (1970) The location of *Escherichia coli* in the pig intestine. *Journal of Medical Microbiology*, **3**, 333–340.

Atkins, A. M., Schofield, G. C. & Reeders, T. (1971) Studies on the structure and distribution of immunoglobulin A-containing cells in the gut of the pig. *Journal of Anatomy*, **109**, 385–395.

Bainter, K. (1973) The physiological role of colostral trypsin inhibitor: experiments with piglets and kittens. *Acta Veterinaria Academiae Scientiarum Hungaricae*, **23**, 247–260.

Balger, G. (1974) Untersuchungen über eine orale Immunisierung mit *E. coli*-Vollantigen bei spf-Ferkeln. *3rd International Pig Society Veterinary Congress, Lyon*. G.35.

Balger, G., Chorherr, S., Sickel, E. & Gieben, D. (1975) Orale, aktive Immunisierung neugeborenes Ferkel gegen *E. coli*: Wirksamkeitsnachweis in Darmligaturtest. *Zentralblatt fur Veterinarmedizin*, B.**22**, 488–498.

Bazin, H., Levi, G. & Doria, G. (1970) Predominant contribution of IgA antibody-forming cells to an immune response detected in extraintestinal lymphoid tissues of germ-free mice exposed to antigen by the oral route. *Journal of Immunology*, **105**, 1049–1051.

Bellamy, J. E. C. 'Neutrophil emigration into the lumen of the porcine small intestine.' Unpublished PhD Thesis, University of Saskatchewan, Canada, 1973.

Bienenstock, J. & Dolezel, J. (1971) Peyer's patches: lack of specific antibody-containing cells after oral and parenteral immunization. *Journal of Immunology*, **106**, 938–945.

Binns, R. M. (1967) Bone marrow and lymphoid cell injection of the pig foetus resulting in transplantation tolerance or immunity, and immunoglobulin production. *Nature*, **214**, 179–181.

Bohl, E. H. (1973) Protection of newborn pigs against TGE. *Ohio Report*, **58**, 50–51.

Bohl, E. H., Gupta, R. K. P., Olquin, M. V. F. & Saif, L. J. (1972) Antibody responses in serum, colostrum, and milk of swine after infection or vaccination with transmissible gastroenteritis virus. *Infection and Immunity*, **6**, 289–301.

Bourne, F. J. (1969) IgA immunoglobulin from porcine serum. *Biochemical and Biophysical Research Communications*, **36**, 138–145.

Bourne, F. J. (1973) The immunoglobulin system of the suckling pig. *Proceedings of the Nutrition Society*, **32**, 205–215.

Bourne, F. J. & Curtis, J. (1973) The transfer of immunoglobulins IgG, IgA and IgM from serum to colostrum and milk in the sow. *Immunology*, **24**, 157–162.

Brandenburg, A. C. & Wilson, M. R. (1973) Immunity to *Escherichia coli* in pigs: IgG immunoglobulin in passive immunity to *Escherichia coli* enteritis. *Immunology*, **24**, 119–127.

Brandtzaeg, P. (1971) Human secretory immunoglobulins. II. Salivary secretions from individuals with selectively excessive or defective synthesis of serum immunoglobulins. *Clinical and Experimental Immunology*, **8**, 69–85.

Brandtzaeg, P. (1974) Mucosal and glandular distribution of immunoglobulin components. Immunohistochemistry with a cold ethanol-fixation technique. *Immunology*, **26**, 1101–1114.

Burdon, D. W. (1973) The bactericidal action of Immunoglobulin A. *Journal of Medical Microbiology*, **6**, 131–139.

Butler, J. E. (1969) Bovine immunoglobulins: A review. *Journal of Dairy Science*, **52**, 1895–1909.

Butler, J. E. (1971) Review of the bovine immunoglobulins. **54**, 1315–1316.

Butler, J. E. (1974) Immunoglobulins of the mammary secretions. In *Lactation III*, ed. Lawson, B. L. & Smith, V. R., pp. 217–255. London: Academic Press.

Butler, J. E. & Maxwell, C. F. (1972) Preparation of bovine immunoglobulins and free secretory component and their specific antisera. *Journal of Dairy Science*, **55**, 151–164.

Butler, J. E., Kiddy, C. A., Maxwell, C. F., Hylton, M. B. & Asofsky, R. (1971) Synthesis of immunoglobulins by various tissues of the cow. *Journal of Dairy Science*, **54**, 1323–1325.

Butler, J. E., Maxwell, C. F., Pierce, C. S., Hylton, M. B., Asofsky, R. & Kiddy, C. A. (1972) Studies on the relative synthesis and distribution of IgA and IgG₁ in various tissues and body fluids of the cow. *Journal of Immunology*, **109**, 38–46.

Butler, W. T., Rossen, R. D. & Waldmann, T. A. (1967) The mechanism of appearance of immunoglobulin A in nasal secretions in man. *Journal of Clinical Investigation*, **46**, 1883–1893.

Campbell, B., Porter, R. M. & Petersen, W. E. (1950) Plasmacytosis of the bovine udder during colostrum secretion and experimental cessation of milking. *Nature*, **166**, 913.

Cebra, J. J. (1969) Immunoglobulins and immunocytes. *Bacteriological Reviews*, **33**, 159–171.

Chamberlain, A. G., Perry, G. C. & Jones, R. E. (1965) Effect of trypsin inhibitor isolated from sows' colostrum on the absorption of γ-globulin by piglets. *Nature*, **207**, 429.

Chapman, H. A., Johnson, J. S. & Cooper, M. D. (1974) Ontogeny of Peyer's patches and immunoglobulin-containing cells in pigs. *Journal of Immunology*, **112**, 555–563.

Cohen, I. R. and Norins, L. C. (1968) Antibodies of the IgG, IgM and IgA classes in newborn and adult sera reactive with Gram-negative bacteria. *Journal of Clinical Investigation*, **47**, 1053–1062.

Cooper, G. N. and Turner, K. (1969) Development of IgM memory in rats after antigenic stimulation of Peyer's patches. *Journal of the Reticuloendothelial Society*, **6**, 419–434.

Crabbé, P. A., Carbonara, A. O. & Heremans, J. F. (1965) The normal human intestinal mucosa as a major source of plasma cells containing γA-immunoglobulin. *Laboratory Investigation*, **14**, 235–248.

Crabbé, P. A., Nash, D. R., Bazin, H., Eyssen, H. & Heremans, J. F. (1969) Antibodies of the IgA type in intestinal plasma cells of germfree mice after oral and parenteral immunization with ferritin. *Journal of Experimental Medicine*, **130**, 723–738.

Craig, S. W. & Cebra, J. J. (1971) Peyer's patches. An enriched source of precursors for IgA-producing immunocytes in the rabbit. *Journal of Experimental Medicine*, **134**, 188–200.

Crandall, R. B., Cebra, J. J. & Crandall, C. A. (1967) The relative proportions of IgG-, IgA- and IgM-containing cells in rabbit tissues during experimental trichinosis. *Immunology*, **12**, 147–158.

Curtain, C. C., Clarke, B. L. & Dufty, J. H. (1971) The origins of the immunoglobulins in the mucous secretions of cattle. *Clinical and Experimental Immunology*, **8**, 335–344.

Curtis, J. & Bourne, F. J. (1971) Immunoglobulin quantitation in sow serum, colostrum and milk and the serum of young pigs. *Biochimica et Biophysica Acta*, **236**, 319–332.

Curtis, J. & Bourne, F. J. (1973) Half-lives of immunoglobulins IgG, IgA and IgM in the serum of newborn pigs. *Immunology*, **24**, 147–155.

Dalton, R. G., Fisher, E. W. & McIntyre, W. I. M. (1960) Antibiotics and calf diarrhoea. *Veterinary Record*, **72**, 1186–1194.

Deutsch, H. F. & Smith, V. R. (1957) Intestinal permeability to proteins in the newborn herbivore. *American Journal of Physiology*, **191**, 271–276.

Duguid, J. P. (1968) The function of bacterial fimbriae. *Archivum Immunologiae et Therapiae Experimentalis*, **16**, 173–188.

Duncan, J. R., Wilkie, B. N. & Winter, A. J. (1972) Natural and immune antibodies for *Vibrio fetus* in serum and secretions of cattle. *Infection and Immunity*, **5**, 728–733.

Eidelman, S. & Davis, S. D. (1968) Immunoglobulin content of intestinal mucosal plasma-cells in Ataxia Telangiectasia. *Lancet*, **i**, 884–886.

El Nageh, M. M. (1970) Étude chez le veau nouveau-né de l'absorption intestinale des anticorps et autres proteines et de leur élimination urinaire. *Annales Médicine Veterinaire*, **111**, 370–404.

Eskeland, T. & Brandtzaeg, P. (1974) Does J chain mediate the combination of 19S IgM and dimeric IgA with the secretory component rather than being necessary for their polymerization? *Immunochemistry*, **11**, 161–163.

Esteves, M. B. & Binaghi, R. A. (1972) Antigenic similarities among mammalian immunoglobulins. *Immunology*, **23**, 137–145.

Felsenfeld, O., Greer, W. E., Kirtley, B. & Jiricka, Z. (1968) Cholera studies on non-human primates. Pt. 8. Comparison of methods for the enumeration of immunologically active cells and early immune globulin, precipitin, vibriocidin and antitoxin formation. *Transactions of the Royal Society of Tropical Medicine and Hygiene*, **62**, 278–284.

Franěk, F., Řiha, I. & Šterzl, J. (1961) Characteristics of γ-globulin, lacking antibody properties in new-born pigs. *Nature*, **189**, 1020–1022.

Freter, R. (1962) Detection of coproantibody and its formation after parenteral and oral immunization of human volunteers. *Journal of Infectious Diseases*, **111**, 37–48.

Freter, R., & Gangarosa, E. G. (1963) Oral immunization and production of coproantibody in human volunteers. *Journal of Immunology*, **91**, 724–729.

Fubara, E. S. & Freter, R. (1973) Protection against enteric bacterial infection by secretory IgA antibodies. *Journal of Immunology*, **111**, 395–403.

Gay, C. C. (1971) Problems of immunization in the control of E. coli infection. *Annals of the New York Academy of Sciences*, **176**, 336–339.

Gay, C. C., Anderson, N., Fisher, E. W. & McEwan, A. D. (1965) Gamma globulin levels and neonatal mortality in market calves. *Veterinary Record*, **77**, 148–149.

Genco, R. J. & Taubman, M. A. (1969) Secretory γA-antibodies induced by local immunization. *Nature*, **221**, 679–681.

Girard, J. P. & Kalbermatten, A. de (1970) Antibody activity in human duodenal fluid. *European Journal of Clinical Investigation*, **1**, 188–195.

Götze, O. & Müller-Eberhard, H. J. (1971) The C3 activator system: an alternate pathway of complement activation. *Journal of Experimental Medicine*, **134**, 90s–108s.

Griscelli, C., Vassalli, P. & McCluskey, R. T. (1969) The distribution of large dividing lymph node cells in syngeneic recipient rats after intravenous injection. *Journal of Experimental Medicine*, **130**, 1427–1451.

Gyles, C. L., Stevens, J. B. & Craven, J. A. (1971) A study of *Escherichia coli* strains isolated from pigs with gastro-intestinal disease. *Canadian Journal of Comparative Medicine*, **35**, 258–266.

Hall, J. G. & Smith, M. E. (1970) Homing of lymph-borne immunoblasts to the gut. *Nature*, **226**, 262–263.

Halpern, M. S. & Koshland, M. E. (1970) Novel subunit in secretory IgA. *Nature*, **228**, 1276–1278.

Hardy, R. N. (1969a) The break-down of [131I]γ-globulin in the digestive tract of the new-born pig. *Journal of Physiology*, **205**, 435–451.

Hardy, R. N. (1969b) Proteolytic activity during the absorption of [^{131}I]γ-globulin in the new-born calf. *Journal of Physiology*, **205**, 453–470.

Heremans, J. F., Crabbé, P. A. & Masson, P. L. (1966) Biological significance of exocrine gamma-immunoglobulin. *Acta Medica Scandinavica*, **179**, Suppl. 445, 84–88.

Hill, I. R. & Porter, P. (1974) Studies of bactericidal activity to *Escherichia coli* of porcine serum and colostral immunoglobulins and the role of lysozyme with secretory IgA. *Immunology*, **26**, 1239–1250.

Hill, I. R., Kenworthy, R. & Porter, P. (1970a) The effect of dietary lactobacilli on intestinal and urinary amines in pigs in relation to weaning and post-weaning diarrhoea. *Research in Veterinary Science*, **11**, 320–326.

Hill, I. R., Kenworthy, R. & Porter, P. (1970b) The effect of dietary lactobacilli on *in-vitro* catabolic activities of the small-intestinal microflora of newly weaned pigs. *Journal of Medical Microbiology*, **3**, 593–605.

Hill, K. J. (1956) Gastric development and antibody transference in the lamb, with some observations on the rat and guinea pig. *Quarterly Journal of Experimental Physiology*, **41**, 421–432.

Ingram, D. G. & Malcomson, M. E. (1970) Antibodies to *Escherichia coli* in young calves; O antigens, *American Journal of Veterinary Research*, **31**, 61–69.

Ingram, P. L. & Lovell, R. (1960) Infection by *Escherichia coli* and Salmonella. *Veterinary Record*, **72**, 1183–1186.

Jones, G. W. & Rutter, J. M. (1972) Role of the K88 antigen in the pathogenesis of neonatal diarrhoea caused by *Escherichia coli* in piglets. *Infection and Immunity*, **6**, 918–927.

Keller, R., Dwyer, J. E. Oh, W. & D'Amodio, M. (1969) Intestinal IgA neutralising antibodies in newborn infants following poliovirus immunization. *Pediatrics*, **43**, 330–338.

Kenworthy, R. (1974) Digestibility and balance studies of gnotobiotic pigs undergoing acute intestinal infection with *Escherichia coli*. *Research in Veterinary Science*, **16**, 208–215.

Kenworthy, R. & Allen, W. D. (1966) The significance of *Escherichia coli* to the young pig. *Journal of Comparative Pathology*, **76**, 31–44.

Kenworthy, R. & Crabb, W. E. (1963) The intestinal flora of young pigs with reference to early weaning, *Escherichia coli* and scours. *Journal of Comparative Pathology*, **73**, 215–228.

Kohler, E. M. (1967) Studies of *Escherichia coli* in gnotobiotic pigs. V. Evaluation of the effects of oral and parenteral administration of immune serum. *Canadian Journal of Comparative Medicine (and Veterinary Science)*, **31**, 283–289.

Kohler, E. M. (1972) Pathogenesis of neonatal enteric colibacillosis of pigs. *Journal of the American Veterinary Medical Association*, **160**, 574–582.

Kohler, E. M. & Bohl, E. H. (1966) Studies of *Escherichia coli* in gnotobiotic pigs. III. Evaluation of orally administered specific antisera. *Canadian Journal of Comparative Medicine (and Veterinary Science)*, **30**, 233–237.

Kriebel, G. W., Jr, Kraft, S. C. & Rothberg, R. M. (1969) Locally produced antibody in human gastrointestinal secretions. *Journal of Immunology*, **103**, 1268–1275.

Laskowski, M., Kassell, B. & Hagerty, G. (1957) A crystalline trypsin inhibitor from swine colostrum. *Biochimica et Biophysica Acta*, **24**, 300–305.

Lawton, A. R., Asofsky, R. & Mage, R. G. (1970) Synthesis of secretory IgA in the rabbit. III. Interaction of colostral IgA fragments with T-chain. *Journal of Immunology*, **104**, 397–408.

Lawton, A. R., Asofsky, R., Hylton, M. B. & Cooper, M. D. (1972) Suppression of immunoglobulin class synthesis in mice. I. Effects of treatment with antibody to μ-chain. *Journal of Experimental Medicine*, **135**, 277–297.

Lecce, J. G. (1966) Glucose milliequivalents eaten by the neonatal pig and cessation of intestinal absorption of large molecules (closure). *Journal of Nutrition*, **90**, 240–244.

Lecce, J. G., Matrone, G. & Morgan, D. O. (1961) Porcine neonatal nutrition: absorption of unaltered nonporcine proteins and polyvinyl pyrrolidone from the gut of piglets and the subsequent effect on the maturation of the serum protein profile. *Journal of Nutrition*, **73**, 158–166.

Logan, E. F. & Penhale, W. J. (1971) Studies on the immunity of the calf to Colibacillosis. I. The influence of colostral whey and immunoglobulin fractions on experimental. *E. coli* septicaemia. *Veterinary Record*, **88**, 222–228.

Mach, J.P. (1970) *In vitro* combination of human and bovine free secretory component with IgA of various species. *Nature*, **228**, 1278–1282.

Mach, J.-P. & Pahud, J.-J. (1971) Secretory IgA, a major immunoglobulin in most bovine external secretions. *Journal of Immunology*, **106**, 552–563.

Mach, J.-P., Pahud, J.-J. & Isliker, H. (1969) IgA with 'secretory piece' in bovine colostrum and saliva. *Nature*, **223**, 952–954.

Mattioli, C. A. & Tomasi, T. B. (1973) The life span of IgA plasma cells from the mouse intestine. *Journal of Experimental Medicine*, **138**, 452–460.

McClelland, D. B. L., Samson, R. R., Parkin, D. M. & Shearman, D. J. C. (1972) Bacterial agglutination studies with secretory IgA prepared from human gastrointestinal secretions and colostrum. *Gut*, **13**, 450–458.

McEwen, A. D. (1950) The resistance of the young calf to disease. *Veterinary Record*, **62**, 83–93.

Mestecky, J., Zikan, J. & Butler, W. T. (1971) Immunoglobulin M and secretory immunoglobulin A: presence of a common polypeptide chain different from light chains. *Science*, **171**, 1163–1165.

Miller, E. R., Harman, B. J., Ullrey, D. E., Schmidt, J., Luecke, R. W. & Hoefer, J. A. (1962) Antibody absorption, retention and production by the baby pig. *Journal of Animal Science*, **21**, 309–314.

Miniats, O. P. & Gyles, C. L. (1972) The significance of proliferation and enterotoxin production by *Escherichia coli* in the intestine of gnotobiotic pigs. *Canadian Journal of Comparative Medicine*, **36**, 150–159.

Miniats, O. P., Mitchell, L. & Barnum, D. A. (1970) Response of gnotobiotic pigs to *Escherichia coli*. *Canadian Journal of Comparative Medicine*, **34**, 269–276.

Mochmann, H., Ocklitz, H. W., Hering, L., Schmidt, E. F. & Richter, H. (1971) The influence of dosage and boostering upon the effectiveness of oral immunization against dyspepsia coli infections in the active mouse protection test. *Zentralblatt für Bakteriologie Parasitenkunde Infektions-krankheiten und Hygiene (Abteilung I)*, **216**, 24–31.

Moon, H. W. (1969) Enteric colibacillosis in the newborn pig: problems of diagnosis and control. *Journal of the American Veterinary Medical Association*, **155**, 1853–1859.

Nagy, L. K., Penn, C. W., & Mackenzie, T. (1974) Studies of immunity of Coli-enteritis in the pig. *Research in Veterinary Science*, **17**, 215–221.

Nordbring, F. & Olsson, B. (1958) Electrophoretic and immunological studies on sera of young pigs. II. The effect of feeding bovine trypsin inhibitor with porcine colostrum on the absorption of antibodies and immune globulins. *Acta Societatis Medicorum Upsaliensis*, **63**, 25–40.

Ogra, P. L. & Karzon, D. T. (1969) Distribution of poliovirus antibody in serum, nasopharynx and alimentary tract following segmental immunization of lower alimentary tract with poliovaccine. *Journal of Immunology*, **102**, 1423–1430.

Ørskov, I. & Ørskov, F. (1966) Episome-carried surface antigen K88 of *Escherichia coli*. I. Transmission of the determinant of the K88 antigen and influence on the transfer of chromosomal markers. *Journal of Bacteriology*, **91**, 69–75.

Owen, B. V., Bell, J. M., Williams, C. M. & Oakes, R. G. (1961) Effects of porcine immune globulin administration on the survival and serum protein composition of colostrum deprived pigs reared in a non-isolated environment. *Canadian Journal of Animal Science*, **41**, 236–252.

Penhale, W. J., Logan, E. F., Selman, I. E., Fisher, E. W. & McEwan, A. D. (1973) Colostral immunity to colibacillosis in the calf. *Annales de Recherches Vétérinaires*, **4**, 223–231.

Pierce, A. E. (1962) Antigens and antibodies in the newly born. *Colston Paper*, **13**, 189–206.

Poger, M. E. & Lamm, M. E. (1974) Localization of free and bound secretory component in human intestinal epithelial cells. A model for the assembly of secretory IgA. *Journal of Experimental Medicine*, **139**, 629–642.

Porter, P. (1969a) Transfer of immunoglobulins IgG, IgA and IgM to lacteal secretions in the parturient sow and their absorption by the neonatal piglet. *Biochimica et Biophysica Acta*, **181**, 381–392.

Porter, P. (1969b) Porcine colostral IgA and IgM antibodies to *Escherichia coli* and their intestinal absorption by the neonatal piglet. *Immunology*, **17**, 617–626.

Porter, P. (1971a) The porcine secretory IgA antibody system. *Acta Veterinaria Brno Supplement 2*, **2**, 59–65.

Porter, P. (1971b) Immunoglobulin IgA in bovine mammary secretions and serum of the neonatal calf. *Biochimica et Biophysica Acta*, **236**, 664–674.

Porter, P. (1972) Immunoglobulins in bovine mammary secretions. Quantitative changes in early lactation and absorption by the neonatal calf. *Immunology*, **23**, 225–238.

Porter, P. (1973a) Studies of porcine secretory IgA and its component chains in relation to intestinal absorption of colostral immunoglobulins by the neonatal pig. *Immunology*, **24**, 163–176.

Porter, P. (1973b) Intestinal defence in the young pig. A review of the secretory antibody systems and their possible role in oral immunization. *Veterinary Record*, **92**, 658–664.

Porter, P. (1973c) The functional role of secretory antibody systems in early development of the pig and the calf. *Proceedings of the Nutrition Society*, **32**, 217–222.

Porter, P. (1973d) Functional heterogeneity of the bovine immune system. *Journal of the American Veterinary Medical Association*, **163**, 789–794.

Porter, P. & Allen, W. D. (1970) Intestinal IgA in the pig. *Experentia*, **26**, 90–92.

Porter, P. & Hill, I. R. (1970) Serological changes in immunoglobulins IgG, IgA and IgM and *Escherichia coli* antibodies in the young pig. *Immunology*, **18**, 565–573.

Porter, P. & Kenworthy, R. (1969) A study of intestinal and urinary amines in pigs in relation to weaning. *Research in Veterinary Science*, **10**, 440–447.

Porter, P., Kenworthy, R. & Thomson, I. (1975) Oral on germ-free and gnotobiotic pigs. II. Serum proteins and antibodies. *Journal of Comparative Pathology and Therapeutics*, **80**, 233–241.

Porter, P. & Noakes, D. E. (1970) Immunoglobulin IgA in bovine serum and external secretions. *Biochimica et Biophysica Acta*, **214**, 107–116.

Porter, P., Kenworthy, R. & Thomson, I. (1975) Oral immunization and its significance in the prophylactic control of enteritis in the preruminant calf. *Veterinary Record*, **97**, 24–28.

Porter, P., Noakes, D. E. & Allen, W. D. (1970a) Secretory IgA and antibodies to *Escherichia coli* in porcine colostrum and milk and their significance in the alimentary tract of the young pig. *Immunology*, **18**, 245–257.

Porter, P., Noakes, D. E. & Allen, W. D. (1970b) Intestinal secretion of immunoglobulins and antibodies to *Escherichia coli* in the pig. *Immunology*, **18**, 909–920.

Porter, P., Noakes, D. E. & Allen, W. D. (1972) Intestinal secretion of immunoglobulins in the preruminant calf. *Immunology*, **23**, 299–312.

Porter, P., Kenworthy, R., Holme, D. W. & Horsfield, S. (1973) *Escherichia coli*. antigens as dietary additives for oral immunization of pigs: trials with pig creep feeds. *Veterinary Record*, **92**, 630–636.

Porter, P., Kenworthy, R., Noakes, D. E. & Allen, W. D. (1974) Intestinal antibody secretion in the young pig in response to oral immunization with *Escherichia coli*. *Immunology*, **27**, 841–853.

Prokešová, L., Kostka, J., Rejnek, J. & Trávníček, J. (1970) Further evidence of active synthesis of immunoglobulins in precolostral germfree piglets. *Folia Microbiologica, (Praha)*, **15**, 337–340.

Rejnek, J., Trávníček, J., Kostka, J., Šterzl, J. & Lanc, A. (1968) Study of the effect of antibodies in the intestinal tract of germ-free baby pigs. *Folia Microbiologica*, **13**, 36–42.

Richardson, A. K. & Kelleher, P. C. (1970) The 11-S sow colostral immunoglobulin. Isolation and physico-chemical properties. *Biochimica et Biophysica Acta*, **214**, 117–124.

Rothberg, R. M., Kraft, S. C. & Farr, R. S. (1967) Similarities between rabbit antibodies produced following ingestion of bovine serum albumin and following parenteral immunization. *Journal of Immunology*, **98**, 386–395.

Roy, H. B., Palmer, J., Shillam, K. W. G., Ingram, P. L. & Wood, P. C. (1955) The nutritive value of colostrum for the calf. 10. The relationship between the period of time that a calfhouse has been occupied and the incidence of scouring and mortality in young calves. *British Journal of Nutrition*, **9**, 11–20.

Rubin, W., Fauci, A. S., Sleisenger, M. H., Jeffries, G. H., and Margolis, S. (1965) Immunofluorescent studies in adult celiac disease. *Journal of Clinical Investigation*, **44**, 475–485.

Rutter, J. M. & Jones, G. W. (1973) Protection against enteric disease caused by *E. coli* – a model for vaccination with a virulence determinant. *Nature*, **242**, 531–533.

Sabin, A. B., Michaels, R. H., Ziring, P., Krugman, S. & Warren, J. (1963) Effect of oral poliovirus vaccine in newborn children. II. Intestinal resistance and antibody response at 6 months in children fed type I vaccine at birth. *Pediatrics*, **31**, 641–650.

Saif, L. J., Bohl, E. H. & Gupta, R. K. P. (1972)

Isolation of porcine immunoglobulins and determination of immunoglobulin classes of transmissible gastroenteritis viral antibodies. *Infection and Immunity*, **6**, 600–609.

Smith, H. W. (1962) Observations on the aetiology of neonatal diarrhoea (scours) in valves. *Journal of Pathology and Bacteriology*, **84**, 147–168.

Smith, H. W. & Crabb, W. E. (1956) The faecal bacterial flora of animals and man; its development in the young. *Journal of Pathology and Bacteriology*, **82**, 53–66.

Smith, H. W. & Halls, S. (1968) The production of oedema disease and diarrhoea in weaned pigs by the oral administration of *Escherichia coli*: factors that influence the course of the experimental disease. *Journal of Medical Microbiology*, **1**, 45–59.

Smith, H. W. & Linggood, M. A. (1970) Transfer factors in *Escherichia coli* with particular regard to their incidence in enteropathogenic strains. *Journal of General Microbiology*, **62**, 287–299.

Smith, H. W. & Linggood, M. A. (1971) Observations on the pathogenic properties of the K88, Hly, and Ent plasmids of *Escherichia coli* with particular reference to porcine diarrhoea. *Journal of Medical Microbiology*, **4**, 467–485.

Smith, H. W. & Linggood, M. A. (1972) Further observations on *Escherichia coli* enterotoxins with particular regard to those produced by atypical piglet strains and by calf and lamb strains: the transmissible nature of these enterotoxins and of AK antigen possessed by calf and lamb strains. *Journal of Medical Microbiology*, **5**, 243–250.

Smith, R. H., Hill, W. B. & Sissons, J. W. (1970) The effect of diets containing soya products on the passage of digesta through the alimentary tract of the pre-ruminant calf. *Proceedings of the Nutrition Society*, **29**, 6A.

Sojka, W. J. (1965) *Escherichia coli* in domestic animals and poultry. *The Commonwealth Bureau of Animal Health*, **7**, 1–230.

Sojka, W. J. (1971) Enteric diseases in newborn piglets, calves and lambs due to *Escherichia coli* infection. *Veterinary Bulletin*, **41**, 509–522.

Sojka, W. J. (1973) Enteropathogenic *E. coli* in man and farm animals. *Canadian Institute of Food Science and Technology Journal*, **6**, 52–63.

South, M. A., Cooper, M. D., Wollheim, F. A., Hong, R. & Good, R. A. (1966) I. Studies of the IgA system on the transport and immunochemistry of IgA in the saliva. *Journal of Experimental Medicine*, **123**, 615–627.

Speer, V. C., Brown, H., Quinn, L. & Catron, D. V. (1959) The cessation of antibody absorption in the young pig. *Journal of Immunology*, **83**, 632–634.

Šterzl, J., Kostka, J., Riha, I. & Mandel, L. (1960) Attempts to determine the formation and character of γ-globulin and of natural and immune antibodies in young pigs reared without colostrum. *Folia Microbiologica (Praha)*, **5**, 29–45.

Steward, M. W. (1971) Resistance of rabbit secretory IgA to proteolysis. *Biochimica et Biophysica Acta*, **236**, 440–449.

Stirm, S., Ørskov, F., Ørskov, I. & Birch-Andersen, A. (1967) Episome-carried surface antigen K88 of *Escherichia coli*. III. Morphology. *Journal of Bacteriology*, **93**, 740–748.

Stobo, J. D. & Tomasi, T. B. (1966) A low molecular weight immunoglobulin antigenically related to 19S IgM. *Journal of Clinical Investigation*, **46**, 1329–1337.

Svendsen, J. & Bienenstock, J. (1972) Isolation of 11-S IgA from porcine milk. *Biochimica et Biophysica Acta*, **263**, 775–778.

Svendsen, J., Wilson, M. R. & Ewert, E. (1972) Serum protein levels in pigs from birth to maturity and in young pigs with and without enteric colibacillosis. *Acta Veterinaria Scandinavica*, **13**, 528–538.

Svendsen, J., Larson, J. L., Bille, M. & Nielsen, M. C. (1974) Post weaning *E. coli* diarrhoea in pigs. *3rd International Pig Society Veterinary Congress, Lyon*. D.7.

Thompson, R. A., Asquith, P. & Cooke, W. T. (1969) Secretory IgA in the serum. *Lancet*, **ii**, 517–519.

Tlaskalová, H., Kamarýtová, V., Mandel, L., Prokešová, L., Kruml, J., Lanc, A. & Miler, I. (1970) The immune response of germ-free piglets after peroral monocontamination with living *Escherichia coli* Strain 086. *Folia Microbiologica (Praha)*, **16**, 177–187.

Tomasi, T. B. (1967) The gamma-A globulins: first line of defense. *Hospital Practice*, **2**, 26–35.

Tomasi, T. B. & Calvanico, N. (1968) Human secretory A. *Federation Proceedings*, **27**, 617.

Tomasi, T. B., Tan, E. M., Solomon, A. & Prendergast, R. A. (1965) Characteristics of an immune system common to certain external secretions. *Journal of Experimental Medicine*, **121**, 101–124.

Uhr, J. W. & Vitetta, E. S. (1974) Cell surface immunoglobulin. VIII. Synthesis, secretion and cell surface expression of immunoglobulin in murine thoracic duct lymphocytes. *Journal of Experimental Medicine*, **139**, 1013–1018.

Vaerman, J.-P. 'Studies on IgA immunoglobulin in man and animals.' Unpublished Thesis, Université Catholique de Louvain, 1970.

Vaerman, J.-P. & Heremans, J. F. (1970) Origin and molecular size of immunoglobulin-A in the mesenteric lymph of the Dog. *Immunology*, **18**, 27–38.

Vaerman, J.-P., Heremans, J. F. & Van Kerckhoven, G. (1969) Identification of IgA in several mammalian species. *Journal of Immunology*, **103**, 1421–1423.

Waldman, R. H., Spencer, C. S. & Johnson, J. E., III. (1972) Respiratory and systemic cellular and humoral immune responses to influenza virus vaccine administered parenterally or by nose drops. *Cellular Immunology*, **3**, 294–300.

Wernet, P., Breu, H., Knop, J. & Rowley, D. (1971) Antibacterial action of specific IgA and transport of IgM, IgA and IgG from serum into the small intestine. *Journal of Infectious Diseases*, **124**, 223–226.

White, F., Wenham, G., Sharman, G. A. M., Jones, A. S., Rattray, E. A. S. & MacDonald, I. (1969) Stomach function in relation to a scour syndrome in piglets. *The British Journal of Nutrition*, **23**, 847–858.

Wilson, M. R. (1972a) The influence of preparturient intramammary vaccination on bovine mammary secretions. Antibody activity and protective value against *Escherichia coli* enteric infections. *Immunology*, **23**, 947–955.

Wilson, M. R. (1972b) Role of immunity in the control of neonatal colibacillosis in pigs. *Journal of the American Veterinary Medical Association*, **160**, 585–590.

Wilson, M. R. & Hohmann, A. W. (1974) Immunity to *Escherichia coli* in pigs: Adhesion of enteropathogenic *Escherichia coli* to isolated intestinal epithelial cells. *Infection and Immunity*, **10**, 776–782.

Wilson, M. R. & Svendsen, J. (1971) Immunity to *Escherichia coli* in pigs. The role of milk in protective immunity to *E. coli* enteritis. *Canadian Journal of Comparative Medicine*, **35**, 239–243.

Wilson, M. R., Duncan, J. R., Heistand, F. & Brown, P. (1972) The influence of preparturient intramammary vaccination on immunoglobulin levels in bovine mammary secretions. *Immunology*, **23**, 313–320.

Wilson, R. A. 'The immunobiology of calf scours.' Unpublished Thesis, Montana State University, 1973.

Wood, P. C. (1955) The epidemiology of white scours among calves kept under experimental conditions. *Journal of Pathology and Bacteriology*, **70**, 179–193.

World Health Organization (1972) Oral enteric bacterial vaccines. *World Health Organization Technical Report Series*, **500**.

15. Immunological aspects of gastrointestinal cancer

S. N. Booth and P. W. Dykes

INTRODUCTION

The immunological relationship between tumour and host is currently under close study both in man and in experimental animals. In the gastrointestinal tract the problem appears particularly provocative with malignancy appearing in several disorders which show gross immunological changes. Such disorders include pernicious anaemia, coeliac disease, ulcerative colitis and Crohn's disease, and it is possible that studies which relate to the development of tumours from the benign process might throw light not only on carcinogenesis in general but also on the aetiology of the primary condition.

Evidence for tumour antigenicity and the specificity of immune responses has been well reviewed (Lewis, 1972; Hellström and Hellström, 1974) and includes reports of spontaneous tumour regression, the disappearance of metastases after resection of the primary tumour, and the occasionally unexpected response of certain neoplasms to inadequate chemotherapy or radiotherapy. Also recent studies in patients treated with long-term immunosuppressive therapy have revealed an increased incidence of neoplasia (Penn, 1974), just as individuals with primary immunodeficiency states have an incidence of neoplasia roughly 10 000 times that of the general age-matched population (Harris and Bagai, 1972). In addition it has been suggested that the peaks of neoplasia, which occur in infancy and in old age, can in part be accounted for by diminished immunological surveillance at the extremes of life (Gatti and Good, 1970). A difficulty in interpreting information from these studies lies in the special types of tumour involved, which include acute leukaemias, lymphoma, neuroblastoma, hypernephroma, melanoma and choriosarcoma. The case for an immunological reaction against commoner gastrointestinal tumours is based on less direct observations, such as the correlation between histological appearances and the clinical course. Thus sinus histiocytosis in local lymph nodes is considered to represent an immunological reaction to cancer, and has been shown to correlate with prolonged survival in patients with gastric and colonic carcinomata even regardless of the presence of nodal metastases (Black, Opler and Speer, 1956; Wartman, 1959). The prognostic significance of lymphocytic infiltration of tumours has been examined inconclusively in man (Thackray, 1964; Tanaka, Cooper and Anderson, 1970), but in studies of murine sarcomas, Russell and Cochrane (1974) have shown regression of the lesion to be directly related to the degree of mononuclear cell infiltration.

This chapter considers firstly the problem of antigenic specificity of tumours, secondly information relating to tumour-associated antigenic substances in gastrointestinal neoplasia, and lastly the evidence for host immune reactions both humoral and cellular. The implications of this information on the development of immunotherapy programmes are examined as well as the small volume of evidence currently available.

ANTIGENIC VARIATION IN GASTROINTESTINAL NEOPLASIA

Although the concept of antigenic change during neoplastic transformation was suggested in the early part of this century, it was not until the 1950s and the development of syngeneic animal strains, that neoantigen formation was established in chemically induced animal tumours (Foley, 1953; Prehn and Main, 1957). These antigens have been shown to be specific for each induced tumour; they are located on the cell surface, and have the capacity to induce rejection of transplanted tumours in previously immunized animals. They have thus been called tumour-specific transplantation antigens (TSTA).

In addition to these specific antigens, tumour-associated substances exist which are common to many tumours of the same type and in experimental animals have been particularly associated with virally induced lesions. These antigens are also found in early foetal tissue and have thus been designated oncofoetal antigens (Alexander, 1972). Although such substances have in certain instances been shown to induce rejection of transplanted tumours, they are more commonly detected in serum by immunoassay procedures using xenogeneic antisera and are therefore not necessarily truly antigenic. Their presence in minute concentration in apparently normal tissue casts further doubt on their tumour specificity and it is currently more correct to consider them as tumour-related substances. Cross-reaction may exist between some of these substances and TSTAs

(Thompson and Alexander, 1973), although specific differences do exist (Baldwin, Glaves and Vose, 1974). It is probable that TSTA is confined to the cell membrane, whereas oncofoetal antigens are also found in the superficial cytoplasm. Why embryonal antigens apparently disappear from normal tissues and then return, possibly by de-repression of existing synthetic mechanisms (Gold and Freedman, 1965a), has not been established.

Another important antigenic variation in neoplasia is the phenomenon of deletion of normal tissue antigens (Penn, 1974). Burnett considered this loss had an important bearing on the behaviour of the tumour, either by enhancing dissemination through a diminution of normal cellular adhesion at the primary site, or by allowing growth of tumour cells at the metastatic site (Burnett, 1957).

Antigenic deletion in relation to gastrointestinal neoplasia is well documented (Nairn, Fothergill, McEntegart and Richmond, 1962; Burtin, von Kleist and Sabine, 1971), and a correlation has been demonstrated between the loss of normal colonic membrane antigen (CMA) and the reappearance of the carcinoembryonic antigen (CEA) in gastrointestinal cancers.

Evidence for the existence of neoantigens in humans largely derives from a search for tumour-related substances and antibodies to them in blood, together with in-vitro studies of leucocyte reaction to tumour cells and their products. Tumour specificity has been looked for by absorption of antisera with extracts of normal tissues, but cross-reactivity remains a perpetual problem, and most apparently tumour-specific substances described in humans have subsequently been shown to be present in normal tissues at very much lower concentrations. Such substances are carcinoembryonic antigen (CEA) and α foetoprotein (αFP), and the other substances discussed below.

CARCINOEMBRYONIC ANTIGEN – CEA

Gold and Freedman (1965) chose colonic cancer for this type of study because of its early discrete localization. Mucosal tissue more than 10 cm from the edge of the tumour was considered normal and was used to absorb antisera raised in rabbits to a saline tumour extract. At least 2 apparently tumour-specific antigens were detected and reactions of identity were obtained with 12 individual colonic tumours. Although present in other endodermal systems the antigen was absent from all normal adult tissues examined including normal stomach, colon and liver, but was found to be present in foetal gut, liver and pancreas during the first two trimesters of pregnancy, thus suggesting the term carcinoembryonic antigen.

Several authors have confirmed the apparent anti-

genic heterogeneity of CEA (von Kleist and Burtin, 1969b; Kleinman, Harwell and Turner, 1971), and a wide range of substances with CEA activity have been extracted from human urine (Nery, James, Barsoum and Bullman, 1974). An antigenic relationship exists between CEA and a glycoprotein of smaller molecular size present in perchloric acid extracts of certain normal tissues (von Kleist, Chavanel and Burtin, 1972; Mach and Pusztaszeri, 1972). This latter substance is commonly termed non-specific cross-reacting antigen (NCA) and its presence may account for the second precipitin line obtained in some CEA preparations.

TISSUE LOCALIZATION AND DISTRIBUTION

Immunofluorescent studies have shown CEA to be localized in the free borders of the malignant mucosal cell, especially where it is adjacent to the glandular lumen. Electron-microscopy using a specific antiserum conjugated to ferritin has further demonstrated localization in the glycocalyx and the cell membrane (Gold, Krupey and Ansari, 1970).

The colonic cancer specificity originally attributed to CEA has subsequently been seriously challenged and ultimately discarded. Prior absorption of antisera with extracts of normal colonic mucosa inhibits the precipitin reaction between CEA and antibody, suggesting that normal colon contains CEA though in much lower concentrations (Martin and Martin, 1970). Furthermore CEA has now been isolated from a variety of non-gastrointestinal cancerous tissues (Khoo, Warner, Lie and Mackay, 1973; Pusztaszeri and Mach, 1973).

With the development of sensitive radioimmunoassays for CEA, a CEA reactive substance has been detected in serum from normal individuals (Laurence et al., 1972; Booth, King, Leonard and Dykes, 1973), and extracts of pooled normal plasma have revealed a glycoprotein which is immunologically indistinguishable from CEA (Chu, Reynoso and Hansen, 1972). CEA-like material has also been found in normal and inflammatory tissue (Pusztaszeri and Mach, 1973; Kupchik and Zamcheck, 1972; Burtin, Martin, Sabine and von Kleist, 1972; Martin and Martin, 1972). On the basis of these observations CEA must therefore be regarded as a tumour-associated substance rather than one which is tumour specific. CEA concentrations measured in perchloric acid extracts of colonic carcinomata and normal colonic mucosa have been reported as 2–230 ng/g and 1–8 ng/g respectively (Martin and Martin, 1972).

NATURE, PROPERTIES AND METABOLISM

The initial demonstration of the solubility of CEA in perchloric extract strongly suggested α glycoprotein composition. Subsequent studies have confirmed this and shown the molecule to be water-soluble with an electrophoretic mobility similar to a β globulin (Krupey,

Gold and Freedman, 1968). Speculation continues as to whether or not CEA is a single molecule and variants have been described (Ichiki, Wenzel, Quirin, Lange and Eveleigh, 1976). Whilst most CEA preparations from metastatic colonic carcinomata have single peaks on ultracentrifugation and sedimentation coefficients in the range 6.9S to 8.0S, suggesting molecular homogeneity, other reports describe multiple peaks and sedimentation coefficients outside this range (Krupey et al., 1968; Coligan, Lautenschleger, Egan and Todd, 1972).

The chemical composition of the CEA molecule also appears to vary between preparations, although the principal amino acid constituents undoubtedly include aspartic acid, proline, glutamic acid, serine, leucine and threonine, whilst methionine is universally absent (Terry, Henkart, Coligan and Todd, 1972). The importance of the molecular structure has been emphasized by Westwood and Thomas (1975), who showed the importance of the disulphide bonds in maintaining immunological identity. The carbohydrate portion of the CEA molecule is characterized by absence of galactosamine and by the presence of mannose. The preparation of immunologically active heterosaccharides of CEA by polystyrene sulphonic acid hydrolytic degradation now suggests that N-acetyl glucosamine is of major importance in the immunoreactive site of CEA, although the pure sugar is not itself immunoreactive (Banjo, Gold, Gehrke, Freedman and Krupey, 1974).

Much confusion still exists concerning the structure of the CEA molecule, but Coligan, Henkart, Todd and Terry (1973) have provided evidence for CEA being a heterogeneous molecular collection with cross-reacting antigenic determinants. Despite the clear demonstration of heterogeneity, it has been possible to establish an international standard which has now been used for inter-laboratory comparisons in many countries (Laurence, Turberville, Anderson and Neville, 1975).

Gold and Freedman (1965) originally suggested that embryonic antigens such as CEA are necessary to maintain the viability of incompletely differentiated cells, and that during the process of cellular differentiation and specialization, repression of these primitive cellular components occurs. During carcinogenesis, de-differentiation and de-repression take place, leading to the reappearance of CEA.

The finding of the blood group A reactive site on the CEA molecule led to the suggestion that CEA is an incompletely synthesized blood group antigen (Simmons and Perlmann, 1973). Carbohydrate analysis does not, however, provide support for this hypothesis since N-acetyl galactosamine, the key immunoreactive constituent of A antigen, is absent in the majority of CEA preparations.

The cellular localization of CEA suggests it to be a secretory product of the cell (Denk, Tappeiner,

Eckerstorfer and Holzner, 1972), and its association with the intracytoplasmic mucus of gastric carcinoma signet ring cells suggests that CEA is an abnormal mucus glycoprotein. Such glycoproteins derived from mucus have been demonstrated in gastrointestinal tumours (Schrager, 1972). However, comparison of the distribution of CEA and a perchloric acid soluble mucus associated antigen has revealed that the production of CEA is independent of mucus secretion (Tappeiner, Denk, Eckerstorfer and Holzner, 1973). CEA has also been described as a sialoglycoprotein synthesized in the liver in increased amounts in malignant disease (Apfel and Peters, 1969), but it is undoubtedly produced by human colonic cancer cell lines in tissue culture (Burtin, Buffe, von Kleist, Wolff and Wolff, 1970), and it seems unlikely that hepatic synthesis plays an important role in its production. The metabolism of radio-labelled CEA has been studied in dogs and rabbits and the plasma disappearance curve appears to resolve into two sections, suggesting two major molecular subgroupings (Shuster, Silverman and Gold, 1973).

CLINICAL APPLICATIONS

Any tumour antigen released intact into accessible body fluids is of potential importance as a possible aid to cancer diagnosis. Gold's group (Thomson, Krupey, Freedman and Gold, 1969), employing a radioimmunoassay for CEA in perchloric acid extracts of serum, found that 35 of 36 patients with colo-rectal carcinomata had CEA levels in excess of their normal range (0–2.5 ng/ml). The values all fell to normal after complete surgical resection of the tumour. The high proportion of positive results in colo-rectal cancer was confirmed by Moore, Kupchik, Marcon and Zamcheck (1971), but raised levels were also found in patients with non-neoplastic diseases, particularly alcoholic cirrhosis. The second major radioimmunoassay method employs separation of antibody-bound CEA from free antigen by zirconyl phosphate gel (Z-gel), and positive results have again been recorded in non-malignant disease, particularly chronic renal failure, chronic respiratory disease and ulcerative colitis (Lo Gerfo, Krupey and Hansen, 1971).

A major disadvantage of both ammonium sulphate precipitation and the Z-gel radioimmunoassays is the requirement of prior extraction with perchloric acid from relatively large quantities of serum. A double antibody radioimmunoassay performed on whole serum or plasma and completed within 24 hours was developed by Egan, Lautenschleger, Coligan and Todd (1972) and has been extensively evaluated (Laurence et al., 1972; Booth et al., 1973).

Results from these assays are summarized in Table 15.1. Elevated CEA levels are found in approximately 70 per cent of patients with gastrointestinal malignant

Table 15.1 Comparison of results of radioimmunoassay of CEA[a]

Method Disease	Ammonium sulphate precipitates				Z-gel		Double antibody	
	(1)	(2)	(3)	(4)	(5)	(6)	(7)	(8)
Neoplasia								
Colon/rectum	97	91	64	68	86	83	69	71
Stomach	–	3/3	3/5		73	2/5	2/5	61
Pancreas	–	100	4/7	4/4	2/2	3/3	3/3	100
Lung	–	6/8	1/1	67	77	7/10	70	43
Breast	–	0/1	50	45	63	–	48	31
Total non-GI	0	46	51	–	70	39	44	36
Non-neoplastic								
Peptic ulcer		–	–		0	–	33	14
Inflammatory bowel disease	0	1/8	30	43	30	–	32	10
Cirrhosis		45	48		0	–	4/5	55
Chronic bronchitis		–	–	–	11	–	45	2/7

[a] Results are expressed as percentage of patients showing elevated levels.
(1) Thomson, Krupey, Freedman and Gold (1969).
(2) Moore, Kupchik, Marcon and Zamcheck (1971).
(3) Joint National Cancer Institute of Canada/American Cancer Society Investigation (1972).
(4) Mach *et al.* (1973).
(5) Lo Gerfo, Krupey and Hansen (1971).
(6) Reynoso *et al.* (1972).
(7) Laurence *et al.* (1972).
(8) Booth, King, Leonard and Dykes (1973).

disease and 40 per cent of patients with other malignant lesions. A major set-back has been the failure of the CEA test to differentiate clearly between neoplastic and non-neoplastic disease; this is particularly disappointing in clinical situations where the distinction is a common problem. Raised values in non-neoplastic disease are not the result of shared antigenic determinants with a glycoprotein of smaller molecular size present in normal tissues (NCA) (von Kleist, Chavanel and Burtin, 1972; Mach and Pusztaszeri, 1972), nor are they related to interference in the assay from non-specific serum glycoproteins (Crawley *et al.*, 1974).

CEA estimation is of some value in determining the extent of tumour spread (Fig. 15.1). The CEA levels have been analysed with respect to the tumour stage in colonic, gastric and breast carcinomata. A minority of patients without lymph node involvement (Group 1) have raised values. Where spread has occurred to the local lymph nodes (Group 2), the proportion rises, and where generalized dissemination occurs (Group 3), 92 per cent are positive. In many of these the level was greater than 100 ng/ml.

Although the overlap between values obtained in normals and in disease states makes the test of little value for cancer screening, Stevens, MacKay and Cullen (1976) have shown that when high CEA values are unexpectedly found in normal persons, careful follow-up indicates a several-fold increase in cancer incidence.

Positive CEA results have been recorded in between 10 per cent and 30 per cent of patients with non-neoplastic bowel disease (Fig. 15.2). Patients with ulcera-

tive colitis and to a lesser extent Crohn's disease carry a risk of malignant change, hence an important question has been whether elevated levels are indicative of a pre-

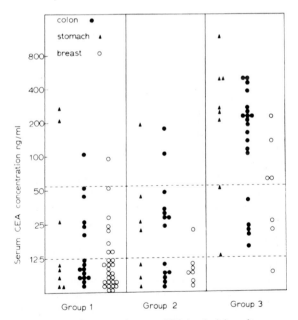

Fig. 15.1 Comparison of serum CEA levels (plotted logarithmically) and tumour dissemination. Normal range 0–12.5 ng/ml. Group 1 – localized tumours without lymph node metastases. Group 2 – tumours with local lymph node metastases. Group 3 – tumours with spread to liver, lung, or bone. (Booth, King, Leonard and Dykes, 1973) – reproduced by courtesy of the Editor of *Gut*.)

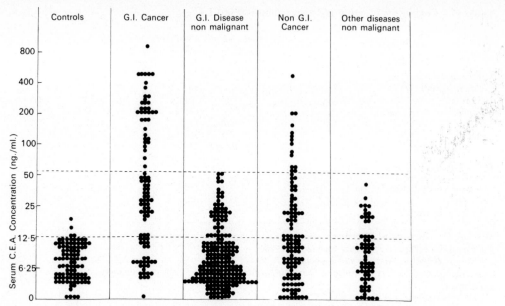

Fig. 15.2 CEA values in normal individuals and in patients with cancer and intestinal disease. (Booth, King, Leonard and Dykes, 1974 – reproduced by courtesy of the Editor of *Scandinavian Journal of Gastroenterology.*)

malignant state or an occult carcinoma. Although some results have been encouraging (Khoo, Hunt and Mackay, 1973; Moore, Kantrowitz and Zamcheck, 1972), in a recent large series of over 300 patients in whom CEA levels were monitored over a 12-month period, elevated values were found to relate more frequently to exacerbation of disease than to neoplasia. Thus this test is unlikely to assist the clinician as a screening test for a complicating carcinoma (Booth, King, Leonard and Dykes, 1974b).

The application of CEA estimation to diagnostic clinical practice has therefore often been disappointing. A prospective evaluation in patients with clinical features of gastrointestinal disease has shown that the test adds little, if anything, to current techniques in the diagnosis of gastric or colo-rectal malignant disease (Booth, 1975). However, results in patients with obstructive jaundice, iron deficiency anaemia, or features of pancreatic disease in which the suspicion of malignancy arose, showed better separation between different diagnostic groups and more information is necessary to clarify the possible usefulness of the test here.

The highest CEA levels occur in association with metastatic disease, especially to the liver (Steele, Cooper, Mackay, Losowsky and Goligher, 1974; Booth *et al.*, 1974a). Pre-operative elevations in blood levels have also been suggested as a valuable prognostic index in apparently operable patients, but the bulk of evidence is against this (Booth *et al.*, 1974a; Mackay *et al.*, 1974) and pathological staging correlates much more closely with ultimate prognosis than does CEA.

A more valuable use for the assay appears to be in the follow-up of patients apparently successfully treated for carcinoma where the serum CEA concentration is normal some months after the operation. Rising values have been observed (Fig. 15.3) in association with the development of secondary deposits from carcinoma of the colon (Booth *et al.*, 1974a; Sorokin *et al.*, 1974; Mach *et al.*, 1974; Mackay *et al.*, 1974), breast (Steward, Nixon, Zamcheck and Aisenberg, 1974), and female genital tract (Khoo and Mackay, 1974), commonly preceding

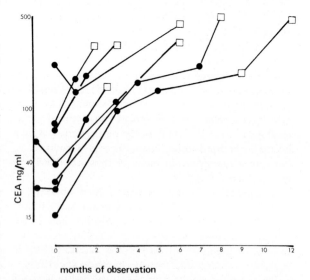

months of observation

Fig. 15.3 Rising CEA values in patients surgically treated for colonic cancer who later developed cancer. (No clinical evidence of cancer – ●; clinical evidence of recurrence – □.)

clinical abnormality by up to 18 months. A fall in CEA concentration as the result of chemotherapy has been observed to correlate with clinical remission (Skarin, Delwiche, Zamcheck, Lokich and Frei, 1974), an observation which may become of considerable clinical value.

More recently Plow and Edgington (1975) have isolated and characterized an apparent isomeric species of CEA which they call CEA-S. Subsequently they detected elevated CEA-S levels in 80 per cent of patients with gastrointestinal cancer, with less than 1 per cent elevation in patients without neoplasia (Edgington, Astarita and Plow, 1975). These results, which compare with the original studies from Montreal (Thomson, Krupey, Freedman and Gold, 1969), have yet to be confirmed by other workers, though a further report of a more specific CEA comes from Rogers, Searle and Bagshawe (1976).

Clinical studies on CEA concentration have not only been directed towards serum and plasma but CEA has also been quantitated in urine and increased values found in patients with bladder carcinomata, and occasionally in urine infection (Hall et al., 1972). Also CEA has been detected in the faeces of cancer patients by immunodiffusion (Freed and Taylor, 1972), but the occurrence of CEA-like activity in the faeces of some normal individuals is obviously a severe limitation and precludes diagnostic value (Elias, Holyoake and Chu, 1974). In patients with neoplastic pleural and ascitic effusions, the concentration of CEA in effusion fluid may be several times the serum concentration. Thus fluid CEA levels used in conjunction with cytology may significantly improve the diagnostic value of examining effusion fluid (Booth, Lakin, Dykes, Burnett and Bradwell, 1977).

Injected radio-labelled CEA-specific antisera localizes to human colonic carcinomata grafted into hamsters (Primus, Wang, Goldenberg and Hansen, 1973) and into nude mice (Mach, Carrel, Merenda, Sordat and Cerottini, 1974). External body scanning can then detect the tumour via its localized radio-labelled antiserum. From the preliminary results it was apparent that large tumours did not take up labelled antibody as well as small lesions, possibly because of large amounts of circulating antigen. Labelled tumour antibodies have also been used in man to localize tumours with some limited success (Quinones, Mizejewski and Beierwaltes, 1971).

ALPHA FOETOPROTEIN – AFP

The second major tumour-associated macromolecule in human cancer, alpha foetoprotein (AFP) also has an oncofoetal specificity. Abelev, Perova, Khramkova, Postnikova and Irlin (1963) first reported that an alpha-1-globulin, known to be present in the serum of foetal but not adult mice, was antigenically identical to a protein synthesized by mouse hepatoma. A similar protein was subsequently observed in the blood of 2 patients with primary liver cancer and was found to cross-react with a monospecific antiserum against a component of human foetal serum (Tatarinov, 1965). Subsequent studies have confirmed the presence of AFP in the foetus and in association with hepatic tumours of many mammalian species (Gitlin and Boesman, 1966).

SYNTHESIS OF AFP

Alpha foetoprotein is synthezised at an early stage in embryonic life and by the 8th week of gestation AFP and albumin are present in approximately equal concentrations, approximately 250–500 ng/100 ml (Andreoli and Robbins, 1962). Thereafter the albumin concentration rises and the AFP level remains constant until midterm when it declines to become undetectable by immonodiffusion at the time of delivery (Masopust, Kithier, Fuchs, Kotal and Radl, 1967).

The major sites of AFP synthesis in embryonic life appear to be the liver and yolk sac (Abelev and Bakirov, 1967). Immunofluorescent microscopy has shown AFP to be associated with the hepatocyte and no staining is detectable in relation to haemopoietic cells, bile ducts or Kuppfer cells (Enggl'gardt, Shipova, Grusev, Jasova and Ter-Grigorova, 1969; Chu, Lin, Yoshida, Chu and Lin, 1974).

No direct evidence has been obtained of AFP synthesis in man, but Kew and his colleagues (1973) have reported elevated serum AFP levels in almost all patients with viral hepatitis. In most cases AFP levels reached a peak late in the illness when other indices of hepatocellular damage were returning to normal, a finding compatible with increasing AFP synthesis during regeneration.

PROPERTIES AND FUNCTIONS OF AFP

The AFP of man is an alpha-1-globulin with a molecular weight of 64 000 and a sedimentation coefficient of 4·5 (Nishi, 1970). Only a small amount of the molecule appears to consist of carbohydrate (Ruoshlahti, Seppälä, Pihko and Vuopio, 1971). The physical properties of AFP are very similar to those of albumin and the two proteins are extremely difficult to separate except by immunological means (Abelev, 1971).

The role of AFP in foetal life is not clear. Presumably it acts as a substitute for albumin until the serum albumin concentration reaches adult levels (Uriel, de Nechaud and Dupiers, 1972). Early studies of serum AFP concentrations in foetal life employed immunodiffusion, a relatively crude method of measurement with a lowest detectable concentration of 1 μg/ml. With the development of more sensitive methods of detection, such as immunoautoradiography and radioimmunoassay, it has recently been established that AFP persists in the serum into adult life, albeit in minute quantities in the region of 1–6 ng/ml (Chayvialle and Ganguli, 1973). It is, therefore, likely that AFP being present in early foetal life is entirely accepted as a self-antigen by the immune system and its presence in the tumour is concentration dependent and not antigenically specific. There are no published studies of immunological reactions to AFP in man, but AFP has been shown to reduce lymphocyte transformation to phytohaemagglutinin (PHA) in man and in the rat (Caldwell, Stevenson and Thompson, 1973). Ziegenfuss (1973) has therefore suggested that transfusion of hepatitis antiserum (containing antibodies to Australia antigen) and lymphocytes sensitized to Australia antigen might reduce this immunological suppression and be of possible value as immunotherapy for hepatocellular carcinoma.

CLINICAL STUDIES

Abelev (1971) has reviewed the clinical data and the results of AFP determinations by immunodiffusion available on more than 1000 patients with primary cancer of the liver and a synopsis of these results is given in Table 15.2. Approximately 70 per cent of patients with primary hepatomas have AFP detectable by immunodiffusion, whereas a negligible proportion of patients with cholangiocellular carcinoma, non-hepatic neoplasia and non-neoplastic liver disease have positive results. Although very few patients with metastatic liver cancer in the original series had elevated AFP levels, more recent studies have revealed positive results in gastric, pancreatic and prostatic cancer metastatic to the liver (O'Conor, Tatarinov, Abelev and Uriel, 1970; Mehlman, Bulkley and Wiernik, 1971).

Considerable variation in the proportion of positive results in hepatocellular cancer has been reported from different areas of the world. Thus in the native populations of South Africa and Senegal where there is a high incidence of primary liver cancer, over 80 per cent of hepatomas are associated with positive AFP levels (Hull, Carbone, Moertel and O'Conor, 1970). The proportion of positive results from Western European countries, however, is approximately 50 per cent, although the rate is higher in patients of African origin. Race may not be the major factor in this difference, for it has been noted that AFP concentrations are higher in younger patients and that the African groups are younger than the European (Mawas, Buffe and Burtin, 1970; Vogel, Primack, McIntire, Carbone and Anthony, 1974).

Even with hepatoma there remains a variable proportion of patients with negative AFP levels by immunodiffusion and more sensitive techniques have therefore been devised in an attempt to increase the diagnostic yield. An immunoautoradiographic method has recently been described with a sensitivity of 50 ng/ml; subjected to this technique 75 per cent of patients, AFP negative by immunodiffusion, have raised levels (Abelev et al., 1971). However, the disadvantage of increased sensitivity is an increase in the incidence of elevated values in other conditions. Thus 98 per cent of women after 15 weeks of gestation have elevated levels, and positive results were also recorded in 14 per cent of patients with metastatic liver cancer and 13 per cent with acute viral hepatitis.

Radioimmunoassays have been developed which are capable of detecting AFP in a concentration as low as 1 ng/ml (Ruoslahti and Seppälä, 1971; Kohn and Weaver, 1974). This sensitive technique detects AFP in the serum of normal adults, the level appearing to rise slightly with age. In addition to secondary carcinoma and viral hepatitis, raised AFP levels by radioimmunoassay may occur in ataxia telangiectasia (Waldmann and McIntire, 1972), childhood cirrhosis (Nayak, Malaviya, Chawla and Chandra, 1972) and rarely in certain gastric carcinomata (Bourreille, Metayer, Sauger, Matray and Fondimare, 1970; Kozower, Fawaz, Mitler and Kaplar, 1971). Despite the increased sensitivity, however, AFP levels within the normal range are encountered in about 10 per cent of patients with hepatocellular carcinomata. There appears to be little relationship to the degree of cellular differentiation (Purves, Bersohn and Geddes, 1970; Abelev et al., 1971), but successful tumour resection may be associated with a fall in AFP concentration (Abelev, 1971).

Table 15.2 The incidence of positive AFP results by immunodiffusion in man. (From the data reviewed by Abelev, 1971)

Country	Hepatoma	Cholangiocellular carcinoma	Metastatic liver carcinoma	Non-neoplastic liver disease	Non-hepatic neoplasia
U.S.S.R.	78.5	2·2	0·4	0·3	0
France	60	0	0·4	0	–
U.S.A.	45	0	0	0	0
U.K.	43	0	0	0	–
South Africa (Bantu)	82	–	–	0	–
Senegal	80	–	–	0	2·9
Total (World; including data not listed above)	69	1·37	0·6	0·25	0·9

In anencephaly and spina bifida there is leakage of serum foetal proteins into the amniotic fluid. The concentration of AFP in maternal blood (Seller, Singer, Coltart and Campbell, 1974) and amniotic fluid (Harris et al., 1974) may thus rise dramatically and be of value in diagnosis or as an indication for termination of pregnancy.

Thus the principal role of serum AFP estimation still appears to be as an aid to the diagnosis of primary hepatocellular carcinoma. Caution must, however, be exercised in the interpretation of marginally elevated results using the more sensitive tests, and equally, negative results should not be relied upon to exclude the diagnosis. In addition the test may be of value as an index of hepatic regeneration after acute hepatic necrosis and as an index of foetal abnormality or distress during pregnancy.

OTHER TUMOUR-ASSOCIATED MACROMOLECULES

FOETAL SULPHOGLYCOPROTEIN ANTIGEN (FSA)

Foetal sulphoglycoprotein antigen (FSA) can be detected in human foetal gastrointestinal tissue from the 7th month of gestation, yet it disappears within the first year of extra-uterine life (Häkkinen, Korhonen and Saxen, 1968). FSA has been reported in the gastric juice of a high proportion of patients with gastric carcinomata, but the antigen may occasionally occur in association with other diseases, including benign peptic ulceration (Häkkinen and Viikari, 1969). Immunological cross-reactivity between CEA and FSA has been demonstrated (Häkkinen, 1972).

Other gastric juice antigens have been described in association with gastric malignancy, but their relationship with CEA or FSA is not known (Deutsch, Apffel, Mori and Walker, 1973; Patterson, Cain, Stoebner and Fox, 1971).

ONCOFOETAL PANCREATIC ANTIGEN

Using the relatively crude technique of immunodiffusion, an antigen extracted from human foetal pancreas has been detected in the sera of 36 of 37 patients with pancreatic carcinoma. The antigen was absent from the sera of patients with other intestinal carcinomata, hepatoma, acute and chronic pancreatitis, and patients with non-neoplastic obstructive jaundice (Banwo, Versey and Hobbs, 1974). These results are promising and initial development using an immunoelectrophoretic method has characterized a number of sub-fractions, but confirmation of these findings is required.

NON-SPECIFIC CROSS-REACTING ANTIGEN (NCA)

Mention has already been made of a perchloric acid soluble glycoprotein of approximate molecular weight 50 000 daltons with similar properties to and shared antigenic determinants with CEA. This antigen, termed non-specific cross-reacting (NCA), is found in many organs, including lung, spleen and normal colonic mucosa. NCA can be detected in cancerous gastrointestinal mucosa and in the serum of cancer patients. A radioimmunoassay for NCA has been developed, but the results are not cancer specific (Darcy, Turberville and James, 1973).

MEMBRANE-ASSOCIATED TISSUE AUTOANTIGEN (MTA)

This recently characterized antigen is also soluble in perchloric acid and has an alpha electrophoretic mobility. It is a glycoprotein with a molecular weight of 30 000–40 000 daltons, but it has no antigenic relationship with CEA or NCA (von Kleist, King and Burtin, 1974). MTA is present in colo-rectal carcinomata and in their hepatic metastases; it can also be found in foetal colonic mucosa, but may occur in small amounts in normal mucosa. An interesting finding, however, is that MTA appears to be autoantigenic (Burtin, 1974). There have to date been no published reports of serum MTA levels in patients.

Many other cancer-associated substances have been described but are at the moment without practical use. They have been well reviewed by Laurence and Neville (1973). A further approach to the search for a specific cancer-related substance has been the examination of multiple indices, for example levels of serum enzymes and other substances. Promising results have been described (Bullen, Cooper, Turner, Neville, Giles and Hall, 1977; Bradwell, Burnett, Ford and Newman, 1976), but confirmation of the value of this approach is required.

IMMUNOLOGICAL CHANGES IN HUMAN GASTROINTESTINAL CANCER

HUMORAL IMMUNITY

Humoral factors with apparent antitumour activity have been described in association with a wide variety of human tumours using several methods of antibody detection (Lewis, 1972; Graham and Graham, 1955; Finney, Byers and Wilson, 1960). Graham and Graham (1955) demonstrated detectable antibodies to a tumour extract in 25 per cent of cancer patients, but the validity of many of these early reports is questionable because of doubts about the cancer specificity of the antigens used. Thus von Kleist and Burtin (1966) showed that whilst the majority of patients with colonic carcinomata had apparently cancer-specific antibodies, absorption studies disclosed that precipitating and haemagglutinating activity was also directed against extracts of normal colonic tissue. Several groups have now reported humoral immunity to colo-rectal tumours (Hodkinson and Taylor, 1969; Nairn *et al.*, 1971), and that such responses may be transient in nature (Odili and Taylor, 1971).

More success has followed the search for specific antibodies in association with malignant melanoma and Lewis *et al.* (1969) have demonstrated that 80 per cent of patients with a localized lesion had circulating antibodies. Absorption studies using normal skin, melanin and liver did not remove the reactive immunoglobulin (Phillips and Lewis, 1970), thus going a long way to confirm tumour specificity. Lewis (1972) has further suggested that these antibodies disappear prior to the clinical appearance of secondary deposits. This phenomenon appears unrelated to the total mass of tumour present, and more recent work from the same group (Hartmann, Lewis, Proctor and Lyons, 1974) indicates the presence of anti-antibodies and argues that these might be responsible for this antibody disappearance.

The possibility of a humoral immune response to the recognized gastrointestinal tumour antigens has received much attention. Alexander (1972) emphasized that foetal antigens such as CEA and AFP are tumour associated rather than specific. Thus their presence in minute quantities in later foetal and extra-uterine life ensures their acceptance as self and thus prevents an immune response in the tumour-bearing host. On the other hand, foetal antigens common to very early embryonal tissues may be capable of stimulating antibody production if they disappear before the development of immunological competence in the foetus.

Gold (1967) tested the sera of a large number of subjects for anti-CEA activity using a semi-purified CEA preparation and a modification of the bis-diazotized benzidine (BDB) haemagglutination technique. Haemagglutinating activity was found in the sera of 70 per cent of patients with non-metastatic digestive tract cancer, but in none of the patients in whom dissemination had occurred. Anti-CEA activity was also demonstrated in the serum of the majority of pregnant and post-partum women studied, although only two subjects in a control group with non-neoplastic diseases and none of the normal controls had positive results.

Although Haverback and Dyce (1972) have provided some small support for the presence of anti-tumour antibodies, Collatz, von Kleist and Burtin (1971) were unable to demonstrate CEA antibodies by passive haemagglutination, immunoabsorption or immunofluorescence. Positive results in some patients were found to be due to antibodies directed against normal tissue proteins in the perchloric acid extracts of tumour, and as Gold also used only semi-purified tumour extracts, it was felt that doubt must exist as to the cancer-specific nature of his antibodies. Similarly antibody activity against CEA could not be demonstrated using the Z-gel radioimmunoassay (Lo Gerfo, Herter and Bennett, 1972).

Gold, Freedman and Gold (1972), in a further study using a radioimmunoelectrophoretic test, concluded that although there was some cross-reactivity between CEA and anti-A-antibody, at least some pregnant women and patients with digestive tract malignancy do have anti-CEA antibodies which did not cross-react. Similar results have been obtained by MacSween (1975).

The existence of CEA–anti-CEA complexes have been questioned and they have been postulated as a cause for the nephrotic syndrome complicating a disseminated colonic carcinoma (Costanza, Pinn, Schwartz and Nathanson, 1973). King, Leonard and Dykes examined both CEA positive and negative sera from patients with colonic cancer for the presence of such complexes. They lowered the pH to dissociate any complexes present, added radio-labelled CEA, and readjusted the pH to 7·4. Using the precipitating second antibody employed in the standard radioimmunoassay (Egan, Lautenschleger, Coligan and Todd, 1972) they then looked for radioactivity in the precipitate. The results showed complete absence of such activity, thus providing good evidence against the presence of complexes in the original sera, and their existence is currently under considerable doubt. Thus with respect to humoral reactions to CEA there is currently little evidence that they do in fact occur, a conclusion entirely consistent with the presence of CEA in normal serum and other normal tissues.

The demonstration of small amounts of AFP in the serum of normal adults, and FSA in gastric juice during the first year of life, similarly argues strongly against these macromolecules being potentially antigenic. The observation of antibodies to the membrane-associated tissue autoantigen (MTA) in colo-rectal carcinomata is of interest, but requires confirmation (Burtin, 1974).

CELL-MEDIATED IMMUNITY

The immunological cell-mediated response to tumours can be either antibody dependent or independent. As the result of experiments undertaken at the beginning of this century, it was demonstrated that tumour immunity could be transferred passively by injection of blood cells from an immune animal into a non-immune subject of the same species (Bashford, Murray, Cramer and Russell, 1908). Syngeneic animal strains had not been developed at this time and these studies did not differentiate between transplantation and umour-specific immunity. Thus it was a further 50 years before Michison (1955) firmly established the role of cell-mediated immunity in the rejection of animal tumours and since that time a large body of evidence has accumulated which shows these reactions do occur in the presence of malignant tumours in man (Klein, 1970).

Non-specific cell-mediated immunity

In addition to these specific responses to a given tumour, the general level of cellular responsiveness has been extensively studied. Catalona and Chretien (1973) have shown diminished skin reactions to dinitrochlorobenzene (DNCB) in patients with non-lymphoid tumours, but failed to demonstrate any difference between those whose disease was localized and those with dissemination. Hughes and Mackay (1965), using intradermal injections of tuberculin, showed a normal response in the presence of localized disease, but a marked reduction in reactivity following spread to local nodes or distant metastases. Indeed suppression of cellular reactivity in the presence of advanced metastatic disease has been widely reported (Gross, 1965; Twomey, Catalona and Chretien, 1974) and furthermore a relationship has also been demonstrated between low peripheral blood lymphocyte counts and advanced tumours (Bone and Lauder, 1974).

A more direct test of the competence of cellular immunity in cancer patients is the capacity to reject transplanted tissue, and in fact delayed rejection of tumour transplants and of normal skin homografts has been clearly demonstrated in patients with advanced malignant disease (Grace and Kondo, 1958; Southam and Moore, 1958; Itoh and Southam, 1964).

The response of lymphocytes in culture to the non-specific mitogen phytohaemagglutinin (PHA) is now generally considered to correlate with the function of the T-lymphocyte, the major effector cell of the cellular immune system. Thus lymphocyte transformation in response to PHA has been studied in a wide variety of human tumours (Garrioch, Good and Gatti, 1970; Sample, Gertner and Chretien, 1971), and Guillou, Brennan and Giles (1973) have reported similar results in patients with gastrointestinal cancer. They further showed that the cellular response was at least in part affected by serum factors as has been shown in other situations, e.g. coeliac disease (Maclaurin, Cooke and Ling, 1971). Edwards, Rowland and Lee (1973) demonstrated that portal venous serum from cancer patients has a much greater effect on this response than peripheral venous serum and suggested that the tumour was releasing an inhibitory substance.

The PHA response of lymphocytes from cancer patients is however, diminished even after washing and culture in homologous serum, suggesting that T-lymphocytes are either quantitatively or qualitatively abnormal in patients with malignant disease. Evidence to support selective T-cell depletion in gastrointestinal cancer has not been found (Guillou, 1974) and it thus seems likely that the T-lymphocytes are intrinsically abnormal, possibly already inhibited by bound tumour antigen. Whatever the mechanism involved, it is apparent that the defect in lymphocyte responsiveness is a reversible one

and is related to the presence of tumour tissue (McIllmurray and Langman, 1973).

Specific cell-mediated immunity

Initiation of delayed hypersensitivity to DNCB and the lymphocyte response to PHA test the general competence of the cellular immune system but give no indication of a response to specific antigens. Cellular immune responses to specific gastrointestinal tumour-associated antigens have been investigated using a variety of techniques, including delayed cutaneous hypersensitivity, lymphocyte transformation, leucocyte migration inhibition, colony inhibition and lymphocyte cytotoxicity.

Delayed cutaneous hypersensitivity reactions to cell-free extracts of autologous tumours have been reported in patients with a variety of neoplastic diseases (Fass, Ziegler, Heberman and Kiryabwire, 1970; Hughes and Lytton, 1964). Hollinshead, Glew, Bunnag, Gold and Heberman (1970) demonstrated delayed hypersensitivity reactions to a soluble membrane-associated antigen of autologous tumour cells in a large proportion of patients with carcinomata of the colon and rectum. Although negative reactions were observed with similar preparations of normal colonic mucosa, the skin-reactive antigen was found in the digestive-tract epithelial cells of first and second trimester foetuses. Purification and fractionation of the extract by polyacrylamide gel electrophoresis demonstrated its independence from CEA (Hollinshead et al., 1972).

Tumour-specific antigens have been shown to stimulate lymphocyte transformation in patients with malignant melanoma (Jehn, Nathanson, Schwartz and Skinner 1970), thus supporting the existence of specific cell-mediated immunity to tumour extracts. Similar attempts in gastrointestinal malignancy using CEA have been unsuccessful (Lejtenyi, Freedman and Gold, 1971).

One of the most widely used tests of cell-mediated immunity has been the lymphocytotoxicity test first applied to human tumours by Hellström, Hellström, Pierce and Yang (1968) and Hellström, Hellström, Sjögren and Warren (1971). Damage has also been demonstrated to foetal intestinal cells in culture, suggesting the importance of an oncofoetal antigen (Hellström, Hellström and Shepard, 1970). Similar results were obtained in patients with carcinoma of the bladder by O'Toole, Perlmann, Unsgaard, Mobergery and Edsmyr (1972) who demonstrated a reduction in cytotoxicity in more advanced and widespread cancers, an observation supported by Bean, Pees, Fogh, Crabstald and Oettgen (1974) using a radioisotope modification of the test. In cancer of the uterine cervix, however, Saksela and Meyer (1973) were unable to demonstrate any difference between the patients with invasive and non-invasive tumour, and this question requires further study. Chemically induced tumours result in the production of neoantigen characterized by a high degree of specificity so that cross-reaction between tumours is uncommon (Baldwin, 1973), whereas in virally induced tumours the reaction is more commonly type specific with some cross-reaction also with foetal and cellular antigens (Coggin, Ambrose and Anderson, 1970). Contradictory information has appeared as to whether the operative cell in this reaction is a T- or B-lymphocyte (de Vries, Cornain and Rümke, 1972; Wybran, Hellström, Hellström and Fudenberg, 1974), but it seems likely that antibody-dependent lymphocytotoxicity plays an important role in tumour immunity (Stolfi, Stolfi, Fugman and Martin, 1974). Animal studies by Fisher, Saffer and Fisher (1974) showed higher concentrations of cytotoxic lymphocytes in regional lymph nodes related to experimental tumours, and the cells were shown to disappear several months after removal of the tumours or in the final stages before death. Embleton (1973) has demonstrated cytotoxicity in patients with colonic cancer, a phenomenon inhibited by serum and tumour extracts (Nind, Matthews, Pihl, Rollard and Nairn, 1975). Recently normal lymphocytes have been shown to have similar cytotoxic properties (Pross and Baines, 1976) and the significance of this phenomenon remains an open question.

Lymphocytes from animals immunized against specific antigen will on further exposure to that antigen respond by releasing a variety of lymphokines, including macrophage inhibitory factor (MIF) and leucocyte inhibitory factor (LIF) (Pick and Turk, 1972). Tests involving LIF have been widely applied to patients suffering from cancer (Wolburg, 1971; Anderson, Bjerrum, Bendixen, Schiødt and Dissing, 1970; Cochran, Spilg, Mackie and Thomas, 1972) and inhibition clearly demonstrated in a wide variety of tumours. Guillou and Giles (1973) have reported the results of leucocyte migration inhibition studies in patients with colo-rectal cancer using an antigen prepared by perchloric acid extraction of colonic tumours. Of 22 cancer subjects 15 showed significant inhibition of migration when cultures were carried out in homologous AB serum, whereas only 6 showed inhibition when the tests were performed in autologous serum. Since the preparation of antigen involved the extraction of colonic carcinomata with perchloric acid, it was considered that the cell-mediated immune response might be directed against CEA. On the other hand, Straus, Rule, Grotsky, Janowitz and Glade (1972) have used a CEA containing meconium antigen in the leucocyte migration inhibition test, and failed to demonstrate any inhibition of migration in carcinoma patients.

McIllmurray, Price and Langman (1974) have indicated tumour specificity for the leucocyte migration test and Black, Leis, Shore and Zachrau (1974) showed a relationship between leucocyte migration and tumour

staging in studies using autologous breast cancer as antigen. Their data also indicated more inhibition to autologous antigen than to homologous antigen, but this question is still open to doubt (Cochran et al., 1974). A similar test using migration of a lymphocyte–monocyte mixture has given extremely promising results (Bull, Leibach, Williams and Helms, 1973) with good differentiation between cancerous patients on the one hand and normal and non-cancerous on the other.

Other tests being applied in this field include the macrophage electrophoretic mobility test (MEM) described by Field and Caspary (1972) and more recently applied by Pritchard, Moore, Sutherland and Joslin (1973). Good results using a leucocyte adherence test by Halliday, Maluish and Isbister (1974) have unfortunately not been confirmed (Armitstead and Gowland, 1976).

Early difficulties in obtaining reproducible results in the cytotoxicity assay prompted Currie and Basham (1972) to extensively wash lymphocytes before carrying out in-vitro testing. They demonstrated a considerable increase in the proportion of positive reactions suggesting the attachment to cells of inhibitory factors. It is clear that different groups of factors exist and the position has been greatly clarified by Baldwin, Price and Robins (1973), who defined an inhibitory substance as one which affects primarily the effector cell, i.e. the lymphocyte, whereas a blocking factor is one which attaches to and affects the target or cancer cell. Such interference was first demonstrated in human patients by Hellström, Sjögren, Warner and Hellström (1971), who have since provided evidence for a role of antigen–antibody complexes in this context (Hayami, Hellström and Hellström, 1974). Robins and Baldwin (1974) have also produced evidence for antibodies and antigens being involved in this reaction in addition to complexes and the final definition of the role and specificity of blocking remains to be established. The possibility that such inhibition might play an important clinical role has been established by studies in mice, where reinjection of thoracic duct lymphocytes washed free of lymph produced clear inhibition of tumour growth (Noonan, Gardner, Clunie, Isbister and Halliday, 1974). The immune relationship between solid tumours and their hosts is complex and poorly understood, and much further information is required (Stevenson and Lawrence, 1975).

IMMUNOTHERAPY

The suggestion that a patient may be cured of his cancer by successfully mobilizing his own immune defences against it, is neither new nor currently very promising. Currie (1972) in a review of 80 years of immunotherapy analysed recorded attempts into active, passive and adoptive immunization for both specific and non-specific stimulants. Though a plethora of techniques and protocols have been used, very little has been achieved, and it appears to be more sensible to consider appropriate animal models which most closely parallel the clinical question under consideration before human studies begin. A universal finding in animals has been the failure of immunotherapy in the presence of large volumes of tumour tissue (Levy, Whitney, Smith and Panno, 1974), thus most human studies taking place in the presence of advanced metastatic disease, frequently in moribund patients, face an almost insuperable hurdle. Recent studies in acute myeloid leukaemia (Powles *et al.*, 1973) have shown promise in this regard, immunization commencing at the completion of successful chemotherapy when the tumour burden was at a minimum and success appeared most probable. Similarly successful studies in gastrointestinal cancer are more likely to follow surgical excision (Rios and Simmons, 1974) than at a terminal stage with widespread dissemination (Graham and Graham, 1959; Taylor and Odile, 1972). In addition the combination of chemotherapy and immunotherapy (Davies, Buckham and Manstone, 1974) appears in animals to be a more successful form of treatment and also forms part of the current human leukaemia programme.

Non-specific immune stimulants introduced to leukaemia research by Mathé *et al.* (1969) have been widely applied in experimental cancer therapy, particularly in the form of bacterial products such as BCG and *Corynebacterium parvum*. Baldwin *et al.* (1974) have established that BCG must come into contact with the tumour for maximum effect and Likhite (1974) achieved successful tumour rejection in rats simply by injecting a *Corynebacterium* extract directly into a tumour mass. In man, similar results have been obtained using BCG in cutaneous deposits from colonic cancer (Bast, Zbar, Borsos and Rapp, 1974).

Passive and adoptive immune support has also been extensively studied in animals, and some effect shown by antibodies (Order, Kirkman and Knapp, 1974) and by lymphocytes and transfer factor (Krementz *et al.*, 1974). Antibodies have also been used simply as a localizing carrier of toxic substances, e.g. chlorambucil (Davies and O'Neill, 1973) and destructive enzymes (Shearer *et al.*, 1974). Such antisera against colonic cancer have shown immune reactivity against CEA and raise the possibility of including CEA in any immunotherapy programme.

It is to be hoped that the principles emerging from animal experimentation in immunotherapy will eventually produce positive results in human cancer which the current work in leukaemia foreshadows. For the moment the major contribution which immunology makes to human oncology is in providing a new understanding of the relationship between host and lesion, in assessing prognosis, and in the development of various diagnostic tests. It may reasonably be hoped that refinement of the present tests and those under development will make significant changes to patient care within the next decade and that further tentative explorations will be made of immunotherapy in certain special situations.

SUMMARY AND CONCLUSIONS

The introduction of the principles and techniques of immunology to gastrointestinal cancer has therefore raised many more problems than it has solved. Cancer-related antigens have been found and studied in hepatic, gastric and colonic tumours, but attempts to prove cancer-specificity have been unsuccessful. Nevertheless, immune reactions by the host against the invading lesion do occur and particularly in colonic disease are under increasing scrutiny. Both antibody and cell-mediated immunity against the tumour have been well documented, more usually to crude antigenic material, and it is probable that such studies will tell us much about the aetiology and pathogenesis of malignant disease. Why cancer appears more commonly at some sites and less at others is at the moment quite unclear but could have immunological implications. Localization of different types and groups of immune cells could be significant, and it is notable that Peyer's patches occur at a site where cancer is rare. Colonic cancer on the other hand is relatively common, and its incidence is higher still in the presence of chronic inflammatory disease. Perhaps the reason lies less in the wall than in the lumen, and bacterial products and steroid derivatives of bile salts have been postulated as the cause (Burkitt, 1971).

Whatever the explanation, study of the immune mechanisms will undoubtedly provide much help in elucidating the development of the lesion. The hope of developing useful diagnostic tests has been only partially fulfilled, but their value and importance in follow-up rather than early diagnosis is now established. A realistic immunotherapy programme is not a current possibility, but remains a continuing long-term goal.

REFERENCES

Abelev, G. I. (1971) Alpha-fetoprotein in ontogenesis and its association with malignant tumours. *Advances in Cancer Research*, **14**, 295–358.

Abelev, G. I. & Bakirov, R. D. (1967) *In vitro* synthesis of serum embryonic antigens by the liver. *Voprosy Meditsinskoi Khimii (Moskova)*, **13**, 378–383.

Abelev, G. I., Perova, S. D., Khramkova, N. I., Postnikova, Z. A. & Irlin, I. S. (1963) Production of embryonal α-globulin by transplantable mouse hepatomas. *Transplantation*, **1**, 174–180.

Abelev, G. I., Tsvetkov, V. S., Biriulina, T. I., Elgoit, D. A., Olovnikov, A. M., Grusev, A. I., Yazova, A. K., Perova, S. D., Rubtsov, I. V., Kantorovich, B. A., Tur, V., Khasanov, A. I. & Levina, D. M. (1971) Evaluation of the use of highly sensitive methods for the determination of alpha-fetoprotein in the diagnosis of hepatocellular cancer and teratoblastoma. *Biulleten Eksperimental'noi Biologii i Meditsiny (Muskova)*, **71**, 75–81.

Alexander, P. (1972) Foetal 'antigens' in cancer. *Nature*, **235**, 137–140.

Anderson, V., Bjerrum, O., Bendixen, G., Schiødt, T. & Dissing, I. (1970) Effect of autologous mammary tumour extracts on human leukocyte migration *in vitro*. *International Journal of Cancer*, **5**, 357–363.

Andreoli, M. & Robbins, J. (1962) Serum proteins and thyroxine-protein interaction in early human fetuses. *Journal of Clinical Investigation*, **41**, 1070–1077.

Apffel, C. A. & Peters, J. H. (1969) Tumors and serum glycoproteins. The Symbodies. *Progress in Experimental Tumour Research*, **12**, 1–54.

Armitstead, P. R. & Gowland, G. (1976) The leucocyte adherence inhibition test in cancer of the large bowel. *British Journal of Cancer*, **32**, 568–573.

Baldwin, R. W. (1973) Immunological aspects of chemical carcinogenesis. *Advances in Cancer Research*, **18**, 1–75.

Baldwin, R. W., Glaves, D. & Vose, B. M. (1974) Differentiation between the embryonic and tumour specific antigens on chemically induced rat tumours. *British Journal of Cancer*, **29**, 1–10.

Baldwin, R. W., Price, M. R. & Robins, R. A. (1973) Significance of serum factors modifying cellular immune responses to growing tumours. *British Journal of Cancer*, **28**, Suppl. 1, 37–47.

Baldwin, R. W., Cook, A. J., Hopper, D. G. & Pimm, M. V. (1974) Radiation-killed BCG in the treatment of transplanted rat tumours. *International Journal of Cancer*, **13**, 743–750.

Banjo, C., Gold, P., Gehrke, C. W., Freedman, S. O. & Krupey, J. (1974) Preparation and isolation of immunologically active glycopeptides from carcinoembryonic antigen (CEA). *International Journal of Cancer*, **13**, 151–163.

Banwo, O., Versey, J. & Hobbs, J. R. (1974) New oncofetal antigen for human pancreas. *Lancet*, **i**, 643–645.

Bashford, E., Murray, J. A., Cramer, W. & Russell, S. (1908) Third scientific report of the Imperial Cancer Research Fund.

Bast, R. C., Jr, Zbar, B., Borsos, T. & Rapp, H. J. (1974) BCG and cancer. *New England Journal of Medicine*, **290**, 1458–1469.

Bean, M. A., Pees, H., Fogh, J. E., Grabstald, H. & Oettgen, H. F. (1974) Cytotoxicity of lymphocytes from patients with cancer of the urinary bladder: detection by a ^{3}H-proline microcytotoxicity test. *International Journal of Cancer*, **14**, 186–197.

Black, M. M., Opler, S. R. & Speer, F. D. (1956) Structural representations of tumor–host relationships in gastric carcinoma. *Surgery, Gynaecology and Obstetrics*, **102**, 599–603.

Black, M. M., Leis, H. P., Jr, Shore, B. & Zachrau, R. E. (1974) Cellular hypersensitivity to breast cancer. Assessment by a leucocyte migration procedure. *Cancer*, **33**, 952–958.

Bone, G. & Lauder, I. (1974) Cellular immunity, peripheral blood lymphocyte count and pathological staging of tumours in the gastrointestinal tract. *British Journal of Cancer*, **30**, 215–221.

Booth, S. N. 'An evaluation of carcinoembryonic antigen in clinical medicine.' Unpublished MD Thesis, University of Birmingham, 1975.

Booth, S. N., King, J. P. G., Leonard, J. C. & Dykes, P. W. (1973) Serum carcinoembryonic antigen in clinical disorders. *Gut*, **14**, 794–799.

Booth, S. N., King, J. P. G., Leonard, J. C. & Dykes, P. W. (1974b) The significance of elevation of serum carcinoembryonic antigen (CEA) levels in inflammatory diseases of the intestine. *Scandinavian Journal of Gastroenterology*, **9**, 651–656.

Booth, S. N., Lakin, J., Dykes, P. W., Burnett, D. & Bradwell, A. R. (1977) Cancer-associated proteins in effusion fluids. *Journal of Clinical Pathology*, **30**, 537–548.

Booth, S. N., Jamieson, G. C., King, J. P. G., Leonard, J. C., Oates, G. D. & Dykes, P. W. (1974a) Carcinoembryonic antigen in management of colorectal carcinoma. *British Medical Journal*, **iv**, 183–187.

Bourreille, J., Metayer, P., Sauger, F., Matray, F. & Fondimare, A. (1970) Existence d'alpha foeto protéine au cours d'un cancer secondaire du foie d'origine gastrique. *Presse Médicale*, **78**, 1277–1278.

Bradwell, A. R., Burnett, D., Ford, C. & Newman, C. (1976) Serial measurements of plasma proteins for maintaining patients with carcinoma of the lung. *Clinical Science and Molecular Medicine*, **52**, 18P.

Bull, D. M., Leibach, J. R., Williams, M. A. & Helms, R. A. (1973) Immunity to colon cancer assessed by antigen-induced inhibition of mixed mononuclear cell migration. *Science*, **181**, 957–959.

Bullen, B. R., Cooper, E. H., Turner, R., Neville, A. M., Giles, G. R. & Hall, R. (1977) Cancer markers in patients receiving chemotherapy for colorectal cancer. In press.

Burkitt, D. P. (1971) Epidemiology of cancer of the colon and rectum. *Cancer*, **28**, 3–13.

Burnett, M. (1957) Cancer – A biological approach. *British Medical Journal*, **i**, 779–786 & 841–847.

Burtin, P. (1974) Membrane antigens of the colonic tumors. *Cancer*, **34**, 829–834.

Burtin, P., von Kleist, S. & Sabine, M. C. (1971) Loss of a normal colonic membrane antigen in human cancers of the colon. *Cancer Research*, **31**, 1038–1041.

Burtin, P., Martin, E., Sabine, M. C. & von Kleist, S. (1972) Immunological study of polyps of the colon. *Journal of the National Cancer Institute*, **48**, 25–29.

Burtin, P., Buffe, D., von Kleist, S., Wolff, E. & Wolff, E. (1970) Demonstration of the carcinoembryonic antigen specific for digestive cancers in human tumors maintained in organotypic culture. *International Journal of Cancer*, **5**, 88–95.

Caldwell, J. L., Severson, C. D. & Thompson, J. S. (1973) Human alpha-fetoprotein: embryonic alpha globulin with *in vitro* immunosuppressive activity. *Federation Proceedings*, **32**, 979.

Catalona, W. J. & Chretien, P. B. (1973) Abnormalities of quantitative dinitrochlorobenzene sensitization in cancer patients: correlating with tumor stage and histology. *Cancer*, **31**, 353–356.

Chayvialle, J. A. P. & Ganguli, P. C. (1973) Radioimmunoassay of alpha-fetoprotein in human plasma. *Lancet*, **i**, 1355–1357.

Chu, T. M., Reynoso, G. & Hansen, H. J. (1972) Demonstration of carcinoembryonic antigen in normal human plasma. *Nature*, **238**, 152–153.

Chu, M. L., Lin, W., Yoshida, T. O., Chu, S. H. & Lin, T. (1974) Demonstration of alpha-fetoglobulin in hepatoma tissue by fluorescent antibody technique. *Cancer*, **34**, 268–273.

Cochran, A. J., Spilg, W. G. S., Mackie, R. M. & Thomas, C. E. (1972) Postoperative depression of tumour directed cell mediated immunity in patients with malignant disease. *British Medical Journal*, **iv**, 67–70.

Cochran, A. J., Grant, R. M., Spilg, W. G., Mackie, R. M., Ross, C. E., Hoyle, D. E., & Russell, J. M. (1974) Sensitization to tumour-associated antigens in human breast carcinoma. *International Journal of Cancer*, **14**, 19–25.

Coggin, J. H., Ambrose, K. R. & Anderson, N. G. (1970) Fetal antigen capable of inducing transplantation immunity against SV40 hamster tumor cells. *Journal of Immunology*, **105**, 524–526.

Coligan, J. E., Henkart, P. A., Todd, C. W. & Terry, W. D. (1973) Heterogeneity of the carcinoembryonic antigen. *Immunochemistry*, **10**, 591–599.

Coligan, J. E., Lautenschleger, J. T., Egan, M. L. & Todd, C. W. (1972) Isolation and characterization of carcinoembryonic antigen. *Immunochemistry*, **9**, 377–386.

Collatz, E., von Kleist, S. & Burtin, P. (1971) Further investigations of circulating antibodies in colon cancer patients: on the autoantigenicity of the carcinoembryonic antigen. *International Journal of Cancer*, **8**, 298–303.

Cooper, E. H., Turner, R., Steele, L., Neville, A. M. & Mackay, A. M. (1975) The contribution of serum enzymes and carcinoembryonic antigen to the early diagnosis of metastatic colorectal cancer. *British Journal of Cancer*, **31**, 111–117.

Constanza, M. E., Pinn, V., Schwartz, R. S. & Nathanson, L. (1973) Carcinoembryonic antigen–antibody complexes in a patient with colonic carcinoma and and nephrotic syndrome. *New England Journal of Medicine*, **289**, 520–523.

Crawley, J. M., Northam, B. E., King, J. P. G., Leonard, J. C., Booth, S. N. & Dykes, P. W. (1974) The effect of serum protein concentrations on the specificity of the radioimmunoassay of carcinoembryonic antigen in malignant neoplasia and non-neoplastic disease. *Journal of Clinical Pathology*, **27**, 130–134.

Currie, G. A. (1972) Eighty years of immunotherapy: A review of immunological methods used for the treatment of human cancer. *British Journal of Cancer*, **26**, 141–153.

Currie, G. A. & Basham, C. (1972) Serum mediated inhibition of the immunological reactions of the patient to his own tumour: a possible role for circulating antigen. *British Journal of Cancer*, **26**, 427–438.

Darcy, D. A., Turberville, C. & James, R. (1973) Immunological study of carcinoembryonic antigen (CEA) and a related glycoprotein. *British Journal of Cancer*, **28**, 147–160.

Davies, D. A. L. & O'Neill, G. L. (1973) *In vivo* and *in vitro* effects of tumour specific antibodies with chlorambucil. *British Journal of Cancer*, **28**, Suppl. 1, 285–298.

Davies, D. A. L., Buckham, S. & Manstone, A. J. (1974) Protection of mice against syngeneic lymphomata. II. Collaboration between drugs and antibodies. *British Journal of Cancer*, **30**, 305–311.

Denk, H., Tappeiner, G., Eckerstorfer, R. & Holzner, J. H. (1972) Carcinoembryonic antigen (CEA) in gastrointestinal and extragastrointestinal tumors and its relationship to tumor cell differentiation. *International Journal of Cancer*, **10**, 262–272.

Deutsch, E., Apffel, C. A., Mori, H. & Walker, J. E. (1973) A tumor associated antigen in gastric cancer secretions. *Cancer Research*, **33**, 112–116.

de Vries, J. E., Cornain, S. & Rümke, P. (1974) Cytotoxicity of non-T versus T lymphocytes from melanoma patients and healthy donors on short- and long-term cultured melanoma cells. *International Journal of Cancer*, **14**, 427–434.

Dykes, P. W., Leonard, J. C., Speirs, C. & King, J. P. G. (1975) Lymphocyte cytotoxicity against colonic cancer cells in gastrointestinal disease. (Unpublished.)

Edgington, T. S., Astarita, R. W. & Plow, E. F. (1976) Association of an isomeric species of carcinoembryonic antigen with neoplasia of the gastrointestinal tract. *New England Journal of Medicine*, **293**, 103–107.

Edwards, A. J., Rowland, G. F. & Lee, M. R. (1973) Reduction of lymphocyte transformation by a factor produced by gastrointestinal cancer. *Lancet*, **i**, 687–689.

Egan, M. L., Lautenschleger, J. T., Coligan, J. E. & Todd, C. W. (1972) Radioimmune assay of carcinoembryonic antigen. *Immunochemistry*, **9**, 289–299.

Elias, E. G., Holyoke, E. D. & Chu, T. M. (1974) Carcinoembryonic antigen (CEA) in feces and plasma of normal subjects and patients with colorectal carcinoma. *Diseases of Colon and Rectum*, **17**, 38–41.

Embleton, M. J. (1973) Significance of tumour associated antigens on human colonic carcinomata. *British Journal of Cancer*, **28**, Suppl. 1, 142–152.

Enggl'gardt, N. V., Shipova, L. Ia., Grusev, A. I., Jasova, A. K. & Ter-Grigorova, E. N. (1969) Obnaruzhenie alpha-F-globulina na srezakh pecheni embrinona cheloveka i novorozhdennykh myshei s pomoshch'iu fliuorestsiruishchikh antitel. *Biulleten Eksperimental'noi Biologii i Meditsiny* (*Moskova*), **68**, 62–64.

Fass, L., Ziegler, J. L., Herberman, R. B. & Kiryabwire, J. W. M. (1970) Cutaneous hypersensitivity reactions to autologous extracts of malignant melanoma cells. *Lancet*, **i**, 116–118.

Field, E. J. & Caspary, E. A. (1972) Lymphocyte sensitization in advanced malignant disease: a study of serum lymphocyte depressive factor. *British Journal of Cancer*, **26**, 164–173.

Finney, J. W., Byers, E. H. & Wilson, R. H. (1960) Studies in tumor auto-immunity. *Cancer Research*, **20**, 351–356.

Fisher, B., Saffer, E. & Fisher, E. R. (1974) Studies concerning the regional lymph node in cancer. IV. Tumor inhibition by regional lymph node cells. *Cancer*, **33**, 631–636.

Foley, E. J. (1953) Antigenic properties of methylchloranthrene-induced tumors in mice of the strain of origin. *Cancer Research*, **13**, 835–837.

Freed, D. L. J. & Taylor, G. (1972) Carcinoembryonic antigen in faeces. *British Medical Journal*, **i**, 85–87.

Garrioch, D. B., Good, R. A. & Gatti, R. A. (1970) Lymphocyte response to P.H.A. in patients with non-lymphoid tumours. *Lancet*, **i**, 618.

Gatti, R. A. & Good, R. A. (1970) Aging, immunity and malignancy. *Geriatrics*, **25**, 158–168.

Gitlin, D. & Boesman, M. (1966) Serum α-fetoprotein, albumin, and γG-globulin in the human conceptus. *Journal of Clincal Investigation*, **45**, 1826–1838.

Gold, P. (1967) Circulating antibodies against carcinoembryonic antigens of the human digestive system. *Cancer*, **20**, 1663–1667.

Gold, P. & Freedman, S. O. (1965) Demonstration of tumor-specific antigens in human colonic carcinomata by immunological tolerance and absorption techniques. *Journal of Experimental Medicine*, 121, 439–462.

Gold, J. M., Freedman, S. O. & Gold, P. (1972) Human anti-CEA antibodies detected by radioimmunoelectrophoresis. *Nature (New Biology)*, 239, 60–62.

Gold, P., Krupey, J. & Ansari, H. (1970) Position of the carcinoembryonic antigen of the human digestive system in ultrastructure of tumor cell surface. *Journal of the National Cancer Institute*, 45, 219–222.

Grace, J. T., Jr & Kondo, T. (1958) Investigations of host resistance in cancer patients. *Annals of Surgery*, 148, 633–641.

Graham, J. B. & Graham, R. M. (1955) Antibodies elicited by cancer in patients. *Cancer*, 8, 409–416.

Graham, J. B. & Graham, R. M. (1959) The effect of vaccine on cancer patients. *Surgery, Gynaecology and Obstetrics*, 109, 131–138.

Gross, L. (1965) Immunological defect in aged population and its relationship to cancer. *Cancer*, 18, 201–204.

Guillou, P. Unpublished MD Thesis, Leeds University, 1974.

Guillou, P. J. & Giles, G. R. (1973) Inhibition of leucocyte migration by tumour-associated antigens of the colon and rectum. *Gut*, 14, 733–738.

Guillou, P. J., Brennan, T. G. & Giles, G. R. (1973) Phytohaemagglutinin stimulated transformation of peripheral and lymph-node lymphocytes in patients with gastro-intestinal cancer. *British Journal of Surgery*, 60, 745–749.

Häkkinen, I. (1972) Immunological relationship of the carinoembryonic antigen and the fetal sulfoglycoprotein antigen. *Immunochemistry*, 9, 1115–1119.

Häkkinen, I. & Viikari, S. (1969) Occurrence of fetal sulphoglycoprotein antigen in the gastric juice of patients with gastric diseases. *Annals of Surgery*, 169, 277–281.

Häkkinen, I., Korhonen, L. K. & Saxen, L. (1968) The time of appearance and distribution of sulphoglycoprotein antigens in the human foetal alimentary canal. *International Journal of Cancer*, 3, 582–592.

Hall, R. R., Laurence, D. J. R., Darcy, D., Stevens, U., James, R., Roberts, S. & Neville, A. M. (1972) Carcinoembryonic antigen in the urine of patients with urothelial carcinoma. *British Medical Journal*, iii, 609–611.

Halliday, W. J., Maluish, A. & Isbister, W. H. (1974) Detection of anti-tumour cell mediated immunity and serum blocking factors in cancer patients by the leucocyte adherence inhibition test. *British Journal of Cancer*, 29, 31–35.

Harris, J. & Bagai, R. C. (1972) Immune deficiency states associated with malignant disease in man. *Medical Clinics of North America*, 56, 501–514.

Harris, R., Jennison, R. F., Barson, A. J., Laurence, K. M., Ruoslahti, E. & Seppälä, M. (1974) Comparison of amniotic-fluid and maternal serum alpha-fetoprotein levels in the early antenatal diagnosis of spina bifida and anencephaly. *Lancet*, i, 429–433.

Hartmann, D., Lewis, M. G., Proctor, J. W. & Lyons, H. (1974) *In-vitro* interactions between antitumour antibodies and anti-antibodies in malignancy. *Lancet*, ii, 1481–1483.

Haverback, B. J. & Dyce, B. J. (1972) Tumour antigen (CEA) in gastric adenocarcinoma masked by a binding substance, likely an antibody. *Gastroenterology*, 62, 760.

Hayami, M., Hellström, I., Hellström, K. E. & Lannin, D. R. (1974) Further studies on the ability of regressor sera to block cell-mediated destruction of Rous sarcomas. *International Journal of Cancer*, 13, 43–53.

Hellström, I., Hellström, K. E. & Shepard, T. H. (1970) Cell-mediated immunity against antigens common to human colonic carcinomas and fetal gut epithelium. *International Journal of Cancer*, 6, 346–351.

Hellström, I., Hellström, K. E., Pierce, G. E. & Yang, J. P. S. (1968) Cellular and humoral immunity to different types of human neoplasms. *Nature*, 220, 1352–1354.

Hellström, I., Hellström, K. E., Sjögren, H. O. & Warner, G. A. (1971) Demonstration of cell mediated immunity to human neoplasms of various histological types. *International Journal of Cancer*, 7, 1–6.

Hellström, I., Sjögren, H. O., Warner, G. A. & Hellström, K. E. (1971) Blocking of cell-mediated tumour immunity by sera from patients with growing neoplasms. *International Journal of Cancer*, 7, 226–237.

Hellström, K. E. & Hellström, I. (1974) Lymphocyte mediated cytotoxicity and blocking serum activity to tumor antigens. *Advances in Immunology*, 18, 209–277.

Hodkinson, M. & Taylor, G. (1969) Autoimmune responses to human tumour antigens. *British Journal of Cancer*, 23, 510–514.

Hollinshead, A., Glew, D., Bunnag, B., Gold, P. & Herberman, R. (1970) Skin-reactive soluble antigen from intestinal cancer-cell membranes and relationship to carcinoembryonic antigens. *Lancet*, i, 1191–1195.

Hollinshead, A. C., McWright, C. G., Alford, T. C., Glew, D. H., Gold, P. & Heberman, R. B. (1972) Separation of skin reactive intestinal cancer antigen from the carcinoembryonic antigen of Gold. *Science*, 177, 887–889.

Hughes, L. E. & Lytton, B. (1964) Antigenic properties of human tumours: delayed cutaneous hypersensitivity reactions. *British Medical Journal*, i, 209–212.

Hughes, L. E. & Mackay, W. D. (1965) Suppression of the tuberculin response in malignant disease. *British Medical Journal*, ii, 1346–1348.

Hull, E. W., Carbone, P. P., Moertel, C. G. & O'Conor, G. (1970) Serum α-fetoprotein in the U.S.A. *Lancet*, i, 779–780.

Ichiki, A. T., Wenzel, K. L., Quirin, Y. P., Lange, R. D. & Eveleigh, J. (1976) Immunochemical studies of carcinoembryonic antigen (CEA) variants. *British Journal of Cancer*, 33, 273–278.

Itoh, T. & Southam, C. M. (1964) Isoantibodies to human cancer cells in cancer patients following cancer homotransplants. *Journal of Immunology*, 93, 926–936.

Jehn, U. W., Nathanson, L., Schwartz, R. S. & Skinner, M. (1970) *In vitro* lymphocyte stimulation by a soluble antigen from malignant melanoma. *New England Journal of Medicine*, 283, 329–333.

Joint National Cancer Institute of Canada/American Cancer Society Investigation (1972) A collaborative study of a test for carcinoembryonic antigen (CEA) in the sera of patients with carcinoma of the colon and rectum. *Canadian Medical Association Journal*, 107, 25–33.

Kew, M. C., Purves, L. R. & Bersohn, I. (1973) Serum alpha-fetoprotein levels in acute viral hepatitis. *Gut*, 14, 939–942.

Khoo, S. K. & Mackay, E. V. (1974) Carcinoembryonic antigen by radioimmunoassay in the detection of recurrence during long-term follow up of female genital cancer. *Cancer*, 34, 542–548.

Khoo, S. K., Hunt, P. S. & Mackay, I. R. (1973) Studies of

carcinoembryonic antigen activity of whole and extracted serum in ulcerative colitis. *Gut*, **14,** 545–548.

Khoo, S. K., Warner, N. L., Lie, J. T. & Mackay, I. R. (1973) Carcinoembryonic antigenic activity of tissue extracts: a quantitative study of malignant and benign neoplasms, cirrhotic liver, normal adult and fetal organs. *International Journal of Cancer*, **11,** 681–687.

King, J. P. G., Leonard, J. C. & Dykes, P. W. An examination for the presence of CEA-anti CEA complexes in the plasma of colonic cancer patients. In preparation.

Klein, G. (1970) Immunological factors affecting tumour growth. *British Medical Journal*, **iv,** 418.

Kleinman, M. S., Harwell, L. & Turner, M. D. (1971) Studies of colonic carcinoma antigens. *Gut*, **12,** 1–10.

Kohn, J. & Weaver, P. C. (1974) Serum-alpha-fetoprotein in hepatocellular carcinoma. *Lancet*, **ii,** 334–337.

Kozower, M., Fawaz, K. A., Miller, H. M. & Kaplan, M. M. (1971) Positive alpha-fetoglobulin in a case of gastric carcinoma. *New England Journal of Medicine*, **285,** 1059.

Krementz, E. T., Mansell, P. W. A., Hornung, M. O., Samuels, M. S., Sutherland, C. A. & Benes, E. N. (1974) Immunotherapy of malignant disease: the use of viable sensitized lymphocytes or transfer factor prepared from sensitized lymphocytes. *Cancer*, **33,** 394–401.

Krupey, J., Gold, P. & Freedman, S. O. (1968) Physicochemical studies of the carcinoembryonic antigens of the human digestive system. *Journal of Experimental Medicine*, **128,** 387–398.

Kupchik, H. Z. & Zamcheck, N. (1972) Carcinoembryonic antigen(s) in liver disease. (II) Isolation from human cirrhotic liver and serum and from normal liver. *Gastroenterology*, **63,** 95–101.

Laurence, D. J. R. & Neville, A. M. (1973) *British Journal of Cancer*, **28,** Suppl. 1, 198, 239.

Laurence, D. J. R., Turberville, C., Anderson, S. G. & Neville, A. M. (1975) First British Standard for carcinoembryonic antigen (CEA) *British Journal of Cancer*, **32,** 295–299.

Laurence, D. J. R., Stevens, U., Bettelheim, R., Darcy, D., Leese, C., Turberville, C., Alexander, P., Johns, E. W. & Neville, A. M. (1972) Role of plasma carcinoembryonic antigen in diagnosis of gastrointestinal, mammary, and bronchial carcinoma. *British Medical Journal*, **iii,** 605–609.

Lejtenyi, M. C., Freedman, S. O. & Gold, P. (1971) Response of lymphocytes from patients with gastrointestinal cancer to the carcinoembryonic antigen of the human digestive system. *Cancer*, **28,** 115–120.

Levy, J. G., Whitney, R. B., Smith, A. G. & Panno, L. (1974) The relationship of immune status to the efficacy of immunotherapy in preventing tumour recurrence in mice. *British Journal of Cancer*, **30,** 289–296.

Lewis, M. G. (1972) Circulating humoral antibodies in cancer. *Medical Clinics of North America*, **56,** 481–499.

Lewis, M. G., Ikonopisov, R. L., Nairn, R. C., Phillips, T. M., Fairley, G. H., Bodenham, D. C. & Alexander, P. (1969) Tumour-specific antibodies in human malignant melanoma and their relationship to the extent of the disease. *British Medical Journal*, **iii,** 547–552.

Likhite, V. V. (1974) Rejection of tumors and metastases in Fischer 344 rats following intratumor administration of killed *Corynebacterium parvum*. *International Journal of Cancer*, **14,** 684–690.

Lo Gerfo, P., Herter, F. P. & Bennett, S. J. (1972) Absence of circulating antibodies to carcinoembryonic antigen in patients with gastrointestinal malignancies. *International Journal of Cancer*, **9,** 344–348.

Lo Gerfo, P., Krupey, J. & Hansen, H. J. (1971) Demonstration of an antigen common to several varieties of neoplasia. *New England Journal of Medicine*, **285,** 138–141.

Mach, J. P. & Pusztaszeri, G. (1972) Communication to the Editors. Carcinoembryonic antigen (CEA): demonstration of a partial identity between CEA and a normal glycoprotein. *Immunochemistry*, **9,** 1031–1034.

Mach, J.-P., Carrel, S., Merenda, C., Sordat, B. & Cerottini, J.-C. (1974) *In vivo* localisation of radiolabelled antibodies to carcinoembryonic antigen in human colon carcinoma grafted into nude mice. *Nature*, **248,** 704–706.

Mach, J.-P., Jaeger, Ph., Bertholet, M. M., Ruegsegger, C.-H., Loosli, R. M. & Pettavel, J. (1974) Detection of recurrence of large bowel carcinoma by radioimmunoassay of circulating carcinoembryonic antigen (CEA). *Lancet*, **ii,** 535–540.

Mach, J.-P., Pusztaszeri, G., Dysli, M., Kapp, F., de Haan, B. B., Loosli, R. M., Grob, P. & Isliker, H. (1973) Dosage radio-immunologique de l'antigène, carcinoembryonnaire (CEA) dans le plasma de malades atteint de carcinomes. *Schweizensche. Med. Woch.*, **103,** 365–371.

Mackay, A. M., Patel, S., Carter, S., Stevens, U., Laurence, D. J. R., Cooper, E. H. & Neville, A. M. (1974) Role of serial plasma CEA assays in detection of recurrent and metastatic colorectal carcinomas. *British Medical Journal*, **iv,** 382–385.

Maclaurin, B. P., Cooke, W. T. & Ling, N. R. (1971) Impaired lymphocyte reactivity against tumour cells in patients with coeliac disease. *Gut*, **12,** 794–800.

MacSween, J. M. (1975) The antigenicity of carcinoembryonic antigen in man. *International Journal of Cancer*, **15,** 246–252.

Martin, F. & Martin, M. S. (1970) Demonstration of antigens related to colonic cancer in the human digestive system. *International Journal of Cancer*, **6,** 352–360.

Martin, F. & Martin, M. S. (1972) Radioimmunoassay of carcinoembryonic antigen in extracts of human colon and stomach. *International Journal of Cancer*, **9,** 641–647.

Masopust, J., Kithier, K., Fuchs, V., Kotal, L. & Radl, J. (1967) Fetoprotein: a specific α_1-globulin of human fetuses. Its ontogenesis and importance for pathology. In *Intrauterine Dangers to the Foetus*, ed. Horsky, J. & Stembera, Z. K., pp. 30–35. Amsterdam: Excerpta Medica Foundation.

Mathé, G., Amiel, J. L., Schwarzenberg, L., Schneider, M., Cattan, A., Schlumberger, J. R., Hayat, M. & de Vassal, F. (1969) Active immunotherapy for acute lymphoblastic leukaemia. *Lancet*, **i,** 697–699.

Mawas, C., Buffe, D. & Burtin, P. (1970) Influence of age on α-fetoprotein incidence. *Lancet*, **i,** 1292.

McIllmurray, M. B., Gray, M. & Langman, M. J. S. (1973) Phytohaemagglutinin-induced lymphocyte transformation in patients before and after resection of large intestinal cancer. *Gut*, **14,** 541–544.

McIllmurray, M. B., Price, M. R. & Langman, M. J. S. (1974) Inhibition of leucocyte migration in patients with large intestinal cancer by extracts prepared from large intestinal tumours and from normal colonic mucosa. *British Journal of Cancer*, **29,** 305–311.

Mehlman, D. J., Bulkley, B. H. & Wiernik, P. H. (1971) Serum alpha-fetoglobin with gastric and prostatic carcinomas. *New England Journal of Medicine*, **285,** 1060–1061.

Michison, N. A. (1955) Studies on the immunological

response to foreign tumor transplants in the mouse. *Journal of Experimental Medicine*, 102, 157–177.

Moore, T. L., Kantrowitz, P. A. & Zamcheck, N. (1972) Carcinoembryonic antigen (CEA) in inflammatory bowel disease. *Journal of the American Medical Association*, 222, 944–947.

Moore, T. L., Kupchik, H. Z., Marcon, N. & Zamcheck, N. (1971) Carcinoembryonic antigen assay in cancer of the colon and pancreas and other digestive tract disorders. *American Journal of Digestive Diseases*, 16, 1–7.

Nairn, R. C., Fothergill, J. E., McEntegart, M. G. & Richmond, H. G. (1962) Loss of gastro-intestinal-specific antigen in neoplasia. *British Medical Journal*, i, 1791–1793.

Nairn, R. C., Nind, A. P. P., Guli, E. P. G., Davies, D. J., Rolland, J. M., McGiven, A. R. & Hughes, E. S. R. (1971) Immunological reactivity in patients with carcinoma of colon. *British Medical Journal*, iv, 706–709.

Nayak, N. C., Malaviya, A. N., Chawla, V. & Chandra, R. K. (1972) α-fetoprotein in Indian childhood cirrhosis. *Lancet*, i, 68–69.

Nery, R., James, R., Barsoum, A. L. & Bullman, H. (1974) Isolation and partial characterization of macromolecular urinary aggregates containing carcinoembryonic antigen-like activity. *British Journal of Cancer*, 29, 413–424.

Nind, A. P. P., Matthews, N., Pihl, E. A. V., Rollard, J. M. & Nairn, R. C. (1975) Analysis of inhibition of lymphocyte cytotoxicity in human colon carcinoma. *British Journal of Cancer*, 31, 620–629.

Nishi, S. (1970) Isolation and characterization of a human fetal α-globulin from the sera of fetuses and a hepatoma patient. *Cancer Research*, 30, 2507–2513.

Noonan, F. P., Gardner, M. A. H., Clunie, G. J. A., Isbister, W. H. & Halliday, W. J. (1974) Control of tumor growth in mice by thoracic duct drainage. Relationship to blocking factor in lymph. *International Journal of Cancer*, 13, 640–649.

O'Conor, G. T., Tatarinov, Y. S., Abelev, G. I. & Uriel, J. (1970) A collaborative study for the evaluation of a serologic test for primary liver cancer. *Cancer*, 25, 1091–1098.

Odili, J. L. & Taylor, G. (1971) Transience of immune responses to tumour antigens in man. *British Medical Journal*, iv, 584–586.

Order, S. E., Kirkman, R. & Knapp, R. (1974) Serologic immunotherapy: results and probable mechanism of action. *Cancer*, 34, 175–183.

O'Toole, C., Perlmann, P., Unsgaard, B., Moberger, G. & Edsmyr, F. (1972) Cellular immunity to human urinary bladder carcinoma. I. Correlation to clinical stage and radiotherapy. *International Journal of Cancer*, 10, 77–91.

Patterson, M., Cain, G. D., Stoebner, R. C. & Fox, J. (1971) Immunological test for gastric malignancies. *Gastroenterology*, 60, 791.

Penn, I. (1974) Occurrence of cancer in immune deficiencies. *Cancer*, 34, 858–866.

Phillips, T. M. & Lewis, M. G. (1970) A system of immunofluorescence in the study of tumour cells. *Revue Européene d'Études Cliniques et Biologiques*, 15, 1016–1020.

Pick, E. & Turk, J. L. (1972) The biological activities of soluble lymphocyte products. *Clinical and Experimental Immunology*, 10, 1–23.

Plow, E. F. & Edgington, T. S. (1975) Isolation and characterisation of a homogeneous isogenous isomeric species of carcinoembryonic antigen (CEA-S). *International Journal of Cancer*, 15, 748–761.

Powles, R. L., Crowther, D., Bateman, C. J. T., Beard, M. E. J., McElwain, T. J., Russell, J., Lister, T. A.,

Whitehouse, J. M. A., Wrigley, P. F. M., Pike, M., Alexander, P. & Hamilton Fairley, G. (1973) Immunotherapy for acute myelogenous leukaemia. *British Journal of Cancer*, 28, 365–376.

Prehn, R. T. & Main, J. M. (1957) Immunity to methylcholanthrene-induced sarcomas. *Journal of the National Cancer Institute*, 18, 769–778.

Primus, F. J., Wang, R. H., Goldenberg, D. M. & Hansen, H. J. (1973) Localization of human GW-39 tumors in hamsters by radiolabeled hetero-specific antibody to carcinoembryonic antigen. *Cancer Research*, 33, 2977–2982.

Pritchard, J. A. V., Moore, J. L., Sutherland, W. H. & Joslin, C. A. F. (1973) Evaluation and development of the macrophage electrophoretic mobility (MEM) test for malignant disease. *British Journal of Cancer*, 27, 1–9.

Pross, H. F. & Baines, M. G. (1976) Spontaneous human lymphocyte mediated cytotoxicity against tumour target cells. 1. The effect of malignant disease. *International Journal of Cancer*, 18, 593–604.

Pusztaszeri, G. & Mach, J. P. (1973) Carcinoembryonic antigen (CEA) in non-digestive cancerous and normal tissues. *Immunochemistry*, 10, 197–204.

Purves, L. R., Bersohn, I. & Geddes, E. W. (1970) Serum alpha-feto-protein and primary cancer of the liver in man. *Cancer*, 25, 1261–1270.

Quinones, J., Mizejewski, G. & Beierwaltes, W. H. (1971) Choriocarcinoma scanning using radiolabeled antibody to chorionic gonadotrophin. *Journal of Nuclear Medicine*, 12, 69–75.

Reynoso, G., Chu, T. M., Holyoke, D., Cohen, E., Nemoto, T., Wang, J.-J., Chuang, J., Guinan, P. & Murphy, G. P. (1972) Carcinoembryonic antigen in patients with different cancers. *Journal of the American Medical Association*, 220, 361–365.

Rios, A. & Simmons, R. L. (1974) Active specific immunotherapy of minimal residual tumor: excision plus neuraminidase-treated tumor cells. *International Journal of Cancer*, 13, 71–81.

Robins, R. A. & Baldwin, R. W. (1974) Tumour-specific antibody neutralization of factors in rat hepatoma-bearer serum which abrogate lymph-node-cell cytotoxicity. *International Journal of Cancer*, 14, 589–597.

Rogers, G. T., Searle, F. & Bagshawe, K. D. (1976) Carcinoembryonic antigen isolation of a sub-fraction with high specific activity. *British Journal of Cancer*, 33, 357–362.

Ruoslahti, E. & Seppälä, M. (1971) Studies of carcino-fetal proteins. III. Development of a radioimmunoassay for α-fetoprotein. Demonstration of α-fetoprotein in serum of healthy human adults. *International Journal of Cancer*, 8, 374–383.

Ruoslahti, E., Seppälä, M., Pihko, H. & Vuopio, P. (1971) Studies of carcino-fetal proteins. II. Biochemical comparison of α-fetoprotein from human fetuses and patients with hepatocellular cancer. *International Journal of Cancer*, 8, 283–288.

Russell, S. W. & Cochrane, C. G. (1974) The cellular events associated with regression and progression of murine (Moloney) sarcomas. *International Journal of Cancer*, 13, 54–63.

Saksela, E. & Meyer, B. (1973) Cell-mediated cytotoxicity against HeLa cells in patients with invasive or preinvasive cervical cancer. *Journal of the National Cancer Institute*, 51, 1095–1102.

Sample, W. F., Gertner, H. R. & Chretien, P. B. (1971) Inhibition of phytohemagglutinin-induced *in vitro* lymphocyte transformation by serum from patients with carcinoma. *Journal of the National Cancer Institute*, **46**, 1291–1297.

Schrager, J. (1972) Comparative study of the principal gastric glycoproteins isolated from gastric aspirates of normal, neoplastic, and foetal gastric mucosae. *Gut*, **13**, 856–857.

Seller, M. J., Singer, J. D., Coltart, T. M. & Campbell, S. (1974) Maternal serum-alpha-fetoprotein levels and prenatal diagnosis of neural-tube defects. *Lancet*, **i**, 428–429.

Shearer, W. T., Turnabaugh, T. R., Coleman, W. E., Aach, R. D., Philpott, G. W. & Parker, C. W. (1974) Cytotoxicity with antibody-glucose oxidase conjugates specific for a human colonic cancer and carcinoembryonic antigen. *International Journal of Cancer*, **14**, 539–547.

Shuster, J., Silverman, M. & Gold, P. (1973) Metabolism of human carcinoembryonic antigen in xenogeneic animals. *Cancer Research*, **33**, 65–68.

Simmons, D. A. R. & Perlmann, P. (1973) Carcinoembryonic antigen and blood group substances. *Cancer Research*, **33**, 313–322.

Skarin, A. T., Delwiche, R., Zamcheck, N., Lokich, J. J. & Frei, E. (1974) Carcinoembryonic antigen: clinical correlation with chemotherapy for metastatic gastrointestinal cancer. *Cancer*, **33**, 1239–1245.

Sorokin, J. J., Sugarbaker, P. H., Zamcheck, N., Pisick, M., Kupchik, H. Z. & Moore, F. D. (1974) Serial carcinoembryonic antigen assays: use in detection of cancer recurrence. *Journal of the American Medical Association*, **228**, 49–53.

Southam, C. M. & Moore, A. E. (1958) Induced immunity to cancer cell homografts in man. *Annals of the New York Academy of Sciences*, **73**, 635–653.

Steele, L., Cooper, E. H., Mackay, A. M., Losowsky, M. S. & Goligher, J. C. (1974) Combination of carcinoembryonic antigen and gamma glutamyl transpeptidase in the study of the evolution of colorectal cancer. *British Journal of Cancer*, **30**, 319–324.

Stevens, D. P., Mackay, I. R. & Cullen, K. J. (1976) Carcinoembryonic antigen in an unselected elderly population: a four year follow-up. *British Journal of Cancer*, **32**, 147–151.

Stevenson, G. T. & Lawrence, D. J. R. (1975) Report of a workshop on the immune response to solid tumours in man. *International Journal of Cancer*, **16**, 887–896.

Steward, A. M., Nixon, D., Zamcheck, N. & Aisenberg, A. (1974) Carcinoembryonic antigen in breast cancer patients: serum levels and disease progress. *Cancer*, **33**, 1246–1252.

Stolfi, R. L., Stolfi, L. M., Fugmann, R. A. & Martin, D. S. (1974) Specific tumor-induced suppression of lymphocyte activity in the antibody-dependent tumoricidal reaction. *International Journal of Cancer*, **14**, 625–632.

Straus, E., Rule, A., Grotsky, H., Janowitz, H. D. & Glade, P. (1972) *In vitro* migration of leucocytes in the presence of meconium antigen in patients with inflammatory bowel disease and cancer of the colon. *Gastroenterology*, **62**, 817.

Tanaka, T., Cooper, E. H. & Anderson, C. K. (1970) Lymphocyte infiltration in bladder carcinoma. *Revue Européene d'Etudes Cliniques et Biologique*, **15**, 1084–1089.

Tappeiner, G., Denk, H., Eckerstorfer, R. & Holzner, H. J. (1973) Occurrence and localization of the carcino-embryonic antigen (CEA) and of a perchloric acid soluble antigen of normal colonic mucosa in carcinomata and polyps of the large bowel. *Virchows Archiv. Abeteilung A Pathologische Anatomy Pathology*, **360**, 129–140.

Tatarinov, Iu. S. (1965) The content of an embryospecific

α globulin in the serum of human embryos, of new born babies, and of adults in cases of primary carcinoma of the liver. *Voprosy meditsinkoi Khimii (Moskova)*, **11**, 20–24.

Taylor, G. & Odili, J. L. I. (1972) Histological evidence of tumour rejection after active immunotherapy in human malignant disease. *British Medical Journal*, **ii**, 183–188.

Terry, W. D., Henkart, P. A., Coligan, J. E. & Todd, C. W. (1972) Structural studies of the major glycoprotein in preparations with carcinoembryonic antigen activity. *Journal of Experimental Medicine*, **136**, 200–204.

Thackray, A. C. (1964) Seminoma. *British Journal of Urology*, **36**, Suppl., 12–27.

Thomson, D. M. P., Krupey, J., Freedman, S. O. & Gold, P. (1969) The radioimmunoassay of circulating carcinoembryonic antigen of the human digestive system. *Proceedings of the National Academy of Sciences (Washington)*, **64**, 161–167.

Thomson, D. M. P. & Alexander, P. (1973) A cross-reacting embryonic antigen in the membrane of rat sarcoma cells which is immunogenic in the syngeneic host. *British Journal of Cancer*, **27**, 35–47.

Twomey, P. L., Catalona, W. J. & Chretien, P. B. (1974) Cellular immunity in cured cancer patients. *Cancer*, **33**, 435–440.

Uriel, J., de Nechaud, B. & Dupiers, M. (1972) Estrogen-binding properties of rat, mouse and man feto-specific serum proteins: demonstration by immuno-autoradiographic methods. *Biochemical and Biophysical Research Communications*, **46**, 1175–1180

Vogel, C. L., Primack, A., McIntire, K. R., Carbone, P. P. & Anthony, P. P. (1974) Serum alpha-fetoprotein in 184 Ugandan patients with hepatocellular carcinoma. *Cancer*, **33**, 959–964.

von Kleist, S. & Burtin, P. (1966) On the specificity of autoantibodies present in colon cancer patients. *Immunology*, **10**, 507–515.

von Kleist, S. & Burtin, P. (1969) Isolation of a foetal antigen from human colonic tumors. *Cancer Research*, **29**, 1961–1964.

von Kleist, S., Chavanel, G. & Burtin, P. (1972) Identification of an antigen from normal human tissue that cross reacts with the carcinoembryonic antigen. *Proceedings of the National Academy of Sciences of the United States of America*, **69**, 2492–2494.

von Kleist, S., King, M. & Burtin, P. (1974) Characterization of a normal tissular antigen extracted from human colonic tumours. *Immunochemistry*, **11**, 249–253.

Vose, B. M., Moore, M., Schofield, P. F. & Dymock, I. W. Leucocytotoxicity in malignant and non-malignant colonic diseases. Presented for publication.

Waldmann, T. A. & McIntire, K. R. (1972) Serum alpha-fetoprotein levels in patients with ataxia-telangiectasia. *Lancet*, **ii**, 1112–1115.

Wartman, W. B. (1959) Sinus cell hyperplasia of lymph nodes regional to adenocarcinoma of the breast and colon. *British Journal of Cancer*, **13**, 389–397.

Westwood, J. H. & Thomas, P. (1975) Studies on the structure and immunological activity of carcinoembryonic antigen – the role of disulphide bonds. *British Journal of Cancer*, **32**, 708–719.

Wybran, J., Hellström, I., Hellström, K. E. & Fudenberg, H. H. (1974) Cytotoxicity of human rosette-forming blood lymphocytes on cultivated human tumor cells. *International Journal of Cancer*, **13**, 515–521.

Ziegenfuss, J. F. (1973) Immunotherapy for Australia-antigen-associated hepatoma. *Lancet*, **i**, 1365–1366.

16. Alpha heavy chain disease and related small-intestinal lymphomas

William F. Doe

INTRODUCTION

Primary intestinal lymphomas are remarkably prevalent in the Mediterranean region and the Middle East (Ramot, Shahin and Bubis, 1965; Eidelman, Parkins and Rubin, 1966; Al-Bahrani and Bakir, 1971) and have a number of characteristic features. Young patients from underprivileged backgrounds present with a malabsorption syndrome resulting from extensive and diffuse infiltration of the wall of the small intestine, predominantly by plasma cells. Clinical studies suggest evolution from a premalignant cellular infiltrate to frank neoplasia involving more primitive immunoblasts. Since the early stage does not appear to be a truly malignant lymphoma, this disease has been named immunoproliferative small-intestinal disease (IPSID) (WHO Memorandum, 1976). Immunoglobulin fragments, comprising incomplete IgA heavy chains, have recently been found in the sera and secretions of the majority of patients (Seligmann, Mihaesco and Frangione, 1971). This condition, named alpha heavy chain disease (αHCD), is a proliferative disorder of the secretory IgA system in which plasma cells synthesize a protein closely related to the Fc fragment of IgA. It represents the heavy chain disease of IgA and although first described in 1968 (Seligmann, Danon, Hurez, Milhaesco and Peud'homme, 1968; Rambaud *et al.* 1968) its discovery had been predicted by Franklin 4 years earlier when he reported the first case of IgG heavy chain disease (Franklin, Lowenstein, Bigelow and Meltzer, 1964). Since the intestine is the major site of IgA synthesis and secretion (Crabbé and Heremans, 1966; Tomasi, 1972) it is not surprising that in the overwhelming majority of cases of αHCD, the plasma cell infiltrate primarily involves the wall of the small intestine and the mesenteric nodes (Seligmann and Mihaesco, 1973) producing the clinicopathological picture of IPSID. Known exceptions include α HCD apparently confined to the bronchial secretory IgA system producing a respiratory form of the disease (Stoop, Ballieux, Hijmans and Zegers, 1971; Faux, Crain, Rosen and Merler, 1973).

The frequency of α HCD among populations exposed to conditions of poor hygiene (Seligmann, Mihaesco and Frangione, 1971) and evidence for complete remissions induced in early cases by oral antibiotic therapy (Rogé, Druet and Marche, 1970) implicate environmental factors in the pathogenesis of this disorder. Since ingested microorganisms are a powerful proliferative stimulus to the secretory IgA system (Crabbé, Nash, Bazin, Eyssen and Heremans, 1970), the premalignant phase of the disease may represent an aberrant immune response by the secretory IgA system to sustained, topical antigenic stimulation (Seligmann *et al.*, 1971). The study of diffuse primary intestinal lymphomas, therefore, may offer important opportunities to gain an understanding of the pathogenesis of lymphoma in man. Uniquely, the association of a disordered immune response and the development of immunoblastic sarcoma, possibly from the same clone of cells, can be studied in a cell population which synthesizes a distinctive marker protein. Moreover, the implication of environmental agents provides a focus for research into the aetiological factors of human intestinal lymphoma and the prospect that public health measures may have a role in prevention.

CLINICAL FINDINGS

The clinical features of α HCD are remarkably uniform. Patients present with a history suggesting progressive malabsorption of several years' duration. The major symptoms are diarrhoea with the features of steatorrhoea, generalized colicky abdominal pain and weight loss. In those with a heavy protein-losing enteropathy, ankle swelling and ascites may develop. Sustained electrolyte loss may lead to symptoms of polyuria due to kaliopaenic nephropathy (Irunberry *et al.*, 1970; Laroche *et al.*, 1970; Manousos, 1974) and hypocalcaemic tetany (Doe *et al.*, 1972; Bonomo, Dammacco, Marano and Bonomo, 1972). At an advanced stage of the disease perforation or intestinal obstruction may be the presenting feature (Bognel *et al.*, 1972; Doe, 1975).

Physical signs are usually limited to wasting, marked clubbing of fingers and toes and ankle oedema. In some instances abdominal lymphoid masses are palpable but the liver and spleen are not clinically enlarged. Peripheral lymphadenopathy is not a feature of α HCD except in terminal stages. A nasopharyngeal lymphoid tumour was present in one patient who had a history of blood in his saliva (Doe, Henry, Hobbs and Dowling, 1970). At laparotomy the wall of the small intestine is often thickened and mesenteric nodes are enlarged (Laroche *et al.*, 1970). The plasma cell proliferation is almost always confined to the small intestine and mesenteric nodes. Haematological studies show that iron and folic acid deficiency are common in this condition but that haemoglobin levels are usually near normal. White blood cell count and differential are usually normal. Morphologically abnormal plasma cells have been found in the peripheral blood (Doe *et al.*, 1972) and circulating 'reticulum cells' incapable of synthesizing α HCD protein have been reported in the terminal stages (Bognel *et al.*, 1972). Biochemical investigations show reduced levels of plasma potassium, calcium and magnesium. Hypoalbuminaemia associated with a protein-losing enteropathy is a common finding. One striking biochemical feature is the marked increase of alkaline phosphatase present in plasma, usually due to the intestinal isoenzyme of alkaline phosphatase (Ramot and Streifler, 1966; Rambaud *et al.*, 1968; Doe *et al.*, 1972).

Radiological examination of the small intestine reveals diffusely abnormal changes. The proximal bowel is often more severely affected than the distal. The mucosal pattern is coarse and nodular and the contour of the bowel may be irregular. When frank malignancy supervenes, strictures leading to obstruction become apparent (Ramot *et al.*, 1965; Nasr, Haghighi, Bakhshandeh and Haghshenas, 1970; Balikian, Nassar, Shammaa and Shahid, 1969; Doe, Henry and Doyle, 1976). Skeletal surveys do not show any evidence of osteolytic lesions, but hypertrophic osteoarthropathy is an occasional finding (Doe *et al.*, 1972).

Tests of intestinal function reveal malabsorption in both jejunum and ileum and steatorrhoea, suggesting diffuse involvement of the whole length of the small intestine. Evidence of parasitic and protozoan infestation is common. Hookworm, *Trichuris trichuria*, *Trichomonas hominis*, *Giardia lamblia* and Coccidia are among many of the parasites reported (Doe *et al.*, 1972; Novis, Kahn and Bank, 1973; Henry, Bird and Doe, 1974; Salem *et al.*, 1977). No parasitic or bacterial pathogen has been consistently isolated from the stools of α HCD patients. Overgrowth of aerobes and anaerobes has been demonstrated in jejunal fluid in several patients whose steatorrhoea, vitamin B_{12} absorption and ^{14}C glycocholate breath test improved following oral antibiotic therapy (Rambaud, unpublished). These findings suggest that a stagnant loop syndrome may contribute to the malabsorption in some patients with α HCD. In other studies, however, no evidence for a stagnant loop syndrome was observed (Chernov, Doe and Gompertz, 1972).

HISTOLOGY

The small intestinal mucosa presents a characteristic appearance. Villi are shortened and broadened, giving the appearance of total or partial villous atrophy. The basic abnormality is a diffuse dense mononuclear infiltrate of the lamina propria causing wide separation of the crypts of Lieberkühn and obliteration of the villous architecture without significant impairment of the integrity of the surface epithelium (Fig. 16.1). The cellular infiltrate is predominantly plasma cell in type (Fig. 16.2), but the stage of maturation of plasma cells varies in biopsies from different patients. Topographically the infiltrate begins in the upper small intestine and is diffuse and extensive, often involving the entire length of the small intestine. Similar histological appearances are usually seen in biopsies taken at different sites along the small intestine. In many cases the cellular infiltrate is confined to the lamina propria, and bears none of the histological stigmata of malignancy, consistent with the view that a premalignant stage of the disease exists. When infiltration beyond the muscularis mucosa occurs, invasion of the submucosa, destruction of mesenteric lymph node architecture and apparent spread to rectum (Laroche, *et al.*, 1970; Bognel *et al.*, 1972), postnasal space (Doe *et al.*, 1970), bone marrow (Rambaud *et al.*, 1968; Doe *et al.*, 1970) and blood (Doe *et al.*, 1972; Bognel *et al.*, 1972) may occur. These findings, together with the abnormal appearances of the invading cells, clearly establish the malignant potential of α HCD. Extensive histological studies have failed to reveal evidence of amyloid deposition. Ultrastructural studies have confirmed that the plasma cell, or a cell intermediate between the plasma cell and the lymphocyte, is the proliferating cell type in α HCD (Scotto, Stralin and Caroli, 1970; Doe *et al.*, 1972). The rough endoplasmic reticulum is prominent in all but the most immature plasma cells and often shows cisternae distended with granular material.

PROTEIN STUDIES

IMMUNOGLOBULIN ABNORMALITIES

The detection of α HCD protein, essential to the diagnosis of α HCD, may be difficult using routine immunochemical analysis. The serum electrophoretic pattern shows a clear abnormality in only 50 per cent of the cases studied (Seligmann *et al.*, 1975) – a broad band extending from the alpha 2 to the fast gamma region. Albumin and gamma globulin bands are significantly reduced (Fig. 16.3). These findings are quite unlike the sharp, narrow band expected in a monoclonal abnormality. In many sera a mild increase in alpha 2 globulins is the only electrophoretic abnormality seen

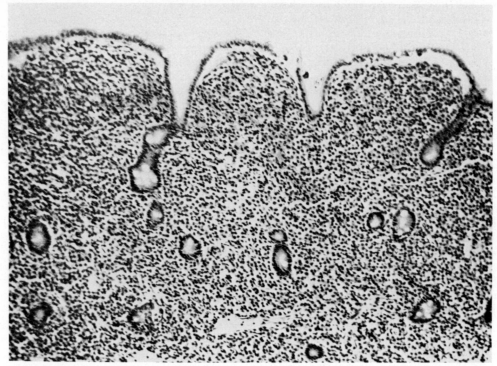

Fig. 16.1 Jejunal biopsy from a patient suffering from alpha chain disease showing flattened villi, crypt sparsity, preservation of surface epithelium and a dense cellular infiltrate.

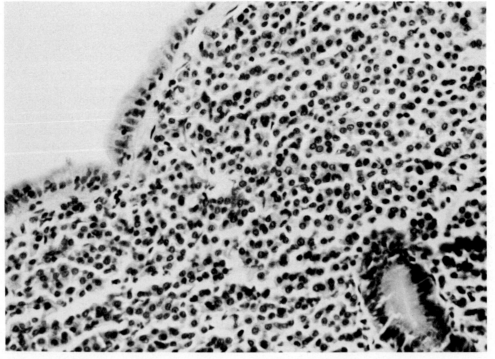

Fig. 16.2 A higher magnification of the jejunal biopsy seen in Figure 16.1. The cellular infiltrate consists largely of immature plasma cells.

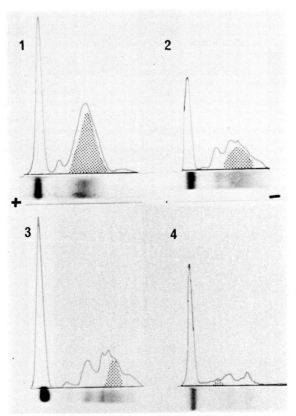

Fig. 16.3 Cellular acetate electrophoresis of sera from 4 cases of alpha chain disease. The alpha chain regions are indicated by dotted areas and are readily seen as a diffuse β–γ hump in patients 1, 2 and 3. In patient 4 no specific abnormality of serum globulins is seen. Note reduction of slow γ globulin levels in sera of all 4 patients. (First appeared in an article by Doe, W. F., in *British Journal of Cancer* (1975), **31**, Suppl. 11, 350–355. Reproduced by kind permission of the author and also the editor of *British Journal of Cancer*.)

(Fig. 16.3). Immunoelectrophoretic analysis of α HCD serum using anti-whole human serum often shows a long precipitin line crossing the albumin and gamma globulin arcs at their extremities. In many cases, however, the presence of α HCD protein is revealed only by antisera to polyclonal IgA, which show a precipitin line of abnormally fast mobility. Exceptionally, a protein fragment of unusually slow electrophoretic mobility is observed (Seligmann *et al.*, 1971). No correspondingly abnormal arc develops against anti-kappa or anti-lambda light chain antisera. While α HCD protein levels of over 4 g per cent have been estimated in the serum of several patients (Seligmann *et al.*, 1968; Doe, 1970), the polymerized state of α HCD protein in serum (Seligmann *et al.*, 1968), and the presence of some normal IgA, prevent accurate measurement of α HCD protein levels in serum using standard radial immunodiffusion techniques (Doe *et al.*, 1972). Serum IgM

and IgG levels are usually low. Although a protein-losing enteropathy may contribute to depressed serum immunoglobulin levels, there is a disproportionate reduction in IgG and IgM levels relative to serum albumin, suggesting that immunosuppression by the proliferating plasma cell mass, analogous to that seen in myeloma, is also a factor (Doe *et al.*, 1972).

Selected antisera specific for IgA and containing antibodies which recognize the conformational specificity of Fab, reveal antigenic deficiencies in α HCD sera. These antisera produce a precipitin line against whole IgA which spurs over α HCD serum and can be used as the basis of a diagnostic test for α HCD protein (Seligmann *et al.*, 1968). Since such antisera are not readily obtainable, a simple, rapid test has been developed which is suitable for multiple samples and which does not require the use of highly specialized antisera (Doe *et al.*, 1972). This method, modified from the one described by Radl (1970), uses both the absence of light chains and the fast mobility of α HCD protein as the basis for its detection. Serum, urine or secretions are electrophoresed into agarose containing both anti-kappa and anti-lambda light chain antisera. Normal immunoglobulins are precipitated close to the origin by the anti-light chain antisera, but α HCD protein, being devoid of light chains, is free to migrate and develops as a characteristically long anodal arc (Doe *et al.*, 1972) (Fig. 16.4). In some instances, IgA myeloma proteins, especially those containing lambda light chains, fail to precipitate with anti-light chain antisera (Osterland and Chaplin, 1966). A detection technique for α HCD protein wholly dependent on failure to precipitate with anti-light antisera may therefore be liable to false positives with some IgA myeloma proteins. The use of electrophoretic mobility as an additional identifying feature, as in the Radl technique (1970), is therefore desirable. In all doubtful cases the pathological protein should be purified, reduced and alkylated to allow direct proof of the absence of light chains by polyacylamide gel electrophoresis or gel filtration.

Alpha heavy chain protein is readily detected in concentrated intestinal fluid from α HCD patients. Indeed, as passage of IgA into the intestinal fluid is the predominant secretory route for IgA synthesized in the intestinal lamina propria, α HCD protein may occasionally be detected more easily in intestinal fluid than in serum. Electrophoretic patterns and immunoelectrophoretic analyses of intestinal fluid are similar to those seen in serum (Seligmann *et al.*, 1969). Polymerization of α HCD protein in serum prevents its filtration at the glomerulus in large quantities, but the aberrant protein is detectable in concentrated urine. Bence-Jones proteinuria is not observed in α HCD. Alpha heavy chain protein is usually absent from pure parotid saliva. In both intestinal fluid and in urine, α HCD protein is bound to secretory component (Seligmann et al., 1969). J chain, the peptide associated with polymerized immunoglobulin molecules, has been found in all the α HCD proteins purified to date (Seligmann and Mihaesco, 1974).

Several exceptions to the typical pattern have been described. A complete IgA myeloma has been reported in 2 patients suffering from IPSID and, in one case, Bence-Jones proteinuria was detected. Gamma heavy chain disease was demonstrated in the serum and intestinal biopsy of a further patient whose clinico-

quarters of the alpha heavy chain (Dorrington, Mihaesco and Seligmann, 1970). The molecular weight of the monomeric polypeptide subunit varied from 29 000 to 34 000 daltons (Dorrington et al., 1970), allowing for the variable but high carbohydrate content of α HCD protein.

Anti-light chain antisera do not precipitate α HCD protein nor is the precipitation reaction between anti-light chain antisera and Bence-Jones protein inhibited by this protein. Moreover, isolated α HCD protein does not recombine with free light chains (Seligmann et al.,

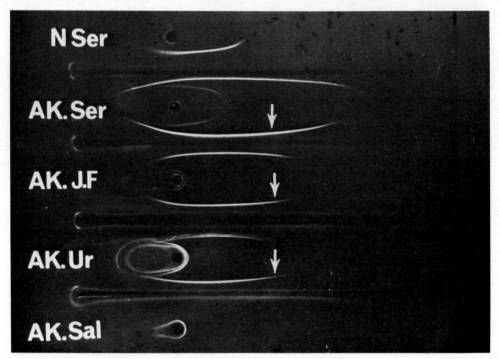

Fig. 16.4 Immunoselection plates detecting free alpha chain protein (arrows) in serum (Ser), concentrated jejunal fluid (JF) and concentrated urine (Ur) from an alpha chain disease patient (AK). No free alpha chain was present in this patient's pure parotid saliva (Sal). Normal serum control (N Ser) shows only a precipitin arc due to normal immunoglobulin. (First appeared in an article by Doe et al. (1972) in *Gut* (1972), **13**, 947–957. Reproduced by kind permission of the authors and the editor of *Gut*.)

pathological picture was characteristic of IPSID (Seligmann, 1975b). Moreover in 2 cases of α HCD a homogeneous IgG component was found in addition to α HCD protein (Seligmann, 1975a, unpublished).

Alpha heavy chain protein shows a remarkable propensity for polymerization. Analytical ultracentrifugation reveals dimers with a sedimentation coefficient of 4S and larger polymers up to 11S in size. Polymers are bound to each other by both –SH and non-covalent bonds (Seligmann et al., 1969). Purified α HCD proteins, when mildly reduced and alkylated and then submitted to Sephadex G200 filtration in 6M guanidine HCl in acetic acid, produce basic polypeptide subunits of 3.2S representing greater than half and less than three-

1969). As noted above, the failure of α HCD protein to precipitate with anti-light chain antisera is not absolute proof of the absence of light chains. There is, however, direct evidence to show that α HCD protein is devoid of light chains. Urea–acid–starch gel electrophoresis of the reduced and alkylated protein shows a diffuse heavy chain band but no light chain bands (Seligmann et al., 1968). Early antigenic analysis and immunochemical findings strongly suggested that α HCD protein includes the entire Fc portion of IgA (Seligmann et al., 1969). The heavy–light peptide is missing and sequencing of the eight COOH-terminal amino acid residues provided a sequence almost identical to that described for the alpha chain COOH-terminus of IgA_1 by Grey, Abel and

Zimmerman (1971). In addition, the hinge peptide was shown to be present in all eight alpha chain proteins tested and analysis of the hinge peptide isolated from one α HCD protein (Seligmann *et al.*, 1971) showed a similar composition to that already described for IgA₁ myeloma protein (Grey *et al.*, 1971). The NH₂-terminal region, however, shows considerable heterogeneity and attempts to obtain an NH₂-terminal sequence using an automated sequencer have been unsuccessful (Seligmann *et al.*, 1971; Wolfenstein-Todel, Mihaesco and Frangione, 1974). Studies of the α HCD protein Def showed that after a short segment, probably representing a portion of the variable region, there is a gap corresponding to the C_{H1} constant domain, the constant part of the Fd fragment. Normal sequence is then resumed, beginning at a valine residue in the hinge region which contains a partly duplicated fragment and the inter-heavy chain disulphide bridges. The remainder of the heavy chain sequence is apparently normal apart from a single substitution at position 12 (Wolfenstein-Todel *et al.*, 1974). Synthesis of α HCD protein, therefore, appears to involve an internal deletion affecting both the V_H and the C_{H1} regions of the alpha heavy chain, which are under independent genetic control, resulting in a fragment consisting of the entire Fc fragment of IgA plus a portion of the variable region. Despite repeated attempts, no antisera specific for individual proteins have been raised, presumably due to the absence of much of the hypervariable region responsible for idiotypic determinants.

The heterogeneity of the NH₂-terminus may be attributable to limited postsynthetic proteolysis of this region such as has been described for the amber and ochre alkaline phosphatase nonsense mutants of *Escherichia coli* (Suzuki and Garen, 1969; Natori and Garen, 1970). In these mutants, incomplete proteins exhibit increased susceptibility to cytoplasmic degradation following release from the ribosome (Natori *et al.*, 1970). A similar intracellular proteolysis has been postulated to explain the heterogeneity of the NH₂-terminus of α HCD protein (Buxbaum and Preud'homme, 1972). Alternatively postsynthetic cleavage could be extracellular. In a case of gamma heavy chain disease (γ HCD), in which N-terminal heterogeneity is also characteristic, the nascent γ HCD protein produced in synthetic studies had a molecular weight of 36 000 whereas the molecular weight of the serum γ HCD protein was reduced to 28 000 daltons (Buxbaum *et al.*, 1972).

There are two subclasses of IgA recognized by an antigenic distinction which resides in the Fc region of the heavy chains. All 41 α HCD proteins tested belong to the IgA₁ subclass (Seligmann, 1975), a surprising finding since 30–40 per cent of normal secretory IgA is subclass 2 (Grey, Abel, Yount and Kunkel, 1968).

This finding, together with the amino acid substitution in position 12 of protein Def, suggests that α HCD proteins may be monoclonal despite their N-terminal heterogeneity. In the absence of the variable regions of light and heavy chains the essential criteria of monoclonality, i.e. shared idiotypic specificity and antibody activity, cannot be tested. This question may be approachable by attempting to isolate light chain messenger RNA (mRNA) from α HCD synthesising cells and translating the mRNA in a cell-free system (WHO Memorandum, 1976).

CELL STUDIES

Culture of jejunal mucosal biopsy specimens from α HCD patients in medium containing ¹⁴C labelled amino acids has established that α HCD protein is synthesized by the mucosa during the period of organ maintenance (Seligmann *et al.*, 1968). Radioimmunoelectrophoretic analysis of proteins synthesized *in vitro* by cells teased from mesenteric nodes demonstrated the production of labelled α HCD proteins. No free labelled light chains were found (Seligmann *et al.*, 1969). Studies of nascent immunoglobulin subunits, during culture of cells synthesizing α HCD protein, demonstrated that the absence of light chains is due to failure of expression of genes coding for light chains and not to failure of light chain, heavy chain assembly (Buxbaum *et al.*, 1972). The possibility that absence of light chain synthesis results from failure of translation rather than transcription is testable by studies directed at detecting the presence of light chain messenger RNA.

Immunofluorescence studies of intestinal mucosa and mesenteric nodes using monospecific anti-IgA revealed intense intercellular staining but weak and variable staining in the cytoplasm of cells composing the cellular infiltrate. Staining for light chains kappa and lambda was negative except for the occasional brightly fluorescing cell which was presumably synthesizing normal immunoglobulin. No membrane-bound immunoglobulin was detected on the surface of α HCD protein synthesizing cells teased from mesenteric nodes (Preud'homme and Seligmann, 1972) or cultured from the jejunal mucosal infiltrate (Doe, Agnesdottir and Valdimarsson, 1974).

COURSE OF THE DISEASE

Little is known about the natural history of α HCD. There appears to be an early 'benign' stage lasting years and characterized by diffuse, extensive infiltration of the small intestine resulting in malabsorption and weight loss. The cellular infiltrate consists largely of mature plasma cells and remains confined to the lamina propria. During this period α HCD protein is readily detectable in the serum and intestinal fluid. Whether this phase is truly benign, however, is open to question. There is a monoclonal expansion of aberrant plasma cells secreting increasing amounts of a disordered immunoglobulin fragment, suggesting latent neoplasia. The differentiated appearance of the cellular infiltrate of the intestinal wall and the scarcity of mitoses do not necessarily militate against malignancy since in other clearly malignant disorders, such as chronic lymphocytic leukaemia and Waldenstrom's macroglobulinaemia, the proliferating cells are normal in appearance. Karyotypic studies of plasma cells taken from the intestinal infiltrate during the benign phase may help resolve this question. Clinically, the recognition of α HCD in its early stage may be important. In four instances, remission of α HCD has been reported following sustained therapy with broad-spectrum antibiotics alone (Roge et al., 1970; Monges et al., 1974; Rambaud, 1976).

Information on the course of α HCD is limited to two cases who were observed over a long period following early diagnosis during the 'benign' phase. In these patients, remission followed vigorous cytotoxic therapy combined with steroids and antibiotics, but subsequently progression to invasive malignancy occurred in each patient (Bognel et al., 1972; Doe, 1975). In one, following a 'benign stage' lasting over 3 years, there was invasion of the wall of the small intestine and mesenteric nodes by a plasmacytic sarcoma leading to intestinal obstruction and perforation. During the terminal phase, α HCD protein was no longer detectable in serum and undifferentiated 'reticulum cells' were found in the small intestine, mesenteric nodes, liver and blood (Bognel et al., 1972). In the second patient there was a sustained remission lasting 18 months. Later, overt malignancy of the small intestine ultimately developed causing intestinal obstruction. In addition, multiple polypoid tumors were found along the length of the gastrointestinal tract. One such polyp formed the apex of an intussusception. The histological appearance of the neoplasms was that of a primitive plasma cell tumour (Doe, 1975).

The nature and origins of the neoplastic cells seen during the malignant phase of α HCD and their relationship to the plasma cell infiltrate characterizing the earlier 'benign' stage remains unsettled. The terminal reticulum cell sarcoma or primitive plasma cell tumour may represent a malignant transformation of the clone of plasma cells synthesizing α HCD protein (Rambaud and Matuchansky, 1973). Alternatively the terminal neoplasia may arise from an unrelated clone, perhaps as a consequence of an immunodeficient state caused by α HCD (Rappaport, Ramot, Huhu and Park, 1972).

RELATIONSHIP TO 'MEDITERRANEAN' LYMPHOMAS

Early reports of α HCD (Rambaud et al., 1968) emphasized its similarity to the diffuse primary intestinal lymphomas first reported in Israel (Ramot et al., 1965, Eidelman et al., 1966) and named 'Mediterranean' lymphoma. This condition has since been described in many countries outside the Mediterranean area, including Iran (Nasr et al., 1970), Iraq (Al-Bahrani and Bakir, 1971), South Africa (Novis et al., 1971), Pakistan (Doe et al., 1972), Cambodia and Argentina (Seligmann, 1975), and has therefore been renamed immunoproliferative small-intestinal disease (IPSID). Initial reports of 'Mediterranean' lymphoma did not include protein studies, but subsequent reports have shown α HCD protein in the sera of some patients, especially in those who showed a purely plasmacytic infiltration of the small intestine (Rappaport et al., 1972). Recent evidence suggests that the majority of these primary, diffuse intestinal lymphomas, causing malabsorption in underprivileged populations, begin as an apparently benign infiltration of the small intestine with plasma cells, which synthesize α HCD protein. Firstly, as mentioned above, two α HCD patients have been observed over several years to progress from an apparently benign stage of α HCD to a malignant intestinal lymphoma identical to so-called 'Mediterranean' lymphoma. Secondly, retrospective study of intestinal biopsy specimens from a group of 20 patients suffering from 'Mediterranean' lymphoma revealed that in 16 cases a diffuse plasma cell infiltrate was present in association with reticulum cell sarcoma, Hodgkin's disease or unclassifiable lymphoma (Rappaport et al., 1972). The remaining 4 patients' biopsy specimens showed a purely plasmacytic proliferation in the small intestine without histological evidence of malignancy. Furthermore the history of prolonged intestinal malabsorption in these patients strongly suggested that plasma cell infiltration preceded development of lymphoma. Unfortunately no protein studies were performed on sera from these patients. Thirdly, α HCD protein has been found in the sera of several cases of 'Mediterranean' lymphoma classified histologically as reticulum cell sarcoma (Ramot and Huhu, 1975).

These findings suggest that a great many, if not all, cases of diffuse 'Mediterranean' lymphoma represent the late malignant phase of α HCD. Failure to detect α HCD protein in some cases of 'Mediterranean' lymphoma may reflect the insensitivity of techniques used, or the advanced, undifferentiated stage of the malignancy. Resolution of this important problem will await careful prospective studies of α HCD.

EPIDEMIOLOGY

Intestinal α HCD affects populations of diverse ethnic and geographic origins (Seligmann *et al.*, 1973) but rarely affects Caucasians. Although early reports of this disorder concerned patients living in the Mediterranean region (Rambaud *et al.*, 1968; Laroche *et al.*, 1970; Irunberry *et al.*, 1970), cases have now been reported in Bangladesh (Doe *et al.*, 1970), Pakistan, Iran (Doe *et al.*, 1972), Turkey (Doe, 1975), Cambodia (Rambaud *et al.*, 1970), Colombia (Pittman *et al.*, 1971), Argentina (Seligmann *et al.*, 1973) and South Africa (Novis *et al.*, 1973). To date, there has been a single case report of intestinal α HCD affecting a Caucasian. This report describes a Finnish boy whose colon and terminal ileum were involved by α HCD (Savilahti and Brandtzaeg, 1973). Some ethnic patterns have been observed. In Israel, Arabs and first or second generation Jewish immigrants from Middle-Eastern and North African countries are affected, but Jews of European or American origin are spared (Ramot *et al.*, 1965). Similarly in South Africa, Cape-Coloureds and mulattoes are susceptible, but apparently the more numerous Bantu population in that country are not (Novis, *et al.*, 1973).

A striking feature of this disorder is the age of the patients affected. The great majority of patients are between 10 and 30 years old, an age incidence in marked contrast to that of multiple myeloma and intestinal lymphoma occurring in Western Europe. In a review of 27 patients there was no sex predominance (Seligmann *et al.*, 1971).

The general incidence of α HCD is not clearly defined although certain regional patterns are suggested by available clinical data. Limited surveys of the small-intestinal mucosal appearance in the general population have been performed. In a small group of rural Iranian villagers, and in autopsy series from Iran and Iraq, histological changes were described, but their relationship to IPSID and α HCD has not been determined (Haghighi, 1976, unpublished; Dutz, Asvadi, Sadri and Kohout, 1971). Normal histology, however, was reported in a similar small survey of the general population from low socio-economic groups in Lebanon (Nasrallah and Nassar, 1976, unpublished).

AETIOLOGY

The clear predilection of α HCD for underprivileged populations suggests that environmental factors may be important in its pathogenesis. One common factor among susceptible populations of differing ethnic origins is their exposure to an environment of poor hygiene (Seligmann *et al.*, 1971). Studies conducted in Israel show that chronic gastrointestinal infection and diarrhoea are common among the Arab population and that Arab children have significantly higher mean serum levels of IgA and IgM compared to Jewish children of European origin (Ramot *et al.*, 1975). Since orally ingested microorganisms are a powerful proliferative stimulus to the secretory IgA system (Crabbé *et al.*, 1970), the early phase of α HCD could represent an aberrant humoral immune response following sustained topical antigenic stimulation of the intestinal mucosa. The stimulating microorganisms may be specific or non-specific. Investigation of possible specific environmental agents, however, has been unrewarding. Limited bacteriological, parasitic and virological studies have not revealed evidence for a specific agent associated with α HCD, but antigenic stimulation may have occurred many years before α HCD becomes manifest clinically. Unfortunately the absence of the Fab region for α HCD protein precludes its use for recognition of putative antigenic stimuli. A further possible role for an environmental factor causing α HCD is that of an oncogenic virus interfering with genetic control of IgA synthesis (Rambaud, *et al.*, 1973). In summary, little progress has been made in determining the role of antigenic stimulation in the pathogenesis of α HCD but, as noted above, it is of great interest that in a number of cases apparently complete remissions have occurred following therapy with antibiotics alone. Why such environmental stimuli should be associated with α HCD rather than IgA myeloma remains unexplained.

There are, however, several possible pathogenic mechanisms. Cells synthesizing α HCD protein may be present in small numbers in normal subjects and have a tendency to undergo malignant proliferation when the secretory immune system is very active such as in chronic intestinal antigenic stimulation (Rambaud *et al.*, 1973). Although α HCD protein has not been detected in normal subjects, gamma heavy chain disease protein, its analogue in IgG heavy chain disease, has been identified recently in normal human plasma (Lam and Stevenson, 1973). This suggests that α HCD could begin as a proliferation of a pre-existent clone of α HCD protein-secreting cells. Alternatively somatic mutation could give rise to a cell that synthesizes an essential component of the α heavy chain which allows it to enter physiologically into the gut-associated lymphoid system, and subsequently home into and selectively proliferate in the lamina propria under abnormal microenvironmental conditions (WHO Memorandum, 1976). Another hypothesis would be that the apparent requirement for an external environmental stimulus may reflect an underlying immunodeficiency; either a defect resulting in increased host susceptibility to infection or a basic defect in the host's ability to terminate the cellular proliferative response to the stimulating signal. The latter defect would represent a loss of the major negative feedback control of proliferation of the B-cell plasma-cytic system, namely specific antibody which normally is an inhibitor of further antibody production. As α HCD protein lacks effective antigen binding sites, α HCD patients may be unable to produce effective antibodies in response to intestinal antigenic challenge and there-fore may lack negative feedback control of B-cell plasma-cytic proliferation. The second means of control of B-cell proliferation is the suppressor T-cell. Deficiency of suppressor T-cell precursors could provide a second explanation for loss of control of B-cell proliferation in this disease (WHO Memorandum, 1976).

The relative importance of genetic predisposition to α HCD is unknown. Although limited family studies have failed to reveal evidence of a heritable trait for this condition (Novis, Bank and Young, 1973; Ramot et al., 1975) a search for genetic markers including HLA and Ia antigens may help identify predisposed subjects. In 'Mediterranean' lymphoma and α HCD the presence of significant amounts of the intestinal isoenzyme of alkaline phosphatase in serum appears to be a genetic marker

(Ramot et al., 1966; Doe et al., 1972) and warrants further study.

CONCLUSION

Alpha HCD is a prevalent condition among many under-privileged populations whose susceptibility may in part be due to a chronic antigenic stimulation of the secretory immune response perhaps affecting genetically predis-posed subjects. The elucidation of the sequence of events that produces a hyperplastic, aberrant immune response, characterized clinically by a severe malabsorp-tion syndrome and the synthesis of an abnormal frag-ment of IgA related to the Fc piece and responsive to antibiotic therapy, may offer a revealing insight into the aetiology of intestinal lymphomas. The natural history of α HCD, progressing from this early, apparently pre-malignant, stage into a frankly malignant immunoblastic sarcoma suggests that this disorder may serve as a model for the study of the oncogenesis of lymphoma in man.

REFERENCES

Al-Bahrani, Z. R. & Bakir, F. (1971) Primary intestinal lymphoma. *Annals of the Royal College of Surgeons of England*, **49**, 103–113.

Balikian, J., Nassar, V. T. Shammaa, M. & Shahid, M. (1969) Primary lymphomas of the small intestine including the duodenum. A roentgen analysis of twenty-nine cases. *American Journal of Roentgenology, Radium Therapy and Nuclear Medicine*, **107**, 131–141.

Bognel, J. C., Rambaud, J. C., Modiglianai, R., Matuchansky, C., Bognel, C., Bernier, J. J., Scotto, J., Hautefeuille, P., Mihaesco, E., Hurez, E., Preud'homme, J. L. & Seligmann, M. (1972) Étude clinique anatomo-pathologique et immunochimique d'un nouveau cas de maladie des chaines alpha suivi pendant cinq ans. *Revue Européenne D'Études Cliniques et Biologiques*, **17**, 362–374.

Bonomo, L., Dammaco, F., Marano, R. & Bonomo, G. M. (1972) Abdominal lymphoma and alpha chain disease. *American Journal of Medicine*, **52**, 73–86.

Buxbaum, J. N. & Preud'homme, J. L. (1972) Alpha and gamma heavy chain diseases in man: intracellular origin of the aberrant polypeptides. *Journal of Immunology*, **109**, 1131–1137.

Chernov, A., Doe, W. F. & Gompertz, D. (1972) Intrajejunal volatile fatty acids in the stagnant loop syndrome. *Gut*, **13**, 103–106.

Crabbé, P. A. & Heremans, J. F. (1966) Étude immunohistochimique des plasmocytes de la muqueuse intestinale humaine normale. *Revue Française d'Études Cliniques et Biologiques*, **11**, 484–492.

Crabbé, P. A., Nash, D. R., Bazin, H., Eyssen, H. & Heremans, J. F. (1970) Immunohistochemical observations on lymphoid tissues from conventional and germ-free mice. *Laboratory Investigation*, **22**, 448–457.

Doe, W. F. (1970) Unpublished.

Doe, W. F. (1975) Alpha chain disease. Clinicopathological features and relationship to so-called Mediterranean lymphoma. *British Journal of Cancer*, **31**, Suppl. II, 350–355.

Doe, W. F., Agnesdottir, G., Valdimarsson, H. (1974) Unpublished.

Doe, W. F., Henry, K. & Doyle, F. H. (1976) Radiological and histological findings in six patients with alpha-chain disease. *British Journal of Radiology*, **49**, 3–11.

Doe, W. F., Hobbs, J. R., Henry, K. & Dowling, R. H. (1970) Alpha chain disease. *Quarterly Journal of Medicine*, **39**, 619–620.

Doe, W. F., Henry, K., Hobbs, J. R., Avery Jones, F., Dent, C. E. & Booth, C. C. (1972) Five cases of alpha chain disease. *Gut*, **13**, 947–957.

Dorrington, K. J., Mihaesco, E. & Seligmann, M. (1970) Molecular size of 3 alpha chain disease proteins. *Biochimica et Biophysica Acta*, **221**, 647–649.

Dutz, W., Asvardi, S., Sadri, S. & Kohout, E. (1971) Intestinal lymphoma and sprue: a systematic approach. *Gut*, **12**, 804–810.

Eidelman, S., Parkins, A. & Rubin, C. (1966) Abdominal lymphoma presenting as malabsorption. A clinicopathologic study of 9 cases in Israel and a review of the literature. *Medicine*, **45**, 111–137.

Fauz, J. A., Crain, J. D., Rosen, F. S. & Merler, E. (1973) An alpha heavy chain abnormality in a child with hypogammaglobulinaemia. *Clinical Immunology and Immunopathology*, **1**, 282–290.

Franklin, E. C., Lowenstein, J. Bigelow, B. & Meltzer, M. (1964) Heavy chain disease. A new disorder of serum γ globulins. Report of the first case. *American Journal of Medicine*, **37**, 332–350.

Grey, H. M., Abel, C. A. & Zimmerman, B. (1971) Structure of IgA proteins. *Annals of the New York Academy of Sciences*, **190**, 37–48.

Grey, H. M., Abel, C. A., Yount, W. J. & Kunkel, H. G. (1968) A subclass of human γA-globulins (γA2) which lacks the disulphide bonds linking heavy and light chains. *Journal of Experimental Medicine*, **128**, 1223–1236.

Haghighi, P. (1976) Unpublished results.

Henry, K., Bird, R. G. & Doe, W. F. (1974) Intestinal

coccidiosis in a patient with alpha chain disease. *British Medical Journal*, **i**, 542–543.

Irunberry, J., Benallegue, A., Illoul, G., Timsit, G., Abbadi, M., Benabdalla, H. S., Boucekkine, T., Ould-Aoudia, J. P. & Colonna, P. (1970) Trois cas de maladie des chaines alpha observés en Algérie. *Nouvelle Revue Française d'Hematologie*, **10**, 609–616.

Lam, C. W. K. & Stevenson, G. T. (1973) Detection in normal plasma of immunoglobulin resembling the protein of γ-chain disease. *Nature*, **246**, 419–421.

Laroche, C., Seligmann, M., Merillon, H., Turpin, G., Marche, C., Cerf, M., Lemaigre, G., Forest, M. & Hurez, D. (1970) Nouvelle observation d'une maladie des chaines lourdes alpha au cours d'un lymphome abdominal de type Méditerranéen avec tuberculose isolée des ganglions mésenteriques et pelvispondylite. *Presse Médicale*, **78**, 55–59.

Manousos, O. N. (1974) Personal communication.

Manousos, O. N., Economidou, J. C., Georgiadou, D. E. Pratsika-Ougourloglou, K. G., Hadziyannis, S. J., Merikas, G. E., Henry, K. & Doe, W. F. (1974) Alpha chain disease with clinical, immunological and histological recovery. *British Medical Journal*, **ii**, 409–412.

Monges, H., Aubert, L., Chamlian, A., Remacle, J. P., Bernard, D., Mathieu, B. & Cougard, A. (1974) *Archives Françaises des Maladies de L'Appareil Digestif* (in press).

Nasr, K., Haghighi, P., Bakhshandeh, K. & Haghshenas, M. (1970) Primary lymphoma of the upper small intestine. *Gut*, **11**, 673–678.

Nasrallah, S. & Nassar, V. (1976) Unpublished.

Natori, S. & Garen, A. (1970) Molecular heterogeneity in the amino-terminal region of alkaline phosphatase. *Journal of Molecular Biology*, **49**, 577–588.

Novis, B. H., Bank, S. & Young, G. (1973) Alpha chain disease. *Lancet*, **ii**, 498.

Novis, B. H., Kahn, L. B. & Bank, S. (1973) Alpha chain disease in sub-Saharan Africa. *American Journal of Digestive Diseases*, **18**, 679–688.

Novis, B. H., Bank, S., Marks, I. N., Selzer, G., Kahn, L. & Sealy, R. (1971) Abdominal lymphoma presenting with malabsorption. *Quarterly Journal of Medicine*, **40**, 521–540.

Osterland, C. K. & Chaplin, H. (1966) Atypical antigenic properties of a γA myeloma protein. *Journal of Immunology*, **96**, 842–848.

Pittman, F. E., Osserman, E. F., Bolands, O. M., Lotero, H. R., Duque, E. E., Pittman, J. C. & Tripathy, K. (1971) Alpha heavy chain disease. The first proven case detected in the Western Hemisphere. *Gastroenterology*, **60**, 792 (Abs.).

Preud'homme, J. L. & Seligmann, M. (1972) Surface bound immunoglobulins as a cell marker in human lymphoproliferative diseases. *Blood*, **40**, 777–794.

Radl, J. (1970) Light chain typing of immunoglobulins in small samples of biological materials. *Immunology*, **19**, 137–149.

Rambaud, J. C. & Matuchansky, C. (1973) Alpha chain disease. Pathogenesis and relation to Mediterranean lymphoma. *Lancet*, **i**, 1430–1432.

Rambaud, J. C. Unpublished.

Rambaud, J. C., Bognel, C., Prost, A., Bernier, J. J., Lequintrec, Y., Lambling, A., Danon, F., Hurez, D., Seligmann, M. (1968) Clinicopathological study of a patient with Mediterranean type of abdominal lymphoma and a new type of IgA abnormality (α chain disease). *Digestion*, I, 321–336.

Rambaud, J. C., Matuchansky, C., Bognel, J. C., Bognel, C., Bernier, J. J., Scotto, J., Perol, C., Ferrier, J. P., Mihaesco, E., Hurez, D. & Seligmann, M. (1970) Nouveau cas de maladie des chaînes alpha chez un Eurasien. *Annales de Médecine Interne*, **121**, 135–148.

Ramot, B. & Hulu, N. (1975) Primary intestinal lymphoma and its relation to alpha heavy chain disease. *British Journal of Cancer*, **31**, Suppl. II, 343–349.

Ramot, B. & Streifler, C. (1966) Raised serum alkaline phosphatase. *Lancet*, **ii**, 587.

Ramot, B., Shahin, N. & Bubis, J. J. (1965) Malabsorption syndrome in lymphoma of small intestine. *Israel Journal of Medical Science*, **1**, 221–226.

Rappaport, H., Ramot, B., Hulu, N. & Park, J. K. (1972) The pathology of so-called Mediterranean abdominal lymphoma with malabsorption. *Cancer*, **29**, 1502–1511.

Roge, J., Druet, P. & Marche, C. (1970) Lymphome Méditerranéen avec maladie des chaînes alpha triple rémission clinique, anatomique et immunologique. *Pathologie-Biologie*, **18**, 851–858.

Salem, P. A., Nassar, V. H., Shahid, M. J., Hajj, A. A., Alami, S. Y., Balikian, J. B. & Salem, A. A. (1977) 'Mediterranean abdominal lymphoma' or immunoproliferative small intestinal disease. *Cancer*, **40**, 2941–2947.

Savilahti, E. & Brandtzaeg, P. (1973) An atypical case of alpha chain disease. *Scandinavian Journal of Immunology*, **2**, 322 (Abs.).

Scotto, J., Stralin, H. & Caroli, J. (1970) Ultrastructural study of two cases of α chain disease. *Gut*, **11**, 782–788.

Seligmann, M. (1975a) Unpublished.

Seligmann, M. (1975b) Immunochemical, clinical and pathological features of α chain disease. *Archives of Internal Medicine*, **135**, 78–82.

Seligmann, M. & Mihaesco, E. (1974). Current knowledge on alpha chain disease. In *Advances in Experimental Medicine and Biology*, ed. Mestecky, J. & Lawton, A. R., Vol. 45, pp. 365–372. New York: Plenum Press.

Seligmann, M., Mihaesco, E. & Frangione, B. (1971) Studies on alpha chain disease. *Annals of the New York Academy of Sciences*, **190**, 487–500.

Seligmann, M., Danon, F., Hurez, D., Mihaesco, E. & Preud'homme, J. L. (1968) Alpha chain disease: a new immunoglobulin abnormality. *Science*, **162**, 1396–1397.

Seligmann, M., Mihaesco, E., Hurez, D., Mihaesco, C., Preud'homme, J. L. & Rambaud, J. C. (1969) Immunochemical studies in four cases of alpha chain disease. *Journal of Clinical Investigation*, **48**, 2374–2389.

Stoop, J. W., Ballieux, R. E., Hijmans, W. & Zegers, B. J. M. (1971) Alpha chain disease with involvement of the respiratory tract in a Dutch child. *Clinical and Experimental Immunology*, **9**, 625–635.

Suzuki, T. & Garen, A. (1969) Fragments of alkaline phosphatase from nonsense mutants. I. Isolation and characterization of fragments from amber and ochre mutants. *Journal of Molecular Biology*, **45**, 549–566.

Tomasi, T. B. (1972) Secretory immunoglobulins. *New England Journal of Medicine*, **287**, 500–506.

Wolfenstein-Todel, C., Mihaesco, E. L. & Frangione, B. (1974) 'Alpha chain disease' Protein Def: internal deletion of a human immunoglobulin A$_1$ heavy chain. *Proceedings of the National Academy of Sciences USA*, **71**, 974–978.

World Health Organisation Memorandum on alpha chain disease and related small-intestinal lymphoma (1976) *Bulletin of the World Health Organisation*, **54**, 615–624.

17. Myelomatosis, amyloidosis, Whipple's disease, tropical sprue and intestinal lymphangiectasia

M. R. Haeney

INTRODUCTION

The gastrointestinal tract is one of the most important sites of potential interaction between environmental antigens and the individual's immune apparatus. It is therefore not surprising that lymphoid tissue accounts for approximately one-quarter of the intestinal mucosal mass (Ch. 1). Recently, the physiological and pathological interactions between the intestinal immune system and environmental antigens have been intensively investigated. This interest stems from several observations. Firstly, is the finding of an increased incidence of gastrointestinal symptoms in patients with primary immunodeficiency syndromes (Ch. 9); thus it was expected that studies of patients with humoral or cellular defects would allow evaluation of the relative importance of antibody and cell-mediated mechanisms in intestinal defence. Secondly, other disorders of the immune system, e.g. multiple myeloma, can be associated with immune suppression and by the same token develop gastrointestinal symptoms. Hence, studies of the intestine in such conditions could also be relevant to an understanding of immunologically dependent mucosal integrity. Thirdly, primary amyloidosis, in which there is tissue deposition of immunoglobulin fragments, and to a lesser extent secondary amyloidosis, may cause intestinal disease but usually by non-immune mechanisms related to amyloid deposits. Fourthly, investigation of certain gastrointestinal diseases, e.g. Whipple's disease, suggested that they could have as their basis subtle immune defects. However, in these conditions, individual exposure to a specific environmental antigen also seems necessary for the patient to develop clinical disease. Whipple's disease is rare, but commoner gastrointestinal diseases, including Crohn's disease, ulcerative colitis (Ch. 7), coeliac disease (Ch. 6) and possibly tropical sprue, may have a similar pathogenesis. Lastly, it has also become apparent that other gastrointestinal diseases, e.g. intestinal lymphangiectasia, can secondarily lead to immune incompetence on the basis of excessive loss of immunoglobulins and/or lymphocytes from the damaged mucosa (Strober, Wochner, Carbone and Waldmann, 1967).

The quality and relative sophistication of the immunological data on the above syndromes and diseases vary enormously. In certain instances the information is the subject of a chapter in this book. This chapter considers (1) myelomatosis and the intestine, (2) gastrointestinal amyloidosis, (3) Whipple's disease, (4) tropical sprue and (5) intestinal lymphangiectasia. Studies of these diseases, although less extensive than, for example, Crohn's disease and ulcerative colitis, have nevertheless helped in the further understanding of gastrointestinal immunophysiology.

1. MYELOMATOSIS AND THE INTESTINE

The diagnosis of multiple myeloma requires two of the following criteria to be satisfied: (1) abnormal plasma cells in the bone marrow, (2) positive radiological findings of myelomatosis, (3) a monoclonal immunoglobulin in the serum, or urine, or both (Galton and Peto, 1968; Medical Research Council, 1971; Medical Research Council, 1973). Although myelomatosis may involve several organ systems, symptomatic involvement of the gastrointestinal tract is rare. In a major review of the presenting features of myeloma, no mention was made of diarrhoea (Osserman, 1959), but occasional reports have documented infiltration of the gastrointestinal tract by solitary plasmacytomas and also in multiple myeloma (Goldstein and Poker, 1966; Tangun, Saracbasi, Inceman, Danon and Seligmann, 1975). Conversely, cases have been described in which ulcerative colitis was accompanied by plasmacytosis (Fadem, 1952; Bernstein and Dixon, 1964).

ILLUSTRATIVE CASE HISTORY

F.K., a 63-year-old Pakistani male, resident in England since 1969, presented in April 1974 with a 6-month history of bloody diarrhoea. Other than evidence of weight loss, clinical examination was normal. Sigmoidoscopy to 17 cm showed a uniformly oedematous, hyperaemic mucosa with mucus and contact bleeding. The stool was fluid and contained blood. Faecal excretions of fat, lactic acid, sodium and nitrogen were raised, but absorption of xylose and vitamin B_{12} was normal. Serum immunoglobulin estimations were as follows: IgG 15.9 g/l (NR 6.00–16.00), IgA 2.41 g/l (NR 0.75–

5.20), IgM 0.86 g/l (NR 0.30–1.80). Serum immuno-electrophoresis showed a monoclonal IgG band. Bence-Jones protein (type kappa) was present in the urine. No osteolytic lesions were detected on a skeletal survey. Bone marrow histology and immunofluorescence showed 18–20 per cent of IgG-staining plasma cells, some abnormal in form, while fewer than 1 per cent IgM- and IgA-staining cells were present. Multiple upper jejunal diverticula were seen on a barium follow-through examination, while a barium enema showed a poorly

scopy has been normal. A second patient with a similar picture has also been seen (Haeney, Ross, Thompson and Asquith, 1977).

CLINICAL FEATURES OF INTESTINAL MYELOMATOSIS

Haemorrhagic colitis, ileocolitis and proctitis have been recorded among the gastrointestinal complications of leukaemia (Prolla and Kirsner, 1964), lymphoma (Nugent, Zuberi, Bulan and Legg, 1972) and lympho-sarcoma (Cornes, Smith and Southwood, 1961;

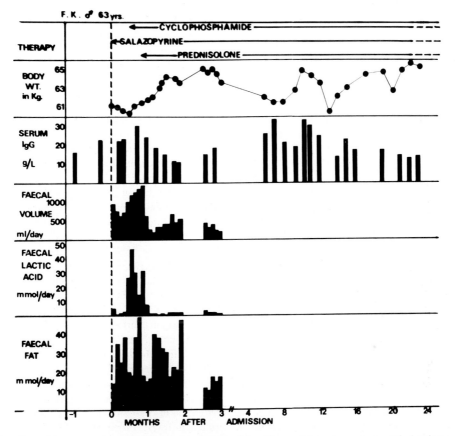

Fig. 17.1 The effect of immunosuppressive therapy on intestinal function and the serum paraprotein level over a 2-year period.

distensible rectum and loss of mucosal pattern in the sigmoid colon. A biopsy taken at 15 cm showed non-specific changes, with infiltration by lymphocytes and polymorphs, but the plasma cells appeared normal, and a normal ratio of Ig-staining plasma cells was seen. There was no evidence of amyloid on specific staining. Over the ensuing 6 weeks, the patient's serum IgG paraprotein level reached 30 g/l, and there was a progressive fall of serum IgA and IgM. He was started on standard doses of cyclophosphamide and prednisolone, with improvement in his diarrhoea and a reduction in the serum para-protein (Fig. 17.1). On treatment, repeated sigmoido-

Myerson, Myerson, Muller, DeLuca and Lawson, 1974). However, major reviews of proven myelomatosis and other monoclonal immunoglobulin disorders have not included proctosigmoiditis as a significant clinical feature (Osserman, 1959; Owen, Pitney and O'Dea, 1959; Michaux and Heremans, 1969; Williams, Bailly and Howe, 1969; Axelsson and Hällen, 1972; Zawadzki and Edwards, 1972; Talerman and Haije, 1973). Histo-logical infiltration of the gastrointestinal tract by myeloma cells may nevertheless occur. In a review of the literature, Goldstein and Poker (1966) recorded 46 cases of plasma cell neoplasia involving the gastrointestinal tract, of which 36 were solitary plasmacytomas and 10 were cases of multiple myeloma diagnosed from necropsy material. All segments of the gastrointestinal tract, with the possible exception of the oesophagus, have been shown to be the site of plasmacytomas, and both solitary and multiple sites of involvement have been reported. The majority of these cases are unaccompanied by monoclonal paraproteinaemia and Bence-Jones proteinuria (Goldstein and Poker, 1966). Typically, the patients with gastric plasmacytoma had either a long history suggestive of chronic peptic ulcer culminating in pyloric obstruction, or a short history of weight loss, anorexia and vomiting, leading to a clinical diagnosis of gastric carcinoma. With plasma cell tumours of other parts of the intestine, abdominal pain, obstruction and bleeding have been the predominant features.

Very few instances of intestinal involvement in myelomatosis have been reported (Goldstein and Poker, 1966; Marano, Dammacco, Pastore and Schiraldi, 1970; Tangun, Saracbasi, Inceman, Danon and Seligmann, 1975), in contrast to the relatively common extramedullary involvement of other organs (Hayes, Bennett and Heck, 1952; Pazmantier and Azar, 1969). Small-intestinal infiltration by myeloma cells may produce a sprue-like syndrome, with weight loss, diarrhoea, and malabsorption of fat and other test substances. The jejunal biopsies have shown diffuse massive lamina propria infiltration by plasma cells, but villous architecture has been reported as normal (Tangun, Saracbasi, Inceman, Danon and Seligman, 1975) and on the other hand as showing subtotal villous atrophy (Marano, Dammacco, Pastore and Schiraldi, 1970). Conversely, transient paraproteinaemia – that is, homogeneous immunoglobulinaemia suddenly appearing in the serum and disappearing within weeks or months – has been documented in a single case of tropical sprue (Young, 1969) and of coeliac disease (Peña, Nieuwkoop, Schuit, Hekkens and Haex, 1976), while benign essential paraproteinaemia, usually IgG, has been reported in unspecified cases of steatorrhoea and diarrhoea (Cooke, 1969).

The only documentation of an association between myeloma and procto-sigmoiditis is that by Haeney, Ross, Thompson and Asquith (1977) who have described two patients with evidence of IgG monoclonal gammopathy and Bence-Jones proteinuria who fulfilled the diagnostic criteria of myelomatosis. Both patients presented with haemorrhagic proctosigmoiditis. There was no evidence of myelomatous infiltration of the gastrointestinal tract, nor was there any evidence of amyloidosis. Other authors have reported the presence of benign essential paraproteinaemia, usually IgG, in patients with ulcerative colitis (Cooke, 1969). Bernstein and Dixon (1964) cite a case of ulcerative colitis,

initially diagnosed as myelomatosis on the basis of bone marrow plasmacytosis, but the other criteria needed to make a diagnosis of myeloma were not satisfied.

CONCLUSION

Whilst the aetiology of many gastrointestinal diseases remains obscure, knowledge of the immunological phenomena associated with these conditions continues to grow. As with other chronic diseases, it is still not possible to say whether the immunological abnormalities are the cause of the intestinal disease or secondary to the inflammation present in the intestine. In this respect, the association of plasma cell dyscrasias and intestinal disease highlights the intimate relationship between local intestinal immunity, local antigenic stimulation and immune surveillance mechanisms.

2. GASTROINTESTINAL AMYLOIDOSIS

The term amyloidosis denotes the presence, in various organs and tissues, of an amorphous substance possessing certain histochemical, immunological and physical features (Pruzanski and Katz, 1976). Characteristically, amyloid stains with congo red (Bennhold, 1922) and exhibits green birefringence in polarized light (Missmahl, 1957). Under the electron-microscope, it has a primarily fibrillar structure (Cohen and Calkins, 1959), the fibrils showing a typical β-pleated-sheet appearance in X-ray diffraction analysis (Eanes and Glenner, 1968). The amyloid substance interferes with physiological processes by replacing normal tissue and so affecting organ function. Several attempts have been made to classify amyloidosis on clinical (Cohen, 1967; Missmahl, 1969), histological or aetiological grounds (Glenner, Terry and Isersky, 1973). It now seems desirable to use two classifications: (1) clinicopathological, according to the site of organ involvement, but with emphasis on heredito-familial background and associated conditions (Pruzanski and Katz, 1976), and (2) immunochemical, according to the composition of the amyloid and the presence or absence of certain amyloid-related substances in the blood (Glenner, Terry and Isersky, 1973; Katz and Pruzanski, 1976; Rimon, 1976).

In the clinicopathological classification, amyloidosis is no longer divided into various patterns of organ or tissue involvement because attempts to classify it in this way have been largely unsuccessful (Isobe and Osserman, 1974). It is generally true, however, that in 'primary generalized' amyloidosis the tongue, heart, gastrointestinal tract, muscles, joints, nerves and skin are most commonly affected, whereas in the 'secondary' type the kidneys, liver, spleen and adrenal glands are mainly involved. A marked overlap between these two groups results in 'mixed' patterns (Isobe and Osserman, 1974; Pruzanski and Katz, 1976).

The immunochemical classification is based on two major types of amyloid-fibril proteins – one related to immunoglobulins and the other not. In primary amyloidosis, or amyloid associated with plasma cell dyscrasias, direct proof of the immunoglobulin origin of amyloid fibrils has been obtained from peptide mapping and amino acid sequence analysis. The major protein constituent of the fibrils is homologous with the variable region of light chains (V_L), or the intact light chain, or both (Glenner, Terry and Isersky, 1973). Antisera to κ-type amyloid fibril proteins showed partial identity with most Bence-Jones κ proteins tested but not with λ proteins and vice versa. Thus antisera were reacting with the antigenic determinants located in the V_L regions, or were detecting conformational determinants since reactivity could be abolished by reduction and alkylation of the fibrils (Franklin and Zucker-Franklin, 1972). Husby, Natvig and Sletten (1974) isolated a single polypeptide chain from the amyloid fibril proteins of a patient with primary amyloidosis that showed sequence homology with λ Bence-Jones protein. The patient's serum contained a protein antigenically related to the amyloid-fibril protein. Antisera to the protein did not react with other amyloid preparations or with immunoglobulins or their fragments. In most cases of secondary amyloidosis, as well as in familial Mediterranean fever, the major component of amyloid fibrils is a non-immunoglobulin protein, AA (Benditt, Eriksen, Hermodson and Ericsson, 1971). Nevertheless, Husby, Sletten, Michaelsen and Natvig (1973) demonstrated this protein in some amyloid fibrils from patients with primary amyloidosis and plasma cell dycrasias. It appears, therefore, that some amyloid preparations have common constituents of both immunoglobulin and non-immunoglobulin origin. Finally, a serum component, SAA, antigenically related to the non-immunoglobulin protein AA, may be a circulating precursor of amyloid fibrils (Husby and Natvig, 1974).

In addition to the fibrillary component, amyloid deposits contain small quantities of a glycoprotein that is antigenically identical with a constituent of normal plasma, namely the P component. It is composed of 5 globular subunits with a pentagonal structure (Skinner, Cohen, Shirahama and Cathcart, 1974).

GASTROINTESTINAL FEATURES IN AMYLOIDOSIS

Amyloid frequently occurs in the gastrointestinal tract. Symmers (1956) estimated the incidence at 70 per cent in 145 patients with 'primary' disease, while Dahlin (1949) found a 55 per cent incidence in 27 patients with the 'secondary' form. All estimates are obviously minimum figures and depend on the thoroughness of the search. Thus at autopsy, amyloid infiltration of the intestinal tract has been demonstrated in 68 out of 70 cases of systemic amyloidosis (Gilat, Revach and Sohar, 1969). In life, positive rectal biopsies have been obtained in 75 per cent of 200 patients with amyloidosis (Blum and Sohar, 1962), while jejunal biopsy has also been reported as a safe and useful technique (Green, Higgins, Brown, Hoffman and Somerville, 1961; Pettersson and Wegelius, 1972).

IMPAIRED MOTOR ACTIVITY

Amyloid may alter the peristaltic activity of any part of the gastrointestinal tract. Oesophageal motility is rarely affected (Gilat and Spiro, 1968), but impaired gastric peristalsis has been more frequently reported (Golden, 1945; Intriere and Brown, 1956; Gilat and Spiro, 1968; CPC, *American Journal of Medicine*, 1974). Deranged small- and large-bowel motility may lead to constipation or diarrhoea. Diarrhoea severe enough to simulate ulcerative colitis has been noted (Casad and Bocian, 1965; Cherenkoff, Costopoulos and Bain, 1972), while there are several records of intestinal pseudo-obstruction (Gilat and Spiro, 1968; Legge, Wollaeger and Carlson, 1970). Factors causing impaired peristaltic activity include amyloid infiltration of the muscular layers of the bowel wall, infiltration of nerve fibres or ganglia in the intestine and narrowing of the vasa nervorum (Gilat and Spiro, 1968).

VASCULAR PROBLEMS

Infarction and perforation

Amyloid is largely deposited in blood vessels. Gilat, Revach and Sohar (1969) found that in 'secondary' amyloidosis and amyloid associated with familial Mediterranean fever, amyloid was deposited in the inner coat of small blood vessels, while in 'primary' amyloidosis and plasma cell dyscrasias, it was found in the outer coat of small and medium blood vessels, corresponding to the classification of amyloid into perireticular and pericollagenous types respectively (Heller, Missmahl, Sohar and Gafni, 1964). As amyloid deposition continues, the blood supply is progressively impaired, perhaps leading to segmental ischaemic enteritis or colitis, ulceration, or finally to intestinal infarction with or without perforation (Brody, Wertlake and Laster, 1964; Brom, Bank, Marks, Milner and Baker, 1969; Seliger, Krassner, Berenbaum and Miller, 1971; Cherenkoff, Costopoulos and Bain, 1972; Mallory, Struthers and Kern, 1975).

Bleeding

Jarnum (1965) reported 18 patients with amyloidosis who had significant gastrointestinal bleeding. Sometimes the bleeding lesion can be identified as an ulcer, but more often either no single lesion is found or else diffuse bleeding is encountered (Gilat and Spiro, 1968; Mallory, Struthers and Kern, 1975).

Other vascular complications

Jarnum (1965) has suggested that vascular insufficiency leads to increased transudation of protein into the bowel lumen. Other authors have confirmed protein-losing enteropathy in patients with amyloidosis (Gilat and Spiro, 1968).

MALABSORPTION

The presence of malabsorption in some patients with amyloidosis has been well established (Beddow and Tilden, 1960; Herskovic, Bartholomew and Green, 1964; Babb, Alarcón-Segovia, Diessner and McPherson, 1967; Gilat and Spiro, 1968; Pettersson and Wegelius, 1972; Ravid and Sohar, 1974). In the majority of cases, the patients had advanced disease. Intestinal malabsorption as the initial clinical manifestation of amyloidosis is rare (Ravid and Sohar, 1974). Massive amyloid deposits causing mucosal destruction (Beddow and Tilden, 1960), vascular insufficiency (Gilat, Revach and Sohar, 1969; Pettersson and Wegelius, 1972; Ravid and Sohar, 1974) and the stagnant bowel syndrome secondary to impaired peristalsis (Scheerer, Schwartz, Pierre, Reed and Linman, 1964) appear to be the most likely explanation of the malabsorption.

CONCLUSION

Amyloid involving the gastrointestinal tract may be deposited anywhere in the mucosa, blood vessels, nerves or muscular layers. It causes derangement of bowel function by direct infiltration or by producing secondary ischaemic changes. The fascination of amyloidosis lies in the recent demonstration that amyloid has a heterogeneous composition primarily of immunoglobulin or non-immunoglobulin origin. Normal plasma constituents antigenically related to amyloid proteins may be circulating precursors of amyloid. The relative importance of these plasma factors, local factors and the way in which they interact in amyloid formation remains to be elucidated.

3. WHIPPLE'S DISEASE

Whipple's disease (intestinal lipodystrophy) characteristically involves the small bowel, lymph nodes and joints, but it can also affect the liver, spleen, heart, brain and other organs. The disease is rare, some 248 patients being reported up to 1974, of whom only 33 were female (Miksche, Blümcke, Fritsche, Küchemann, Schüler and Grözinger, 1974). Histologically, the disease is characterized by the presence of periodic acid–Schiff (PAS) staining macrophages in affected tissues. Electron-microscopy of the small intestine shows this PAS-positive material to be the phagocytosed remains of cell walls of numerous bacillary bodies located in an extracellular position in the lamina propria (Yardley and Hendrix, 1961).

CLINICAL FEATURES

The majority of patients present with weight loss, malabsorption, abdominal pain, recurrent pyrexia and lymphadenopathy, often preceded by a migratory polyarthropathy. Less frequent features include skin pigmentation, cardiac involvement, pleuropericarditis, peritonitis, amyloidosis and neuropsychiatric syndromes (Maizel, Ruffin and Dobbin, 1970; Miksche, Blümcke, Fritsche, Küchemann, Schüler and Grözinger, 1974). Paulley (1952) first reported that the disease responded to antibiotics and since then a number of drugs have been tried and found effective (Miksche, Blümke, Fritsche, Küchemann, Schüler and Grözinger, 1974). Clinical improvement occurs within days, arthralgia ceases within weeks, while laboratory values usually return to normal within 6–9 months. Histological recovery may not occur for at least 2 years, but electron-microscopy shows earlier improvement (Oliva, González Campos, Navarro and Mogena, 1972).

ILLUSTRATIVE CASE HISTORY

E.C., a 54-year-old Caucasian female, presented with a sero-negative, non-erosive polyarthropathy and Raynaud's phenomenon. Four years later she developed vague abdominal pain, episodic diarrhoea, night sweats and axillary lymphadenopathy. Investigation showed anaemia, peripheral lymphocytopaenia, steatorrhoea and malabsorption of xylose, iron and vitamin B_{12}. Hepatitis B with persistent HBs antigenaemia was a later complication. Dissecting microscopy of a proximal jejunal biopsy demonstrated the classical 'club-shaped' villi of Whipple's disease (Fig. 17.2). On light microscopy (Fig. 17.3), the characteristic dense infiltration of PAS-positive macrophages in the lamina propria was easily seen. Prior to treatment, although the percentage of B-cells in the peripheral blood (as assessed by EAC rosettes and surface immunofluorescence) was normal, the absolute values were reduced. Serum immunoglobulin and complement levels were normal. A notable feature was her impaired cell-mediated immunity: the numbers of circulating T-cells (E rosettes) were low, there was cutaneous anergy to a number of antigens, and impaired peripheral lymphocyte activation by various mitogens and antigens. Finally, splenic atrophy was found at laparotomy. On treatment with cotrimoxazole, there was a dramatic clinical and morphological improvement (Fig. 17.4), and the peripheral lymphocyte counts returned to normal. However, skin

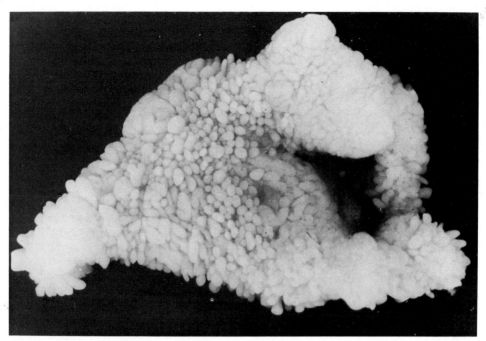

Fig. 17.2 The dissecting microscope appearance of the jejunal biopsy in Whipple's disease, showing swollen 'club-shaped' villi ($\times$ 25).

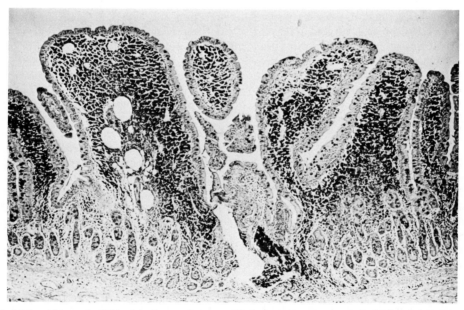

Fig. 17.3 A jejunal biopsy in Whipple's disease showing villi distended by characteristic PAS-staining macrophages in the lamina propria ($\times$ 90).

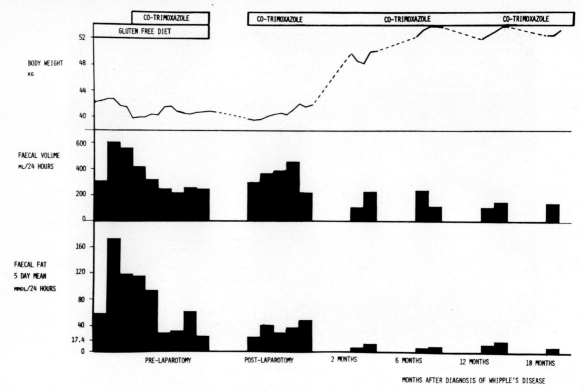

Fig. 17.4 The clinical responsiveness of Whipple's disease to 18 months of chemotherapy with cotrimoxazole.

tests remained unchanged and *in-vitro* lymphocyte transformation was still depressed, suggesting that the cellular defect was primary. In support of this theory was the lack of improvement on Levamisole, a drug which allegedly activates functionally defective T-cells (Biniaminov and Ramot, 1975); no significant improvement in the patient's *in-vitro* lymphocyte responsiveness or cutaneous anergy occurring after 4 months' therapy (Haeney and Ross, 1978).

IMMUNE STATUS IN WHIPPLE'S DISEASE

Many isolated aspects of immune status have been reported in Whipple's disease, but what is badly needed is a much more comprehensive evaluation of immunological reactivity in a reasonably large series of patients, both before and after treatment. This should include morphological examination of lymphoid tissues, functional assessment of the reticuloendothelial system, measurements of serum and secretory immunoglobulins including specific antibody production, and specific and non-specific tests of lymphocyte function and cell-mediated immunity.

Lymphoid cells of the intestinal mucosa in untreated Whipple's disease

In contrast to well-documented studies in, for example, coeliac disease (Asquith, 1974; Ferguson, 1976), few

reports have quantitated the numbers of intraepithelial lymphocytes and lamina propria cells in Whipple's disease. Raised intraepithelial lymphocyte counts were noted in 1 patient (Montgomery and Shearer, 1974). With respect to cells in the lamina propria of the small intestine, several groups of workers (Dobbin and Ruffin, 1967; Maxwell, Ferguson, McKay, Imrie and Watson, 1968; Douglas, Crabbé and Hobbs, 1970; Cochran, Cook, Gallagher and Peacock, 1973) have commented on the scarcity of lymphocytes and plasma cells. Results of immunofluorescent staining of jejunal biopsies differ; Douglas, Crabbé and Hobbs (1970) and Groll, Valberg, Simon, Eidinger, Wilson and Forsdyke (1972) noted a uniform decrease in plasma cells of each immunoglobulin class. In contrast, others (Cerf, Hurez, Marche and Debray, 1970; Barbier, Balasse-Ketelbant, Kennes, Menu, Platteborse and Parmentier, 1975) have found IgA-staining cells to be mainly affected.

The reticuloendothelial system

In view of the characteristic macrophage infiltration of involved organs it is surprising that there have been no detailed studies to test the functional integrity of the reticuloendothelial (RE) system. Nevertheless, there is an isolated report of impaired macrophage adherence to glass in a patient with Whipple's disease (CPC, *New England Journal of Medicine*, 1971). With respect to gross assessment of the RE system, the spleen is usually normal in size (Maizel, Ruffin and Dobbins, 1970), although splenomegaly has been documented in at least 6 patients (Reizenstein, 1958; Martel and Hodges, 1959; Ross, Gialanella and Kealey, 1960; Schlein, Herman and Gallinek, 1961; Hecker and Reid, 1962; Lundberg and Linder, 1963), and there is a single reference to splenic atrophy (Haeney and Ross, 1978).

Humoral immunity

In the serum, no clear-cut pattern of pre-treatment immunoglobulin levels has emerged in Whipple's disease (Table 17.1). Four cases of hypogammaglobulinaemia have been reported (Sandor and Kozmer, 1957; Martel and Hodges, 1959; Anton, 1961; Cochran, Cooke, Gallagher and Peacock, 1973), while Berens, Cohen and Schwabe (1969) described a patient with isolated IgM deficiency. Of the remaining cases, the majority have shown a high normal or elevated IgA, a normal or slightly reduced IgG and a normal IgM. Post-treatment levels have tended to return to normal except IgM, which has been reported as depressed (Maxwell, Ferguson, McKay, Imrie and Watson, 1968; Groll, Valberg, Simon, Eidinger, Wilson and Forsdyke, 1972; Barbier, Balasse-Ketelbant, Kennes, Menu, Platteborse and Parmentier, 1975) or elevated (Pastor and Geerken, 1973). Whereas serum IgA levels are either normal or high, in the intestinal secretions, low or low normal levels of IgA are usual (Debray, Leymarios, Matuchansky, Marche, Hurez and Cerf, 1969; Cerf, Hurez, Marche and Debray, 1970; Douglas, Crabbé and Hobbs, 1970; Maizel, Ruffin and Dobbins, 1970), reflecting the reduced numbers of mucosal IgA cells. Studies of serum complement activity have been normal both before and after treatment (Martin, Vilseck, Dobbins, Buckley and Tyor, 1972; Haeney and Ross, 1978).

Specific serum antibody activity appears to have been studied in only 2 patients. Maxwell, Ferguson, McKay, Imrie and Watson (1968) found low serum antibody titres to *Streptococcus* and *Salmonella* in a patient studied after 15 months' antibiotic therapy. In the 2nd patient, the effect of diphtheria and tetanus immunization was investigated (Groll, Valberg, Simon, Eidinger, Wilson and Forsdyke, 1972). Prior to treatment, the patient had no antibodies to tetanus or diphtheria, as measured by tanned red-cell agglutination (there was no known history of prior exposure to either antigen); in the post-treatment stage, following immunization, antibody synthesis to diphtheria was normal, but subnormal to tetanus toxoid until 2 booster injections had been given.

Cell-mediated immunity

In contrast to the marginal changes in humoral immunity found in Whipple's disease, the cellular findings have been more impressive.

Peripheral lymphocytes

Before treatment, lymphocytopaenia is a consistent finding (CPC, *New England Journal of Medicine*, 1971; Groll, Valberg, Simon, Eidinger, Wilson and Forsdyke, 1972; Pastor and Geerken, 1973; Haeney and Ross, 1978), with both T- and B-cells being equally affected (Barbier, Balasse-Ketelbant, Kennes, Menu, Platteborse and Parmentier, 1975; Haeney and Ross, 1978). Peripheral lymphocyte counts return to normal usually within the first 3 months of treatment (Groll, Valberg, Simon, Eidinger, Wilson and Forsdyke, 1962; Haeney and Ross, 1978).

Skin tests

With one exception, skin tests on untreated patients have shown depressed or absent responses (Table 17.1). The exception was a patient described by Buchholtz, Maintz and Otto (1974) who had a positive delayed hypersensitivity (DH) response to the single antigen tested (PPD). All other patients had impaired reactivity to a panel of 3–5 antigens (CPC, *New England Journal of Medicine*, 1971; Groll, Valberg, Simon, Eidinger, Wilson and Forsdyke, 1972; Pastor and Geerken, 1975; Barbier, Balasse-Ketelbant, Kennes, Menu, Platteborse and Parmentier, 1975; Haeney and Ross, 1978): *Candida*, mumps, PPD, streptokinase-streptodornase (SK-SD) and trichophyton. In contrast, opinion is divided as to whether or not cutaneous reactivity is restored following treatment. Three patients with negative skin tests converted to positive when the Whipple's disease was treated (CPC, *New England Journal of Medicine*, 1971; Groll, Valberg, Simon, Eidinger, Wilson and Forsdyke, 1972; Pastor and Geerken, 1973), while in 2 others there was no improvement in the depressed (Barbier, Balasse-Ketelbant, Kennes, Menu, Platteborse and Parmentier, 1975) or absent (Haeney and Ross, 1978) responses. The most extensive study of skin reactivity in Whipple's disease is that of Martin, Vilseck, Dobbins, Buckley and Tyor (1972); in their relatively large series of 7 patients with treated disease, both immediate and delayed cutaneous hypersensitivity responses to a total of 23 bacterial, fungal or viral antigens were investigated. Immediate hypersensitivity was depressed in 6 of the 7 patients, while reactivity at 48 hours and 72 hours was significantly impaired compared with control patients and 5 of the 7 subjects were anergic. In summary, of the total of 12 patients reported here, 9 had persistently depressed DH reactions on treatment and this is despite clinical recovery.

Lymphocyte transformation

In-vitro lymphocyte transformation to various mitogens and antigens has been examined both before and during therapy (Table 17.1). The methods employed have not been recorded in some reports, neither has there been a

Table 17.1 Results of immunological investigations in patients with Whipple's disease

Reference	Number of patients studied	Serum immunoglobulins			Before treatment Serum complement	Peripheral lymphocyte count	Skin tests	Lymphocyte Mitogens
		IgG	IgA	IgM				
Sandor and Kozmer (1957)	1	Hypogammaglobulinaemia						
Martel and Hodges (1959)	1	Hypogammaglobulinaemia						
Anton (1961)	1	Hypogammaglobulinaemia						
Maxwell, Ferguson, McKay et al. (1968)	1							
Berens, Cohen and Schwabe (1969)	1	N	N	O				
Debray, Leymarios, Matuchansky et al. (1969)	1		↑					↓
Watson, Maxwell and Ferguson (1969)	2							
Cerf, Hurez, Marche et al. (1970)	4	N (4)	↑↑(3)	N (3)				↓
Douglas, Crabbé and Hobbs (1970)	1	N	↑↑	N				
CPC, New England Journal of Medicine (1971)	1	↓	N	N		↓	−	
Groll, Valberg, Simon et al. (1972)	1	↑	↑↑	↑		↓	−	↓
Martin, Vilseck, Dobbins et al. (1972)	2/7[a]	N	N	N	N			
Cochran, Cook, Gallagher et al. (1973)	1	↓↓	↓↓	↑				
Pastor and Geerken (1973)	1	↓	N	N		↓	−	
Buchholtz, Maintz and Otto (1974)	1	N	N	N	C3↓		+	
Lamberty, Varela, Font et al. (1974)	1	N	↑	↓				
Barbier, Balasse-Ketelbant, Kennes et al. (1975)	1	↓	↑↑	↓			±	↓
Haeney and Ross (1978)	1	N	N	N	N	↓	−	↓

[a] Numbers of patients studied before and after treatment respectively.
N = Normal.
↓ or ↑ = Varying degrees of depression or elevation of the parameters studied.
± = Marginally significant change.
− = No response.
Bracketed figures = Number of patients studied where this is less than the total studied as per column 1.

uniform method of expressing the results. Nevertheless, there is complete agreement that lymphocyte responsiveness to the non-specific stimulant phytohaemagglutinin (PHA) is impaired in untreated patients, compared with control subjects (Debray, Leymarios, Matuchansky, Marche, Hurez and Cerf, 1969; Cerf, Hurez, Marche and Debray, 1970; Groll, Valberg, Simon, Eidinger, Wilson and Forsdyke, 1972; Barbier, Balasse-Ketelbant, Kennes, Menu, Platteborse and Parmentier, 1975; Haeney and Ross, 1978). Since PHA stimulates the majority of T-cells (Ling and Kay, 1975), the results indicate a quantitative or qualitative pre-treatment defect in T-cell function. In the case described by Haeney and Ross (1978) there was also lowered lymphocyte stimulation by pokeweed mitogen (PWM), a plant extract considered to stimulate both T- and B-lymphocytes (Ling and Kay, 1975). Lymphocyte activation by specific antigens had also been impaired in the 3 patients studied (Debray, Leymarios, Matuchansky, Marche, Hurez and Cerf, 1969; CPC, New England Journal of Medicine, 1974; Haeney and Ross, 1978). Following therapy, using PHA as the mitogen, 13 of a total of 15 patients studied have shown depressed responsiveness (Table 17.1) (Maxwell, Ferguson, McKay, Imrie and Watson, 1968; Watson, Maxwell and Ferguson, 1969; Groll, Valberg, Simon, Eidinger, Wilson and Forsdyke, 1972; Martin, Vilseck, Dobbins, Buckley and Tyor, 1972; Barbier, Balasse-Ketelbant, Kennes, Menu, Platteborse and Parmentier, 1975; Haeney and Ross, 1978), and in the 2 subjects with normal responses, no pre-treatment values are available (CPC, New England Journal of Medicine, 1971; Pastor and Geerken, 1973).

transformation	Serum immunoglobulins			Serum complement	*After treatment*		Lymphocyte transformation	
					Peripheral lymphocyte count	Skin tests		
Antigens	IgG	IgA	IgM				Mitogens	Antigens
	N	N	↓		↑		↓	
↓	N	N	N				↓	
↓	N	N	N		N	+	N	N
	N	N	↓		N	±	↓	
	N	N	N		N	−	↓	
	N	N	↑		N	+	N	
	N	N	N					
	N	↑	↓			±	↓	
↓	N	N	N	N	N	−	↓	↓

One patient has shown improved transformation to *Candida* and streptokinase-streptodornase (SK-SD) but not PPD on treatment (CPC, *New England Journal of Medicine*, 1971) while another has shown no improvement to *Candida*, PPD or tetanus toxoid (Haeney and Ross, 1978). In the latter case, there was still no significant improvement in the patient's lymphocyte transformation responsiveness to mitogens/antigens or in cutaneous anergy after 4 months of additional Levamisole therapy.

Allograft rejection

Rejection of tissues transplanted into allogeneic recipients is generally regarded as an example of cell-mediated immunity (Medawar, 1958), and T-cells appear to be primarily responsible for initiating the response. Graft rejection is impaired in animals with selective congenital, acquired or experimental T-cell defects, e.g. nude mice with thymic dysplasia (Pantelouris, 1971). Gross, Valberg, Simon, Eidinger, Wilson and Forsdyke (1972) skin grafted a patient with Whipple's disease. In the pre-treatment phase, there was no sign of rejection for 4 months and then the graft was rejected over the next 3 months, contrasting sharply with the normal median survival time for allogeneic skin grafts of 10–12 days. Following antibiotics, a second graft was placed on the patient. Although this graft was taken from a different donor, the 2 grafts shared histocompatibility antigens. The second graft showed no evidence of rejection for 4 weeks and was then rejected over 10 days. The marked delay in rejection in the pre-treatment phase and the increased (but still abnormal) rejection rate after treatment again suggest that in Whipple's disease there is a defect in T-cell function which is only partially reversible by antibiotics.

Production of migration-inhibition factor

Lymphokines are poorly characterized, soluble, non-antibody products of lymphocyte activation by specific antigens (Ch. 3). One such lymphokine, migration-inhibition factor (MIF) affects the *in-vitro* migration of normal macrophages from capillary tubes. With certain qualifications, this test has been accepted as an *in-vitro* correlate of cellular immunity (David and David, 1972). Barbier, Balasse-Ketelbant, Kennes, Menu, Platteborse and Parmentier (1975) reported a patient with Whipple's disease who, before treatment, had a positive MIF response to *Candida* despite a negative *Candida* skin test. After treatment, inhibition of migration was more marked, but the skin test remained negative. Dissociation of skin reactivity and *in-vitro* lymphocyte function tests is well recognized in other situations (David and David, 1972) and hence is, in itself, unlikely to be of any significance. However, in the case cited, there was more marked inhibition following treatment and this could indicate improved cellular reactivity. One other patient was shown to have absent MIF production to SK-SD, with impaired lymphocyte transformation and cutaneous anergy to that antigen prior to treatment (CPC, *New England Journal of Medicine*, 1971).

CONCLUSION

Any hypothesis regarding the aetiology of Whipple's disease must take into account its rarity, its predilection for male Caucasians, the predominant involvement of the gastrointestinal tract, and the bacilliform particles found in the intestine and other organs. It was Whipple (1907) who first postulated bacterial infestation as the likely cause of intestinal lipodystrophy. Since 1960, organisms, all with the same ultrastructural appearance, have been regularly observed in affected tissues (Maizel, Ruffin and Dobbins, 1970), but no single type has been consistently isolated. Recently, Clancy, Tomkins, Muckle, Richardson and Rawls (1975) reported that a cell-wall-deficient form of an α-haemolytic *Streptococcus* was grown from a prolonged monolayer cell culture of a lymph node taken from a patient with Whipple's disease. Serological cross-reactivity was shown between the organism and the material within Whipple's disease macrophages. *In-vitro* studies characterized the organism as a facultative intracellular parasite that caused the accumulation of PAS-positive material within cells. Parenteral injection of this organism into a rabbit induced a systemic disease characterized by the accumulation of PAS-positive material

within macrophages. These results, if confirmed, strongly suggest that a pathogenic bacterium is one essential aetiological factor in Whipple's disease.

However, the changes in immunological reactivity found in Whipple's disease suggest that host factors are also important. Antibody-dependent mechanisms are unlikely to be relevant as humoral immune responsiveness is only slightly altered and reverts to normal on treatment. This contrasts with the markedly depressed cell-mediated immune reactions which have, in the majority of cases, persisted despite clinically successful therapy, suggesting that the cellular defect is primary. The abnormality appears to be one affecting T-cells; such a defect could predispose to infection by the previously mentioned pathogenic bacterium and could help to explain the sex and racial differences. The additional observation of abundant macrophage infiltration of affected organs also needs to be explained. It may represent either a compensatory or an unmoderated response of intact macrophages.

Cooperation between macrophages and lymphocytes is well recognized and appears to be important both in the induction of immune response (Mosier and Coppelson, 1968) and for optimal effector function against invading microorganisms (North, 1974). Adaptive changes which enable host macrophage populations to express immunity are mediated by a population of immunologically committed lymphocytes produced in response to infection (North, 1974). In Whipple's disease, the postulated T-cell defect could also be accompanied by an inability of the macrophages to digest bacteria and/or process bacterial antigens. In this context, it is a pity that there are no detailed *in-vitro* studies of macrophage function in such patients. A relative failure of lymphocyte effector mechanisms involving T-cells, but not B-cells, could lead to excessive reliance on macrophage phagocytosis. Meltzer (1976) has shown that the peritoneal macrophages of conventionally housed, T-cell-deficient, nude mice were more tumouricidal and more responsive to chemotactic stimuli than macrophages from normal mice and normal litter mates of nude mice. Responses of macrophages from these nude mice were equivalent to responses of macrophages from BCG-infected normal mice. In contrast, macrophages from germ-free nudes were not tumouricidal *in vitro*, suggesting that environmental stimuli induce activation even in the absence of T-cells. The unique macrophage infiltrate seen in Whipple's disease could therefore be the result of a T-cell defect. As the microorganisms persist in spite of the large numbers of macrophages, it suggests that the organisms themselves are more resistant to macrophage inactivation than other bacteria. There is experimental evidence for this hypothesis. Thymectomized, irradiated and bone-marrow-reconstituted mice can develop anti-*Listeria* immunity, due to a residual population of competent T-cells which is large enough to generate that immunity (North, 1974). In contrast, similarly prepared mice fail to develop immunity to systemic infection with *Mycobacterium tuberculosis* (North, 1974). The discrepancy is probably a reflection of the degree of macrophage activation required to destroy each parasite, since it is known that the tubercle bacillus is more resistant to inactivation by macrophages than is *Listeria*. Consequently, the host may need to develop a much higher level of macrophage activation to express antituberculous immunity than to express anti-*Listeria* immunity and this may require the production of a large number of committed T-cells – a number that cannot be realized in T-cell-deficient mice.

Summarizing, in Whipple's disease, the patients have defective T-cell function and appear to be infected with a microorganism, possibly the cell-wall deficient α-haemolytic *Streptococcus* recently proposed by Clancy, Tomkins, Muckle, Richardson and Rawls (1975). Defective production of specifically committed T-cells results in insufficient macrophage activation to eliminate a relatively resistant organism, although there is a compensatory increase in non-specific macrophage accumulation and phagocytosis. It is the latter that results in the characteristic infiltrate which is the hallmark of the disease.

4. TROPICAL SPRUE

Tropical sprue has been defined as a syndrome of intestinal malabsorption of unknown aetiology, occurring in residents of, or visitors to, certain areas of the tropics, and characterized by malabsorption of 2 or more test substances (Klipstein and Baker, 1970; Baker, 1971; Lindenbaum, 1973). The term tropical sprue is thus a diagnosis of exclusion in a patient with documented malabsorption, in whom all other known causes are excluded. While it is probable that tropical sprue, as presently defined, is a syndrome rather than a disease (Lindenbaum, 1973) it is increasingly recognized that the natural history and clinical features of the disease are modified in different population groups by factors such as the duration of residence in the tropics, the adequacy of the available diet, the state of nutrition of the individual, the nature of the small-intestinal flora and possibly by genetic differences (Baker and Mathan, 1971).

CLINICAL FEATURES

A number of recent review articles are available (Klipstein, 1970; Baker, 1971; Wellcome Trust Collaborative Study, 1971; Lindenbaum, 1973). Classically, the patients with tropical sprue present with a history of chronic diarrhoea and evidence of multiple deficiency states, such as glossitis, angular stomatitis, anaemia and hypoproteinaemia. Investigation shows steatorrhoea and malabsorption of folate, vitamin B_{12}, xylose, salt and water, radiological changes and characteristic but non-specific, jejunal morphological abnormalities. However, many patients may present with only one of the complications of malabsorption, such as anaemia, without overt gastrointestinal symptoms. In many areas, investigation of apparently healthy subjects reveals a high prevalence of minor abnormalities of intestinal structure and function (Klipstein, 1970; Schenk, Klipstein and Tomasini, 1972; Lindenbaum, Harmon and Gerson, 1972; Haghighi and Nasr, 1975). There is clearly a whole spectrum of tropical intestinal disease, ranging from the person with fully developed sprue to the asymptomatic patient with mild biopsy changes. Some investigators believe that this spectrum represents differing manifestations of the same disease while others believe that the various subgroups of patients probably represent separate disease entities (Baker and Mathan, 1972). Tropical sprue may be a syndrome with multiple aetiologies, but circumstantial evidence favours a virus as the causative agent (Baker, 1971). In this respect, the recent finding of pleomorphic fringed particles resembling ortho-myxoviruses and corona-viruses in 90 per cent of stools from South Indian children and adults raises the question of whether these particles are causally related to the intestinal abnormalities of the area (Mathan, Mathan, Swaminathan, Yesudoss and Baker, 1975).

IMMUNOLOGICAL FINDINGS IN PATIENTS WITH TROPICAL SPRUE

In marked contrast to Whipple's disease and intestinal lymphangiectasia, tropical sprue can assume epidemic proportions (Baker and Mathan, 1971) and yet no thorough assessments of humoral and cell-mediated immune function are available. The commonly reported features are summarized in Table 17.2.

Lymphoid cell population of the jejunal mucosa
Elevated numbers of intraepithelial (IE) lymphocytes were thought to be present by Klipstein and Falaiye (1969) and by Baker (1971). However, Montgomery and Shearer (1974) quantitated these cells in absolute terms. The range seen in 12 patients with tropical sprue was 20–96 IE lymphocytes per 100 epithelial cells, compared with a range of 7–22 in 20 normal subjects. The 3 highest counts were in subjects with at least a 6-month history of sprue, but in the remainder, there was no relationship between the IE lymphocyte count and the length of history. In the same study, the degree of elevation of IE lymphocyte counts was similar to that found in patients with adult coeliac disease (Montgomery and Shearer, 1974). Although the identification and function of intraepithelial lymphocytes is a subject of con-

Table 17.2. Immunological findings in patients with untreated tropical sprue

Reference	Number of patients	Inter-epithelial lymphocytes	Jejunal mucosa — Lamina propria cells	Jejunal mucosa — Immuno-fluorescence	Serum immunoglobulins — IgG	Serum immunoglobulins — IgA	Serum immunoglobulins — IgM
Jarnum, Jeejeebhoy and Singh (1968)	8				↓ (6) ↑ (1) N (1)	O (2) ↑ (1) N (5)	 ↑ (2) N (6)
Klipstein and Falaiye (1969)	33	↑	Increase in lymphocytes, plasma cells and eosinophils		↓ (20)	↓ (10)	↓ (13)
Maldonado and Sanchez (1969)	65			IgA > > IgM > IgG in 6 patients	↓ (2) ↑ (4) N (59) Group means = normal	O (1) ↑ (5) N (59)	 ↑ 3 N (62)
Brunser, Eidelman and Klipstein (1970)	9		Increased cellularity, plasma cells predominant	IgA > > IgM > IgG	N	N	N
Douglas, Crabbé and Hobbs (1970)	3			Normal density of Ig-bearing cells IgA > > IgM > IgG	↓ (1) N (2)	↓ (1) ↑ (1) N (1)	↓ (1) ↑ (1) N (1)
Samuel, Singh and Jarnum (1970)	28				↓ (1) ↑ (4) N (23)	O (2) ↑ (9) N (17)	↓ (12) ↑ (5) N (11)
Baker (1971)	N.S	↑	Increased numbers of lymphocytes, plasma cells and histiocytes				
Schenk, Klipstein and Tomasini (1972)	51			Normal distribution (14) ↑A ↑G ↑M (7) ↑A ↑G (12) ↑A (10) ↑G (8)			
Haeney, Montgomery and Schneider (1974)	2				↑ (2) N (1)	↑ (1)	N (2)
Montgomery and Shearer (1974)	12	↑↑	Total cells increased. No significant increase in lymphocytes. Plasma cells increase × 3				
Misra, Malhotra, Malaviya and Saha (1976)	25				↑ Group means vs. controls	N	↑

Bracketed figures = Number of patients studied where this is less than the total studied as per column 1.
N = Normal.
0 = Absent.
↓ or ↑ = Varying degrees of depression or elevation of the parameters studied.
N.S. = Not stated.

troversy, recent evidence in T-deprived mice suggests that intraepithelial lymphocytes are effector T-cells and a manifestation of ongoing cell-mediated immunity to intraluminal antigens (Parrott and de Sousa, 1973; Guy-Grand, Griscelli and Vassalli, 1974; Guy-Grand, Griscelli and Vassalli, 1975; Marsh, 1975a, 1975b). The elevated counts in patients with tropical sprue imply that cellular immunity may also be important in this condition.

Subjective analysis of the lamina propria cells has shown increases, with plasma cells and lymphocytes predominating (Klipstein and Falaiye, 1969; Brunser, Eidelman and Klipstein, 1970; Baker, 1971). Montgomery and Shearer (1974) confirmed that there was an absolute increase in total cells in tropical sprue ($16·6 \times 10^3$ cells/mm²) compared with normal controls ($11·0 \times 10^3$ cells/mm²). Plasma cells, but not lymphocytes, were significantly higher in sprue patients ($3·85 \times 10^3$ cells/mm²) than in controls ($1·12 \times 10^3$ cells/mm²). In relation to the duration of disease, with increased chronicity, there was a progressive increase in the plasma cell density. Although lymphocytes were initially increased in varying degrees, they tended to fall with time, especially after 6 months. No significant changes were detected among other cell types in the lamina propria. These findings contrast with those of Rubin and Dobbins (1965), who considered that lymphocytes were more predominant than plasma cells. Montgomery and Shearer (1974) suggest that sprue is a dynamic process and that with evolution of the sprue illness, the initially high lymphocyte population may be replaced by plasma cells, which come to dominate the picture in chronic cases.

Using fluorescein-conjugated antisera to human immunoglobulins, all workers have reported normal proportions of IgA-, IgM- and IgG-staining cells (Maldonado and Sanchez, 1969; Brunser, Eidelman and Klipstein, 1970; Douglas, Crabbé and Hobbs, 1970; Schenk, Klipstein and Tomasini, 1972).

Serum immunoglobulin levels

There has been no clear-cut pattern of immunoglobulin levels in patients with untreated tropical sprue (Table 17.2). In different series, serum IgG has been high (Haeney, Montgomery and Schneider, 1974; Misra, Malhotra, Malaviya and Saha, 1976), normal (Maldonado and Sanchez, 1969; Brunser, Eidelman and Klipstein, 1970; Samuel, Singh and Jarnum, 1970) or low (Jarnum, Jeejeebhoy and Singh, 1968; Klipstein and Falaiye, 1969). Serum IgA has usually been normal (Jarnum, Jeejeebhoy and Singh, 1968; Maldonado and Sanchez, 1969; Brunser, Eidelman and Klipstein, 1970; Samuel, Singh and Jarnum, 1970; Misra, Malhotra, Malaviya and Saha, 1976) with the exception of occasional patients with none (Jarnum, Jeejeebhoy and Singh, 1968; Maldonado and Sanchez, 1969; Samuel, Singh and Jarnum, 1970) or low levels (Klipstein and Falaiye, 1969). While serum IgM has been reported as depressed in 33–43 per cent of patients in some series (Klipstein and Falaiye, 1969; Douglas, Crabbé and Hobbs, 1970), equally there are reports of normal (Jarnum, Jeejeebhoy and Singh, 1968; Maldonado and Sanchez, 1969) or elevated levels (Misra, Malhotra, Malaviya and Saha, 1976).

Other findings

Douglas, Weetman and Haggith (1976), using autologous radio-labelled blood lymphocytes, have shown that 1 patient with tropical sprue had an increased enteric loss of lymphocytes compared with control values. Confirmation of this finding is needed in other patients.

In view of the similarities between tropical sprue and coeliac disease, it is of interest that tropical enteropathy, like coeliac disease, may also predispose to lymphoma formation (Haghighi and Nasr, 1975). Baker and Mathan (1971) document 3 patients who, 5 or more years after the onset of diarrhoea and malabsorption, developed malignant lymphomas of the intestine.

CONCLUSION

The available evidence, both direct and circumstantial, favours an infective agent, probably a virus, in the pathogenesis of tropical sprue. Until the agent(s) can be more positively identified, then immunological studies of tropical sprue will be seriously hampered. The results of serum immunoglobulin levels are unimpressive. However, the increased numbers of plasma cells in the more chronic cases (Montgomery and Shearer, 1974) suggest the involvement of humoral mechanisms in perpetuating the disease. Hence, studies using *in-vitro* culture of intestinal biopsies to evaluate immunoglobulin synthesis could be rewarding.

There has been no investigation of non-specific and specific cell-mediated immunity in tropical sprue. Schwartz (1974) has hypothesized that lymphomas result from impaired immunoregulation of lymphoid tissue. Thus, unchecked proliferation of lymphoid cells in response to persistent antigenic stimulus (e.g. an infectious agent) in patients with inherent defects of suppressor T-cell function may lead to the exuberant growth of B-cells (Schwartz, 1974). The development of malignant lymphomas in tropical sprue could be via this mechanism and suggests that studies of T-cell function should be done. Of major interest are the reports of increased numbers of intraepithelial lymphocytes (putative T-cells) in tropical sprue. Similar observations in coeliac disease have led to the suggestion that the pathogenesis of the mucosal damage is via a cell-mediated reaction to gluten. This mechanism, involving different antigens, may be involved in the aetiology of tropical sprue.

5. INTESTINAL LYMPHANGIECTASIA

Intestinal lymphangiectasia is a disorder of the gastrointestinal tract associated with lymphatic dilatation, loss of lymph into the bowel lumen and a protein-losing enteropathy. The lymphangiectasia, which can be primary or secondary, may be localized to the lamina propria, be generalized (involving lamina propria, submucosa, serosa and mesentery) or affect only the mesentery (Vardy, Lebenthal and Schwachman, 1975). In most cases, the disorder is sporadic and appears to be a congenital (primary) generalized developmental abnormality of central lymphoid channels of unknown aetiology (Waldmann, Stroker and Blaese, 1972). Many patients with intestinal lymphangiectasia have abnormal lymphatics elsewhere in the body which may be clinically apparent or demonstrable by lymphangiography (Pomerantz and Waldmann, 1963). In one series, chylous effusions were present in 45 per cent of patients (Waldmann, Strober and Blaese, 1972). Intestinal lymphangiectasia can also be secondary to other disorders, e.g. constrictive pericarditis or pericardial effusion (Waldmann, Wochner and Strober, 1969), but an association also exists with atrial septal defects (Davidson, Waldmann, Goodman and Gordon, 1961), congenital pulmonary stenosis (Jeejeebhoy, 1962), familial cardiomyopathy (Dölle, Martini and Petersen, 1962) and right heart failure secondary to the carcinoid syndrome (Waldmann, Wochner and Strober, 1969). A significant number of these secondary cases have lymphocytopaenia prior to corrective surgery (Petersen and Ottosen, 1964), suggesting loss of whole lymph into the intestine, while in 2 patients abnormalities of the intestinal lymphatics were demonstrated (Kaihara, Nishimura, Aoyagi, Kameda and Neda, 1963; Petersen and Ottosen, 1964).

One of the fascinating aspects of intestinal lymphangiectasia is the associated immunological deficiency which consists of hypogammaglobulinaemia, lymphocytopaenia, cutaneous anergy, impaired lymphocyte transformation and prolonged allograft survival (Strober, Wochner, Carbone and Waldmann, 1967; Weiden, Blaese, Strober, Block and Waldmann, 1972; Waldmann, Strober and Blaese, 1972; Nelson, Blaese, Strober, Bruce and Waldmann, 1975).

CLINICAL FEATURES

Intestinal lymphangiectasia can present in a variety of ways (Roberts and Douglas, 1976). The major clinical features result from the protein-losing enteropathy, and consist of hypoproteinaemic oedema, pleural effusions and ascites. However, some patients present with infections secondary to the intestinal loss of immunoglobulin and lymphocytes (Strober, Wochner, Carbone and Waldmann, 1967). Gastrointestinal symptoms are usually mild, although intermittent steatorrhoea does occur. Jejunal biopsies and lymphangiography may show dilated central lymphatics and abnormalities of systemic lymphatic vessels respectively (Pomerantz and Waldmann, 1963; Dobbins, 1966; Roberts and Douglas, 1976). Treatment usually consists of a low-fat diet supplemented with medium chain triglycerides (MCT) (Holt, 1964; Ivey, DenBesten, Kent and Clifton, 1969). In the normal intestine, fat increases the flow in the thoracic duct and during fat absorption plasma proteins escape into intestinal lymphatics (Wollin and Jaques, 1973). Beneficial effects of the low-fat, MCT diet are presumably due to a reduction in these events. Other treatments include surgery (Kinmonth and Cox, 1974) and the use of the synthetic plasmin inhibitor, transexamic acid (Kondo, Hosokawa and Masuda, 1975).

ILLUSTRATIVE CASE HISTORY

J.S., a 46-year-old Caucasian female, presented with anorexia, central abdominal pain and the skin lesion of chicken pox. The latter consisted of centripetally distributed crops of non-haemorrhagic vesicles which only remitted after 6 weeks and left severe scarring. Investigations revealed hypoalbuminaemia, a severe protein-losing enteropathy, and mild malabsorption of xylose and fat. Barium studies showed dilatation of the small bowel with thickening of the mucosal folds and sharply defined translucencies due to droplets of secretions. Immunological findings included significant lymphocytopaenia with reduced numbers of T-cells (estimated by E rosettes), and cutaneous anergy to PPD, Candida and trichophyton. Compared to normal controls, there was impairment of in-vitro lymphocyte transformation to phytohaemagglutinin, pokeweed mitogen, PPD and chicken-pox antigens. A varicella complement fixation test was negative. The serum IgG level was reduced, but IgA, IgM and IgE levels were normal. Complement components, C_3 and C_4, were elevated. Although antibodies to Salmonella typhi were initially negative, she became sero-positive following immunization. A diagnostic laparotomy showed a thickened oedematous jejunum with prominent lymphatics and scattered yellow nodules on the serosal and mucosal surface (Fig. 17.5). The dissecting microscope appearance was of chyle-stained leaf-like villi. The characteristic histological appearances of intestinal lymphangiectasia, namely cyst-like, dilated, fat-containing lacteals, were present within the lamina propria and connective tissue core of several villi (Fig. 17.6), but there was no apparent increase in the lymphoid population of the lamina propria.

Following treatment with a low-fat diet (5 g/day), supplemented with medium chain triglycerides (60 g/day), absorption of fat and xylose improved and there was a fall in faecal protein loss with a rise in serum albumin. A peroral jejunal biopsy performed after 3 months' treatment was normal. Nevertheless, hypogammaglobulinaemia, lymphocytopaenia, cutaneous anergy and impaired in-vitro lymphocyte responses remain (Ross, Thompson, Goldsmith and Asquith, 1978).

IMMUNE STATUS IN PATIENTS WITH INTESTINAL LYMPHANGIECTASIA

Lymphoid cells of the intestinal mucosa

A formal quantitative assessment of intraepithelial lymphocytes and lamina propria cells has not been made, but approximately normal numbers of jejunal lymphocytes and plasma cells have been noted in individual cases (McGuigan, Purkerson, Trudeau and Peterson, 1968; Ross, Thompson, Goldsmith and Asquith, 1978). Furthermore, using fluorescein-labelled antisera to

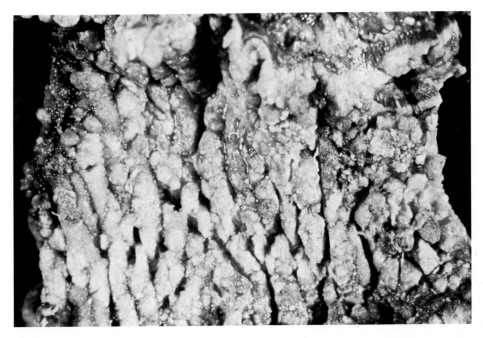

Fig. 17.5 The appearance of abnormal jejunum in intestinal lymphangiectasia exercised at laparotomy, showing a thickened, oedematous mucosa with scattered chyle droplets on the surface of several villi (× 3).

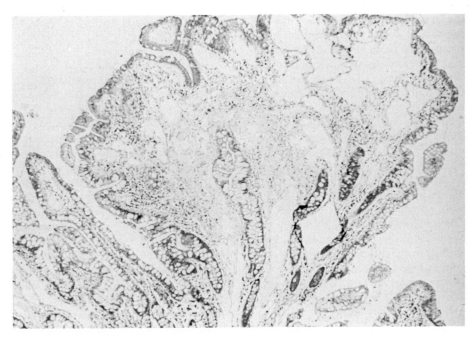

Fig. 17.6 The classical appearance of intestinal lymphangiectasia – cyst-like, dilated lacteals within the lamina propria of the villi (× 90).

human immunoglobulins, normal numbers of cells bearing surface immunoglobulins were found by the same authors. With respect to other studies, in the large series reported by Waldmann, Strober and Blaese (1972), lymphocytes were reduced in the intestinal submucosa and also in peripheral lymph nodes.

Humoral immunity

The more commonly studied parameters of humoral immunity in untreated intestinal lymphangiectasia are summarized in Table 17.3.

Serum immunoglobulins

The majority of reported cases have shown greatly reduced serum IgG concentrations, with a less marked reduction in serum IgA and IgM levels. In one instance, serum and salivary IgA were absent both before and after clinical recovery (Eisner and Bralow, 1968). Normal levels of IgA and IgM (Vardy, Lebanthal and Schwachman, 1975; Ross, Thompson, Goldsmith and Asquith, 1978) and also IgE (Nelson, Blaese, Strober, Bruce and Waldmann, 1975; Ross, Thompson, Goldsmith and Asquith, 1978) have been found in some patients.

Metabolic turnover studies, using purified radio-labelled immunoglobulins, show greatly reduced levels of circulating and total exchangeable immunoglobulins, IgG being more severely affected than IgA and IgM (Strober, Wochner, Carbone and Waldmann, 1967; Waldmann, Strober and Blaese, 1972). Hence, the low serum immunoglobulins are not due to dilution in an increased plasma pool, or to an abnormal distribution among body compartments. In the same studies the synthetic rates of IgG, IgA and IgM were normal or slightly raised. In contrast, the fraction of the intra-vascular pool catabolized per day was increased to 34 per cent for IgG, 59 per cent for IgA and 66 per cent for IgM, compared with normal control values for 7 per cent, 28 per cent and 17 per cent respectively (Strober, Wochner, Carbone and Waldmann, 1967; Waldmann, Strober and Blease, 1972). Thus the commonly reported reductions in the serum concentrations of IgG, IgA and IgM are probably secondary to shortened survival, the proteins most affected being those with the longest half life (Strober, Wochner, Carbone and Waldmann, 1967). This is substantiated by the return of serum IgG levels to normal in some patients following surgical correction of the predisposing lesion (Nelson, Blaese, Strober, Bruce and Waldmann, 1975; Vardy, Lebanthal and Schwachman, 1975), or dietary management (Eisner and Bralow, 1968).

Serum antibody production

Humoral immunity has been further assessed by measuring antibody titres before and after challenge with a variety of antigens. Foshay tularaemia vaccine and the

Vi polysaccharide antigen from *Escherichia coli* were used by Strober, Wochner, Carbone and Waldmann (1967) and Waldmann, Strober and Blaese (1972) because of the unlikelihood of any prior exposure. Specific antibodies were produced although peak titres were not as high as in controls. With the more common antigens, diphtheria toxoid, tetanus toxoid, *Brucella abortus* and pneumococcal polysaccharide I, maximal serum antibody titres were reached at 7 days, the rise in titre ranging from $4 \times$ for tetanus toxoid to $2048 \times$ for pneumococcal polysaccharide I (Nelson, Blaese, Strober, Bruce and Waldmann, 1975). In contrast, Eisner and Bralow (1968) found a poor antibody response to the O and H antigens of *Salmonella typhi* and paratyphi B following immunization, but considered that this might, in part, have been due to variable vaccine potency.

Complement

Pre-treatment complement levels have been infrequently reported. Ross, Thompson, Goldsmith and Asquith (1978) noted elevated C_3 and C_4 levels, in contrast to the normal values of earlier reports (Eisner and Bralow, 1968; Vardy, Lebanthal and Schwachman, 1975).

Cell-mediated immunity

More profound abnormalities have been found in cell-mediated immunity in intestinal lymphangiectasia. The major findings are summarized in Table 17.3.

Peripheral blood lymphocytes

In untreated cases, lymphocytopaenia is a constant feature, and in some series, mean lymphocyte counts are only 30 per cent of normal (Waldmann, Strober and Blaese, 1972). Estimates of the ratio of T- to B-cells (estimated by rosetting techniques and surface immunoglobulins) suggest a preferential depletion of T-lymphocytes and a relative enrichment in the proportion of B-cells (Haywood, 1976; Ross, Thompson, Goldsmith and Asquith, 1978). Douglas, Weetman and Haggith (1976), using ^{51}Cr-labelled autologous peripheral lymphocytes, showed a marked increase in the faecal loss of cells in 5 patients with intestinal lymphangiectasia, and concluded, from indirect evidence, that these were mainly T-cells. This extends a previous report of enteric loss of labelled chylous fluid lymphocytes in this condition (Weiden, Blaese, Strober, Bruce and Waldmann, 1972). Lymphocytopaenia is probably the result of loss of lymphocytes into the gastrointestinal tract from the recirculating lymphoid pool. There is additional support for this hypothesis. Firstly, the protein-losing enteropathies associated with lymphocytopaenia have demonstrable lymphatic abnormalities (Petersen and Hastrup, 1965; Laster, Waldmann, Fenster and Singleton, 1966), whereas the non-lymphocytopaenic forms do not (Hui-

Table 17.3 Immunological findings in untreated intestinal lymphangiectasia

References	Number of patients	Serum immunoglobulin levels				Serum antibody production	Peripheral blood lymphocyte count	Skin tests	DNCB sensitization	Allograft rejection	Lymphocyte transformation by		
		IgG	IgA	IgM	IgE						Mitogens	Antigens	Allogeneic lymphocytes
Strober, Wochner, Carbone and Waldmann (1967)	18	↓↓↓	↓↓	→		+(5)	↓↓	↓↓ (12)	Negative (3)	Absent (4)			
Eisner and Bralow (1968)	1	↓↓↓	0	N		±		Negative			N	↓↓	
McGuigan, Purkerson, Trudeau and Peterson (1968)	1	↓↓↓	↓↓	→		+	↓↓	Negative			N	N	
Waldmann, Strober and Blaese (1972)	25	↓↓↓	↓↓	→		+	↓↓	↓↓ (21)	Negative (10)	Absent (4)	↓↓ (12)	↓↓ (12)	↓↓ (12)
Weiden, Blaese, Strober, Block and Waldmann (1972)	12										↓↓	↓↓	↓↓
Nelson, Blaese, Strober, Bruce and Waldmann (1975)	1	↓↓↓	→	→	N	+	↓↓	Negative	Negative	Absent	↓↓	↓↓	
Vardy, Lebanthal and Schwachman (1975)	15	↓ (4)	N (4)	N or ↓ (4)			→						
Roberts and Douglas (1976)	5	Low N	N	N			→						
Ross, Thompson, Goldsmith and Asquith (1978)	1	↓↓	N	N	N	+	↓↓	Negative			↓↓	↓↓	

Bracketed figures refer to the number of patients studied where this is less than the total studied as per column 1.
N = Normal.
0 = Absent.
↓ or ↑ = Varying degrees of depression or elevation of the parameters studied.

zenga, Wollaeger and Green, 1961; Waldmann, Wochner, Laster and Gordon, 1967). Secondly, in lymphocytopaenic patients, reversal of the protein loss may be associated with reversal of the lymphocytopaenia (Davidson, Waldmann, Goodman and Gordon, 1961; Laster, Waldmann, Fenster and Singleton, 1966; Nelson, Blaese, Strober, Bruce and Waldmann, 1975; Vardy, Lebanthal and Schwachman, 1975). Thirdly, lymphatic fluid containing radio-opaque contrast media, when injected into the foot, has been shown to leak directly into the gastrointestinal tract (Mistilis, Skyring and Stephen, 1965).

Skin tests

(a) *Intradermal*. Cutaneous anergy is present in the majority of subjects studied. Using PPD, mumps, trichophyton and *Candida*, Strober, Wochner, Carbone and Waldmann (1967) found only 17 per cent of their patients reacted to one or more of the antigens, compared with 91 per cent of normal individuals. Extending the studies to a larger series (21 patients) only 2 had a positive delayed skin reaction to any of 7 antigens studied (the 4 already mentioned plus streptokinase-streptodornase, tetanus and diphtheria), while over 97 per cent of normal individuals had positive responses (Waldmann, Strober and Blaese, 1972). Other reports based on individual cases have confirmed these findings (Eisner and Bralow, 1968; McGuigan, Purkerson, Trudeau and Peterson, 1968; Ross, Thompson, Goldsmith and Asquith, 1978). Intradermal skin reactivity following treatment is not so clear-cut, conversion being reported in some cases (Nelson, Blaese, Strober, Bruce and Waldmann, 1975) but not others (Ross, Thompson, Goldsmith and Asquith, 1978).

(b) *Contact sensitization*. Cell-mediated immunity can be assessed by the ability to become sensitized to a group of substituted nitrobenzenes, of which 2,4-dinitrochlorobenzene (DNCB) and 2,4-dinitrofluorobenzene (DNFB) are the most commonly used. Contact sensitization with these compounds depends on their conjugation with skin proteins through covalent bonds (Landsteiner, 1945) and the response to a 2nd (challenge) dose is mediated by T-cells. None of the 10 patients with intestinal lymphangiectasia tested by Waldmann, Strober and Blaese (1972) could be sensitized to DNCB, in contrast to over 95 per cent of the controls. This was confirmed in 4 other untreated cases (Strober, Wochner, Carbone and Waldmann, 1967; Nelson, Blaese, Strober, Bruce and Waldmann, 1975). There are no similar studies of patients during clinical remission.

Allograft survival

Cellular hypersensitivity has been evaluated in a small number of patients by skin transplantation studies (Table 17.3). Skin grafts consisting of a full-thickness 8-mm punch biopsy were transplanted to 4 patients and in all cases the allografts showed no rejection during 2 years of observation. In 2 cases, 2nd grafts from the same donor showed no evidence of rejection over a further period of 1 year (Strober, Wochner, Carbone and Waldmann, 1967; Waldmann, Strober and Blaese, 1972). In 1 patient with intestinal lymphangiectasia secondary to constrictive pericarditis, a skin graft accepted pre-operatively was slowly rejected 4 months after pericardiectomy (Nelson, Blaese, Strober, Bruce and Waldmann, 1975).

Lymphocyte transformation

The already mentioned cutaneous anergy, absent DNCB sensitization and prolonged allograft survival could be the result of reduced numbers of circulating lymphocytes secondary to their enteric loss. However, using *in-vitro* lymphocyte transformation responses to mitogens, antigens and allogeneic lymphocytes, Weiden, Blaese, Strober, Block and Waldmann (1972) showed that the peripheral blood lymphocytes from 12 patients were also qualitatively abnormal. Using equal numbers of lymphocytes from patients and controls, transformation responses to the non-specific mitogens phytohaemagglutinin (PHA), pokeweed mitogen (PWM) and staphylococcal filtrate (SF) were less than 60 per cent of normal. In the presence of the specific antigens streptolysin O, streptokinase-streptodornase, diphtheria toxoid, tetanus toxoid, *Candida albicans* and vaccinia, in only 2 out of 46 determinations of lymphocyte transformation were the results in patients equal to controls, while 32 of the 46 determinations were less than 25 per cent of normal values (Weiden, Blaese, Strober, Block and Waldmann, 1972). These results are similar to those obtained in some other studies (Nelson, Blaese, Strober, Bruce and Waldmann, 1975; Ross, Thompson, Goldsmith and Asquith, 1978), but not in all (Eisner and Bralow, 1968; McGuigan, Purkerson, Trudeau and Peterson, 1968). It is noteworthy that patients with the most deficient *in-vitro* lymphocyte reactivity tend to have the lowest absolute lymphocyte counts, lowest serum albumin concentrations and the highest rates of intestinal protein loss (Weiden, Blaese, Strober, Block and Waldmann, 1972). Following treatment, a gradual return to normal of lymphocyte responsiveness occurs over a period of 6 to 18 months (Nelson, Blaese, Strober, Bruce and Waldmann, 1975). Mean lymphocyte reactivity to allogeneic lymphocytes in a one-way mixed lymphocyte reaction was 27 per cent of control values, and no individual response exceeded 73 per cent of the corresponding control result (Weiden, Blaese, Strober, Block and Waldmann, 1972).

In contrast to the impaired responses of peripheral blood lymphocytes, chylous fluid lymphocytes obtained from 5 patients were more responsive ($3 \times -100 \times$) than corresponding peripheral lymphocytes, and frequently approached or exceeded the degree of stimulation seen in blood lymphocytes from control individuals (Weiden, Blaese, Strober, Block and Waldmann, 1972; Nelson, Blaese, Strober, Bruce and Waldmann, 1975). Thus, patients with untreated intestinal lymphangiectasia have lymphocytes capable of responding normally to stimuli, but in the peripheral blood these responder cells are relatively depleted.

Susceptibility to infection

The increased susceptibility to infections found in patients with impaired immune responsiveness is well documented (Soothill, 1975). In one series of intestinal lymphangiectasia (Strober, Wochner, Carbone and Waldmann, 1967) 2 out of 6 children died, 1 having furunculosis, cellulitis of the abdominal wall and terminal peritonitis, while the other had recurrent episodes of furunculosis, pneumonia, otitis media and urinary tract infection. The remaining 4 patients had no apparent increase in infection. In the same report, of 12 adults, 2 had recurrent respiratory tract infections. Recently, Ross, Thompson, Goldsmith and Asquith (1978) have described a patient who presented with a severe varicella zoster infection (see Case History) and in whom the immunological deficit was only partially improved by dietary therapy.

Risk of malignancy

In view of the changes in immunological reactivity, it is interesting that 3 of the 50 patients known to one group of workers have developed malignancies approximately 3 to 25 years after the initial clinical manifestation of intestinal lymphangiectasia (Waldmann, Strober and Blaese, 1972). One patient developed a reticulum cell sarcoma of the stomach, while 2 patients developed lymphoma, 1 affecting the small intestine, the other initially affecting the breast but with ultimate widespread involvement. Although the numbers are small, the type of malignancy is similar to that seen in patients with congenital immunodeficiency states and in drug-immunosuppressed recipients of organ grafts (Schwartz, 1974).

CONCLUSION

In general, immunodeficiency states may result from decreased synthesis of immunocompetent cells and their products, or from increased catabolism of these immune effectors. Intestinal lymphangiectasia is an example of a hypercatabolic immunodeficiency syndrome resulting from increased exogenous catabolism of immune effectors. The reduced serum immunoglobulin levels

are due to their loss into the gastrointestinal tract, proteins with the longest half life being maximally affected (Strober, Wochner, Carbone and Waldmann, 1967). Humoral immunity is less abnormal than cellular immune mechanisms. Changes in the latter are due to a quantitative reduction in the absolute lymphocyte count following increased enteric loss of lymphocytes (Douglas, Weetman and Haggith, 1976) and to a probable preferential loss of T-cells (Weiden, Blaese, Strober, Block and Waldmann, 1972; Nelson, Blaese, Strober, Bruce and Waldmann, 1975; Douglas, Weetman and Haggith, 1976). Thoracic duct lymph contains several distinct lymphocyte subpopulations. In experimental animals, the majority of duct lymphocytes belong to a pool of thymus-dependent, long-lived cells which recirculate from peripheral blood to lymph via specialized post-capillary venules within peripheral lymphoid tissue (Gowans, 1959; Howard, Hunt and Gowans, 1972). Loss of lymphocytes normally present in thoracic duct lymph would be expected to result in deficiencies of immune function subserved by these cells. Weiden, Blaese, Strober, Block and Waldmann (1972) have made calculations to show the effect of continued losses of lymphocytes on the number of long-lived lymphocytes in the peripheral blood. With a 20 per cent daily loss of lymphocytes from a population initially composed of 80 per cent long-lived cells (half life, 1×10^3 days) and 20 per cent short-lived cells, the ratio would fall from $4:1$ to $1:21$, representing a reduction from 80 per cent to less than 5 per cent of the total lymphocyte pool. Prolonged external thoracic duct drainage in animals and in man results in (1) peripheral blood lymphocytopaenia (Tunner, Carbone, Blaylock and Irvin, 1965; Searcy and Fish, 1970; Tilney, Atkinson and Murray, 1970; Fitts, Majeski, Sharbaugh, Hargest, Graber and Hennigar, 1972; Yu, Peter and Stratton, 1972), (2) depletion of lymphocytes in thymus-dependent areas of peripheral lymphoid tissues (Searcy and Fish, 1970; Fitts, Majeski, Sharbaugh, Hargest, Graber and Hennigar, 1972), (3) cutaneous anergy (Tunner, Carbone, Blaylock and Irvin, 1965; Searcy and Fish, 1970), (4) prolonged allograft survival (McGregor and Gowans, 1964; Tunner, Carbone, Blaylock and Irvin, 1965; Tilney, Atkinson and Murray, 1970) and (5) diminished *in-vitro* proliferative responses of peripheral blood lymphocytes to phytohaemagglutinin (Iversen, 1969; Yu, Peter and Stratton, 1973). Thus, in terms of cell-mediated immunity, intestinal lymphangiectasia appears to be the clinical analogue of animals subjected to prolonged external thoracic duct drainage; the lymphocyte subpopulation which is most affected consists largely of thymus-dependent long-lived cells.

REFERENCES

American Journal of Medicine (1974) Clinico-Pathologic Conference. Infiltrative gastrointestinal disease. *American Journal of Medicine*, 57, 127–134.

Anton, A. T. (1961) Agammaglobulinaemia complicating Whipple's disease – case report. *Ohio State Medical Journal*, 57, 650–652.

Asquith, P. (1974) In *Coeliac Disease, Clinics in Gastroenterology*, ed. Cooke, W. T. & Asquith, P., Vol. 3, No. 1, pp. 213–234, London: W. B. Saunders.

Axelsson, U. & Hällén, J. (1972) A population study on monoclonal gammopathy. *Acta Medica Scandinavica*, 191, 111–113.

Babb, R. R., Alarcón-Segovia, D., Diessner, G. R. & McPherson, J. R. (1967) Malabsorption in rheumatoid arthritis. An unusual complication caused by amyloidosis. *Arthritis and Rheumatism*, 10, 63–70.

Baker, S. J. (1971) Tropical sprue. *British Medical Bulletin*, 28, 87–91.

Baker, S. J. & Mathan, V. I. (1971) Tropical sprue in Southern India. In *Tropical Sprue and Megaloblastic Anaemia (Wellcome Trust Collaborative Study)*, Ch. 8, pp. 198–260. Edinburgh: Churchill Livingstone.

Barbier, P., Balasse-Ketelbant, P., Kennes, B., Menu, R., Platteborse, R. & Parmentier, R. (1975) Whipple's disease. An immunologic and electronmicroscopy study. *Archives Françaises des Maladies de l'Appareil Digestif*, 64, 659–666.

Beddow, R. M. & Tilden, I. L. (1960) Malabsorption syndrome due to amyloidosis of the intestine secondary to lepromatous leprosy: report of a case. *Annals of Internal Medicine*, 53, 1017–1027.

Benditt, E. P., Eriksen, N., Hermodson, M. A. & Ericsson, L. H. (1971) The major proteins of human and monkey amyloid substance: common properties, including unusual N-terminal amino-acid sequences. *Febs Letters*, 19, 169.

Bennhold, H. (1922) Quoted by Hobbs, J. R. (1973), in: An ABC of amyloid. *Proceedings of the Royal Society of Medicine*, 66, 705–710.

Berens, S. C., Cohen, R. A. & Schwabe, A. D. (1969) Diagnostic problems of a partially treated Whipple's disease. Report of a case of isolated deficiency of IgM. *California Medicine*, 110, 477–481.

Bernstein, J. S., & Dixon, D. D. (1964) Ulcerative colitis disguised as multiple myeloma. *American Journal of Digestive Diseases*, 9, 625–633.

Biniaminov, M. & Ramot, B. (1975) *In vitro* restoration by Levamisole of thymus-derived lymphocyte function in Hodgkin's disease. *Lancet*, i, 464.

Blum, A. & Sohar, E. (1962) The diagnosis of amyloidosis: ancillary procedures. *Lancet*, i, 721–724.

Brody, I. A., Wertlake, P. T. & Laster, L. (1964) Causes of intestinal symptoms in primary amyloidosis. *Archives of Internal Medicine*, 113, 512–518.

Brom, B., Bank, S., Marks, I. N., Milner, G. & Baker, P. (1969) Ischaemic colitis, gastric ulceration and malabsorption in a case of primary amyloidosis. *Gastroenterology*, 57, 319–323.

Brunser, O., Eidelman, S. & Klipstein, F. A. (1970) Intestinal morphology of rural Haitians: a comparison between overt tropical sprue and asymptomatic individuals. *Gastroenterology*, 58, 655–668.

Buchholz, K., Maintz, J. & Otto, H. F. (1974) Clinical-immunological and electron microscopic findings in Whipple's disease. *Klinische Wochenschrift*, 52, 672–677.

Casad, D. E. & Bocian, J. J. (1965). Primary systemic amyloidosis simulating acute idiopathic ulcerative colitis. *American Journal of Digestive Diseases*, 10, 63–74.

Cerf, M., Hurez, D., Marche, C. & Debray, C. (1970) The plasma cells of the small intestine in Whipple's disease. *La Presse Médicale*, 78, 2127–2130.

Cherenkoff, R. M., Costopoulos, L. B. & Bain, G. O. (1972) Gastrointestinal manifestations of primary amyloidosis. *Canadian Medical Association Journal*, 106, 567–569.

Clancy, R. L., Tomkins, W. A. F., Muckle, T. J., Richardson, H. & Rawls, W. E. (1975) Isolation and characterization of an aetiological agent in Whipple's disease. *British Medical Journal*, iii, 568–570.

Cochran, M., Cook, M. G., Gallagher, J. C. & Peacock, M. (1973) Hypogammaglobulinaemia with Whipple's disease. *Postgraduate Medical Journal*, 49, 355–358.

Cohen, A. S. (1967) Amyloidosis. *New England Journal of Medicine*, 277, 522–530, 574–583, 628–638.

Cohen, A. S. & Calkins, E. (1959) Electron microscopic observations on a fibrous component in amyloid of diverse origins. *Nature*, 183, 1202–1203.

Cooke, K. B. (1969) Essential paraproteinaemia. *Proceedings of the Royal Society of Medicine*, 62, 777–778.

Cornes, J. S., Smith, J. C. & Southwood, W. F. (1961) Lymphosarcoma in chronic ulcerative colitis with report of 2 cases. *British Journal of Surgery*, 49, 50–53.

Dahlin, D. C. (1949) Secondary amyloidosis. *Annals of Internal Medicine*, 31, 105–119.

David, J. R. & David, R. A. (1972) Cellular hypersensitivity and immunity. Inhibition of macrophage migration and the lymphocyte mediators. *Progress in Allergy*, 16, 300–449.

Davidson, J. D., Waldmann, T. A., Goodman, D. S. & Gordon, R. S. (1961) Protein-losing gastroenteropathy in congestive heart-failure. *Lancet*, i, 899–902.

Debray, C., Leymarios, J., Matuchansky, C., Marche, C., Hurez, D. & Cerf, M. (1969) Aspects immunologiques dans la maladie de Whipple. *Archives Françaises des Maladies de l'Appareil Digestif*, 58, 584–585.

Dobbins, W. O., III (1966) Electron microscopic study of the intestinal mucosa in intestinal lymphangiectasia. *Gastroenterology*, 51, 1004–1017.

Dobbins, W. O., III & Ruffin, J. M. (1967) A light- and electron-microscopic study of bacterial invasion in Whipple's disease. *American Journal of Pathology*, 51, 225–242.

Dölle, W., Martini, G. A. & Petersen, F. (1962) Idiopathic familial cardiomegaly with intermittent loss of protein into the gastro-intestinal tract. *German Medical Monthly*, 7, 300–306.

Douglas, A. P., Crabbé, P. A. & Hobbs, J. R. (1970). Immunochemical studies of the serum, intestinal secretions and intestinal mucosa in patients with adult coeliac disease and other forms of the coeliac syndrome. *Gastroenterology*, 59, 414–425.

Douglas, A. P., Weetman, A. P. & Haggith, J. W. (1976) The distribution and enteric loss of 51 Cr-labelled lymphocytes in normal subjects and in patients with coeliac disease and other disorders of the small intestine. *Digestion*, 14, 29–43.

Eanes, E. D. & Glenner, G. G. (1968) X-ray diffraction studies of amyloid filaments. *Journal of Histochemistry and Cytochemistry*, 16, 673–677.

Eisner, J. W. & Bralow, S. P. (1968) Intestinal lymphangiectasia with immunoglobulin A deficiency. *American Journal of Digestive Diseases*, 13, 1055–1064.

Fadem, R. S. (1952) Differentiation of plasmacytic responses from myelomatous diseases on the basis of bone marrow findings. *Cancer*, 5, 128–137.

Ferguson, A. (1972) Immunological roles of the gastrointestinal tract. *Scottish Medical Journal*, 17, 111–118.

Ferguson, A. (1976) Celiac disease and gastrointestinal food allergy. In *Immunological Aspects of the Liver and Gastrointestinal Tract*, ed. Ferguson, A. & MacSween, R. N. M. Ch. 5, pp. 153–202. Lancaster: MTP Press.

Fitts, C. T., Majeski, J. A., Sharbaugh, R. J., Hargest, T. S., Graber, C. D. & Hennigar, G. R. (1972) Immunosuppression by thoracic duct filtration. *Transplantation*, 14, 236–238.

Franklin, E. C. & Zucker-Franklin, D. (1972) Antisera specific for human amyloid reactive with conformational antigens. *Proceedings of the Society for Experimental Biology and Medicine*, 140, 565–572.

Galton, D. A. G. & Peto, R. (1968) A progress report on the Medical Research Council's therapeutic trial in myelomatosis. *British Journal of Haematology*, 15, 319–320.

Gilat, T. & Spirö, H. M. (1968) Amyloidosis and the gut. *American Journal of Digestive Diseases*, 13, 619–633.

Gilat, T., Revach, M. & Sohar, E. (1969) Deposition of amyloid in the gastrointestinal tract. *Gut*, 10, 98–104.

Glenner, G. G., Terry, W. D. & Isersky, C. (1973) Amyloidosis: its nature and pathogenesis. *Seminars in Haematology*, 10, 65–86.

Golden, A. (1945) Primary systemic amyloidosis of the alimentary tract. *Archives of Internal Medicine*, 75, 413–416.

Goldstein, W. B. & Poker, N. (1966) Multiple myeloma involving the gastrointestinal tract. *Gastroenterology*, 51, 87–93.

Gowans, J. L. (1958) The recirculation of lymphocytes from blood to lymph in the rat. *Journal of Physiology*, 146, 54–69.

Green, P. A., Higgins, J. A., Brown, A. L., Hoffman, H. N. & Somerville, R. L. (1961) Amyloidosis: appraisal of intubation biopsy of the small intestine in diagnosis. *Gastroenterology*, 41, 452–456.

Groll, A., Valberg, L. S., Simon, J. B., Eidinger, D., Wilson, B. & Forsdyke, D. R. (1972) Immunological deficit in Whipple's disease. *Gastroenterology*, 63, 943–950.

Guy-Grand, D., Griscelli, C. & Vassalli, P. (1974) The gut-associated lymphoid system: nature and properties of the large dividing cells. *European Journal of Immunology*, 4, 435–443.

Guy-Grand, D., Griscelli, C. & Vassalli, P. (1975) Peyer's patches, gut IgA plasma cells and thymic function: study in nude mice bearing thymic grafts. *The Journal of Immunology*, 115, 361–364.

Haeney, M. R. & Ross, I. N. (1978) Whipple's disease in a female, with impaired cell-mediated immunity unresponsive to co-trimoxazole and levamisole therapy. *Postgraduate Medical Journal*, 54, 45–50.

Haeney, M. R., Montgomery, R. D. & Schneider, R. (1974) Sprue in the Middle East: five case reports. *Gut*, 15, 377–386.

Haeney, M. R., Ross, I. N., Thompson, R. A. & Asquith, P. (1977) IgG myeloma presenting as ulcerative colitis. *Journal of Clinical Pathology*, 30, 862–867.

Haghighi, P. & Nasr, K. (1975) Tropical sprue: subclinical and idiopathic enteropathy. *Pathology Annual*, 10, 177–203.

Hayes, D. W., Bennett, W. A. & Heck, F. J. (1952)

Extramedullary lesions in multiple myeloma. *Archives of Pathology*, 53, 262–272.

Hayward, A. R. (1976) Quoted in: The distribution and enteric loss of 51 Cr-labelled lymphocytes in normal subjects and in patients with coeliac disease and other disorders of the small intestine. *Digestion*, 14, 29–43.

Hecker, R. & Reid, R. T. W. (1962) Cerebral demyeleination in Whipple's disease. *Medical Journal of Australia*, 1, 211–212.

Heller, H., Missmahl, H. P., Sohar, E. & Gafni, J. (1964) Amyloidosis: its differentiation into peri-reticulin and peri-collagen types. *Journal of Pathology and Bacteriology*, 88, 15–34.

Herskovic, T., Bartholomew, L. G. & Green, P. A. (1964) Amyloidosis and malabsorption syndrome. *Archives of Internal Medicine*, 114, 629–633.

Holt, P. R. (1964) Dietary treatment of protein loss in intestinal lymphangiectasia. The effect of eliminating dietary long chain triglycerides on albumin metabolism in this condition. *Pediatrics*, 34, 629–635.

Howard, J. C., Hunt, S. V. & Gowans, J. L. (1972) Identification of marrow-derived and thymus-derived small lymphocytes in the lymphoid tissue and thoracic duct lymph of normal rats. *Journal of Experimental Medicine*, 135, 200–219.

Huizenga, K. A., Wollaeger, E. E., Green, P. A. & McKenzie, B. F. (1961) Serum globulin deficiencies in non-tropical sprue, with report of two cases of acquired agammaglobulinaemia. *American Journal of Medicine*, 31, 572–580.

Husby, G. & Natvig, J. B. (1974) A serum component related to nonimmunoglobulin amyloid protein AS, a possible precursor of the fibrils. *The Journal of Clinical Investigation*, 53, 1054–1061.

Husby, G., Natvig, J. B. & Sletten, K. (1974) New, third class of amyloid fibril protein. *The Journal of Experimental Medicine*, 139, 773–778.

Husby, G., Sletten, K., Michaelsen, T. E. & Natvig, J. B. (1973) Amyloid fibril protein subunit, 'Protein AS': distribution in tissue and serum in different clinical types of amyloidosis including that associated with myelomatosis and Waldenström's macroglobulinaemia. *Scandinavian Journal of Immunology*, 2, 395–404.

Intriere, A. D. & Brown, C. H. (1956) Primary amyloidosis: report of a case of gastric involvement only. *Gastroenterology*, 30, 833–838.

Isobe, T. & Osserman, E. F. (1974) Patterns of amyloidosis and their association with plasma-cell dyscrasia, monoclonal immunoglobulins and Bence-Jones proteins. *New England Journal of Medicine*, 290, 473–477.

Iversen, J. G. (1969) Phytohaemagglutinin response of recirculating and non-recirculating rat lymphocytes. *Experimental Cell Research*, 56, 219–223.

Ivey, K., DenBesten, L., Kent, T. H. & Clifton, J. A. (1969) Lymphangiectasia of the colon with protein loss and malabsorption. *Gastroenterology*, 57, 709–714.

Jarnum, S. (1965) Gastrointestinal haemorrhage and protein loss in primary amyloidosis. *Gut*, 6, 14–18.

Jarnum, S., Jeejeebhoy, K. N. & Singh, B. (1968) Dysgammaglobulinaemia in tropical sprue. *British Medical Journal*, iv, 416–417.

Jeejeebhoy, K. N. (1962) Cause of hypoalbuminaemia in patients with gastrointestinal and cardiac disease. *Lancet*, i, 343–348.

Kaihara, S., Nishimura, H., Aoyagi, T., Kameda, H. & Neda, T. (1963) Protein-losing gastroenteropathy as cause of hypoproteinaemia in constrictive pericarditis. *Japanese Heart Journal*, **4**, 386–394

Katz, A. & Pruzanski, W. (1976) Newer concepts in amyloidogenesis. *Canadian Medical Association Journal*, **114**, 872–873.

Kinmonth, J. B. & Cox, S. J. (1974) Protein-losing enteropathy in primary lymphoedema: mesenteric lymphography and gut resection. *British Journal of Surgery*, **61**, 589–593.

Klipstein, F. A. (1970) Recent advances in tropical malabsorption. *Scandinavian Journal of Gastroenterology*, **6**, 93–114.

Klipstein, F. A. & Baker, S. J. (1970) Regarding the definition of tropical sprue. *Gastroenterology*, **58**, 717–721.

Klipstein, F. A. & Falaiye, J. M. (1969) Tropical sprue in expatriates from the tropics living in the continental United States. *Medicine (Baltimore)*, **48**, 475–491.

Kondo, M., Hosokawa, K. & Masuda, M. (1975) Treatment of protein-losing gastroenteropathy. *British Medical Journal*, **ii**, 40.

Lamberty, J., Varela, P. Y., Font, R. G., Jarvis, B. W. & Coover, J. (1974) Whipple disease: light and electron microscopy study. *Archives of Pathology*, **98**, 325–330.

Lancet Editorial (1975) Levamisole. *Lancet*, **i**, 151–152.

Landsteiner, K. (1945) *The Specificity of Serological Reactions*. Cambridge, Mass.: Harvard University Press.

Laster, L., Waldmann, T. A., Fenster, L. F. & Singleton, J. W. (1966) Albumin metabolism in patients with Whipple's disease. *Journal of Clinical Investigation*, **45**, 637–644.

Legge, D. A., Wollaeger, E. E. & Carlson, H. C. (1970) Intestinal pseudo-obstruction in systemic amyloidosis. *Gut*, **11**, 764–767.

Lindenbaum, J. (1973) Tropical enteropathy. *Gastroenterology*, **64**, 637–652.

Lindenbaum, J., Harman, J. W. & Gerson, C. D. (1972) Subclinical malabsorption in developing countries. *American Journal of Clinical Nutrition*, **25**, 1056–1061.

Ling, N. R. & Kay, J. E. (1975) *Lymphocyte Stimulation*, 2nd ed. Amsterdam: North Holland Publishing.

Lundberg, G. D. & Linder, W. R. (1963) Whipple's disease with associated splenomegaly and pancytopenia. *Archives of Internal Medicine*, **112**, 207–211.

McGregor, D. D. & Gowans, J. L. (1964) Survival of homografts of skin in rats depleted of lymphocytes by chronic drainage from the thoracic duct. *Lancet*, **i**, 629–632.

McGuigan, J. E., Purkerson, M. L., Trudeau, W. L. & Peterson, M. L. (1968) Studies of the immunologic defects associated with intestinal lymphangiectasia with some observations on dietary control of chylous ascites. *Annals of Internal Medicine*, **68**, 398–404.

Maizel, H., Ruffin, J. M. & Dobbins, W. O., III (1970) Whipple's disease: a review of 19 patients from one hospital and a review of the literature since 1950. *Medicine (Baltimore)*, **49**, 175–205.

Maldonado, N. & Sanchez, N. J. (1969) Immunologic studies in tropical sprue. *American Journal of Gastroenterology*, **52**, 141–149.

Mallory, A., Struthers, J. E. & Kern, F. (1975) Persistent hypotension and intestinal infarction in a patient with primary amyloidosis. *Gastroenterology*, **68**, 1587–1592.

Marano, R., Dammacco, F., Pastore, G. & Schiraldi, O. (1970) A case of IgAL-myelomatosis involving the intestinal tract. *Digestion*, **3**, 294–302.

Marsh, M. N. (1975a) Studies of intestinal lymphoid tissue. I. Electron microscopic evidence of 'blast transformation'

in epithelial lymphocytes of mouse small intestinal mucosa. *Gut*, **16**, 665–674.

Marsh, M. N. (1975b) Studies of intestinal lymphoid tissue. II. Aspects of proliferation and migration of epithelial lymphocytes in the small intestine of mice. *Gut*, **16**, 674–682.

Martel, W. & Hodges, F. J. (1959) The small intestine in Whipple's disease. *American Journal of Roentgenology and Radium Therapy*, **81**, 623–636.

Martin, F. F., Vilseck, J., Dobbins, W. O., III, Buckley, C. E. & Tyor, M. P. (1972) Immunological alterations in patients with treated Whipple's disease. *Gastroenterology*, **63**, 6–18.

Mathan, M., Mathan, V. I., Swaminathan, S. P., Yesudoss, S. & Baker, S. J. (1975) Pleomorphic virus-like particles in human faeces. *Lancet*, **i**, 1068–1069.

Maxwell, J. D., Ferguson, A., McKay, A. M., Imrie, J. C. & Watson, W. C. (1968) Lymphocytes in Whipple's disease. *Lancet*, **i**, 887–889.

Medawar, P. B. (1958) The homograft reaction. *Proceedings of the Royal Society of London*, **149**, 145–166.

Medical Research Council (1971) Myelomatosis: comparison of melphelan and cyclophosphamide therapy. *British Medical Journal*, **i**, 640–641.

Medical Research Council (1973) Report of the first myelomatosis trial. Part I. Analysis of presenting features of prognostic importance. *British Journal of Haematology*, **24**, 123–139.

Meltzer, M. S. (1976) Tumoricidal responses *in vitro* of peritoneal macrophages from conventionally housed and germ-free nude mice. *Cellular Immunology*, **22**, 176–181.

Michaux, J. L. & Heremans, J. F. (1969) Thirty cases of monoclonal immunoglobulin disorders other than myeloma or macroglobulinaemia. *American Journal of Medicine*, **46**, 562–579.

Miksche, L. W., Blümke, S., Fritsche, D., Küchemann, K., Schüler, H. W. & Grözinger, K. H. (1974) Whipple's disease: etiopathogenesis, treatment, diagnosis and clinical course. Case report and review of the world literature. *Acta Hepato Gastroenterologica*, **21**, 307–326.

Misra, R. C., Malhotra, S. K., Malaviya, A. N. & Saha, K. (1976) Serum immunoglobulins in tropical sprue. *Indian Journal of Medical Research*, **64**, 211–217.

Missmahl, H. P. (1957) Quoted by Hobbs, J. R. (1973), in: An ABC of Amyloid. *Proceedings of the Royal Society of Medicine*, **66**, 705–710.

Missmahl, H. P. (1969) Amyloidosis. In *Textbook of Immunopathology*, ed. Miescher, P. A. & Müller-Eberhard, H. J. Vol. II, pp. 421–434. New York: Grune and Stratton.

Mistilis, S. P., Skyring, A. P. & Stephen, D. D. (1965) Intestinal lymphangiectasia. Mechanism of enteric loss of plasma-protein and fat. *Lancet*, **i**, 77–80.

Montgomery, R. D. & Shearer, A. C. I. (1974) The cell population of the upper jejunal mucosa in tropical sprue and postinfective malaborption. *Gut*, **15**, 387–391.

Mosier, D. E. & Coppelson, L. W. (1968) A three-cell interaction required for the induction of the primary immune response in vitro. *Proceedings of the National Academy of Science*, **61**, 542–547.

Myerson, P., Myerson, D., Miller, D., DeLuca, V. A. & Lawson, J. P. (1974) Lymphosarcoma of the bowel masquerading as ulcerative colitis. *Diseases of the Colon and Rectum*, **17**, 710–715.

Nelson, D. L., Blaese, R. M., Strober, W., Bruce, R. M. & Waldmann, T. A. (1975) Constrictive pericarditis, intestinal lymphangiectasia, and reversible immunologic deficiency. *Journal of Pediatrics*, **86**, 548–554.

New England Journal of Medicine (1971) Clinico-Pathological Conference, 35, 1971, **285**, 567–575.

North, R. J. (1975) Cell-mediated immunity and the response to infection. In *Mechanisms of Cell-Mediated Immunity*, ed. McCluskey, R. T. & Cohen, S., Ch. 8, pp. 185–220. New York: John Wiley and Sons.

Nugent, F. W., Zuberi, S., Bulan, M. B. & Legg, M. A. (1972) Colonic lymphoma in ulcerative colitis. *Lahey Clinic Foundation Bulletin*, **21**, 104–111.

Ochs, H. D. & Ament, M. E. (1976) Gastrointestinal tract and immunodeficiency. In *Immunological Aspects of the Liver and Gastrointestinal Tract*, ed. Ferguson, A. & MacSween, R. N. M. Ch. 3, pp. 83–120. Lancaster: MTP Press.

Oliva, H., González Campos, C., Navarro, V. & Mogena, H. H. (1972) Two cases of Whipple's disease showing clinical and morphological similarity. *Gut*, **13**, 430–437.

Osserman, E. F. (1959) Plasma cell myeloma. II. Clinical aspects. *New England Journal of Medicine*, **261**, 952–960.

Owen, J. A., Pitney, W. R. & O'Dea, J. F. (1959) 'Myeloma' serum electrophoretic patterns in conditions other than myelomatosis. *Journal of Clinical Pathology*, **12**, 344–350.

Pantelouris, E. M. (1971) Observations on the immunobiology of 'nude' mice. *Immunology*, **20**, 247–252.

Parrott, D. M. V. & de Sousa, M. A. B. (1974) B-cell stimulation in nude (nu/nu) mice. In *Proceedings of the First International Workshop on Nude Mice*, ed. Rygaard, J. & Povlsen, C. O., pp. 61–69. Stuttgart: Gustav Fischer Verlag.

Pastor, B. M. & Geerken, R. G. (1973) Whipple's disease presenting as pleuropericarditis. *American Journal of Medicine*, **55**, 827–831.

Paulley, J. W. (1952) A case of Whipple's disease (intestinal lipodystrophy). *Gastroenterology*, **22**, 128–133.

Pazmantier, M. W. & Azar, H. A. (1969) Extraskeletal spread in multiple plasma cell myeloma: a review of 57 autopsied cases. *Cancer*, **23**, 167–174.

Peña, A. S., Nieuwkoop, J. V., Schuit, H. R. E., Hekkens, W. Th. J. M. & Haex, A. J. Ch. (1976) Transient paraproteinaemia in a patient with coeliac disease. *Gut*, **17**, 735–739.

Petersen, V. P. & Hastrup, J. (1963) Protein-losing enteropathy in constrictive pericarditis. *Acta Medica Scandinavica*, **173**, 401–410.

Petersen, V. P. & Ottosen, P. (1964) Albumin turnover and thoracic-duct lymph in constrictive pericarditis. *Acta Medica Scandinavica*, **176**, 335–344.

Pettersson, T. & Wegelius, O. (1972) Biopsy diagnosis of amyloidosis in rheumatoid arthritis. Malabsorption caused by intestinal amyloid deposits. *Gastroenterology*, **62**, 22–27.

Pomerantz, M. & Waldmann, T. A. (1963) Systemic lymphatic abnormalities associated with gastrointestinal protein loss secondary to intestinal lymphangiectasia. *Gastroenterology*, **45**, 703–711.

Prolla, J. C. & Kirsner, J. B. (1964) The gastrointestinal lesions and complications of the leukaemias. *Annals of Internal Medicine*, **61**, 1084–1103.

Pruzanski, W. & Katz, A. (1976) Clinical and laboratory findings in primary generalized and multiple-myeloma-related amyloidosis. *Canadian Medical Association Journal*, **114**, 906–909.

Ravid, M. & Sohar, E. (1974) Intestinal malabsorption: First manifestation of amyloidosis in familial Mediterranean fever. *Gastroenterology*, **66**, 446–449.

Reizenstein, P. (1958) Idiopathic steatorrhoea with mesenteric chyladenitis: two cases resembling Whipple's disease. *Gastroenterologia*, **30**, 342–353.

Rimon, A. (1976) The chemical and immunochemical identity of amyloid. *Current Topics in Microbiology and Immunology*, **74**, 1–20.

Roberts, J. H. & Douglas, A. P. (1976) Intestinal lymphangiectasia: the variability of presentation. A study of five cases. *Quarterly Journal of Medicine*, **177**, 39–48.

Ross, I. N., Thompson, R. A., Goldsmith, A. R. & Asquith, P. (1978) Intestinal lymphangiectasia presenting with chicken pox. In preparation.

Ross, J. R., Gialanella, R. & Kealey, O. (1960) Whipple's disease diagnosed by jejunal biopsy; via the oral route. *Lahey Clinic Foundation Bulletin*, **12**, 58–63.

Rubin, C. E. & Dobbins, W. O., III (1965) Peroral biopsy of the small intestine. A review of its diagnostic usefulness. *Gastroenterology*, **49**, 676–697.

Samuel, A. M., Singh, B. & Jarnum, S. (1970) Immunoglobulins in tropical sprue. *Scandinavian Journal of Gastroenterology*, **5**, 129–134.

Sandor, T. & Kozmer, J. (1957) Quoted by Cochran, M., Gallagher, J. C., Cook, M. G. & Peacock, M. (1973) Hypogammaglobulinaemia with Whipple's disease. *Postgraduate Medical Journal*, **49**, 355–358.

Scheerer, P. P., Schwartz, D. L., Pierre, R. V., Reed, E. C. & Linman, J. W. (1964) Gastrointestinal paramyloidosis in plasmacytic myeloma. *Journal of American Medical Association*, **188**, 968–970.

Schenk, E. A., Klipstein, F. A. & Tomasini, J. T. (1972) Morphologic characteristics of jejunal biopsies from asymptomatic Haitians and Puerto Ricans. *American Journal of Clinical Nutrition*, **25**, 1080–1083.

Schlein, P., Herman, M. A. & Gallinek, W. E. (1961) Intestinal lipodystrophy (Whipple's disease). Report of a case diagnosed by peroral biopsy of the small intestine with the Crosby capsule. *Medical Annals of the District of Columbia*, **30**, 400–403.

Schwartz, R. S. (1974) Immunosuppression and neoplasia. In *Progress in Immunology II*, ed. Brent, L. & Holborow, J. Vol. 5, Clinical Aspects II, pp. 229–232. Amsterdam: North Holland Publishing.

Searcy, J. R. & Fish, J. C. (1970) Immunological consequences of lymph lymphocyte depletion. *Review of Surgery*, **27**, 295.

Seliger, G., Krassner, R. L., Beranbaum, E. R. & Miller, F. (1971) The spectrum of roentgen appearance in amyloidosis of the small and large bowel: radiologic-pathologic correlation. *Radiology*, **100**, 63–70.

Skinner, M., Cohen, A. S., Shirahama, T. & Cathcart, E. S. (1974) P-component (pentagonal unit) of amyloid: isolation, characterisation, and sequence analysis. *Journal of Laboratory and Clinical Medicine*, **84**, 604–614.

Soothill, J. F. (1975) Immunity-deficiency states. In *Clinical Aspects of Immunology*, 3rd ed, ed. Gell, P. G. H., Coombs, R. R. A. & Lachmann, P. J., pp. 649–687. Oxford: Blackwell Scientific Publications.

Strober, W., Wochner, R. D., Carbone, P. P. & Waldmann, T. A. (1967) Intestinal lymphangiectasia: a protein-losing enteropathy with hypogammaglobulinaemia, lymphocytopenia and impaired homograft rejection. *Journal of Clinical Investigation*, **46**, 1643–1656.

Symmers, W. St. C. (1956) Primary amyloidosis: a review. *Journal of Clinical Pathology*, **9**, 187–211.

Talerman, A. & Haije, W. F. (1973) The frequency of M-components in sera of patients with solid malignant neoplasms. *British Journal of Cancer*, **27**, 276–282.

Tangun, Y., Saracbasi, Z., Inceman, S., Danon, F. & Seligmann, M. (1975) IgA myeloma globulin and Bence-Jones proteinuria in diffuse plasmacytoma of the small intestine. *Annals of Internal Medicine*, **83,** 673.

Tilney, N. L., Atkinson, J. C. & Murray, J. E. (1970) The immunosuppressive effect of thoracic duct drainage in human kidney transplantation. *Annals of Internal Medicine*, **72,** 59–64.

Tunner, W. S., Carbone, P. P., Blaylock, W. K. & Irvin, G. L., III (1965) Effect of thoracic duct lymph drainage on the immune response in man. *Surgery, Gynecology and Obstetrics*, **121,** 334–338.

Vardy, P. A., Lebanthal, E. & Schwachman, H. (1975) Intestinal lymphangiectasia: a reappraisal. *Paediatrics*, **55,** 842–851.

Verhaegen, H., De Cock, W., De Cree, J., Verbruggen, F., Verhaegen-Declercq, M. & Brugmans, J. (1975) *In vitro* restoration by Levamisole of thymus-derived lymphocyte function in Hodgkin's disease. *Lancet*, **i,** 978.

Waldmann, T. A., Strober, W. & Blaese, R. M. (1972) Immunodeficiency disease and malignancy. Various immunologic deficiencies of man and the role of immune processes in the control of malignant disease. *Annals of Internal Medicine*, **77,** 605–628.

Waldmann, T. A., Wochner, R. D. & Strober, W. (1969) The role of the gastrointestinal tract in plasma protein metabolism. Studies with ^{51}Cr-albumin. *American Journal of Medicine*, **46,** 275–285.

Waldmann, T. A., Wochner, R. D., Laster, L. & Gordon, R. S. (1967) Allergic gastroenteropathy. A cause of excessive gastrointestinal protein loss. *New England Journal of Medicine*, **276,** 761–769.

Watson, W. C., Maxwell, J. D. & Ferguson, A. (1969) Lymphocytes in Whipple's disease. *Proceedings of the Royal Society of Medicine*, **62,** 986–987.

Weiden, P. L., Blaese, R. M., Strober, W., Block, J. B. & Waldman, T. A. (1972) Impaired lymphocyte transformation in intestinal lymphangiectasia: evidence for at least two functionally distinct lymphocyte populations in man. *Journal of Clinical Investigation*, **51,** 1319–1325.

Wellcome Trust Collaborative Study (1971) Discussion. In *Tropical Sprue and Megaloblastic Anaemia (Wellcome Trust Collaborative Study)*, Ch. 10, pp. 269–291. Edinburgh: Churchill Livingstone.

Whipple, G. H. (1907) A hitherto undescribed disease characterised anatomically by deposits of fat and fatty acids in the intestine and mesenteric lymphatic tissues. *Bulletin of the Johns Hopkins Hospital*, **18,** 382–391.

Williams, R. C., Bailly, R. C. & Howe, R. B. (1969) Studies of 'benign' serum M-components. *American Journal of Medical Science*, **257,** 275–293.

Wollin, A. & Jaques, L. B. (1973) Plasma protein escape from the intestinal circulation to the lymphatics during fat absorption. *Proceedings of the Society for Experimental Biology and Medicine*, **142,** 1114–1117.

Yardley, J. H. & Hendrix, T. R. (1961) Combined electron and light microscopy in Whipple's disease – demonstration of 'bacillary bodies' in the intestine. *Bulletin of the Johns Hopkins Hospital*, **109,** 80–98.

Young, V. H. (1969) Transient paraproteins. *Proceedings of the Royal Society of Medicine*, **62,** 778–780.

Yu, D. T., Peter, J. B. & Stratton, J. A. (1973) Lymphocyte dynamics: changes in density profiles and response to phytohemagglutinin of human lymphocytes during prolonged thoracic duct drainage. *Clinical Immunology and Immunopathology*, **1,** 456–462.

Zawadzki, Z. A. & Edwards, G. A. (1972) Non-myelomatous monoclonal immunoglobulinaemia. In *Progress in Clinical Immunology*, ed. Schwartz, R. S., Vol. 1, pp. 105–156. New York: Grune and Stratton.

Index

Entries in Bold type indicate main discussion in text or chapter headings

Alkaline phosphatase
  in alpha heavy chain disease, 307
Allograft rejection
  in animal models of coeliac disease, 136
  in animal models of inflammatory bowel disease, 146
  in lymphangiectasia, 334
  in Whipple's disease, 325–326
Alpha foetoprotein, 293–295
  clinical studies in, 294–295
  properties and function of, 293–294
  synthesis of, 293
Alpha heavy chain disease, 306–314
  aetiology of, 313–314
  clinical features of, 306–307, 311–312
  epidemiology of, 313
  histology in, 307
  infestation in, 307, 313
  Mediterranean lymphoma in, 312
  nutrition, significance in, 306, 313
  protein studies in, 307–311
  treatment of, 307, 312, 313
Alveolitis, allergic
  in coeliac disease, 73
Amoebiasis, 247–249
  see also Entamoeba histolytica infestation
Amyloidosis, 318–320
  in alpha heavy chain disease, 307
  classification of, 318–319
  intestinal motor activity in, 319
  vascular problems in, 319–320
Animal models
  for coeliac disease, 129–137
  for Crohn's disease, 110, 111
  for inflammatory bowel disease, 137–146
  for pernicious anaemia, 55, 58
Antibodies
  autoantibodies, in coeliac disease, 72–75
  autoantibodies, in pernicious anaemia, 57
  bacterial, in ulcerative colitis, 100
  bacteriophage, in coeliac disease, 71–72
  bacteriophage, in ulcerative colitis, 72
  in coccidiosis, 251
  colon, in ulcerative colitis, 98–100
  in Crohn's disease, 107–108
  cytotoxic, in animal models of coeliac disease, 136

cytotoxic, in animal models of inflammatory bowel disease, 143–145
dietary, in coeliac disease, 71
dietary, in food allergy, 202, 203
egg protein, in food allergy, 202
in *Entamoeba histolytica* infestation, 247–248
foods (various), in atopic allergy, 201–206
fish, in atopic allergy, 198
IgE, in nematode infestation, 254
intrinsic factor in pernicious anaemia, 55–58
maternal, in passive immunity in piglet and calf, 269–270
milk, in Crohn's disease, 108
milk, in gastrointestinal diseases, 202
milk, in milk allergy, 190–191
milk, in ulcerative colitis, 101
mucosal, in coeliac disease, 71
parietal cell, in common variable hypogammaglobulinaemia, 156
parietal cell, in pernicious anaemia, 55–58
polio, in coeliac disease, 72
reticulin, in coeliac disease, 72–73
reticulin, in Crohn's disease, 108
reticulin, in ulcerative colitis, 101–102
RNA, in Crohn's disease, 108
tissue, in coeliac disease, 73–74
in ulcerative colitis, 98–102
viral, in ulcerative colitis, 100–101
Antigen handling
  intestinal, mechanism of, 7–8, 20
  in Peyer's patches, 8–9, 221–222
Apes, disease of, resembling inflammatory bowel disease, 139
Aphthous ulceration, 42–43
Arthus reactions
  mechanism of, 17
  in nematode infestation, 253
Ataxia telangiectasia, 172
Atopic food hypersensitivity, 195–201
  see also Food allergy
Auer reaction, in animal models of inflammatory bowel disease, 145
Autacoids, 23
Autoantibodies, role in gastrointestinal disease, 17
Azathioprine, in Crohn's disease, 111–112

B-cells, *see* Lymphocytes, B-cells
Bacterial adhesion
  inhibition, in cholera vibrio, 230–231
  role of secretory IgA antibodies, 6
  significance, in enteric infection, 276–277
Bacterial infection of the intestine, *see* Intestinal microflora; Cholera vibrio; *E. coli*; Salmonella; Shigella
Bacterial inhibition, significance in intestinal infection, 276
Bacterial toxins, significance in intestinal infection, 277–278
Bacterial and viral infections of the gastrointestinal tract, 214–236
Behcet's syndrome, 42, 43
Bence-Jones protein
  in alpha heavy chain disease, 310
  in myelomatosis, 316–317
Bird fancier's lung, in coeliac disease, 73
Breast feeding and intestinal microflora, 235–236
Bronchial lymphoid tissue, relationship to Peyer's patches, 9
Bruton's hypogammaglobulinaemia, 152–154
  see also Lymphocytes, B-cell defect, in X-linked hypogammaglobulinaemia
Bursa of Fabricius, deficiency of, 152

Calves, enteric infection in, its immuno-prophylaxis, 268–282
Calves, maternal immunoglobulins in, 269–270
Candida albicans
  see also Chronic mucocutaneous candidiasis
  in chronic mucocutaneous candidiasis, 167–171
  oral, immunological features in, 44–45
  in severe combined immunodeficiency, 171
Carcinoembryonic antigen, 289–293
  chemical characteristics of, 289–291
  clinical applications of its estimation, 290–293
  in diagnosis of malignancy, 290–293
  tissue localization of, 289
  in ulcerative colitis, 102